Professional's Handbook of

COMPLEMENTARY
&
ALTERNATIVE
MEDICINES

Charles W. Fetrow, PharmD
Juan R. Avila, PharmD

Springhouse Corporation
Springhouse, Pennsylvania

Staff ✎

Senior Vice President, Editorial
Patricia Dwyer Schull, RN, MSN

Publisher
Donna O. Carpenter, ELS

Clinical Director
Ann M. Barrow, RN, MSN, CCRN

Art Director
John Hubbard

Managing Editor
Andrew T. McPhee, RN, BSN

Drug Information Editor
Lisa Truong, RPh, PharmD

Senior Editor
Naina Chohan

Editors
Peter H. Johnson, Patricia Nale

Clinical Editor
Eileen Gallen, RN, BSN

Associate Acquisitions Editor
Louise E. Quinn

Copy Editors
Brenna H. Mayer (manager), Karen C. Comerford, Donna Birdsell, Beth Pitcher

Designers
Arlene Putterman (associate art director), Elaine Kasmer Ezrow, Joseph John Clark, Donald G. Knauss, B.J. Krim, Donna S. Morris, Stephanie Peters

Typographers
Diane Paluba (manager), Joyce Rossi Biletz

Manufacturing
Deborah Meiris (director), Pat Dorshaw (manager), Otto Mezei (book production manager)

Editorial Assistants
Carrie R. Cameron, Carol A. Caputo

Indexer
Barbara Hodgson

℞ A member of the Reed Elsevier plc group

Visit our Web site at http://www.springnet.com

ISSN 1522-0877
ISBN 0-87434-971-0

Contents ✎

Overview & herbal agents

Appendices

About the authors ✑

Charles W. Fetrow, *PharmD*, is the Coordinator of Pharmacokinetics and the Outpatient Anticoagulant and Drug Evaluation Services at St. Francis Medical Center in Pittsburgh, Pa. A member of the American Society of Health-System Pharmacists, Dr. Fetrow teaches pharmacokinetics at St. Francis and at Duquesne University and is a member of the adjunct faculty of the University of Pittsburgh.

Juan R. Avila, *PharmD*, is an Assistant Professor in the Department of Pharmacy Practice at Shenandoah University in Winchester, Va. Dr. Avila previously served as an Assistant Professor at Duquesne University and as a clinical psychiatry pharmacy specialist at St. Francis Medical Center, both in Pittsburgh, Pa. He is a member of the American Association of Colleges of Pharmacy and American Society of Health-System Pharmacists.

Acknowledgments

We would like to express our sincere appreciation to the following individuals for their significant contributions to this project: our wives, Joanne and Crystal, for their enduring patience and understanding; Christine O'Neil and all of our contributors who helped us compile entries; the St. Francis Health Sciences Library staff, especially David Brennan, Brad Long, Mary Lee Fazio, Bob Jewell, and Vi Brown for their essentially perfect retrieval of hard-to-find journal publications; Melanie Patrick, Sara Erberle, and our students, who often found themselves immersed in our projects at a moment's notice; the staff at Springhouse Corporation, especially Pat Schull, Donna Carpenter, Ann Barrow, Andy McPhee, Lisa Truong, Naina Chohan, Louise Quinn, and Carrie Cameron, whose advice, support, patience, and belief in us helped make this book possible; and the medical staffs and personnel of St. Francis Medical Center, Winchester Medical Center, and Shenandoah University, whose continued encouragement and interest in the project provided the fuel that kept our editorial fires burning.

Charles W. Fetrow, PharmD
Juan R. Avila, PharmD

Contributors and consultants 🐾

Special consultant

Christine K. O'Neil, PharmD
Assistant Professor Clinical
Pharmacy
Duquesne University
Clinical Pharmacist
St. Francis Medical Center
Pittsburgh

Reem A. Abo-Zena, PharmD
Pharmacy Practice Resident
The Cleveland Clinic
Foundation
Cleveland

Jorge G. Avila, PharmD
Oncology Pharmacy
Resident
H. Lee Moffitt Cancer
Center & Research Institute
Tampa, Fla.

Erica A. Barnum, PharmD
Pharmacy Resident
Moses H. Cone Memorial
Hospital
Greensboro, N.C.

Cathy L. Bartels, PharmD
Assistant Professor, Director
of Drug Information
School of Pharmacy and
Allied Health Sciences
University of Montana
Missoula

**Stephanie Beckman,
PharmD**
Clinical Pharmacist
Western Missouri Mental
Health Center
Adjunct Clinical Instructor
University of Missouri–
Kansas City

**Hildegarde J. Berdine,
PharmD**
Clinical Assistant Professor
Duquesne University
School of Pharmacy
Pittsburgh

Keith Berndtson, MD
Medical Director
American WholeHealth/
Lincoln Park
American WholeHealth, Inc.
Chicago

Donna Bey, PharmD
Clinical Specialist, Drug
Information
Medical University of South
Carolina Medical Center
Charleston

Riccardo L. Boni, PhD
Assistant Professor of
Pharmaceutical Chemistry
Duquesne University
Mylan School of Pharmacy
Pittsburgh

**Paula McFadden
Bortnichak, MD**
Freelance Medical
Consultant; Psychiatrist
Sparta, N.J.

**Mary L. Brubaker, PharmD,
FASHP, BCPS, BCNSP, CHES**
Clinical Assistant Professor
Northern Arizona
University
Flagstaff

**Hope E. Campbell, PharmD,
BCPS**
Clinical Research
Pharmacist
Vanderbilt University
Medical Center
Nashville, Tenn.

Paula J. Ceh, PharmD
Assistant Professor of
Pharmacy Practice
Butler University
College of Pharmacy and
Health Sciences
Indianapolis

M.L. Champion, PharmD
Clinical Pharmacist
University of Pittsburgh
Medical Center
Southside Hospital

Mary L. Chavez, PharmD
Director of Didactic
Education
Midwestern University
College of Pharmacy–
Glendale (Ariz.)

Umberto Conte, PharmD
Clinical Pharmacist
The Mount Sinai Medical
Center
New York

Jason C. Cooper, PharmD
Assistant Professor Clinical
Specialist, Drug
Information
Medical University of South
Carolina
Charleston

**Virginia L. Cronin, RN, MSN,
MBA**
Associate Professor
Northern Virginia
Community College
Annandale

**Melissa Crouthamel,
PharmD**
Clinical Pharmacist
University of Pittsburgh
Medical Center

Eric Culley, RPh PharmD
Candidate
Duquesne University
Pittsburgh

**Christine M. Damico, MSN,
CPNP**
Pediatric Nurse Practitioner
Central Bucks Pediatric
Associates
Doylestown, Pa.

**Linda M. Dean, RN, MSN,
CRNP, ACRN, CS**
Clinical Nurse Coordinator
MCP Hahnemann, Section
HIV/AIDS Medicine
Partnership Comprehensive
Care Practice
Philadelphia

Brent Ednie, MD
Indiana (Pa.) Hospital
Department of Internal
Medicine

Rachael M. Fantz, PharmD
Psychiatric Pharmacy
Resident
Medical University of South
Carolina
Charleston

Suzanne E. Fecik, PharmD
Clinical Pharmacist
Behavioral Health
Pharmacy
Scripps Mercy Hospital
San Diego

Sandra S. Feldman, PharmD
Pharmacy Practice Resident
Buffalo (N.Y.) General
Hospital

Emily F. Grandey, MD
Internal Medicine
St. Francis Medical Center
Pittsburgh

Michelle A. Gravlin, PharmD
Clinical Pharmacist
Cox Medical Center North
Adjunct Clinical Instructor
University of Missouri-
Kansas City
Springfield

Amy L. Gruel, PharmD
Visiting Faculty
School of Pharmacy &
Allied Health Sciences
University of Montana
Missoula

**Peggi Guenter, RN, PhD,
CNSN**
Editor-in-Chief
*Nutrition in Clinical
Practice*
American Society of
Parenteral and Enteral
Nutrition
Silver Spring, Md.

Stacy L. Haber, PharmD
Clinical Assistant Professor
The University of Arizona
College of Pharmacy
Tucson, Ariz.

**William R. Hamilton,
PharmD**
Assistant Professor
Creighton University
School of Pharmacy and
Allied Health Professions
Omaha

**Fred Harchelroad, MD,
FAAEM, FACMT**
Director, Medical
Toxicology Treatment
Center
Allegheny University
Hospitals: Allegheny
General
Pittsburgh

Jennifer Harkins, RN
Coram Health Care
Winston-Salem, N.C.

Jane Holmes, PharmD
Clinical Coordinator
Pharmacy Services
Allegheny University
Hospitals: Allegheny Valley
Natrona Heights, Pa.

Jamie L. Holowka, PharmD
Clinical Pharmacist
University of Pittsburgh
Medical Center

Pamela A. Hucko, PharmD
Pharmacy Practice Resident
West Virginia University
Hospital
Morgantown

**Anne-Marie Jefferson,
PharmD**
Department of Pharmacy
University Medical Center
Jacksonville, Fla.

T. M. Jenkins, PharmD
Senior Masters of Pharmacy
Administration Resident
The Ohio State University
Medical Center
Columbus

Kirk Jones, PharmD
Clinical Pharmacist
University of Pittsburgh
Medical Center: Beaver
Pittsburgh

April M. King, PharmD
Clinical Pharmacist
In-Home Health, Inc.
Pittsburgh

Robert V. Laux, PharmD
Assistant Professor
Duquesne University
Pittsburgh

Mandy C. Leonard, PharmD
Drug Information Specialist
The Cleveland Clinic
Foundation
Cleveland

David Lippman, MD
Internal Medicine
St. Francis Medical Center
Pittsburgh

Scott F. Long, RPh, PhD
Assistant Professor of
Pharmacology and
Toxicology
School of Pharmacy
Southwestern Oklahoma
State University
Weatherford

Kevin J. Lynch, PharmD
Clinical Manager
Stadtlander's Managed
Services
Pittsburgh

**Barbara L. Martinelli, RPh,
BCNSP, MBA**
Clinical Pharmacist/
Coordinator
Metabolic Support Team
St. Francis Medical Center
Pittsburgh

Laura K. McCoy, MS, PharmD
Manager, Patient Care
Services
Children's Hospital
Columbus, Ohio

Lee Ann McDowell, PharmD
Clinical Pharmacy
Specialist
University of Pittsburgh
Medical Center Health
System

Pamela S. Messer, RN, MSN
Drug Safety Surveillance
Manager
Wyeth-Ayerst
Radnor, Pa.

Brian J. Moore, RPh
Clinical Pharmacist
Ohio State University
Medical Center
Columbus

Heather C. Murren, PharmD
Staff Pharmacist
Magee-Women's Hospital
Pittsburgh

Linda M. Nicolaus, PharmD
Staff Pharmacist
Eckerd Drug, Inc.
Pittsburgh

Brian N. Peters, PharmD
Pharmacy Practice
Resident/Graduate Research
Associate
The Ohio State University
Medical Center
Columbus

T.W. Prasthofer, PhD
Associate Professor,
Biopharmaceutical Sciences
Shenandoah University
School of Pharmacy
Winchester, Va.

Harry S. Rafkin, MD
Head, Clinical Investigation
for Critical Care Medicine
Director, Department of
Research
St. Francis Medical Center
Pittsburgh

Holly Roche, PharmD
Staff Pharmacist
University of Pittsburgh
Medical Center:
Presbyterian
Pittsburgh

Catherine Romanos, PharmD
Pharmacy Practice Resident
Ohio State University
Medical Center
Columbus

J.P. Rose, PharmD
Clinical Pharmacist
Allegheny University
Hospitals: Allegheny
General
Pittsburgh

Paul L. Schiff, Jr., BSc, MSc, PhD
Professor of Pharmaceutical
Sciences
School of Pharmacy
University of Pittsburgh

Pazit Shaked, PharmD
Resident, Pharmacy
Practice
Albert Einstein Healthcare
Network
Philadelphia

Douglas Slain, PharmD
Clinical Fellow
Clinical Instructor
Virginia Commonwealth
University Medical College
Richmond, Va.

Adam Sohnen, MD
Internist, Department of
Internal Medicine
St. Francis Medical Center
Pittsburgh

Joan Stachnik, PharmD, BCPS
Drug Information Specialist
University of Illinois
College of Pharmacy
Chicago

S.B. Tanna, PharmD
Specialty Practice Resident
The Ohio State University
Medical Center
Columbus

S.E. Taylor, PharmD
Critical Care Resident
University of Pittsburgh
Medical Center Health
System

James A. Tjon, PharmD
Drug Information
Pharmacist
University of Pittsburgh
Medical Center

Theresa M. Wadas, RN, MSN, CCRN, CRNP
Nurse Practitioner
Advanced Heart Failure &
Transplant Service
University of Alabama
Hospital
Birmingham

Matthew Wallack, MD
Medical Resident in
Neurology
Wake Forest University
Medical Center
Winston-Salem, N.C.

Mary Grace S. Wilson, PharmD
Staff Pharmacist
Children's Hospital
Pittsburgh

Eric Wright, PharmD
Clinical Pharmacist
VA Pittsburgh Healthcare
System
Clinical Instructor
University of Pittsburgh
School of Pharmacy

Chris A. Yeschke, RPh
Supervisor, Sterile Products
Pharmacy Services
St. Francis Medical Center
Pittsburgh

Foreword ✍

Today, more than 60 million people in the United States use alternative medicines. These agents are being used with increasing frequency by a growing number of patients who seek treatment with largely unproved therapies. Even more of a concern is that nearly three out of four patients who use alternative medicines never mention their use of the agents to their physicians.

Without question, herbal medicines are here to stay. Because so many patients use herbals today, every health care professional—physicians, nurses, nurse practitioners, physician assistants, pharmacists, medical and nursing students, and others involved with drug therapy for patients—needs to know as much as possible about herbal medicines.

Most important, that information needs to be reliable and unbiased. Yet nearly every herbal resource available today offers largely anecdotal data or is so strongly biased for or against herbal medicines that even the most conscientious health care professionals have difficulty discerning fact from myth and answering with any certainty the numerous questions they have about herbal therapy. Could a patient's low hemoglobin be caused by the garlic she's taking? Should a patient taking a prescription antihypertensive medication also be taking mistletoe on his own? What lifesaving actions should you be prepared to take if a patient with asthma uses royal jelly to help lower his cholesterol?

The *Professional's Handbook of Complementary & Alternative Medicines* answers these questions and more. The book not only offers detailed information about more than 300 of the most commonly used herbal medicines but also provides references and an analysis for every entry. Culled from respected scientific sources throughout the world, the references allow you to ascribe whatever weight you feel appropriate to the information contained in each entry. And the analysis offers the authors' insight into the therapeutic usefulness of each herb.

The authors, both widely respected and highly experienced, have pored through hundreds of journal articles and thousands of pages of government documents to compile this most comprehensive reference. You won't find a more detailed, professional resource about herbal medicines anywhere, nor one presented with such a keen eye toward presenting the *facts* about herbals, not the folklore.

No matter your field of expertise, no matter how many patients you care for or provide services to, you'll want to keep the *Professional's Handbook of Complementary & Alternative Medicines* handy—for your sake and your patients'.

Simeon Margolis, MD, PhD
Professor of Medicine and Biological Chemistry
The Johns Hopkins University School of Medicine
Baltimore, MD

Preface 🍂

A patient was once referred to us because she was experiencing unexplained hair loss. Her primary care physician thought the hair loss might be caused by one of the medicines she was taking and thought we might be able to shed some light on her condition. When we asked the patient, whom we'll call Mrs. Emmett, to bring to the clinic all of the medicines she was taking, she asked, "Are you sure you want me to do that?" *Of course,* we answered.

When we saw her again, this pleasant looking lady in her mid-40s was straining to carry a garbage bag nearly filled with medicine bottles, not one of which contained a prescription drug! Over the next 2 hours, Mrs. Emmett described why she was taking each of the dozens of herbal agents she carried in the bag and how she remembered which pills she was supposed to take at which times of the day—in some cases, as many as four times a day.

The breadth of this patient's self-prescribed therapy left us feeling helpless, frustrated, and convinced more than ever of the urgent need to create a clinically sound reference about complementary and alternative medicines that would meet the needs of other health professionals who each day faced their own Mrs. Emmett.

In addition to the many phone calls about traditional medicines we receive each day from nurses and doctors throughout our respective institutions, we've been fielding a growing number of calls from colleagues who have questions about herbal medicines. "What is hawthorn," they ask, "and what do I tell my patient taking it?" "How does mugwort work?" "Does oleander contain ingredients my patient may be allergic to?" Our colleagues, like us, have been frustrated by the lack of clear, readily available information about herbal agents, and that frustration has, in part, fueled our desire to produce this book.

Most accessible data about herbal agents come not from reputable scientific sources but from herb manufacturers themselves or from advocacy literature. Other information may come from foreign journals not readily available in the United States or from animal studies not easily reviewed by clinical practitioners.

We've taken this worldwide, sometimes disjointed array of information and developed it into one cohesive, comprehensive, and scientifically valid reference that examines complementary and alternative medicines with an eye of fairness and openness. Adam Sohnen, M.D., a colleague of ours, once told us to listen to patients in a nonjudgmental way and recognize the negative forces that propel alternative ways of thinking and the positive forces that foster self-improvement. He was right. We need to reinforce the positive efforts patients expend on achieving wellness and at the same time gently direct the patient's enthusiasm toward therapies of proven effectiveness. And while we must never extinguish a patient's hope, we must at the same time take care not to propagate false promises. We believe *Professional's Handbook of Complementary & Alternative Medicines* fulfills these worthwhile goals.

We strongly encourage the continued quest to gather scientifically valid data about alternative medicines that so many patients rely on as part of their treatment. We hope the *Professional's Handbook of Complementary & Alternative Medicines* will help you learn the *facts* about herbal medicines. Only then will your patients receive meaningful information about this subject of growing importance to us all.

Charles W. Fetrow, PharmD
Juan R. Avila, PharmD

How to use *Professional's Handbook of Complementary & Alternative Medicines* 🖎

One of the first books of its kind written specifically for health care professionals, *Professional's Handbook of Complementary & Alternative Medicines* takes a scientific and comprehensive look at complementary and alternative medicines, focusing mainly on herbal agents. The book's features and format are designed to accommodate the wide-ranging needs of health care professionals seeking information about herbal medicines.

An overview chapter explains the history of complementary and alternative medicines and discusses the uses, risks, and regulations of herbal versus traditional medicine. This chapter is followed by a compendium of hundreds of medicinal herbs organized alphabetically by generic name for quick access.

References are placed at the end of each entry so they can be referred to easily. Coverage of each herb is consistent, with clearly marked headings, so you can locate specific information quickly. Special features help enhance knowledge and skills.

● An alert symbol (⚠) calls your attention to warnings, cautions, and other critical information about the use of the herbal agent.

● The "Research findings" logo profiles important studies cited in selected entries; each describes the study, its results, and conclusions.

● A "Folklore" logo contains interesting background information on an herb, such as the history of its use or other facts related to the agent.

● Numerous appendices provide additional information to make the book even more useful.

HERBAL ENTRIES

Each entry provides detailed information about the herb. A guide word at the top of each page identifies the generic herb covered on that page. Each entry is complete in itself and doesn't require turning to other sections of the book for more information. Headings within each entry follow this sequence: generic name, synonyms, common trade names, common forms, source, chemical components, actions, reported uses, dosage, adverse reactions, interactions, contraindications and precautions, special considerations, points of interest (where appropriate), analysis, and references.

Synonyms
In each herbal entry, the generic name is followed by an alphabetized list of its synonyms.

Common trade names
This section is an alphabetical list of the most common trade names associated with the herb. Several commerical agents are produced by different manufacturers and may occur in combination with other agents. The mention of a trade name does not imply endorsement of that product or guarantee its legality.

Common forms

This section lists known preparations available for each agent—for instance, tablets, capsules, extracts, tinctures. Available dosage forms and standardized strengths are listed, if known.

Source

This section provides information about the source plant's botanical name and other data about the occurrence of the agent in nature.

Chemical components

This section summarizes the key chemical composition of the herbal agent and offers data relevant to the herb's reported actions.

Actions

This section describes how the herb is thought to achieve its therapeutic effects, based on in vitro, animal, and human studies. Keep in mind that an herb's action depends on the chemical components of the plant and their concentrations within each product. In addition, results from animal studies don't always apply to humans; therefore, definitive statements about an agent's action in humans should not be made without human clinical trials.

Reported uses

This section describes anecdotal uses of the agent, based on clinical studies with humans and case reports. These uses should not to be considered as recommendations but rather as unproven claims of use. This section also summarizes significant results from key scientific and clinical studies.

Dosage

This section lists the routes and general dosage information for each form of the herb and, where available, in accordance with its reported use. This information has been gathered from herbal literature, anecdotal reports, and available clinical data. However, not all uses have specific dosage information. In fact, consensus on dosage seldom exists. Dosage notations in this section reflect current clinical trends and should not be considered as recommendations of the authors or publisher.

Adverse reactions

This section lists, in alphabetical order, undesirable effects that may follow use of the herb. Some of these effects have not been reported but may theoretically occur, given the chemical composition or action of the agent. Overdose and treatment information is included, as appropriate.

Interactions

This section lists each agent's clinically significant interactions with other drugs or foods. The interaction is followed by the effect of the interaction and then a specific suggestion for avoiding the interaction itself. As with adverse reactions, some interactions have not been proven but are theoretically possible. The interacting drug or food is *italicized* for at-a-glance review.

Contraindications and precautions

This section lists any condition, especially a disease, in which the use of the agent is undesirable, and provides recommendations for cautious use as appropriate.

Special considerations

This section offers helpful information for clinicians, such as monitoring parameters and methods for the prevention and treatment of adverse reactions. Patient-teaching tips that focus on educating the patient about the drug's purpose, preparation, administration, and storage are also included, as are suggestions for promoting patient compliance with the therapeutic regimen and steps the patient can take to prevent or minimize the risk or severity of adverse reactions.

Points of interest

This section includes anecdotal information, historical facts, or other relevant data about selected herbal agents.

Analysis

In this section, the authors evaluate the anecdotal, herbal, and scientific literature and try to separate facts from myths about that herb's reported uses. The analysis summarizes exactly where each agent stands from a scientific point of view and offers recommendations for use or further study, as appropriate.

References

This section covers key clinical studies referred to in the entry. The authors and reviewers conducted an exhaustive review of literature from around the world—including numerous foreign publications and hard-to-find research studies.

A guide to additional references—such as Germany's Commission E monographs—appears at the back of the book and points you toward other reliable sources of information about herbal remedies.

APPENDICES

In the book's appendices, you'll find selected herbal agents with limited clinical data, herbal agents listed as unsafe by the FDA, potentially unsafe plants, herbal agents to avoid during pregnancy, potential drug–herbal agent interactions, selected therapeutic monitoring guidelines, study data on herbal agents by disorder, and a resource list for complementary and alternative medicines. You'll also find an herbal agent information sheet. This reproducible patient-teaching aid may be completed with patient-specific information and given to your patient taking an herbal medicine.

INDEX

The index lists the generic name and synonyms of each herbal agent as well as the indications for which specific dosage information exists.

Abbreviations

Abbreviation	Meaning	Abbreviation	Meaning
ACE	angiotensin-converting enzyme	IU	international unit
		I.V.	intravenous
AIDS	acquired immunodeficiency syndrome	kg	kilogram
		L	liter
ALT	alanine aminotransferase	lb	pound
AST	aspartate aminotransferase	LDL	low-density lipoprotein
		LH	luteinizing hormone
ATP	adenosine triphosphate	m	meter
b.i.d.	twice daily	MAO	monoamine oxidase
BPH	benign prostatic hyperplasia	mcg	microgram
BUN	blood urea nitrogen	mg	milligram
cAMP	cyclic 3', 5' adenosine monophosphate	MI	myocardial infarction
		ml	milliliter
CBC	complete blood count	MRSA	methicillin-resistant *Staphlococcus aureus*
CK	creatine kinase		
CNS	central nervous system	NSAID	nonsteroidal anti-inflammatory drug
COPD	chronic obstructive pulmonary disease	OAM	Office of Alternative Medicine
CSA	Controlled Substance Act		
CSF	cerebrospinal fluid	OTC	over-the-counter
CV	cardiovascular	oz	ounce
DHEA	dehydroepiandrosterone	PABA	para-aminobenzoic acid
DNA	deoxyribonucleic acid	P.O.	by mouth
FDA	Food and Drug Administration	P.R.	by rectum
		PT	prothrombin time
FSH	follicle-stimulating hormone	PTT	partial thromboplastin time
		q.i.d.	four times daily
g	gram	RBC	red blood cell
G	gauge	RDA	recommended daily allowance
GI	gastrointestinal		
G6PD	glucose-6-phosphate dehydrogenase	RNA	ribonucleic acid
		S.L.	sublingual
gtt	drop(s)	t.i.d.	three times daily
H_1	histamine$_1$	TSH	thyroid-stimulating hormone
H_2	histamine$_2$		
HCG	human chorionic gonadrotropin	U	unit
		USP	United States Pharmacopeia
HIV	human immunodeficiency virus	VRE	vancomycin-resistant enterococcus
I.M.	intramuscular		
INR	international normalized ratio	WBC	white blood cell

OVERVIEW
&
HERBAL AGENTS

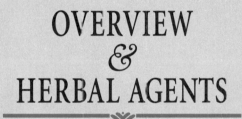

Overview of complementary & alternative medicines

The use of complementary and alternative medicine has become a phenomenon too massive to ignore. Schools are granting doctorates in naturopathy. Among patients who see mainstream health care professionals, one-third use herbal remedies, although many fail to disclose this information to their primary health care provider. In 1997, the herbal industry constituted a $3.2 billion business and continues to grow at 25% annually. In fact, some reports indicate that about 80% of the world's population uses herbs for medicinal purposes.

Despite efforts by health care professionals to keep pace with an ever-growing body of factual medical evidence, share that knowledge with patients, and continue to offer new FDA-approved pharmaceuticals, devices, and procedures at an almost alarming rate, the general public still feels the need to reach out for something extra. In an increasing number of instances, that something is herbal medicine.

Studies indicate that many patients who use alternative medicines and also seek conventional treatment tend to exercise more; be more careful about avoiding fatty foods, tobacco, and alcohol; be more compliant with taking their regular medications, and make lifestyle modifications more readily than patients who seek conventional health care only. Consequently, today's health care professionals need to educate themselves on which complementary and alternative medicines are helpful, which are harmful, which are ineffective, and which lack sufficient data about safety and efficacy. An understanding of phytomedicine and its components is the first step in that education.

Phytomedicine

Of all available complementary or alternative therapies, phytomedicine—the practice of using plants or plant parts to achieve a therapeutic cure—appears to be more than a fad. Phytomedicine has been around for several centuries, perhaps even longer, and is in common use throughout the world. The United States is one of the last nations to embrace phytomedicine.

The National Institutes of Health estimates that, in the United States, approximately one in three people pursue some form of complementary or alternative medical therapy, such as herbal medicine, homeopathy, acupuncture, biofeedback, color therapy, music therapy, hypnotherapy, aromatherapy, Ayurvedic medicine, Bach flower remedies, and a host more. The number of people using these therapies may be even higher among those who have a chronic disease.

Partly in response to the popularity of alternative remedies, the NIH established the Office of Alternative Medicines (OAM), which studies and compiles data on alternative medicines. In other countries, similar committees, such as Commission E in Germany, have reviewed the safety and efficacy of herbs and published the results so that product debates can be resolved.

HISTORY OF PHYTOMEDICINE

Although early Native Americans used plants to treat various maladies, the practice of phytomedicine fell out of favor over the years and has remained for generations largely outside the realm of contemporary American medical practice. Germany, certain Asian countries, and several other nations, including Italy, Spain, the Netherlands, and Belgium, have taken a more aggressive approach.

Herbal medicine in Germany

Germany is famed for its aggressive approach to herbal medicine. By recent estimates, Germany has allowed as many as 700 herbal products to be marketed in its country. Approximately 70% of German health care professionals currently prescribe phytopharmaceuticals to their patients and at the same time support one of the world's largest markets for herbal drugs. Furthermore, Commission E, a branch of the German government similar to the FDA in the United States, has compiled therapeutic monographs for more than 300 herbal medicines. The monographs discuss safety and efficacy of the agents.

Herbal medicine in the United States

Despite a slow start, the commercialized herbal industry in the United States is now booming. More than 500 different herbs are currently marketed in this nation. Mass marketing and media blitzes aimed at health-food stores, supermarkets, and retail pharmacies have prompted rapid growth in the sales of herbal supplements.

Public accessibility to these products has grown tremendously. Herbal and dietary supplements can be purchased at the local mall, drug store, grocery store, or corner convenience store. Herbal agents can be obtained through mail-order catalogs, wholesalers, or even over the Internet.

All available indications suggest that unlimited and unrestricted access to herbal products will continue, herbal manufacturers will flourish, and attempts at regulation or standardization of the industry will prove only marginally effective.

PHARMACOGNOSY

The study of chemicals from natural sources for their medicinal application is termed *pharmacognosy*. The term usually refers to the study of chemical entities in higher plants, such as bushes, shrubs, and trees, and components of lower plants (fungi, molds, yeasts), but land and marine animals, fish, and insects can also serve as potential medicinal agents.

Approximately 250,000 species of flowering plants exist in the world today. Of these, only a small percentage have been adequately studied for pharmacologic activity. Many more valuable agents may lie waiting to be discovered in plants yet to be screened for therapeutic applications.

Determining the species of plant to pursue for pharmacologic activity is often difficult, especially with so many plants to explore. Anecdotal reports of therapeutic efficacy and local medical folklore are usually seen as effective ways to identify potentially therapeutic plant components.

Manufacturing an herbal agent

In most industrialized nations, crude drugs—defined as natural substances collected and dried before manufacturing—are seldom employed as chief therapeutic agents. More commonly, certain components of the plant are identified, removed, modified, and applied therapeutically in a consistent manner.

Many plants can be grown in climates that resemble the plant's native land. Compatibility of the plant to a particular region and the cost of harvesting the plant in that same area determine the availability of crude drugs. In addition, national and international restrictions on the collection of wild plants tend to limit availability of plant resources and drive up the cost of production. These factors also tend to force countries to specialize in producing only certain types of phytomedicinal resources.

Despite the tendency for a country to produce only certain resources, the quality of crude drugs is often questionable. By the time a crude drug arrives at a manufacturing center, it has been subjected to adulteration, deterioration, or contamination. Deliberate adulteration most frequently occurs with expensive natural substances or natural substances in short supply. Mechanical devices may be economical when collecting some plants but may be of little use when collecting others.

Cultivating specific plants ensures a reliable source of the plant with less risk of adulteration. Environmental conditions—temperature, rainfall, length of daylight, altitude, atmosphere, and soil—can dramatically affect the quality and concentration of active plant constituents. The age of the plant can also be an important factor in the quality of active constituents in a crude drug.

Before drying of the plant, insect-infested or disease-infested plant parts should be removed. In this process, called "garbling," unwanted material, such as dirt, debris, and unnecessary plant parts, are removed from the plant before drying and again before packaging and storage.

Drying can last anywhere from a few hours to a few weeks, depending on the relative humidity of the local climate and the physical nature of the plant components. Drying by artificial heat (hot water pipes, stoves, belt dryers) carries the advantage of shorter drying times. Veterans of the process have learned when to halt the drying phase to prevent plant parts from becoming too brittle and dried.

Deterioration of the dried product can occur when the dried plant is exposed to moisture in the surrounding air (usually about 10% to 15%) and sunlight. Some processes introduce sterilization as a way to minimize microbial contamination. Proper storage and preservation must take place to ensure quality of the product until delivery to the manufacturing facility, where the crude drug undergoes a variety of grinding, crushing, extraction, or distillation processes prior to being formed into an herbal pharmaceutical.

Standards of quality

Official standards are critical for ensuring the quality of herbal products. At present, these standards aren't well established. On the forefront of strengthening the official standards lies the European Scientific Cooperative for Phytotherapy, a committee composed of manufacturers of herbal medicines and herbal associations working with European research groups.

Standards that should be addressed include sampling, foreign matter, moisture content, loss of potency from drying, quantitative chemical analysis, ash values, microbial contamination, toxic residues, extractive values, and determinations of volatile oils. The committee is currently developing standards to address these issues.

Regulating the herbal industry

A major contention of herbal medicine advocates is the notion that, because herbal medicines are natural products, they are somehow safer or more effective. However, the vast majority of alternative medicine products are completely unregulated and not yet required to demonstrate safety, efficacy, or quality before becoming commercially available. That scenario differs greatly from the way drugs have been regulated in the past.

Early attempts at regulation

The first attempt by the U.S. government to regulate any medicine—herbal or traditional—was the Food and Drugs Act of 1906, which prohibited the adulteration or misbranding of drugs. The Act focused primarily on the quality of products being marketed but didn't address the safety and efficacy of the medicines themselves. The Food and Drugs Act arose from public pressure imposed upon the government following a series of fraudulent incidents involving patent medicine manufacturers and meatpacking firms.

It wasn't until the late 1930s that the issue of product safety was finally addressed. The FDA had been established by Congress in 1928 but had been granted little authority and even less guidance about how to proceed. Subsequently, in 1937, a newly marketed product, elixir of sulfanilamide, was found to be toxic, and contributed to the deaths of more than 100 people. This tragedy became the impetus for the passage of the Federal Food, Drug, and Cosmetic Act the following year, which mandated that all drugs sold in the United States be proven safe before being marketed.

Having addressed the issues of quality and safety of medicinal products, only the issue of product efficacy remained unregulated. That changed in 1962, when Senators Kefauver and Harris amended the Federal Food, Drug, and Cosmetic Act to require that any drug originating after 1962 be proven both safe and effective before reaching the marketplace.

Current regulations

Currently in the United States, debate continues about what role the FDA should play in regulating and approving alternative medicines. The FDA presently regulates the pharmaceutical industry by requiring manufacturers of new products to file a New Drug Application, which must detail scientifically sound laboratory and clinical trials that demonstrate a drug product's safety and efficacy. These trials can be expensive, so the pharmaceutical industry tends to focus on products it can patent, which exclude naturally occurring products, such as plants and other alternative medicines.

Products approved before 1962 that had shown evidence of safety but lacked evidence of efficacy were "grandfathered in" and allowed to stay on the shelf as long as their manufacturers made no claims of the agents' efficacy. In the late 1980s, the FDA decided to examine these grandfathered drugs and commissioned a study of over-the-counter drugs, including many herbal products. A few herbal products had enough evidence to support claims of both safety and efficacy, but the majority were deemed unsafe or ineffective. In some cases, insufficient data were available to evaluate the agents' effectiveness. Although the FDA lists many herbs as safe, herbal manufacturers can't legally claim therapeutic efficacy of their products without evidence to support the claim.

As the popularity of alternative medicines began to grow, it became clear that some manufacturers in the herbal industry were trying to circumvent the intent of the Federal Food, Drug, and Cosmetic Act. Despite the fact that the manufacturers of herbal medicines couldn't put therapeutic claims directly on the container or label, a myriad of pamphlets, books, and advertisements for the product were available on request or within arm's reach from where the product sat on the shelf. As this practice became more prevalent, the FDA began to intervene, which led to political confrontations between the two sides. The climax of this huge debate yielded the Dietary Supplement, Health, and Education Act, signed into law in October, 1994. The Act defined herbal products as dietary supplements and protected them from regulation as food additives unless the products contained therapeutic claims of efficacy.

For all products introduced before October, 1994, the burden of proof to demonstrate safety was now in the hands of the FDA, not the manufacturer. The Act stipulates that all products introduced after that date must be proven safe by the manufacturer. In addition, information regarding therapeutic claims for herbal products can be disseminated into the marketplace as long as the information is neither misleading nor product-specific and is physically separated from the product and without product stickers affixed to it.

Herbal use and traditional medicine

Health care professionals should look closely at the risks and benefits of herbal medicines, just as they do at the risks and benefits of traditional therapies.

SUPPORTING HERBAL USE

Proponents of herbal medicine tend to cite three main reasons for supporting the use of herbal rather than traditional medicines.

An estimated 25% of today's relied-upon, contemporary pharmaceuticals have originated either in part or entirely from naturally occurring chemicals from plants. Advocates of herbal therapy tend to rely heavily on this fact as support for herbal pharmaceuticals. Herbal constituents or their derivatives have provided therapeutic agents for heart failure, pain, tissue congestion, edema, inflammation, cancer, constipation, hypercoagulable states, and many other diseases. Well-known therapeutic agents derived from herbal sources include capsaicin (red pepper plant), pilocarpine (jaborandi tree), taxol (Pacific yew tree), and warfarin (sweet clover). Examination of these constituents provides a compelling argument for the clinical application of future herbal agents.

Herbal medicine has been around for centuries and is said to be valuable because the philosophies and practices of herbal medicine have not perished. No one knows for sure when or where the first attempt at using a plant to effect a therapeutic cure was conducted. Some references suggest that Neanderthal man might have been one of the first phytomedicine practitioners. Ancient Middle Easterners appear to have been the first to rigorously document the use of plants for various diseases, compiling the first known pharmacopoeia, titled *Materia Medica*. The Greek historian Herodotus recounted how Egyptians worshipped certain plants, believing that some herbs held the secret to a healthy life and longevity. Not to be outdone by the Egyptians, the Greeks also incorporated various plants and flowers into several aspects of Greek mythology.

Plant use and herb worship have grown to become as diverse and as intertwined as the branches of a tree. The overwhelming majority of lay literature directed toward the consumer freely endorses the use of herbal medicines. Various advocacy texts cite anecdotal accounts of so-called cures to promote uses for the plants. There is no lack of legends, folklore, or anecdotal stories to support any herbalist's suggestions. Occasionally, these stories of success with herbs have taken on almost mythical or supernatural proportions.

RISKS

Like modern, tested pharmaceuticals, herbal medicines have some risk associated with their consumption. The fact that a plant is completely natural doesn't necessarily make the use of agents derived from that plant risk-free. Several plants, when consumed in their most natural form, can cause grave illness or even death in humans and animals. Many of these plants are routinely avoided by herbalists, scientists, and the general public because of their risks. However, hundreds of herbs and alternative medicines exist, most of which haven't been studied adequately, particularly in relation to their toxicology.

Adverse reactions to herbal medicines can be directly related to exposure to one or more chemical components of the plant or to an inappropriate or incorrect manufacturing process during the preparation of a dietary or herbal supplement.

Although laws do not require reporting of adverse effects of dietary supplements to the FDA, many adverse effects have been documented. A review of adverse effects reported in the medical literature between 1992 and 1995 highlights cases of hypersensitivity reactions, hepatotoxic reactions, and renal damage associated with various herbal products. One of the more infamous adverse events was associated with the amino-acid L-tryptophan, touted for its ability to reduce pain and promote sleep. During the late 1980s, it was discovered that tablet fillers contained in a few L-tryptophan products caused a rare, but reportedly fatal, syndrome, eosinophilia-myalgia syndrome.

Dietary supplements and weight-loss products containing ephedra alkaloids raised public concern recently owing to a number of adverse effects, such as increased blood pressure, tremors, arrhythmias, seizures, strokes, heart attacks, and death. These effects were documented in several hundred incident reports sent to the FDA between 1993 and 1997.

A study designed to assess the prevalence of herbal product use and its associated morbidity in an adult asthmatic population found an increase in the number of hospitalizations for patients who self-medicated with herbal products and black coffee or tea. In a large retrospective study of admissions to a Taiwanese hospital, it was found that 4% of admissions were related to herbal drug use, ranking herbal medications third among drug categories most responsible for adverse effects.

Inadequate or inappropriate dissemination of information to the public, combined with weak regulation, can lead unwary consumers to use herbal medicines that can cause dangerous adverse reactions. Manufacturers of dietary supplements and herbal drugs spend millions of dollars a year on advertising for their products. Existing regulations for product labeling of herbal supplements fail to provide ample warning of risks to consumers. Many advertisements could be considered misleading or at least of questionable accuracy, despite FDA restrictions to limit manufacturers' claims to those that relate only to proper health maintenance.

In addition, the awesome marketing power of the Internet has a huge potential to magnify the use of herbal products. If the information regarding the marketing of alternative medicines is left unreviewed by government agencies, this can lead to dangerous consequences. Herbal products otherwise unobtainable in the United States have been purchased over the Internet and have been associated with substantial morbidity.

HERBAL REGULATIONS

Dietary supplement and herbal medicine manufacturers are generally not required to submit to the same standards and regulations that apply to major pharmaceutical companies. As a result, the public can face significant dangers related to herbal medicine use.

In the spring of 1998, for instance, the FDA issued a warning regarding an herbal medicine named Sleeping Buddha. Apparently, the product contained an unlabeled sedative, the benzodiazepine estazolam. Fortunately, no adverse reactions from this product were reported. Around the same time, the FDA issued another warning regarding an herb called plantain, a plant that contains digitalis-like glycosides. Consumption of the herb by elderly patients or patients with cardiac disease could cause subsequent cardiac problems. Potential dangers of this sort fall into the category of what are often called extrinsic misadventures. These are usually related to a lack of standardization or to contamination, adulteration, or substitution of the products. They may also be related to a misidentification or misbranding.

The quantity of pharmacologically active chemical components of many plants can vary considerably depending on the time of year during harvest, age of the plant, or method of pollination. Other variables include the amount of water given to the plants, wind, inclement weather, and soil condition.

In addition, consumers may be exposed to a variety of compounds when herbal supplements are ingested. Manufacturers don't always separate active chemical ingredients of the plant. As a result, patients may ingest many different chemicals that occur naturally in the plant, along with the reportedly active constituents.

Additional concerns arise from the notable lack of stability testing of the product. These data are usually not available on the label or anywhere else. Various contaminants—including heavy metals, aspirin, caffeine, theophylline, diuretics, corticosteroids, benzodiazepines, and atropine—have been discovered in reportedly pure herbal products.

LACK OF CONSENSUS

There exists an overwhelming lack of consensus about how an herbal medicine should be used therapeutically. Recommended dosages vary considerably among sources, even among noted advocates in the field. No standards exist for monitoring adverse effects or effectiveness.

The time an individual spends evaluating his response to an herbal supplement could be spent seeking professional medical advice and using proven pharmacotherapy. In cases of severe depression or other severe mental illnesses or in a patient with a life-threatening disease, a delay in seeking professional help could prove the difference between life and death.

ABUSES

Unlike their prescription-only counterparts, herbal medicines can be purchased and consumed freely by virtually anyone. Purchases and use can take place without forethought or advice, without restriction or limitation, without even something as seemingly insignificant as confirming a person's age. In stark contrast, individuals are required to be a certain age before purchasing cigarettes or alcohol. Individuals wishing to purchase these chemicals must further demonstrate proof of the minimum age requirement by displaying a valid driver's license. In general, such identification is required of minors because society believes they are not mature enough and perhaps lack sufficient education to handle the potential dangers and responsibilities that accompany the use of chemicals that can intoxicate, addict, and cause physiologic damage.

Herbal medicines are not without the potential for abuse, the potential to harm, and in some cases, the potential to addict or intoxicate. Perhaps similar legislation should be passed to require consumers wishing to purchase certain herbal agents to provide some kind of identification before such a purchase can be made.

Among many cultures, traditional healers and religious leaders have used psychoactive plants as part of their rituals, yet the perception remains that plants are safe and pose no danger of abuse or dependence. Many plants might have been safely used for hundreds of years in controlled settings such as religious rituals, but when used indiscriminately by the general public, use of these plants can lead to problems.

The leaves of the coca shrub, for instance, have been chewed by the Incas and their descendants for countless generations to help them work in the high altitudes of the Andes. The anxiolytic kava, currently being heavily promoted, has been used in Polynesia for hundreds of years without reported adverse consequences, yet it is now known that the drug increases the effects of alcohol. By itself, kava can lead to intoxicating effects. Kava users continue to consume the agent even after they develop adverse effects, such as the skin reactions that can occur from chronic use.

The abuse potential of a drug may not be identified immediately; most often, it is identified after one or more controlled clinical trials. Unfortunately, herbal products don't have to undergo rigorous trials before being marketed, so problems can be identified only after many people experience a particular adverse effect such as dependence.

Cost

Although herbal medicines tend to be less expensive than their FDA-labeled counterparts, the hidden cost of herbals can be substantial. The cost of delayed effective therapy, treatment of adverse effects and drug interactions, and subsequent hospital admissions adds significantly to the cost of using ineffective herbal remedies in place of more effective traditional therapy. As herbal medicine becomes more popular, and as herbal medicine manufacturers spend increasing amounts of their profit on advertising, the cost of herbals will begin to approach the cost of traditional medicines.

Educating patients about herbal use

A stepwise approach to patient counseling allows health care professionals to carefully broach the subject of alternative therapies with their patients. Patients prescribed traditional medications deserve and are routinely given specific advice about the drugs they're receiving. Patients who use herbal or alternative medicines should be no different.

All patients should be reminded to disclose all medications they take, alternative or otherwise. Health care professionals should routinely include herbal medicines when asking about the patient's drug use and explain that full information about current medications is needed to help prevent or solve problems related to adverse effects or drug interactions. If it doesn't pose a great inconvenience for the patients, they should be asked to bring their medications with them to the health care professional's office. In the event of an adverse reaction, having the containers at hand could provide valuable data about chemical content, brand names, manufacturer names, frequency of dosage, and other important information.

The patient should be told that alternative medicines may be beneficial as well as harmful and that herbal medicines may interact adversely with the patient's existing medications or adversely affect the patient's disease. Using herbals may also lead to significant delays in the time it takes for the patient to enter the mainstream health care system and receive more appropriate and effective therapy for his condition.

Every patient should be aware of the quality of alternative products and the frequent lack of scientific evidence about herbals as compared with more traditional agents. It may be especially relevant to discuss the quality of products produced in the alternative industry versus that of the modern pharmaceutical industry or to offer comparisons between products for both industries with respect to cost, frequency of dosage, or potential adverse effects.

Patients should be instructed to watch for unusual signs or symptoms while taking any medicine, but particularly alternative medicines. These symptoms may in fact represent significant adverse reactions to the herbal medicines or drug interactions between an herbal and a traditional medicine.

Realistic and appropriate therapeutic goals should be discussed with each patient. If patients are unwilling to consider traditional pharmaceuticals, they should at least agree to monitor their goals of therapy along with the health care professional. If, after a sufficient trial of alternative medicine, these goals have not been achieved, the health care professional may be able to persuade the patient to return to more appropriate conventional pharmacotherapy.

Future of herbal medicine

Herbal medicine has evolved distinctly, isolated from the mainstream of modern medicine. The lack of available medical literature and clinical documentation makes it seem as though the growth of herbal medicine has occurred in some parallel universe. Nevertheless, precedent suggests that it may be foolish to ignore promising chemical constituents in the herbal compendium.

Experts in pharmacognosy suggest that only a small percentage of Earth's plants have been thoroughly investigated for their pharmacologic activity. Many of today's dominant pharmaceutical companies appear to have forgotten this fertile reservoir of unique chemical entities and instead concentrate on revisions or spin-offs of existing successful agents and new compounds in biotechnology. Over the years, perhaps we will continue to find that the practice of developing new medicines from plants can help many people and in some cases even bring about the creation of more valuable compounds than those taken directly from the plants themselves. ⌒

ACIDOPHILUS

Common trade names
(Various manufacturers) Bacid, DDS-Acidophilus, Florajen Acidophilus Extra Strength, Kyo-Dophilus, Lactinex (mixed culture of *Lactobacillus acidophilus* and *L. bulgaricus*), MoreDophilus, Probiata, Pro-Bionate, Superdophilus

Common forms
Available in various dosages, in cultures ranging from 500 million to 4 billion viable organisms of *L. acidophilus,* in capsules, granules, powders, softgels, suppositories, tablets, milk, and yogurts.

Source
L. acidophilus is a bacterium that is usually commercially prepared as concentrated, dried, viable cultures. Acidophilus cultures can be found in varying quantities in many dairy products, especially milk and yogurts.

Chemical components
L. acidophilus and other *Lactobacillus* species (*L. bulgaricus, L. catenaforme, L. fermentum, L. jensenii,* and *L. minutus*) are anaerobic, gram-positive, nonsporulating bacilli that typically inhabit the vaginal and GI tracts of mammals. Some evidence suggests that *L. acidophilus* may produce an antibacterial compound that improves the ability of the bacteria to survive in environments that contain competing bacteria. Although usually nonpathogenic, these bacteria have been implicated as possible causes of some infections.

Actions
L. acidophilus may aid digestion and absorption of food nutrients and produce B-complex vitamins and vitamin K. The bacterium normally resides in the GI tract with about 400 other species of bacteria and yeasts. It helps maintain a balance of bacterial diversity and prevent the overgrowth of any single species. As part of the normal GI flora, *L. acidophilus* inhibits growth of other organisms by

competing for nutrients, altering the pH of the environment, or producing bacteriocins, such as hydrogen peroxide, lactic acid, or acetic acid.

Some exogenous antibacterial compounds produced by *L. acidophilus* have been shown to affect the production of interferon. Others may exert antibacterial activity against *Helicobacter pylori* or other intestinal bacteria.

Human studies have demonstrated that the ingestion of *L. acidophilus* reduces the concentration of certain fecal enzymes that promote the formation of carcinogens in the colon. It is not known whether or not this reduction influences the prevalence of colon cancer.

Reported uses

Acidophilus cultures are commonly used to prevent or treat uncomplicated diarrhea, particularly that caused by disruption of normal intestinal flora by antimicrobials. Acidophilus cultures are also claimed to be useful in patients with infectious diarrhea, ulcerative colitis, irritable bowel syndrome, diverticulitis, or *H. pylori*–induced gastric ulcers, though evidence to support those claims is lacking.

Acidophilus may be useful as an aid in the treatment and prevention of bacterial vaginosis and vaginal yeast infections due to *Candida albicans*. However, clinical trials have been inconclusive (Fredricsson et al., 1989).

Limited evidence suggests that acidophilus may offer relief to patients with fever blisters, hives, canker sores, and acne, but these skin conditions are largely self-limiting and results are uncertain.

Attempts to document a cholesterol-lowering effect for acidophilus products in humans have so far proved unsuccessful.

Dosage

Dosage is based on the number of live organisms in a commercial acidophilus culture.

For most reported uses, a daily intake of 1 to 10 billion viable organisms administered in three or four divided doses is often cited as a reasonable regimen.

Adverse reactions

• Possible intestinal flatus initially; usually subsides with continued use.

Interactions

None reported.

Contraindications and precautions

Lactose-sensitive patients may find it difficult to tolerate dairy products containing acidophilus cultures.

Special considerations

• Know that to be effective, acidophilus products must provide viable *L. acidophilus* organisms that can survive the hostile environment of the GI tract. Proper manufacturing techniques, packaging, and storing of the product are necessary to ensure viability. Some manufacturers require refrigeration of their products, depending on which subspecies is used for the parent cultures. Some dairy sources of acidophilus, particularly yogurt and milk, may not contain viable cultures.

• Inform the patient that acidophilus acquired from dairy products may not be a reliable source of cultures because of dramatic temperature fluctuations during transport.

• Advise the patient that acidophilus products are not considered safe and effective by the FDA for use as antidiarrheals.

• Tell the patient to expect some flatus, at least initially. This reaction tends to subside with continued use.

Points of interest

• Many acidophilus products contain questionable levels of *L. acidophilus* content and may contain other bacterial species of questionable benefit. Significant variations in potency and stability have been observed. Products made by the same company but having different lot numbers have been used in clinical trials with conflicting results.

Analysis

Data supporting the use of *L. acidophilus*–containing products as antidiarrheal agents and for maintaining normal levels of intestinal and vaginal bacteria and yeasts stem mainly from in vitro studies and theoretical evidence. Clinical trials in humans have yet to yield many positive results. To further complicate the issue, variability of the quality of acidophilus cultures ingested might have influenced the results of clinical trials. Standardization of these products must be accomplished prior to conducting studies that evaluate the effectiveness of these agents for therapeutic use.

References

Fredricsson, B., et al. "Bacterial Vaginosis Is Not a Simple Ecological Disorder," *Gynecol Obstet Invest* 28:156, 1989.

ACONITE

FRIAR'S CAP, HELMET FLOWER, MONKSHOOD, SOLDIER'S CAP, WOLFSBANE

Common trade names

No commercially prepared products are available in the United States.

Common forms
Available as a tincture, tea, or liniment.

Source
Active components of the drug are obtained from leaves, flowers, and roots of *Aconitum napellus*. An erect perennial herb with tuberous roots, aconite is native to mountainous regions in Europe, Japan, China, India, and North America.

Chemical components
Aconite contains the alkaloids aconitine, picraconitine, aconine, napelline, and others responsible for the plant's primary toxicities. Potency depends on the plant's alkaloid content, which varies with the season and the altitude at which the plant was collected. Leaves and roots are usually richest in alkaloids.

Other components found in the plant include malonic acid, succinic acid, itaconic acid, aconitic acid, sugars, starches, fats, and resin.

Actions
Aconite's action is primarily cardiotoxic because of its effect on the inward sodium channels. The agent causes prolonged cardiac repolarization. As a result, various arrhythmias—primarily ventricular—can occur.

In one study, aconite (0.6 mg/kg) administered intraperitoneally to a rabbit caused damage to the myelin sheath of the visceral pathway, spinal cord, and peripheral nerves (Kim et al., 1991). Picking the flowers or other parts of the *Aconitum napellus* plant can cause toxicity due to absorption of the agent through the skin.

Reported uses
The first reported use of aconite as a therapeutic agent was in tincture preparations in the 1800s. It was believed at that time to be useful for treating neuralgia, headache, inflammation, and fever. Currently, few sources promote use of this plant for any therapeutic use because of its potential for toxicity. Some countries have incorporated aconite into topical liniments, claimed to create congestion in local blood vessels and subsequent redness of the skin.

Some literature suggests use of the agent in the treatment of hypertension.

Animal models have suggested that aconite possesses antitumor, antibacterial, and antifungal activity, but these effects have not been demonstrated in humans.

Dosage
No forms of this plant are recommended for human consumption.

Adverse reactions
- Acidosis
- Bradycardia
- Diarrhea
- Hypersalivation
- Hypokalemia
- Mydriasis and blurred vision
- Nausea
- Numbness of the oral mucosa
- Throat constriction
- Vomiting
- Weakness and paresthesia

⚠ Ventricular tachycardia may occur. Aconite-induced arrhythmias are usually unresponsive to traditional antiarrhythmics, cardioversion, and pacing. In most cases, patients were placed on bypass machines until the arrhythmia resolved on its own or until death occurred (Fitzpatrick et al., 1994; Tai et al., 1992).

⚠ Death has resulted from as little as 5 ml of aconite tincture, 2 mg of pure aconite, 1 g of crude plant parts, or 6 g cured aconite. No known antidote exists.

Interactions
Antiarrhythmics, antihypertensives, other drugs: possible enhanced toxicity. Avoid concomitant use.

Contraindications and precautions
Contraindicated for all conditions, especially in patients with known coronary disease or cardiac dysfunction, arrhythmias, or hemodynamic instability, or in those who have known hypersensitivity to the plants, or who are pregnant or breast-feeding.

Special considerations
- Instruct the patient to avoid consumption of any part of this plant.
- Inform the patient that aconite should remain in the garden. The plant should be handled only with gloves that retard absorption of plant oils through the skin.

Points of interest
- Aconite extract has been implicated in numerous suicides and was once used as a poison for arrows (Fatovich, 1992).
- Feline studies have shown that atropine may antagonize cardiac depressive and hypersalivation effects related to aconite. Human data are inconclusive in this regard.

Analysis
Case reports and available clinical information about aconite toxici-

ty and fatalities clearly illustrate the danger of this drug (But et al., 1994). Aconite currently has no therapeutic value and poses a grave danger to patients who use the agent even in small quantities.

References

But, P., et al. "Three Fatal Cases of Herbal Aconite Poisoning," *Vet Hum Toxicol* 36:212-15, 1994.

Fatovich, D. "Aconite: A Lethal Chinese Herb," *Ann Emerg Med* 21:309-11, 1992.

Fitzpatrick, A. J., et al. "Aconite Poisoning Management with a Ventricular Assist Device," *Anesth Intens Care* 22:714-17, 1994.

Kim, S. H., et al. "Myelo-Optic Neuropathy Caused by Aconite in Rabbit Model," *Jpn J Ophthalmol* 35:417, 1991.

Tai, Y., et al. "Cardiotoxicity After Accidental Herb-Induced Aconite Poisoning," *Lancet* 340:1254-56, 1992.

AGAR

AGAR-AGAR, CHINESE GELATIN, COLLE DU JAPON, E406, GELOSE, JAPANESE GELATIN, JAPANESE ISINGLASS, LAYOR CARANG, VEGETABLE GELATIN

Common trade names
(Available in combination) Agarbil, Agoral, Agoral Plain, Demosvelte-N, Falqui, Lexat, Paragar, Pseudophage

Common forms
Available as a dry powder, in flakes, or in strips.

Source
Agar is an aqueous extract from the cell walls of various species of red marine algae, including *Gelidium cartilagineum, Gracilaria confervoides,* and others.

Chemical components
Agar is composed primarily of the calcium salt of a sulfuric acid ester of the complex polysaccharide agarose-agropectin. The powdered form of agar is soluble in boiling water. The resultant solution gels when cool, even at concentrations as low as 5%.

Actions
The pharmacokinetics of agar have not been well studied in humans. Poorly absorbed from the GI tract, agar promotes fecal bulk and may influence absorption of dietary minerals, proteins, and fat.

In one study, five patients were placed on a high-fiber diet (agar-agar) for 5 days. During that time, protein and fat digestibility was markedly decreased, and fecal excretion of cholesterol increased (Kaneko et al., 1986).

In animal studies, rats fed 10% agar-agar experienced reduced absorption of calcium, iron, zinc, copper, chromium, and cobalt. A marked increase in fecal dry matter indicated that agar was not absorbed (Harmuth-Hoene et al., 1980; Kondo et al., 1996). Other animal studies show that agar decreases protein digestibility and reduces nitrogen retention (Harmuth-Hoene, 1976; Harmuth-Hoene et al., 1979). These effects may result from partial breakdown of agar by intestinal flora and a resultant inhibition of proteolytic enzymes.

Reported uses
Agar has long been used as a culture medium in bacteriology. It is also used as an emulsifying and suspending agent in many pharmaceutical and food products. Agar was formerly used frequently as a bulk-forming laxative. It has been found to be less effective than phototherapy and phenobarbital in the treatment of neonatal hyperbilirubinemia (Vales et al., 1990).

Dosage
As a bulk-forming laxative, 4 to 16 g P.O. once or twice daily.

Adverse reactions
Adverse reactions associated with bulk-forming laxatives include:
• Aspiration, when administered with insufficient liquids
• Bowel obstruction or esophageal obstruction
• Decreased absorption of vitamins, minerals and nutrients (especially calcium, iron, zinc, copper, chromium, and cobalt).

Interactions
Alcohol: dehydration and precipitation of agar from solutions. Avoid concomitant use.
Electrolyte solutions: partial dehydration and decreased viscosity of agar solutions. Avoid concomitant use.
Tannic acid: precipitation of agar from solutions. Avoid concomitant use.

Contraindications and precautions
Contraindicated in patients with impaired consciousness (because of the risk of aspiration) and in pregnant or breast-feeding patients. Use cautiously in patients with a history of esophageal or bowel obstruction or throat or swallowing problems.

Special considerations
• Be aware that bowel obstruction and esophageal obstructions are potential risks.
• Advise the patient to report signs of chest pain, chest tightness or pressure, abdominal pains, regurgitation, vomiting, or difficulty in

swallowing or breathing to their health care provider.

● Warn the patient about the potential for decreased absorption of vitamins and minerals. Products containing agar should be consumed on an empty stomach to minimize this risk.

● Advise the patient to anticipate a change in the bulk and appearance of their stools. If appropriate, offer a stool softener to patients who might have difficulty tolerating the increase in fecal bulk.

Analysis
Because no long-term human studies have assessed the effects of agar on mineral and nutrient absorption and because more effective agents such as psyllium have been developed, products containing agar should not be routinely considered in the treatment of constipation.

References

Harmuth-Hoene, A. E. "The Effect of Non-protein Food Constituents on the Nutritive Value of Radiation-Sterilized Casein," *Int J Vitam Nutr Res* 46:348-55, 1976.

Harmuth-Hoene, A. E., et al. "Effect of Indigestible Polysaccharides on Protein Digestibility and Nitrogen Retention in Growing Rats," *Nutr Metab* 23:399-407, 1979.

Harmuth-Hoene, A. E., et al. "Effect of Dietary Fiber on Mineral Absorption in Growing Rats," *J Nutr* 110:1774-84, 1980.

Kaneko, K., et al. "Effect of Fiber on Protein, Fat and Calcium Digestibility and Fecal Cholesterol Excretion," *J Nutr Sci Vitaminol* 32: 317-25, 1986.

Kondo, H., et al. "Influence of Dietary Fiber on the Bioavailability of Zinc in Rats," *Biomed Environ Sci* 9:204-08, 1996.

Vales, T.N., et al. "Pharmacologic Approaches to the Prevention and Treatment of Neonatal Hyperbilirubinemia," *Clin Perinatol* 17:245-73, 1990.

AGRIMONY

CHURCH STEEPLES, COCKLEBUR, LIVERWORT, PHILANTHROPOS, STICKLEWORT, STICKWORT

Common trade names
Potter's Piletabs (England)

Common forms
Available as tablets or teas.

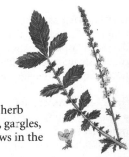

Source
The leaves, stems, and flowers of the dried herb *Agrimonia eupatoria* are used to make teas, gargles, and compresses. Agrimony commonly grows in the Western United States, Europe, and Asia.

Chemical components

Active elements in agrimony include tannins (ellagitannins and trace gallotannins), polysaccharides, silicic and urosolic acids, agrimonolide, flavonoids (luteolin and apigenin), an essential oil, and vitamins B_1, K, and ascorbic acid. The seeds contain oleic, linoleic, and linolenic acids.

Actions

Anecdotal reference to stringent and mild antiseptic properties are reported. In one animal study, agrimony extracts decreased serum glucose levels and slowed the rate of weight loss in mice with streptozotocin-induced diabetes (Swanston-Flatt et al., 1990).

Reported uses

Agrimony is claimed to be useful for many purposes. (See *Agrimony: Fact and fiction*, page 22.) However, few or no human clinical trials involving agrimony have been performed.

Dosage

Little is known about dosages for agrimony for any reported use. One source suggests adding 2 to 4 teaspoons of dried leaves per cup of water to make a tea that can be taken once daily. Other sources suggest use of agrimony in a poultice applied topically to treat sores.

Adverse reactions

• Hypersensitivity and photosensitivity reactions

Interactions

None reported.

Contraindications and precautions

Contraindicated in patients with a history of allergy to plants of the rose family and in pregnant or breast-feeding patients.

Special considerations

• Monitor the patient for dermatologic reactions, especially if the herb is being applied topically.
• Advise the patient that little scientific data about this herb exist.
• Warn the patient to avoid strong sunlight; agrimony may predispose patients to sunburn.

Points of interest

• Agrimony has been used as a dye. It is pale yellow in September and deep yellow later in the year.

Analysis

This plant is not recommended for medicinal use because little information about its safety and effectiveness exists.

References

Swanston-Flatt, S. K., et al. "Traditional Plant Treatments for Diabetes: Studies in Normal and Streptozotocin Diabetic Mice," *Diabetologia* 33:462-64, 1990.

ALLSPICE

CLOVE PEPPER, JAMAICA PEPPER, PIMENTA, PIMENTO

Common trade names

Available as a condiment in various commercial preparations.

Common forms

Available in various forms.
Powdered fruit: 10 to 30 grains
Fluid extract: essential oil
Pimento water (aqua pimentae): contains oil of pimento, 1 fluid oz.

Source

Active chemicals are derived from the dried, unripened berries of a tree (*Pimento officinalis* or *Eugenia pimenta*) native to Central America, Mexico, and the West Indies.

Chemical components

The active components of allspice include eugenol, methyleugenol, and caryophyllene in a volatile oil. Other components include quercetin, glycosides, sesquiterpenes, vitamins (A, C, thiamine, riboflavin, niacin), minerals, tannin, resin, sugar, and gum. The volatile oil can be obtained through distillation of the fruit. The rind of the berries is thought to lead to the greatest medicinal activity.

Actions

Limited data are available on the pharmacokinetic actions of the active ingredients. Two metabolites have been identified: homovanillic acid and homomandelic acid.

In animal models, about 1% of the active ingredient, eugenol, is demethylated. It causes CNS depression and inhibits prostaglandin activity in human colonic tissue. Eugenol has also been claimed to possess antioxidant properties. Eugenol is excreted mostly in the urine.

Allspice is claimed to act as a GI stimulant and an antiflatulent agent. Eugenol is known to increase the activity of certain digestive enzymes including trypsin, a protein-digesting enzyme.

Pimentol, derived from methanol extract of allspice, acts as a hydroxyl radical scavenger in in vitro models. Eugenol's antioxidant properties have been reproduced in a few in vitro studies. Despite this effect, however, some data suggest that eugenol may promote cancer growth (Oya et al., 1997).

Several in vitro studies of allspice provide evidence of antibacterial and antifungal activity (Hitokoto et al., 1980; Moleyar and Narasimham, 1992; Nadal et al., 1973).

In animal studies, ethanolic and aqueous extracts administered I.V. to rats caused dose-related hypotension, CNS depression, analgesia, and hypothermia (Suarez et al., 1997).

Reported uses

The essential oil derived from the allspice berry has been claimed to be therapeutically useful in the treatment of indigestion and flatulence in traditional medicine, but there is little or no clinical data to support these claims.

Other claims of therapeutic usefulness include treatment of diarrhea, fatigue, diabetes, colds, menstrual cramps, and hysterical paroxysms. However, there is no evidence to support these claims. No human clinical trials have been reported in the literature.

Crushed allspice berries have been applied topically to treat bruises and soothe sore joints and muscles. The anesthetic properties of eugenol may be the rationale for this application. Indeed, eugenol is used by dentists as a local anesthetic and antiseptic for teeth and gums.

Dosage

As a vehicle for purgative medicines, 1 to 2 fluid oz (5 parts bruised pimento to 200 parts water, distilled down to 100 parts).

For indigestion, 1 to 2 teaspoons allspice powder per cup of water may be given, up to 3 cups daily.

For flatulence, 2 to 3 drops of allspice oil on sugar may be given.

For toothache pain, 1 to 2 drops of allspice oil may be applied to painful area. Do not administer more often than q.i.d.

For muscle pain, allspice powder may be mixed with enough water to make a paste to be applied topically.

Adverse reactions

• Gastroenteritis
• Nausea
• Rash (contact dermatitis)
• Vomiting
⚠ Seizures (with excessive use)

Interactions

Iron and other minerals: interference with absorption of the minerals. Avoid concomitant use.

Contraindications and precautions

Contraindicated in patients with chronic GI diseases, such as duodenal ulcers, reflux disease, ulcerative colitis, spastic colitis, diverticulosis, or diverticulitis. Also contraindicated in patients with cancer or who are at high risk for cancer. Avoid use in pregnant or breast-feeding patients.

Special considerations

• Monitor the patient using allspice topically for hypersensitivity reactions.
• Inform the patient that eugenol may pose an undetermined potential risk of cancer.
• Advise the patient that some sources recommend that no more allspice should be consumed than an amount normally contained in foods as a condiment.

Points of interest

• Allspice is commonly used as an aromatic spice in foods and to provide flavor in toothpaste and other products. It is regarded as safe for external use by the FDA.

Analysis

With the exception of a few in vitro and animal studies and human toxicology case reports, limited clinical data exist to support the use of allspice for any of its alleged therapeutic uses. Most of the information currently available on this agent is found in the lay literature, not peer-reviewed journals. Allspice and eugenol have been widely used in foods, dental products, and other pharmaceuticals, and can be considered safe for consumption in small quantities. However, controlled clinical trials are needed to explore larger therapeutic claims.

References

Hitokoto, H., et al. "Inhibitory Effects of Spices on Growth and Toxin Production of Toxigenic Fungi," *Appl Environ Microbiol* 39: 818-22, 1980.

Kanerva, L., et al. "Occupational Allergic Contact Dermatitis from Spices," *Contact Dermatitis* 35:157-62, 1996.

Moleyar, V., and Narasimham, P. "Antibacterial Activity of Essential Oil Components," *Int J Food Microbiol* 16: 337-42, 1992.

Nadal, N., et al. "Antimicrobial Properties of Bay and Other Phenolic Essential Oils," *Cosmet Perum* 88:37-38, 1973.

Oya, T., et al. "Spice Constituents Scavenging Free Radical and Inhibiting Pentosidine Formation in a Model System," *Biosci Biotechnol Biochem* 61: 263-66, 1997.

Suarez, U.A., et al. "Cardiovascular Effects of Thanolica and Aqueous Extracts of *Pimenta dioica* in Sprague-Dawley Rats," *J Ethnopharmacol* 5: 107-11, 1997.

ALOE

ALOE BARBADENSIS, ALOE VERA, BARBADOS ALOE, BURN PLANT, CAPE ALOE, CURACAO ALOE, ELEPHANT'S GALL, FIRST-AID PLANT, HSIANG-DAN, LILY OF THE DESERT, LU-HUI, MEDICINE PLANT, MIRACLE PLANT, PLANT OF IMMORTALITY, SOCOTRINE ALOE, VENEZUELA ALOE, ZANZIBAR ALOE

Common trade names

(Various manufacturers; available in combination) All Natural Aloe Vera Gel, Aloe Grande, Alce Vera Gel, Soft Gel Capsules; Aloe Vera Inner Leaf Capsules, Aloe Vera Jelly, Aloe Vera Juice, Aloe Vera Ointment, Aloe Vesta Perineal, Benzoin Compound Tincture, Dermaide Aloe, Skin Gel Aloe Life, Whole Leaf Aloe Vera Juice

Common forms

Capsules: 75 mg, 100 mg, 200 mg aloe vera extract, or aloe vera powder
Gel: 98%, 99.5%, 99.6%, aloe vera gel
Juice: 99.6%, 99.7%, aloe vera juice
Also available as cream, hair conditioner, jelly, juice, liniment, lotion, ointment, shampoo, skin cream, soap, sunscreen, and in facial tissues.

Source

Aloe gel is obtained from the center parenchymatous tissues of the large blade-like leaves of *Aloe vera* (also referred to as *Aloe barbadensis, A. vulgaris* hybrids, *A. africana, A. ferox, A. perryi,* and *A. spicata*). Orally ingested preparations are composed either of the colorless juice from secretory cells located just below the leaf epidermis or a solid yellow latex obtained by evaporating the juice.

Commercial products are available as topical and oral preparations. Topical preparations contain a colorless mucilaginous gel, called aloe gel or aloe vera gel. This gel is sometimes erroneously called "aloe juice." Aloe gel is prepared by a variety of methods, with variable consistencies and stability, although fresh gel from the plant may be preferred.

Chemical components

The chemical composition of aloe varies, depending on the species and the environmental growing conditions. The juice and latex contain hydroanthraquinone derivatives (10-C-D-glucosyl diastereoisomers of aloe-emodin anthrone) including anthraquinone glycosides aloin A and B (formerly known as barbaloin and isobarbaloin, respectively). A reddish black glistening residue known as aloin (a mixture of aloin A and aloin B) is produced when the latex is filtered and dried.

Aloe gel, in contrast, is mostly water. Other gel compounds include bradykininase, a serine carboxypeptidase, magnesium lactate, organic acids, steroids, sugars, vitamins, and the polysaccharides acemannan and glucomannan. Because mechanical separation of gel from latex is not always complete, aloe gel may accidentally contain anthraquinone glycosides from the latex.

Actions

When taken internally, aloin is cleaved by intestinal bacteria and produces a metabolite that irritates the large intestines and stimulates colonic motility, propulsion, and transit time. In addition, aloin causes active secretion of fluids and electrolytes in the lumen and inhibits reabsorption of fluids from the colon. These effects cause a feeling of distention and increased peristalsis. The cathartic effect occurs 8 to 12 hours after ingestion.

When taken externally, besides acting as a moisturizer on burns and other wounds, aloe reduces inflammation, possibly by blocking production of thromboxane A_2, inactivating bradykinin, inhibiting prostaglandin A_2, and inhibiting oxidation of arachidonic acid.

Aloe's antipruritic effect may result from blockage of the conversion of histidine to histamine as a result of the inhibition of histidine decarboxylase. Wound healing is believed to result from increased blood flow to the wounded area.

Some in vitro studies have demonstrated that aloe juice and aloe gel preparations inhibit the growth of bacteria and fungi commonly isolated from wounds and burns (Grindlay and Reynolds, 1986). Other studies have found inconsistent activity in this regard. Conflicting results may be due to variable content of the aloe preparations and deterioration of some of the active compounds. Because the identification and stability of the active components are unknown, the clinical relevance of claims of antibacterial and antifungal effects remains unknown.

Reported uses

Therapeutic claims center on its use externally as a topical gel for minor burns, sunburn, cuts, frostbite, skin irritation, and other dermal wounds and abrasions. Numerous studies have validated these claims by demonstrating that topical application of aloe gel decreases acute inflammation, promotes wound healing, reduces pain, and exerts an antipruritic effect (Heggers et al., 1987).

Internally, the dried latex has been claimed to be useful as a stimulant laxative. Other claims for use of aloe include amenorrhea, asthma, colds, seizures, bleeding, and ulcers. No medical evidence supports the clinical application of aloe for these conditions.

Aloe preparations have also been considered for use in the treatment of acne, AIDS, arthritis, asthma, blindness, bursitis, cancer, colitis, depression, diabetes, glaucoma, hemorrhoids, multiple sclerosis, peptic ulcers, and varicose veins. No well-controlled clinical trials substantiate the use of aloe for any of these disorders.

Dosage

For pruritus, skin irritation, burns, and other wounds (external forms), aloe may be applied liberally as needed. Although internal use is not recommended, some sources suggest 100 to 200 mg aloe or 50 to 100 mg aloe extract P.O., taken in the evening. Information about dosages for aloe juice is lacking.

Adverse reactions

- Accumulation of blood in pelvic region (with large doses)
- Contact dermatitis
- Damage to mucosa of the intestine (may be irreversible)
- Delayed healing of deep wounds due to reduced oxygen permeability (topical forms)
- Harmless brown discoloration of the intestinal mucous membranes and red discoloration of the urine (with frequent use)
- Painful intestinal spasms

⚠ Fluid and electrolyte loss from frequent use; loss of potassium from intestine, leading to reduced serum potassium

⚠ Reflex stimulation of uterine musculature, which may cause spontaneous abortion or premature birth during late pregnancy
⚠ Severe hemorrhagic diarrhea, kidney damage, and possible death from overdose

Interactions

Antiarrhythmics, cardiac glycosides, loop diuretics, other potassium-wasting drugs, steroids, thiazides: increased effects when aloe used internally. Avoid internal use of aloe when taking these drugs.

Contraindications and precautions

External aloe preparations contraindicated in patients known to be hypersensitive to aloe or in those with a history of allergic reactions to plants in the Liliaceae family (garlic, onions, and tulips). Internal use contraindicated in pregnant or breast-feeding patients, during menstruation, in children, and in patients with kidney or cardiac disease (because of the potential for hypokalemia and possible disturbance of cardiac rhythm).

Special considerations

⚠ Know that oral use can cause severe abdominal discomfort and serious hypokalemia and electrolyte imbalance.
⚠ Be aware that unapproved use of aloe vera injections for cancer has been associated with the death of four patients (Anon., 1998). Use of injectable aloe vera preparations or chemical constituents of aloe vera is not recommended.
• Caution the patient against the use of aloe vera gel or aloe vera juice for internal use.

Analysis

Aloe has a long history of popular use, and topical use of aloe is generally considered safe. However, the FDA does not recommend aloe for any specific condition. Fresh aloe may be useful for the treatment of burns and minor tissue injury; however, studies are not well documented. Because aloe laxatives containing anthraquinone produce dramatic cathartic effects, less toxic laxatives should be used. There are no studies supporting the use of aloe juice for internal consumption. Although a recent in vitro study found that aloe-emodin exerts genotoxic activity (Muller et al., 1996), further research is needed regarding its use as an anticancer agent.

References

Anon. "License Revoked for Aloe Vera Use," *Nat Med Law* 1:1-2, 1998.
Grindlay, D., and Reynolds, T. "The Aloe Vera Phenomenon: A Review of the Properties and Modern Uses of the Leaf Parenchyma Gel," *J Ethnopharmacol* 16:117-51, 1986.

Heggers, J.P., et al. "Beneficial Effects of Aloe in Wound Healing," *Phytotherapy Res* 7:S48-S52, 1987.

Muller, S.O., et al. "Genotoxicity of the Laxative Drug Components Emodin, Aloe-Emodin, and Danthron in Mammalian Cells: Topoisomerase II-Mediated," *Mutat Res* 371:165-73, 1996.

AMERICAN CRANESBILL

ALUM BLOOM, ALUM ROOT, AMERICAN KINO, CHOCO-
LATE FLOWER, CROWFOOT, DOVE'S-FOOT, *GERANIUM
ROBERTIANUM*, HERB ROBERT, OLD MAID'S NIGHTCAP,
SHAMEFACE, SPOTTED CRANESBILL, STINKING CRANES-
BILL, STORKSBILL, WILD CRANESBILL, WILD GERANIUM

Common trade names
None known.

Common forms
Available as extracts, decoctions, tinctures, teas, and poultices.

Source
Forms for internal use are prepared using the dried rhizome and leaves of *Geranium maculatum,* a perennial herb found commonly in the Eastern United States and Canada. Topical preparations are usually created using flowers of the plant.

Chemical components
Tannin, which is hydrolyzed to gallic acid, is the principal active ingredient of American cranesbill. It occurs in high concentrations in the dried rhizomes of *Geranium maculatum.*

Actions
Precise mechanisms of action have not been adequately described in primary medical literature.

Reported uses
The internal use of the extract has been claimed to be useful for cancer, inflammation of the lip, leukorrhea, diarrhea, cholera, dysentery, plague, renal bleeding, inflammation of the bladder, menorrhagia, and metrorrhagia, and as a contraceptive.

Claims for external use include stomatitis, burns, sores, sore throat, and hemorrhoids. Modern medical literature has not justified these claims. One recent in vitro study found no antibacterial activity of American cranesbill against organisms that cause cholera (Guevara et al., 1994).

Dosage
Infusion: 1 oz of plant material in 1 pint of water.
Decoction: 1 to 2 teaspoons of the rhizome in 1 cup of water t.i.d.
Tincture: 2 to 4 ml t.i.d.

Adverse reactions
• Hepatotoxicity (with high tannin concentrations)

Interactions
None reported.

Contraindications and precautions
Contraindicated in pregnant or breast-feeding patients.

Special considerations
• Advise the patient to avoid consuming this herb because not enough is known about its effects.
• Advise the patient still wishing to use this herb to report unusual symptoms to a health care professional.

Analysis
Because safety and efficacy data of American cranesbill are unavailable, its use should be avoided.

References
Guevara, J.M., et al., "The In Vitro Action of Plants on *Vibrio cholerae,*" *Rev Gastroenterol Peru* 14:27-31, 1994. Abstract.

ANGELICA

ANGELICA ROOT, ANGELIQUE, DONG QUAI, ENGELWURZEL, GARDEN ANGELICA, HEILIGENWURZEL, ROOT OF THE HOLY GHOST, TANG-KUEI, WILD ANGELICA

Common trade names
(Various manufacturers) The species *Angelica sinensis,* from which this agent gets its name, is known as dong quai or tang-kuei.

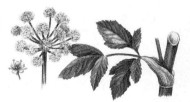

Common forms
Available as fluid extract, tincture, essential oil, or cut, dried, or powdered root.

Source

Active compounds are derived from the roots, fruits, rhizomes, and leaves of many species of *Angelica*, a perennial in the parsley family, which includes *A. acutiloba, A. archangelica, A. atropurpurea, A. dahurica, A. edulis, A. gigas, A. keiskei, A. koreana, A. polymorpha, A. pubescens, A. radix,* and *A. sinensis.*

Chemical components

Various coumarins, (angelicin, osthol, bergapten, imperatorin, oreoselone, oxypeucedanin, umbelliferone, xanthotoxol, and xanthotoxin) have been isolated from different *Angelica* species. The phenolic compound ferulic acid has been obtained from *A. sinensis.* Decursinol angelate is purified from the root of *A. gigas.* Two chalcones (xanthoangelol and 4-hydroxyderricin) are isolated from *A. keiskei.*

Other compounds have been isolated from the roots and fruits of *A. archangelica,* such as terpene hydrocarbons, alcohols, esters, lactones, aliphatic carbonyls, and other aromatic compounds. Polysaccharides, palmitic acid, and the flavonoid archangelenone have also been isolated. Other compounds found in the volatile oils include alpha- and beta-phellandrene, alpha-pinene, alpha-thujene, limonene, beta-carophyllene, linalool, borneol, acetaldehyde, and some macrocyclic lactones.

Actions

Antitumor properties have been noted in several animals. Decursinol angelate has cytotoxic and protein-kinase C activating activities (Ahn et al., 1996). In mice with skin cancer, chalcones from the root extract of *A. keiskei* exhibited potent antitumor properties. Extracts from *A. archangelica* reduced the mutagenic effects of thiotepa in mouse bone marrow cells, and *A. radix* increased the production of tumor necrosis factor in mice.

Anti-inflammatory and analgesic properties have also been noted. Compounds isolated from the roots of *A. pubescens* inhibited centrally and peripherally mediated inflammatory substances.

Coumarin osthole inhibits platelet aggregation in vivo and in vitro (Hoult and Paya, 1996). *A. sinensis* significantly inhibited thromboxane A_2 formation and mildly affected prostaglandin I_2 production in animals compared with aspirin.

Angelica polysaccharide has been shown to promote the proliferation and differentiation of hematopoietic progenitor cells in healthy and anemic mice (Wang and Zhu, 1996).

Coumarins and ferulic acid from *A. dahurica* root have antimicrobial actions (Kwon et al., 1997). Two chalcones isolated from *A. keiskei* also showed antibacterial activity against gram-positive bacteria.

The aqueous extract of *A. sinensis* given I.V. decreased myocardial injury and the incidence of premature ventricular contractions and arrhythmias induced by myocardial reperfusion. Furanocoumarins inhibited the in vitro binding of diazepam to CNS benzodiazepine receptors in rat cells (Bergendorff et al., 1997).

A. sinensis and nifedipine improved pulmonary function and decreased mean arterial pulmonary pressures in chronic obstructive pulmonary disease patients with pulmonary hypertension. *A. polymorpha* has been found to selectively inhibit the production of allergic antibodies in asthmatics.

Uterine stimulant effects on the mouse and relaxation of the trachea in animals have been observed.

Reported uses

This Chinese herb has been claimed to be of therapeutic usefulness for many disorders. It has been called a "cure-all" for gynecologic disorders and been promoted for such conditions as postmenopausal symptoms, menstrual discomfort, and anemia as a result of the agent's purported estrogen-like effects and erythropoietic potential. However, no controlled studies have corroborated these benefits.

In a study of young women with leukorrhagia and insufficient luteal function, angelica root extract, in combination with several other Chinese herbs, regulated the menstrual cycle and reduced the severity of leukorrhagia.

Other claims include angelica's ability to improve circulation in the extremities, to treat headaches and backaches, and to relieve osteoporosis, hay fever, asthma, and eczema.

Most studies on angelica have been conducted on animals, making it difficult to determine therapeutic benefits in humans.

Dosage

No consensus exists. Studies conducted with angelica used various concentrations of extracts, aqueous solutions, and powders, making identification of standardized dosage difficult.

Adverse reactions

• Hypotension from coumarins derived from *A. pubescens* (Hoult and Paya, 1996)

• Photodermatitis and phototoxicity due to effect of furanocoumarins

⚠ Potential increased risk of bleeding when used in combination with drugs such as heparin or warfarin

Interactions

Warfarin: significantly prolonged PT when *A. sinensis* is administered with warfarin. Avoid concomitant use.

Contraindications and precautions

Avoid use in pregnant or breast-feeding patients because of potential stimulant effects on the uterus. Use cautiously in diabetic patients.

Special considerations

● Monitor the patient taking angelica for signs of bleeding—especially if anticoagulants are being taken.

● Advise the patient that using angelica poses a cancer risk.

● Warn the patient to watch for signs of allergic reactions to this plant and to report such reactions promptly to the health care professional.

● Advise the patient to take precautions against direct sun exposure while taking angelica preparations.

Points of interest

● *A. atropurpurea* last appeared in the USP around 1860.

● Concerns have been raised regarding the potential carcinogenic risk of angelica, which led the International Fragrance Commission to recommend a limit of 0.78% angelica root in commercial preparations of suntan lotions.

Analysis

Although angelica is widely used in traditional Chinese medicine, the use of the agent appears supported only by anecdotal evidence. The herb has been studied extensively in animal models, but scientifically valid human studies are lacking. Until more conclusive data are available, it is difficult to justify the therapeutic use of angelica for specific disorders.

References

Ahn K.S., et al. "Decursinol Angelate: A Cytotoxic and Protein Kinase-C Activating Agent from the Root of *Angelica gigas*," *Planta Med* 62:7-9, 1996.

Bergendorff, O., et al. "Furanocoumarins with Affinity to Brain Benzodiazepine Receptors In Vitro," *Phytochemistry* 44:1121-24, 1997.

Hoult, J.R., and Paya, M. "Pharmacological and Biochemical Actions of Simple Coumarins: Natural Products with Therapeutic Potential," *Gen Pharmacol* 27:713-22, 1996.

Kwon, Y.S., et al. "Antimicrobial Constituents of *Angelica dahurica* Roots," *Phytochemistry* 44:887-89, 1997.

Wang, Y., and Zhu, B. "The Effect of Angelica Polysaccharide on Proliferation and Differentiation of Hematopoietic Progenitor Cells," *Chung Hua I Hsueh Tsa Chih* 76:363-66, 1996.

ANISE

ANISEED, ANISE OIL, SWEET CUMIN

Common trade names
(Various manufacturers) Beech Cough Drops, Bronhillor Natural Source Cough Candies & Throat Discs

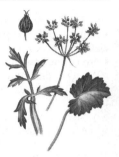

Common forms
Available as an extract, in lozenges, and in teas. Also available in trace quantities as flavoring agents in liqueurs, lozenges, and teas as well as a fragrance in soaps, creams, perfumes, foods, and candies.

Source
Pimpinella anisum, the anise plant, is native to the Mediterranean area. The dried ripe fruit of the plant is referred to as aniseed. Anise oil is extracted from aniseed by steam distillation. Anise oil can also be obtained from the Chinese star anise plant (*Illicium verum*).

Chemical components
Anise extract typically contains 1% to 3% volatile anise oil. The primary constituent of anise oil is anethole (80% to 90%). Other components include alpha-pinene, linalool, anisaldehyde, and methyl chavicol. The composition of anise oil from *I. verum* resembles that obtained from *P. anisum* but also contains trace quantities of safrole and myristicin. Naturally occurring coumarins and sitosterols have been found in tissue cultures of the root of *P. anisum*.

Actions
Despite weak anticonvulsant effects, animal models have failed to justify claims of anise in this therapeutic application. One report suggests that aniseed extract exhibits mild sympathomimetic activity. Mucociliary transport velocity increased when patches of ciliated epithelium of frog esophagus were exposed to anise oil extract. However, another study showed that other volatile oils have more pronounced sympathomimetic effects than does anise oil.

Anise oil has been shown to exert varying effects on tracheal and ileal smooth muscle of the guinea pig (Reiter and Brandt, 1985). Anise oil extract exerts estrogenic, antifungal, and antibacterial properties. Anethole, a component of anise, gives licorice its characteristic flavor and odor (Caldwell and Sutton, 1988).

Reported uses

Therapeutic claims surround the use of this agent as an antispasmodic, anti-asthmatic, antiflatulent agent, cough suppressant, and expectorant. Modern medical literature describing well-designed trials do not confirm any of these therapeutic benefits in humans. The primary use of anise oil remains as a flavoring agent in foods and beverages. It has also been used as an insect repellent and insecticide.

In a Russian study, a combination of volatile oils was given to decrease mental fatigue in a group of aviation flight controllers. Combinations of anise, brandy mint, and lavender were shown to prevent occupation-induced changes in mental capacity and blood content and tension of the cerebrovascular circulation (Leshchinskaia et al., 1983).

Anecdotal reports suggest that anethole ointment has been used to treat lice and scabies (Chandler and Hawkes, 1984).

Dosage

For intestinal gas, 0.1 ml anise oil P.O. t.i.d.

Small quantities of anise are commonly found in cough drops, baked goods, and beverages.

Adverse reactions

● Allergic hypersensitivity and contact dermatitis
● Stomatitis and inflammation of the l p when used in toothpaste
⚠ Nausea, vomiting, seizures and pulmonary edema with ingestion of as little as 1 to 5 ml of anise oil
⚠ Pseudo-Conn's syndrome (hypermineralocorticism) possible after intoxication of anise-based beverage (Trono et al., 1983)

Interactions

Iron: possibly enhanced iron absorption across the intestinal mucosa. A study with rats suggests that anise extract may promote the absorption of iron across the intestinal mucosa (el-Shobaki et al., 1990). However, this effect has not been studied in humans. Avoid concomitant use.

Contraindications and precautions

Contraindicated in pregnancy (potential for estrogenic activity). Use cautiously in patients prone to atopy or contact dermatitis.

Special considerations

● Pure anise oil should not be taken internally except under the supervision of a health care provider.
● Store in a tightly sealed, light-resistant container at room temperature.

• Monitor the patient for weight gain as a result of sodium and water retention.
• Advise the patient against ingesting pure anise oil because of potential toxicity.

Points of interest
• Anise oil is generally considered safe by the FDA.

Analysis
Although ancient medical folklore has suggested many applications for anise oil, actual therapeutic benefits appear limited. Until more data become available, anise should be used only as a flavoring agent and a fragrance. Ingestion of large quantities (at least several milliliters) of anise oil should probably be avoided because of potential gastrotoxicity.

References
Caldwell, J., and Sutton, J.D. "Influence of Dose Size on the Disposition of Trans-methoxy-14C Anethole in Human Volunteers," *Food Chem Toxicol* 26:87-91, 1988.
Chandler, R.F., and Hawkes, D. "Aniseed: Spice, Flavor, Drug," *Can Pharm J* 117:28-29, 1984.
Leshchinskaia, I.S., et al. "Effect of Phytonocides on the Dynamics of the Cerebral Circulation in Flight Controllers During Their Occupational Activity," *Kosm Biol Aviakosm Med* 17:80-83, 1983.
Reiter, M., and Brandt, W. "Relaxant Effects on Tracheal and Ileal Smooth Muscles of the Guinea Pig," *Arzneimittelforschung* 35:408-14, 1985.
el-Shobaki, F.A., et al. "The Effect of Some Beverage Extracts on Intestinal Iron Absorption," *Z Ernahrungswiss* 29:264-69, 1990.
Trono, D., et al. "Pseudo-Conn's Syndrome due to Intoxication with Non-alcoholic Pastis," *Schweiz Med Wochenschr* 113:1092-95, 1983.

ARNICA

ARNICA FLOWERS, ARNICA ROOT, COMMON ARNICA, LEOPARD'S BANE, MEXICAN ARNICA, MOUNTAIN ARNICA, MOUNTAIN DAISY, MOUNTAIN TOBACCO, SNEEZEWORT, WOLF'S BANE

Common trade names
Arnicaid, Arnica Spray, Arniflora (Gel)

Common forms
Available as a spray for topical application and in tablets, teas, gels, tinctures, creams (preferred in Europe), ointments, and sublingual preparations. Creams typically contain 15% arnica oil; salves should contain 20% to 25% arnica oil.

Source

Active components are usually extracted from the flowers and root-stocks of *Arnica montana, A. fulgens, A. sororia,* and *A. cordofolia.* Mexican arnica is derived from *Heterotheca inuloides.* Certain species of *Arnica* are native from Alaska to the Western United States and Mexico. Others are native to Europe and Siberia.

Chemical components

Arnica's active ingredients are thought to be flavonoid glycosides and sesquiterpenoid lactones, including arnisterol (arnidiol), anthoxanthine, faradiol, helenalin, dihydrohelenalin, and choline. Arnica also contains a group of polysaccharides with a content of 65% to 100% galacturonic acid and 0.5% to 1% volatile oils, tannins, and resins.

Actions

Four sesquiterpenoids isolated from *H. inuloides* in one study demonstrated antibacterial activity in vitro. One compound exhibited gram-positive antibacterial activity and minimal bactericidal concentrations of 12.5 mcg/ml against methicillin-resistant *Staphylococcus aureus* (Kubo et al., 1994).

An *A. montana* extract has been shown to increase phagocytosis in mice (Wagner and Jurcic, 1991).

In a Dutch study, most arnica flavonoids demonstrated moderate to low cytotoxicity in vitro when compared to cisplatin. Helenalin, a sesquiterpene lactone, displayed the strongest cytotoxicity (Willuhn et al., 1994). Another study apparently found a quicker recovery from carbon tetrachloride–induced toxic liver injury in rats when the rats were given a preparation of phenolic compounds of *A. montana.*

An in vitro study found that helenalin and dihydrohelenalin inhibited platelet function in humans. Another study in healthy human volunteers failed to find significant effects on blood clotting parameters immediately following administration of an arnica extract (Baillargeon et al., 1993).

In vitro studies have documented an anti-inflammatory effect for some components of arnica (Schaffner, 1997).

Reported uses

Arnica is claimed to be useful for relieving muscle and joint aches and is frequently cited in herbal literature as being able to promote wound healing. In veterinary medicine, the agent is classified as a counterirritant, an effect most likely related to the isomeric alcohol component of arnica.

Analgesic effects failed to be verified in a double-blind study of arnica, metronidazole, and a placebo among postoperative dental patients (Kaziro, 1984). (See *Analgesic effects of arnica,* page 38.)

RESEARCH FINDINGS

Analgesic effects of arnica

A study involving 118 patients with impacted wisdom teeth examined a tincture of *Arnica montana* for its analgesic and wound healing abilities (Kaziro, 1984). Random assignment of metronidazole 400 mg, arnica 200 centisemal dilutions in neutral tablets, or placebo was given b.i.d. to subjects after having their teeth extracted. The subjects were also given a regularly scheduled narcotic analgesic.

Double-blind assessment of pain as measured by visual analogue scale, trismus (mouth-opening), edema, and wound healing was conducted in all patients in each group at postoperative days 4 and 8. On day 4, pain relief scores were not significantly different. On day 8, results indicated a statistically significant difference in analgesia in favor of metronidazole when compared with either arnica or placebo.

Metronidazole was also more effective than either arnica or placebo in its ability to prevent swelling and promote healing. Arnica was not favored in any of the outcome measurements. In fact, the investigators found that arnica seemed to increase pain and edema. Although this study found differences favoring the use of metronidazole, the statistical test used is questionable for the data evaluated. Results should be assessed with that caution in mind.

Similarly, a homeopathic dose of arnica was tested against a placebo in a population of postoperative abdominal hysterectomy patients. No significant difference was found between the two groups (Hart et al., 1997). In a small study of marathon runners, another formulation of arnica failed to produce statistically significant benefits in muscle stiffness, laboratory measurements of muscle injury, or healing time of muscle injuries.

Dosage
No consensus exists. Homeopathic doses (trace quantities) appear to be most popular.

Adverse reactions
• Allergic dermatitis (with topical use)
• Gastroenteritis
• Hepatic failure
• Nervous disorders
⚠ Cardiac toxicity, arrhythmias, hypertension
⚠ Muscular weakness, collapse, and death
⚠ Nausea, vomiting, organ damage, coma, and possibly death in

children from ingestion of arnica flowers or roots. Induce emesis and gastric lavage to remove undigested contents. Supportive care may be necessary.

Interactions
Antihypertensive agents: possible reduced effectiveness of antihypertensive agents. Avoid concomitant use.

Contraindications and precautions
Avoid use in pregnant patients because of the risk of uterine oxytocic activity and lack of knowledge about its teratogenic potential.

Special considerations
• Do not apply arnica to abraded skin or open wounds.
• Keep arnica preparations out of the reach of children.
• Explain to the patient that when taken orally or applied to an open wound, arnica may cause hypertension, cardiotoxicity, vertigo, and renal dysfunction due to activity of sesquiterpene lactones and components of the essential oil.
• Advise the patient to avoid prolonged topical use because of the potential for allergic hypersensitivity reaction.

Points of interest
• Arnica has been approved by the German Commission E as a topical agent with effective anti-inflammatory, analgesic, and antibacterial properties. The FDA, however, has classified arnica as an unsafe herb.

Analysis
Despite interesting in vitro studies and exciting possibilities for use of this agent, clinical trials have failed to document therapeutic benefits of arnica. External use is discouraged because of the risk of allergic reactions.

The results of well-conducted clinical trials that verify a favorable risk-benefit ratio are needed before therapeutic applications can be considered.

References
Baillargeon, L., et al. "The Effects of *Arnica montana* on Blood Coagulation: A Randomized, Controlled Trial," *Can Fam Physician* 39:2362-67, 1993.

Hart, O. et al. "Double-Blind, Placebo-Controlled, Randomized Clinical Trial of Homeopathic Arnica C30 for Pain and Infection After Total Abdominal Hysterectomy," *J R Soc Med* 90:73-78, 1997

Kaziro, G.S. "Metronidazole and *Arnica montana* in the Prevention of Postsurgical Complications: A Comparative Placebo-Controlled Trial," *Br J Oral Maxillofac Surg* 22:42-49, 1984.

Kubo, I., et al. "Antimicrobial Agents from *Heterotheca inuloides*," *Planta Med* 60:218-21, 1994.

Schaffner, W. "Granny's Remedy Explained at the Molecular Level: Helenalin Inhibits NF-kappa B," *Biol Chem* 378:935, 1997. Editorial.

Wagner, H., and Jurcic , K. "Immunologic Studies of Plant Combination Preparations: In Vitro and In Vivo Studies on the Stimulation of Phagocytosis," *Arzneimittelforschung* 10:1072-76, 1991.

Willuhn, G., et al. "Cytotoxicity of Flavonoids and Sesquiterpene Lactones from *Arnica* Species Against GLC4 and the COLO 320 Cell Lines," *Planta Med* 60:434-37, 1994.

AVENS

BENEDICT'S HERB, CITY AVENS, CLOVE ROOT, COLEWORT, GEUM, GOLDY STAR, HERB BENNET, WAY BENNET, WILD RYE, WOOD AVENS

Common trade names
Few or no commercially prepared products are available in the United States.

Common forms
Available as a tincture or tea.

Source
The drug is a volatile oil extracted from the dried herb, rhizome, or root of *Geum urbanum*, a member of the Rose family (Rosaceae).

Chemical components
The volatile oil contains primarily eugenol, along with tannins, gum, and resin. The roots contain gallic acid, caffeic acid, and chlorogenic acid.

Actions
The mechanism for eugenol's anti-inflammatory activity is thought to involve the potent inhibition of cyclooxygenase. Other factors may be involved as well, including inhibition of prostaglandin production (Tunon et al., 1995).

Reported uses
Avens is claimed to have astringent, anti-inflammatory, antiseptic, tonic, and aromatic properties. In earlier times, avens was used as a treatment for plague, stomach ills, and insect bites. More recently, folk medicine has claimed that the extract is effective in the treatment of diarrhea, dysentery, leukorrhea, sore throat, chills, intermittent fever, wounds, chronic hemorrhage, gastric irritation, and headache. Modern medical literature does not justify these claims.

Dosage

Various dosages have been used: 1 dram (fluid extract of the herb), ½ to 1 dram (fluid extract of the root), or 15 to 30 grains as a tonic (powdered herb or root) P.O. t.i.d.

Adverse reactions

None reported.

Interactions

None reported.

Contraindications and precautions

Avoid use in pregnant or breast-feeding patients.

Special considerations

• Advise the patient that little scientific information exists concerning pharmacologic actions of this herb, and that other pharmaceutical remedies such as NSAIDs have known risks and benefits.
• Advise the patient who still wishes to consume avens to report unusual symptoms to his health care professional.

Points of interest

• Avens has been revered in Europe since the 12th century. Some people believe it has the power to ward off evil spirits and deter poisonous creatures.

Analysis

In vitro data suggest only potential efficacy as an anti-inflammatory agent, compared to available NSAIDs; however, data on safety and randomized, controlled trials evaluating efficacy are necessary before use of this drug can be considered.

References

Tunon, H., et al. "Evaluation of Anti-inflammatory Activity of Some Swedish Medicinal Plants: Inhibition of Prostaglandin Biosynthesis and PAF-Induced Exocytosis," *J Ethnopharmacol* 48:61-76, 1995.

BALSAM OF PERU
BLACK BALSAM, INDIAN BALSAM, MYROXYLON

Common trade names
None known.

Common forms
Many commercial products, such as shampoos, conditioners, lotions, and salves, contain small quantities of balsam of Peru.

Source
Balsam of Peru is obtained from a boiled extract of battered and scorched tree bark of *Myroxylon pereirae* (*M. balsamum*). The balsam of Peru tree, a legume, grows in Florida, Central America, and Peru.

Chemical components
Balsam of Peru is 50% to 65% cinnamein, a volatile oil, and 20% to 28% resin. Cinnamein is composed of benzyl cinnamate, benzoic acid esters, cinnamic acid esters (such as styracin), benzyl alcohol, and the ester form of the alcohol peruviol, often considered equivalent to nerolidol (a sesquiterpene alcohol). Styrene, vanillin, and coumarin occur as trace components. The resin contains cinnamic and benzoic acids.

Actions
Balsam of Peru is reported to possess mild antiseptic and antibacterial properties and is claimed to promote skin growth.

Reported uses
This agent has been claimed to be useful as an expectorant, an antihemorrhoidal agent, an anthelmintic, a pediculocide, and an anticancer agent. Balsam of Peru is also used in topical preparations to treat wounds, indolent ulcers, scabies, diaper rash, hemorrhoids, anal pruritus, bedsores, dandruff, and other skin problems. Dentists have used balsam of Peru in dental impression media and to treat postextraction alveolitis, commonly called dry socket.

Dosage
One source suggests 1.8- to 3-mg suppositories P.R.

Adverse reactions
• Contact dermatitis (possibly related to cinnamein, with frequent use)
• Systemic toxicity in infants following application on nipples of breast-feeding mother

Interactions
Compounds containing sulfur: separation of the resin component from the balsam. Avoid concomitant use.

Contraindications and precautions
Use cautiously with patients prone to contact dermatitis. Avoid use in pregnant or breast-feeding patients.

Special considerations
• Advise the patient to watch for allergic reactions to topical forms of this agent.
• Inform the patient that little information exists to support therapeutic claims for internal use of this agent.
• Advise the female patient to avoid use of herb during pregnancy or when breast-feeding.

Points of interest
• Balsam of Peru has a pleasing odor and vanilla-like flavor, which make it useful in pharmaceutical preparations and shampoos and conditioners. It can also be found in small quantities (0.0015%) in chocolate candies, baked goods, gelatins, puddings, frozen dairy desserts, and other food products.
• Balsam of Peru is nearly insoluble in water but soluble in alcohol, chloroform, and glacial acetic acid.
• Germany allows use of this agent for a number of dermatologic conditions.

Analysis
Contact dermatitis reactions limit use of this agent. Little scientific evidence exists to support the agent for medicinal purposes. Balsam of Peru will probably remain in use only as a fragrance in the pharmaceutical and cosmetic industries.

References
"Peruvian Balsam," in *Remington's Pharmaceutical Sciences.* Easton, Pa.: Mack Publishing Co., 1990.
"Peruvian Balsam," in *The United States Dispensatory.* Philadelphia: Lippincott-Raven Pubs., 1993.

BARBERRY

BERBERRY, COMMON BARBERRY, EUROPEAN BARBERRY,
JAUNDICE BERRY, OREGON GRAPE, PEPPERRIDGE BUSH,
SOUR-SPINE, SOWBERRY, TRAILING MAHONIA,
WOOD SOUR

Common trade names
Oregon Grape Root

Common forms
Available as 400-mg tablets and as liquid, extract, and tea.

Source
Barberry comes from the roots, wood, and bark of *Mahonia vulgaris*
and *M. aquifolium* (also known as *Berberis aquifolium* and *B. vulgaris*),
plants that have edible, red-orange, fruitlike berries. *Mahonia*
species are native to europe and some parts of North America and
have long been used as landscape shrubs.

Chemical components
Barberry species contain tannins and many isoquinoline alkaloids,
including berberine, berbamine, oxycanthine, jatrorrhizine, bervulcine,
magnoflorine, and columbamine.

Actions
Berberine, the most extensively studied component of barberry, may
possess sedative, anticonvulsant, and anthelmintic properties. Berberine
has demonstrated in vitro antibacterial activity against several
species. This activity exceeds that of chloramphenicol. Berberine also
exerts local anesthetic effects when injected subcutaneously.

An ethanolic extract of *B. vulgaris* has shown anti-inflammatory
activity in in vitro and animal studies. Other alkaloid isolates of the
plant have been found to be less potent in their anti-inflammatory
effects than the total ethanol extract (Ivanovska and Philipov, 1996).

A few of the isoquinoline alkaloids exert uterine stimulating effects
in animals (Farnsworth et al., 1975). Other studies have shown
hypotensive and antiarrhythmic effects with berbamine and antiarrhythmic
activity with berberine.

Reported uses
Barberry is claimed to be of therapeutic usefulness as an antidiarrheal
agent, an antipyretic, a cough suppressant, and an agent for
the amelioration of jaundice.

Berberine had been used as an astringent in various ophthalmologic
preparations but is rarely used in these forms today. Berberine has

been shown to be more effective than a placebo in resolving vibrio cholerae–induced diarrhea. However, it had no benefit over placebo in patients with diarrhea due to other causes (Maung et al., 1985).

Dosage

In one study, a dosage of 400 mg daily was used (Maung et al., 1985).

Adverse reactions

- Confusion
- Diarrhea
- Nephritis
- Potential for spontaneous abortion related to uterine stimulant effect (animal data)
- Stupor

⚠ Some references suggest that symptoms of poisoning from this plant may appear as diarrhea, nephritis, confusion, and stupor. Toxic dosage is unknown.

Interactions

None reported.

Contraindications and precautions

Contraindicated in pregnancy because of risk of spontaneous abortion. Use cautiously in women of childbearing age.

Special considerations

- Monitor for signs and symptoms of poisoning and alert primary health care professional if such signs or symptoms occur.
- Warn the patient against consuming large quantities of barberry; potentially toxic chemicals are contained in the plant.
- Advise the patient that little evidence exists for medicinal uses of the barberry plant.
- Warn the female patient to avoid use of herb during pregnancy.

Points of interest

- Berberine gives the rootwood of the barberry plant its characteristic bright golden-yellow color.
- Berberine salts derived from barberry have been used as an ingredient in eyedrops and eye washes.

Analysis

More evidence needs to be collected before barberry or its components can be considered useful for therapeutic application. Berberine, the most investigated component of the extract, is no longer commonly used in ophthalmic preparations. This compound needs further evaluation as an antidiarrheal agent before it can be recommended for acute diarrhea.

References

Farnsworth, N.R., et al. "Potential Value of Plants as Sources of New Antifertility Agents. I," *J Pharm Sci* 64:535-98, 1975.

Ivanovska, N., and Philipov, S. "Study on the Antiinflammatory Action of *Berberis vulgaris* Root Extract, Alkaloid Fractions, and Pure Alkaloids," *Int J Immunopharmacol* 10:553-61, 1996.

Maung, K.U., et al. "Clinical Trial of Berberine in Acute Watery Diarrhea," *BMJ* 291:1601, 1985.

BASIL

COMMON BASIL, GARDEN BASIL, HOLY BASIL, SWEET BASIL

Common trade names
None known.

Common forms
Available as a tea and chopped or powdered leaves.

Source
The crude drug is derived from the leaves of *Ocimum basilicum* (sweet or common basil) or *O. sanctum* (holy basil), members of the mint family (Labiatae).

Chemical components
The active components of basil include linalool, methyl chavicol (estragol), and eugenol. Other components include monoterpenes (such as cineol, ocimene, geraniol, and camphor), sesquiterpenes, and phenylpropanes such as methyl cinnamate.

Actions
In human trials, *O. sanctum and O. album* significantly lowered urine glucose and fasting and postprandial blood glucose in 40 patients with non-insulin-dependent diabetes mellitus. Total cholesterol was also slightly decreased (Agrawal et al., 1996).

Animal studies have revealed some peripherally mediated analgesic effects of the fixed oil of *O. sanctum* (Singh and Majumdar, 1995). Another trial in guinea pigs found antiasthmatic and antiinflammatory properties in extracts from fresh leaves and the essential oils of the leaves of *O. sanctum* (Singh and Agrawal, 1991). In studies with rats, components of *O. basilicum* (flavonoid glycosides, methanol extracts, and aqueous extracts) were found to have antiulcer effects (Akhtar et al., 1992).

Reported uses

Basil is claimed to possess anti-inflammatory, hypoglycemic, analgesic, antiulcerogenic, and antiseptic properties.

Dosage

The dosage reported in one trial was 2.5 g of fresh dried leaf powder once daily (Agrawal et al., 1996). A tea can be made by placing 2.5 g of fresh dried leaf powder in ½ cup water, straining, and drinking once or twice daily as needed.

Adverse reactions

• Hepatocarcinoma. Estragole is a known hepatocarcinogen in animals.
• Hypoglycemia

Interactions

Insulin, sulfonylureas, other antidiabetic agents: may enhance hypoglycemic effects. Avoid concomitant use.

Contraindications and precautions

Avoid use in pregnant or breast-feeding patients because of potential for increased menstrual flow and the mutagenic effects of estragole. Use cautiously in diabetic patients.

Special considerations

• Monitor the diabetic patient for symptoms of hypoglycemia if they consume basil in quantities that exceed amounts typically used for foods.
• Instruct the patient to avoid long-term use of this agent because of its potential mutagenic effect.
• Advise the female patient to avoid use of herb during pregnancy or when breast-feeding.

Points of interest

• Cultivation practices and soil variations can significantly change the chemical composition of basil.

Analysis

Few human studies examine the effects of basil for medicinal purposes. However, one study showed significant reductions in blood glucose levels, which led the investigators to comment on basil's usefulness in the treatment of non-insulin-dependent diabetes mellitus (Agrawal et al., 1996). Although the results of this small study are suggestive, results have yet to be duplicated in a large, controlled trial. Claims of efficacy in other diseases have not been substantiated in human trials.

References

Agrawal, P., et al. "Randomized Placebo Controlled, Single-Blind Trial of Holy Basil Leaves in Patients with Non-Insulin-Dependent Diabetes Mellitus," *Int J Clin Pharmacol Ther* 34:406-09, 1996.

Akhtar, M.S., et al. "Antiulcerogenic Effects of *Ocimum basilicum* Extracts, Volatile Oils and Flavonoid Glycosides in Albino Rats," Int J Pharmacognosy 30:97-104, 1992.

Brinker, F. *The Toxicology of Botanical Medicines,* rev. 2nd ed. Sandy, Oreg.: Eclectic Medicinal Publications, 1996.

Dey, B.B., and Chaundhuri, M.A. "Essential Oil of *Ocimum sanctum* and Its Antimicrobial Activity," *Indian Perfum* 28:82-86, 1984.

Singh, S., and Agrawal, S.S. "Antiasthmatic and Anti-inflammatory Activity of *Ocimum sanctum,*" Int J Pharmacognosy 29:306-10, 1991.

Singh, S., and Majumdar, D.K. "Analgesic Activity of *Ocimum sanctum* and Its Possible Mechanism of Action," *Int J Pharmacognosy* 33:188-92, 1995.

BAY

BAY LAUREL, BAY LEAF, BAY TREE, SWEET BAY

Common trade names

Various manufacturers provide the entire leaf or crushed leaves as a condiment. No known medicinal products.

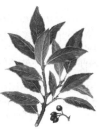

Common forms

Available as leaves, berries, extracts, and essential oils.

Source

Leaves and berries of *Laurus nobilis,* a small tree native to the Mediterranean, are commonly used to obtain bay. Another species of bay tree grows in California; its product is more bitter and is used primarily for extracts.

Chemical components

The volatile oil contains eugenol, alpha-pinene, linalool, sabinene, limonene, piperidine, cineole, camphene, phenylhydrazine, and geraniol. Other constituents include costunolide, laurenobiolide, catechins, proanthocyanidins, launobine, boldine, reticuline, isodomesticine, neolitsine, and nandergine.

Actions

Eugenol acts as a sedative in rodents. Cineole has shown antibacterial activity against vibrio parahaemolyticus. In mice, costunolide has shown a hepatic microsomal enzyme inductive effect on liver glutathione s-transferase enzyme (Wada et al., 1997). Other studies with mice suggest chemotherapeutic effects (Rao and Hashim, 1995).

Reported uses

Because of the plant's strong aromatic qualities, herbalists have claimed that bay leaves are useful for common colds. Additional claims include use of bay as a stimulant, an antirheumatic, and a diuretic. Bay is often an ingredient in natural toothpastes because of its purported antiseptic properties. Extracted oil has been used to treat muscle sprains and strains.

Dosage

The leaves are most commonly used to season foods and, if whole, are typically removed before consumption. Bay leaves should be thoroughly dried and crushed before ingestion. Bay extracts have been applied topically or used in baths and soaks.

Adverse reactions

- Asthma
- Contact dermatitis (Hausen and Hjorth, 1984)

⚠ GI impaction and perforation. Bay leaves are largely indigestible, have sharp serrated edges, and should not be consumed intact. The leaves can become lodged in the esophagus or intestines and often require surgical removal (Panzer, 1983).

Interactions

Insulin: enhanced hypoglycemic actions (bay leaf extract). Bay increases insulin's effects more than threefold, and therefore may be useful in a diabetic diet. Monitor concomitant use carefully.

Contraindications and precautions

Avoid use in pregnant or breast-feeding patients.

Special considerations

- Warn the patient that the essential oil from bay leaves should not be consumed because of the risk of allergic reaction and asthma attack.
- Warn the patient not to ingest whole, intact bay leaves.
- Advise the female patient to avoid use of herb during pregnancy or breast-feeding.

Points of interest

- Nutritionists recommend bay in diabetic diets for its insulin-potentiating effects.

Analysis

Bay leaf is a popular seasoning but no therapeutic claim for treating diabetes or any other disease can be clinically verified.

References

Hausen, B.M., and Hjorth, N. "Skin Reactions to Topical Food Exposure," *Dermatol Clin* 2:567-78, 1984.

Panzer, P.E. "The Dangers of Cooking with Bay Leaves," *JAMA* 250:164-65, 1983. Letter.

Rao, A.R. and Hashim, S. "Chemopreventive Action of Oriental Food-Seasoning Spices Mixture Garam Masala on DMBA-Induced Transplacental and Translactational Carcinogenesis in Mice," *Nutr Cancer* 23:91-101, 1995.

Wada, K,. et al. "Inductive Effects of Bay Leaf and Its Component Costunolide on the Mouse Liver Glutathione S-Transferase," *Fac Natural Medicines* 51:283-85, 1997.

BAYBERRY

CANDLEBERRY, MYRICA, SOUTHERN WAX MYRTLE, SPICEBUSH, SWEET OAK, TALLOW SHRUB, VEGETABLE TALLOW, WAXBERRY, WAX MYRTLE PLANT

Common trade names
Bayberry Bark

Common forms
Available as 450-mg and 475-mg capsules and as liquid, tea, and extract.

Source
Bayberry is a shrub native to Texas and the Eastern United States. Medicinal extracts are usually obtained from the dried root bark of *Myrica cerifera*.

Chemical components
Various portions of the bayberry plant are rich in tannins. Other compounds include the triterpenes myricadiol, taraxerol, and taraxerone, and the flavonoid glycoside myricitrin. Gum, starch, and an acrid astringent resin also occur. Bayberry wax contains palmitic, myristic, and lauric acid esters.

Actions
The pharmacokinetics of bayberry are incompletely known. Some data suggest that myricadiol exerts mineralocorticoid activity. Myricitrin may stimulate the secretion of bile. Dried bayberry root is reported to possess emetic, antipyretic, and antibiotic effects (Paul et al., 1974). The high tannin content of bayberry bark gives the herb its astringent properties.

Reported uses

Bayberry in tea preparations has been claimed to be useful as a stimulant, an antidiarrheal agent, an emetic, an agent for jaundice, and as a topical agent to promote wound healing.

Dosage

No consensus exists. Most references suggest consumption as a tea.

Adverse reactions

- Allergic rhinitis and hypersensitivity reactions (Jacinto et al., 1992)
- Carcinogenic (Data from studies using rodents are conflicting.)
- Gastric irritation
- Liver damage (possibly related to tannin content)
- Vomiting

Interactions

None reported.

Contraindications and precautions

Avoid ingestion of plant parts because of the high tannin content; tannins are known to cause GI irritation and liver damage. Contraindicated in pregnancy and breast-feeding patients; effects are unknown.

Special considerations

- Monitor the patient for weight gain and hypertension related to sodium and water retention.
- Monitor the patient using bayberry extract for hypersensitivity reactions.
- Advise the female patient to avoid use of herb during pregnancy or breast-feeding.

Points of interest

- Bayberry is best known for its small, bluish white berries, from which the wax is extracted to make fragrances and candles.

Analysis

Little medical evidence exists to support therapeutic claims for bayberry. Hypersensitivity reactions from the pollen extract may limit its use. Bayberry's high tannin content precludes oral use because of the potential for gastric distress and liver damage.

References

Jacinto, C.M., et al. "Nasal and Bronchial Provocation Challenges with Bayberry (*Myrica cerifera*) Pollen Extract," *J Allergy Clin Immunol* 90:312-18, 1992.

Paul, B.D., et al. "Isolation of Myricadiol, Myriciatrin, Taraxerol, and Taxerone from *Myrica cerifera* Root Bark," *J Pharm Sci* 63:958-59, 1974.

BEARBERRY

ARCTOSTAPHYLOS, BEAR'S GRAPE, CROWBERRY,
FOXBERRY, HOGBERRY, KINNIKINNICK, MANZANITA,
MOUNTAIN BOX, ROCKBERRY, UVA-URSI

Common trade names
(Available in combination) Arctuvan, Solvefort, Uroflux, Uvalyst

Common forms
Available as drops, tablet, and tea.

Source
The crude drug is obtained from the dry leaves (not berries) of the
low, trailing evergreen shrub *Arctostaphylos uva-ursi* (also *A. coac-
tylis* and *A. adenotricha*).

Chemical components
Leaves contain hydroquinone derivatives (mainly arbutin), hydroquinone monoglucoside, and small amounts of methylarbutin. Other
compounds include gallotannin, arbutin gallic acid ester, triterpenes,
iridoid glycoside monotropein, piceoside, phenol carboxylic acids
(mainly gallic), paracoumaric flavonoids, and syringic acids.

Actions
Bearberry contains 5% to 15% arbutin, which hydrolyzes when ingested and releases hydroquinone (Jahodar et al., 1978). Hydroquinone is the principal antiseptic and astringent constituent of the
plant (Turi et al., 1997). Ursolic acid (a triterpene derivative) and
isoquercetin (a flavonoid pigment) contribute to the diuretic action
of the extract.

One study in mice indicated that bearberry may counter the
symptoms of diabetes, particularly weight loss, without affecting
glycemic control (Swanston-Flatt et al., 1989). A Japanese study reports that bearberry increases the inhibitory effect of dexamethasone, prednisolone, and indomethacin in inflammatory and allergic
responses (Matsuda et al., 1992).

Reported uses
Bearberry is claimed to be modestly effective as a urinary tract antiseptic and diuretic. It has also been used as a diuretic in veterinary
medicine.

Dosage
Doses of 1 to 10 g daily have been suggested. Doses as high as 20 g
have been reported with no adverse effects; however, toxicity may appear in some patients from as little as 1 g.

Adverse reactions
- Cyanosis
- Green-colored urine
- Nausea
- Vomiting

⚠ Taken in large doses (more than 20 g as single dose), bearberry may cause ringing in the ears, vomiting, seizures, and CV collapse.

Interactions
Diuretics: enhanced electrolyle loss. Avoid concomitant use.
Urinary acidifiers (ascorbic acid, methenamine): inactivation of bearberry in urine. Avoid concomitant use.

Contraindications and precautions
Avoid in pregnant or breast-feeding patients; effects are unknown. Use cautiously in patients taking diuretics; bearberry may promote electrolyte disturbances.

Special considerations
- Alert laboratory technicians conducting urinalyses that the patient's urine may be green because of the effects of bearberry.
- Advise the patient that traditional diuretics should be considered over the use of bearberry.
- Warn the patient taking diuretics that concomitant use of bearberry could lead to excessive electrolyte loss, possibly increasing likelihood of muscle cramps, heart palpitations, dizziness, weakness, or CV collapse.
- Advise the patient that urine may change to a greenish color.
- Advise the female patient to avoid use of herb during pregnancy or when breast-feeding.

Points of interest
- An alkaline pH in the urine is believed necessary before bearberry can act as a urinary tract antiseptic.

Analysis
Inadequate data currently prevent the recommendation of bearberry for any disease state. Further study of this agent and its constituents are needed; bearberry may have potential as a diuretic or anti-inflammatory agent.

References
Jahodar, L., et al. "Investigation of Iridoid Substances in *Arctostaphylos uva-ursi*," *Pharmazie* 33:536-37, 1978.
Matsuda, H., et al. "Effects of Water Extract From *Arctostaphyllos uva-ursi* on the Antiallergic and Anti-inflammatory Activities of Dexamethasone Ointment," *Yakugaku Zasshi* 112:73-77, 1992. Abstract.

Swanston-Flatt, S.K., et al. "Evaluation of Traditional Plant Treatments for Diabetes: Studies in Streptozocin Diabetic Mice," *Acta Diabetol Lat* 26:51-55, 1989.

Turi, M., et al. "Influence of Aqueous Extracts of Medicinal Plants on Surface Hydrophobicity of *E. coli* Strains of Different Origin," *APMIS* 105:956-62, 1997. Abstract.

BEE POLLEN

BUCKWHEAT POLLEN, MAIZE POLLEN, PINE POLLEN, POLLEN PINI, PUHUANG, RAPE POLLEN, SONGHUAFEN, TYPHA POLLEN

Common trade names
(Available in combination) Aller G Formula 25

Common forms
Tablets: 500 mg, 1,000 mg
Capsules: 500 mg, 1,000 mg
Granules: 300 mg
Also available as liquids, candy bars, and wafers.

Source
Bee pollen consists of flower pollen and nectar, mixed with digestive enzymes (saliva) from worker honeybees (*Apis mellifera*). Bee pollen is harvested at the entrance of a beehive as bees travel through a wire mesh, which forces them to brush their legs against a collection vessel. Commercial quantities of pollen can be obtained directly from flowers.

Chemical components
Bee pollen consists of protein, carbohydrates, minerals, and essential fatty acids, comprised largely of alpha-linolenic and linoleic acids. Bee pollen also contains small amounts of vitamin C, B-complex vitamins, and various amino acids, hormones, enzymes, and coenzymes.

Actions
Many nutrients occur in concentrated amounts in bee pollen. Bioflavonoids, for example, function as strong antioxidants within the body and have been shown to reduce cholesterol, strengthen and stabilize capillaries, reduce inflammation, and act as antihistamines, antiallergens, and antivirals.

Effects of bee pollen extract on acetaminophen toxicity in rats were studied. Researchers concluded that early intervention with bee pollen (within 1 hour) could potentially increase survival. All untreated rats died within 24 hours; many of the rats receiving bee pollen survived 72 hours or longer.

Other in vitro tests suggest that bee pollen bioflavonoids may exert antioxidant activity and promote the detoxification of metabolically stressed cells.

Reported uses

Bee pollen has been claimed to be useful for treating allergies, asthma, and impotence. Because of its antioxidant properties, bee pollen has also been claimed to be useful for lowering the risk of cancer and heart disease. Cholesterol- and triglyceride-lowering effects of bee pollen have prompted use of the agent for hypertension, atherosclerosis, varicose veins, hemorrhoids, and a variety of circulatory problems.

Bee pollen has also been suggested as a treatment for prostatitis and other inflammatory conditions. No clinical studies exist to support any of these claims.

Dosage

Most sources suggest 500 to 1,000 mg P.O. t.i.d. 30 minutes before meals.

Adverse reactions

• Allergic reactions, ranging from self-limiting nausea and vomiting to anaphylaxis (Broadhurst, 1997)

Interactions

Insulin, other antidiabetic agents: may promote hyperglycemia in diabetics. Avoid concomitant use of bee pollen with hypoglycemic agents.

Contraindications and precautions

Contraindicated in patients with a known history of atopy or an allergy to pollen or plant products because of the risk of hypersensitivity reactions. Also contraindicated in diabetic patients.

Special considerations

• Refrigerate fresh pollen to maintain its quality.
• Imported pollens are often subject to sterilization techniques during customs inspections, and therefore lack many enzymes and nutrients.

Points of interest

• Bee pollen achieved renewed notoriety during the late 1970s after several famous athletes provided testimony on its behalf.
• Germany allows use of bee pollen as an appetite stimulant.

Analysis

The concept behind manipulating the immune response with bee pollen does not differ appreciably from the allopathic concept of an "allergy shot." Both techniques introduce an allergen into the body, which stimulates an immune response. The difference lies in the fact that because bee pollen must be taken orally (it is largely destroyed during digestion), a patient requires 10,000 times the amount of a typical injected-allergen challenge to elicit an immune response.

Bee pollen products aren't standardized. The agent typically contains pollens from many kinds of plants. Pollen composition varies from week to week and hive to hive. This lack of standardization means that product efficacy varies from one dose to another.

The overall lack of scientific data for bee pollen mandates that therapeutic applications be avoided until appropriate studies are performed.

References

Broadhurst, L. "*Information About Bee Pollen.*" Botanical Medicine Conference. Philadelphia, 1997.

Griffith, H.W. "Bee Pollen," in *The Complete Guide to Vitamins, Minerals, and Supplements.* Tucson, Ariz.: Fisher Books, 1988.

BENZOIN

BENJAMIN TREE, BENZOE, BENZOIN TREE, GUM BENJAMIN, SIAM BENZOIN, SUMATRA BENZOIN

Common trade names

(Various manufacturers; available in combination) Balsam of the Holy Victorious Knight, Friar's Balsam, Jerusalem Balsam, Pfeiffer's Cold Sore Preparation, Turlington's Balsam Of Life, Ward's Balsam,

Common forms

Available as compound benzoin tincture USP, which contains 10% benzoin, 2% aloe, 8% storax, 4% tolu balsam, and 75% to 83% alcohol. Benzoin is also an ingredient in coldsore lotions, creams, and ointments.

Source

Benzoin is a balsamic resin usually obtained by wounding the bark of *Styrax benzoin* trees that are at least 7 years old. Benzoin can also be obtained from the bark of *S. paralleloneurus* and *S. tonkinensis*.

Chemical components

Sumatra benzoin (*S. benzoin*) is composed primarily of benzoic and cinnamic acids and their esters. It also contains small quantities of phenylpropyl cinnamate and benzyl cinnamate, styracin, styrene, benzaldehyde, and vanillin. Sumatra benzoin yields at least 75% of alcohol-soluble extract; Siam benzoin (*S. tonkinensis*) yields at least 90%. In the United States, either extract can be used in compound benzoin tincture.

Actions
Benzoin tinctures possess mild bactericidal properties, but the efficacy and spectrum of these properties are poorly described. Benzoin, which has a characteristic balsamic aroma, also has adhesive properties and mucosal protectant activity.

Reported uses
Benzoin has been used for over 100 years, but most uses are anecdotal and have not been systematically studied. The agent has been applied topically as an antiseptic and as a wound adhesive. A comparative trial of compound benzoin tincture and gum mastic found mastic to be a superior wound adhesive that was better tolerated than benzoin tincture (Lesesne, 1992). Benzoin tincture has been painted on the skin prior to applying adhesive tape for supportive dressings.

The American Dental Association accepts benzoin tincture as a topical mucosal protectant and for symptomatic relief of pain from gingivitis, canker sores, and oral herpetic lesions (Council on Dental Therapeutics, 1984).

Benzoin has been used in cough and cold products for its claimed expectorant properties. Compound benzoin tincture has been added to hot water to create a volatile steam inhalation. However, this may be no more effective than unmedicated water vapor (Covington, 1993).

Dosage
For steam inhalation, approximately 5 ml of compound benzoin tincture added to 1 pint of hot water. Alternatively, place the tincture on a handkerchief for inhalation.
For mucosal protection, in adults and children over age 6 months, a few drops applied topically no more than once every 2 hours. The tincture should be used in infants only under medical supervision.

Adverse reactions
- Allergic reactions
- Asthma (inhalation)
- Contact dermatitis
- Gastritis or GI hemorrhage if ingested (Arys and Awasthi, 1987)
- Urticaria

RESEARCH FINDINGS
Gastritis from benzoin ingestion

This case illustrates the need for patients to follow instructions about administering any medication.

A young man was prescribed compound benzoin tincture as inhalation therapy for symptomatic relief of acute bronchitis. The man mistakenly took the tincture—2 teaspoon b.i.d.—internally instead of by inhalation for 10 days.

He went to the hospital, complaining of gastric symptoms of increasing severity. His symptoms, including a low hemoglobin level and the presence of blood in his stools, were consistent with those occurring with significant blood loss. He was diagnosed with and treated for severe erosive gastritis (Arys and Awasthi, 1987). He recovered uneventfully.

Interactions

None reported.

Contraindications and precautions

Inhalation of benzoin products is contraindicated in patients with reactive airways disease such as asthma. Benzoin is toxic if taken internally. (See *Gastritis from benzoin ingestion*.) Use products containing benzoin cautiously in atopic patients or those prone to contact dermatitis.

Special considerations

• Monitor closely for signs and symptoms of gastritis or GI hemorrhage in patients taking benzoin internally.
• Monitor use of benzoin in infants closely.
⚠ Watch for signs and symptoms of allergic reaction, particularly in atopic individuals.
• Tell the patient that topical use can cause discoloration of the skin and contact dermatitis.
• Advise the patient with asthma, atopy, or contact dermatitis to avoid use.
• Inform the patient that volatile steam inhalation of benzoin isn't effective; unmedicated water vapor may be used instead.

Analysis

Most clinical data regarding the use of benzoin products come from case reports and a long history of use in numerous specialities. As a wound adhesive, alternative products have been shown to be superior to benzoin (Lesesne, 1992). As a skin and mucosal protectant, other agents have been shown to be at least as effective as benzoin and cause fewer allergic reactions (James, 1984). The inhalation of compound benzoin tincture has been used for many years but has never been systematically studied. Inhaled steam is likely to be at least as effective (Covington, 1993). Antiseptics with extensively studied effectiveness are preferred over benzoin tinctures. Clinicians should be aware of the potential risks of allergic reactions, especially in atopic patients.

References

Arys, T.V.S., and Awasthi, R. "Severe GI Haemorrhage Following Accidental Ingestion of Tincture Benzoin Compound," *J Assoc Physicians India* 35:805, 1987.

Council on Dental Therapeutics. *Accepted Dental Therapeutics,* 40th ed. Chicago: American Dental Association, 1984.

Covington, T.R., ed. *Handbook of Nonprescription Drugs,* 11th ed. Washington, D.C.: American Society of Hospital Pharmacists, 1993.

James, W.D. "Allergic Contact Dermatitis to Compound Tincture of Benzoin," *J Am Acad Dermatol* 11:847-50, 1984.

Lesesne, C.B. "The Postoperative Use of Wound Adhesives: Gum Mastic versus Benzoin USP," *J Dermatol Surg Oncol* 18:990, 1992.

BETEL PALM

ARECA NUT, BETAL, BETEL NUT, CHAVICA BETAL, HMARG, MAAG, MARG, PAAN, PAN MASALA, PAN PARAG, PINANG, SUPAI

Common trade names

No known U.S. manufacturers. Betel nuts are sold under various names in ethnic grocery stores in the United States.

Common forms

Available as betel oil, raw leaves, and nuts.

Source

Betel palm is derived from the raw and sweetened leaves and nuts of *Areca catechu,* a member of the Palmaceae (Palm) family. The plant is native to India, China, Indonesia, Sri Lanka, the Philippines, and parts of Africa.

Chemical components

Several compounds have been identified in leaf and nut extract: arecoline (an alkaloid related to tobacco alkaloids such as nicotine), arecaidine, arecaine, arecolidine, guvacine, phenolic compounds, and betel-phenol. A volatile oil from the leaves contains chavicol, chaibetol, cadinene, and allylpyrocatechol.

Actions

Arecoline, a parasympathomimetic (cholinergic) and sympatho-mimetic agent, produces CNS and respiratory stimulation, facial flushing, and elevated temperatures. It also exerts mild psychoactive properties. Betel-phenol and chavicol are counterirritants and salivary stimulants.

Reported uses

Approximately 200 million people throughout the Pacific rim, Southeast Asia, India, and Indonesia chew betel nuts and leaves. Betel is used as a mild stimulant and digestive aid. An oily extract of leaves containing phenolic compounds is claimed to be useful for respiratory symptoms and as a gargle for sore throats and cough. Arecoline is a veterinary cathartic and anthelmintic.

Dosage

The betel nut is generally sweetened with lime (calcium hydroxide), wrapped in the leaf of the betel vine, and chewed, similar to the American habit of chewing tobacco. Chewing the "quid," as the chewing of betel nuts is termed, can take as long as 15 minutes. Users may chew as many as 15 quids daily. Chewing betel leaves and betel nuts releases a highly variable quantity of arecoline.

Adverse reactions

- CNS stimulation
- Exacerbation of asthma
- Facial flushing
- Fever
- Gingivitis, peridontitis (with prolonged use)
- Red staining of teeth and oral cavity (with prolonged use)
- Resorption of oral calcium and osteomyelitis (dentition) (with prolonged use; related to lime)

⚠ Dizziness, nausea, vomiting, diarrhea, seizures (with excessive chewing, similar to toxicity experienced from excessive nicotine use; Ko et al., 1995; Merlidhar and Upmanyu, 1996).

⚠ Risk of oral and esophageal cancers with prolonged oral use

Interactions

Alcohol: increased risk of oral cancer. Avoid concomitant use.
Antiglaucoma agents: possible enhanced or decreased effects. Monitor use of betel palm products in patients taking antiglaucoma agents. Avoid concomitant use.
Atropine, propranolol: abolished temperature-elevating effects and enhanced CNS effects of arecoline. Avoid concomitant use (Chu, 1995).

Beta blockers, calcium channel blockers, digoxin: possible enhanced heart rate–reducing effects. Avoid concomitant use.

Contraindications and precautions
Arecoline use, arecaidine use, or betel chewing is contraindicated in patients prone to developing oral leukoplakia, fibrosis, or cancer, particularly cancer of the esophagus or squamous cell carcinoma. Avoid use of betel palm products in pregnant or breast-feeding patients (Babu et al., 1996).

Special considerations
• Ask the patient of Asian or Indian descent regarding his use of this product; betel chewing may be a habit considered innocuous to him.
• Monitor the patient for signs and symptoms of excessive autonomic stimulation, including GI stimulation, cramps, diarrhea, vomiting, hypersalivation, pallor, cold sweats, miosis, blurred vision, bradycardia, hypertension, fasciculations, voluntary muscle paralysis, hallucinations, tachycardia, constipation, mydriasis, and hyperthermia (sympathomimetic). The patient may present with a wide variety of these symptoms.
• Warn the patient that mouth and esophageal cancers have been associated with prolonged betel nut chewing.
• Advise the female patient to avoid use of herb during pregnancy or when breast-feeding.

Analysis
Betel nut chewing in Asia and Indonesia has been compared to tobacco or alcohol use in the West; both substances are legal but potentially harmful. An effort has been made in Canada to outlaw the importation of all betel products but has been met with resistance (Huston, 1991). As with tobacco, there appears to be no appropriate medicinal use for betel.

References
Babu, S., et al. "Oral Fibrosis Among Teenagers Chewing Tobacco, Areca Nut, and Pan Masala," *Lancet* 343:692, 1996. Letter: Comment.

Chu, N.S. "Betel Chewing Increases the Skin Temperature: Effects of Atropine and Propranolol," *Neurosci Lett* 194:130-32, 1995.

Huston, B. "Betel Nuts." Bureau of Food Regulatory, International and Intraagency Affairs, Health Canada. Field Compliance Guide. Citation 1991-01. Ottawa, Canada.

Ko, Y.C., et al. "Betel Quid Chewing, Cigarette Smoking and Alcohol Consumption Related to Oral Cancer in Taiwan," *J Oral Pathol Med* 24:450-53, 1995.

Merlidhar, V., and Upmanyu, G. "Tobacco Chewing, Oral Submucous Fibrosis and Anaesthetic Risk" *Lancet* 347:1840, 1996. Letter.

BETHROOT

BIRTHROOT, COUGH ROOT, GROUND LILY, INDIAN BALM, INDIAN SHAMROCK, JEW'S HARP, PURPLE TRILLIUM, SNAKE BITE, SQUAW ROOT, STINKING BENJAMIN, TRILLIUM, TRILLIUM PENDULUM, WAKE-ROBIN

Common trade names
(Available in combination) Trillium Complex

Common forms
Available as powder, powdered root, and fluid extract.

Source
The active agents of bethroot are derived from the dried rhizomes, roots, and leaves of *T. erectum*, a low-lying perennial member of the Lily family (Liliaceae), which grows in Canada and Eastern and Central United States.

Chemical components
The chemical composition of *T. erectum* is not well documented. The plant is reported to contain tannic acids, oxalates, a cardiotonic glycoside similar to convallamarin, and a saponin called trillarin (a diglycoside of diosgenin). Diosgenin may be chemically converted to pregnenolone and progesterone.

Actions
Bethroot is reported to have astringent, antiseptic, tonic, expectorant, and local irritant properties, most likely due to its tannic acid content. This plant is also reported to act as a uterine stimulant, which may be attributed to the diosgenin component. (See *Origins of bethroot names.*) Some components of other *Trillium* species have antifungal properties (Hufford, 1988).

Reported uses
Trillium Complex is used in Australia to treat menorrhagia. The dried rhizome is still used by some herbalists as a uterine stimulant. Bethroot is known as a popular cure for snakebite, bleeding, and skin irritations. It has been used as an astringent to reduce topical irritation, bleeding, and diarrhea, and as a tonic expectorant.

Dosage
Various dosages have been used, including 1 tablespoon of powder in a pint of boiling water taken "freely in wineglassful doses," or 1 dram of powdered root P.O. t.i.d. or 30 minims of fluid extract as an astringent or tonic expectorant.

FOLKLORE
Origins of bethroot names

Some plants have common names that reflect age-old uses. Bethroot, for example, is also known as birthroot because it was used by Native Americans to reduce postpartum bleeding. The plant acquired another name—stinking benjamin—from the fact that its dark purple flowers give off an aroma resembling rotting flesh. Following the early doctrine that "like cures like," the plant was applied to gangrenous wounds in an attempt to halt the infection.

Adverse reactions
- GI irritation, vomiting (oxalates and saponins)
- Potential cardiotoxicity (convallamarin-like glycoside)

Interactions
Cardiac agents: possible interference with actions of cardiac agents. Avoid concomitant use.

Contraindications and precautions
Avoid use in pregnant patients because of reported uterine stimulant properties.

Special considerations
- Monitor for GI irritation and nausea. Treat symptomatically if these effects occur and consider discontinuation of herb.
- Caution the patient taking drugs for a cardiac condition to avoid use of bethroot because of its potential to influence cardiac function.
- Advise the female patient to avoid use of herb during pregnancy.

Analysis
Bethroot has been used as a folk remedy to promote parturition, control postpartum bleeding, and to treat snake bites, skin irritation, and many other problems, but there is little clinical or scientific evidence to support these claims. The chemistry and dosage range of bethroot have been poorly documented. Controlled animal and human studies are needed before bethroot or any of its constituents can be considered medically useful.

References
Hufford, C.D., et al. "Antifungal Activity of *Trillium grandiflorum* Constituents," *J Nat Prod* 51:94-96, 1988.

BETONY

BISHOPSWORT, WOOD BETONY

Common trade names
Wood Betony

Common forms
Available as capsules and tea.

Source
Betony is derived from the flowers and leaves of *Stachys officinalis.* The plant grows in Europe, Northern Africa, and Siberia.

Chemical components
In addition to tannins (which constitute 15% of betony), betony contains stachydrine, betaine, betonicine, flavonoid glycosides, and phenylethanoid glycosides.

Actions
Studies in Russia suggest that some flavonoid glycosides in the plant can lower blood pressure. Tannins give the plant astringent and antidiarrheal properties. Some components of betony have been found to be toxic to some animals (Lipkan et al., 1974).

Reported uses
Folklore suggests many therapeutic applications for betony. Modern claims are made for use of this agent in asthma, bronchitis, heartburn, seizures, palpitations, wounds, kidney disease, diarrhea, roundworm infestation, stomach aches, toothaches, and more. Modern scientific studies have failed to verify any of these claims.

Dosage
Betony is mostly taken as an infusion or a tea.

Adverse reactions
• GI irritation (related to tannins)
• Liver damage (related to tannins)

Interactions
Antihypertensive agents: enhanced effects. Avoid concomitant use.

Contraindications and precautions
Contraindicated in pregnant patients because of the risk of uterine stimulation.

Special considerations
• Advise the patient to use the herb cautiously because of the potential for liver damage and GI discomfort due to high tannin content.
• Advise the female patient to avoid use of herb during pregnancy.

Analysis
Despite various claims, available evidence does not support use of this agent for any therapeutic application.

References
Lipkan, G.N., et al. "Primary Evaluation of the Overall Toxicity and Anti-inflammatory Activity of Some Plant Preparations, *Farm Zh* 1:78-81, 1974.

BILBERRY

BILBERRIES, BOG BILBERRIES, EUROPEAN BLUEBERRIES, HUCKLEBERRIES, WHORTLEBERRIES

Common trade names
(Various manufacturers) Bilberry Extract, Bilberry Vegicap

Common forms
Available as capsules (60 mg, 80 mg, 120 mg, 450 mg), liquid, tincture, fluid extract, and dried roots, leaves, and berries.

Source
The active components of bilberry are extracted by a drying process from *Vaccinium myrtillus.* On occasion, a hydroalcoholic extraction of the leaf is prepared.

Chemical components
Bilberry extracts are composed of about 25% anthocyanosides, 1.5% to 10% tannins, and small percentages of flavonoids, plant acids, and pectins. There are more than 15 naturally occurring anthrocyanosides in bilberry.

Actions
The pharmacokinetics of *V. myrtillus* anthocyanosides (VMA) or *V. myrtillus* extract (VME) have been studied in male rats. VMA is thought to undergo both renal and biliary elimination (Morazzoni et al., 1991). The anthocyanosides are thought to be the active components, producing reductions in vascular permeability and tissue edema in some animals. Studies with animals suggest that VME decreases vascular permeability by interacting with collagen in vascular epithelium.

In addition, VMA is also thought to aid microvascular blood flow by intensifying arteriolar rhythmic diameter changes. Leaf extracts reduced triglyceride levels in diabetic rats immediately after feeding, possibly through increased triglyceride lipoprotein catabolism.

An in vitro study indicates that VME exerts potent antioxidant effects and a protective effect on low density lipoproteins (Laplaud et al., 1997).

Studies with animals have shown that anthocyanosides speed up regeneration of visual purple in the retina, allowing better adaptation to darkness and light (Alfieri and Sole, 1964). Anthocyanosides decrease excessive platelet aggregation in rat models (Morazzoni and Magistretti, 1986). The anthocyanoside myrtillin in bilberry causes hypoglycemia, although the mechanism is unclear. In rats, bilberry anthocyanosides exerts preventative and curative antiulcer actions (Criston and Magistretti, 1986).

Reported uses
This agent is claimed to be useful in treating visual and circulatory problems. A human study conducted in the 1960s concluded that bilberry had a positive effect on night vision in normal subjects (Jayle et al., 1965). Anecdotally, bilberry has also been used to treat glaucoma, cataracts, diabetic retinopathy, macular degeneration, varicose veins, and hemorrhoids.

Dosage
The dosage of bilberry varies considerably; standardized products consisting of 25% anthocyanoside content should be used.
To improve night vision, 60 to 120 mg of bilberry extract P.O. daily.
For visual and circulatory problems, 240 to 480 mg P.O. daily in two or three divided doses.

Adverse reactions
⚠ Toxic reactions. Long-term consumption of large doses of bilberry leaves can be poisonous. Doses of 1.5 g/kg/day or higher may be fatal.

Interactions
Anticoagulants, other antiplatelet agents: inhibition of platelet aggregation, potentially enhancing the risk of bleeding if used concurrently. Monitor patient.
Disulfiram: disulfiram reaction may occur if herbal product contains alcohol. Avoid concurrent use.

Contraindications and precautions

Contraindicated in pregnant and breast-feeding patients. Use cautiously in patients taking anticoagulants.

Special considerations

● Monitor the patient for signs and symptoms of bleeding if the patient is taking an anticoagulant.

● Warn the patient taking disulfiram not to take liquid extracts or tinctures containing alcohol.

Points of interest

● During World War II, British pilots ingested bilberry preserves to enhance their night vision. Native Americans used bilberry teas and tinctures to treat symptoms of diabetes.

Analysis

The use of bilberry extracts for treating vascular leakage and edema appears intriguing, but inadequate human clinical trial data exist to substantiate efficacy in this area. Little is known regarding the toxicity profile of bilberry, except that dosages exceeding 480 mg daily may be dangerous.

References

Alfieri, R., and Sole, P. "Influence des anthocyanosides adminstres par voie parenteraler sur l'adaptoelectroretinogramme du lapin," *CR Soc Biol* 158:2338, 1964.

Criston, A., and Magistretti, M.J. "Antiulcer and Healing Activity of *V. myrtillus* Anthocyanosides," *Il Farmacio* 42:29-43, 1986.

Jayle, G.E., et al. "Study Concerning the Action of Anthocyanoside Extracts of *Vaccinium myrtillus* on Night Vision," *Ann Ocul* (Paris) 198:56-62, 1965.

Laplaud, P.M., et al. "Antioxidant Action of *Vaccinium myrtillus* Extract on Human Low Density Lipoproteins in Vitro: Initial Observations," *Fundam Clin Pharmacol* 11:35-40, 1997. Abstract.

Morazzoni, P., and Magistretti, M.J. "Effects of *V. myrtillus* Anthocyanosides on Prostacyclin-like Activity in Rat Arterial Tissue," *Fitoterapia* 57:11-14, 1986.

Morazzoni, P., et al. "*Vaccinium myrtillus* Anthocyanosides Pharmacokinetics in Rats," *Arzneimittelforschung* 41:128-31, 1991.

BIRCH

BIRCH TAR OIL, BIRCH WOOD OIL, BLACK BIRCH, CHERRY BIRCH, SWEET BIRCH OIL, WHITE BIRCH

Common trade names

None known.

Common forms

Available as essential oil (bark, wood), dried bark, and tea.

Source

Active compounds of birch are derived from the dried bark and twigs of the birch species *Betula alba (B. pendula), B. verrucosa, B. pubescens,* and *B. lenta.* Several birch species are native to Eastern North America, Europe, and parts of Russia.

Chemical components

Destructive distillation of the bark of *B. alba* yields birch tar oil, turpentine oil, isomeric hydrocarbons, guaiacol, cresol, creosol, pyrocatechol, phenol, xylenol, and betulin. Flavonoids, hyperoside, avicularin, galactosyl-3 myricetol, glucuronyl-3 quercetol, and quercetin occur in the dried leaves. Sweet birch oil is produced by steam distillation of the water-softened bark of *B. lenta.* Methyl salicylate is liberated in the process. Sweet birch oil is composed almost entirely of methyl salicylate.

Actions

Methyl salicylate has anti-inflammatory, antipyretic, and analgesic properties. Hemostatic function in animals has been shown to be affected by the thromboplastic agents presumably found in *B. pendula.* The mechanism of action resembles that of human tissue thromboplastin (Kudriashov et al., 1986). In other animal studies, birch has been shown to exert diuretic properties (Bisset, 1994).

Reported uses

Claims for this agent include relief of headaches and other analgesic effects, treatment of various acute and chronic skin disorders, and treatment of kidney stones and GI disorders. Essential oils are claimed to act against rheumatism, gout, tuberculous cervical lymphadenitis, bladder infections, and neuralgias. In veterinary medicine, essential oil of birch wood has been used to treat various skin diseases (Budavari et al., 1996).

Dosage

Extracts or teas can be made by steeping 2 to 3 g of the bark in boiling water for 10 to 15 minutes; the infusion may be ingested several times daily.

Adverse reactions

• Acute contact dermatitis from exposure to birch leaves or sap (Lahti and Hannuksela, 1980)
• Allergic rhinitis due to pollen allergens
• Cross-sensitization with other plant allergens, such as celery and mugwort pollen (Vallier et al., 1988)

Interactions
None reported.

Contraindications and precautions
Contraindicated in pregnant and breast-feeding patients. Use cautiously in patients with seasonal allergic rhinitis or known hypersensitivity to plant allergens.

Special considerations
• Monitor for signs and symptoms of allergic reaction, particularly in patients with allergies to celery, mugwort, or other plants.
⚠ Warn patient to keep birch preparations out of the reach of children. Sweet birch oil is composed of 98% methyl salicylate. Methyl salicylate has been shown to be fatal to children when applied topically to the skin. Poisonings have been reported with as little as 4.7 g of methyl salicylate, applied topically.
• Advise the patient that topical preparations may cause irritation of the skin and mucous membranes. Encourage the patient to report new or unusual dermatologic manifestations.
• Advise the female patient to avoid use of herb during pregnancy or when breast-feeding.

Points of interest
• Betulin is currently being evaluated for its antitumor properties.
• In Germany, leaves of *B. pendula* are used as a diuretic during irrigation therapy for urinary tract infections.

Analysis
Chemical composition from birch possess some interesting properties. However, until more clinical research becomes available, these agents have no role in modern medicine. The risk of hypersensitivity reactions makes OTC use a cause for concern.

References
Bisset, N.G., ed. *Herbal Drugs and Phytopharmaceuticals.* Boca Raton, Fla.: CRC Press, 1994.

Budavari, S., et al., eds. *The Merck Index*, 12th ed. Whitehouse Station, N.J.: Merck and Co., Inc., 1996.

Kudriashov, B.A., et al. "Hemostatic System Function as Affected by Thromboplastic Agents from Higher Plants," *Nauchnye Doki Vyss Shkoly Biol Nauki* 4:58-61, 1986.

Lahti, A., and Hannuksela, M. "Immediate Contact Allergy to Birch Leaves and Sap," *Contact Dermatitis* 6:464-65, 1980.

Vallier, P., et al. "A Study of Allergens in Celery with Cross-Sensitivity to Mugwort and Birch Pollens," *Clin Allergy* 18:491-500, 1988.

BISTORT
ADDERWORT, COMMON BISTORT, EASTER LEDGES,
EASTER MANGIANT, KNOTWEED, ODERWORT,
OSTERICK, PATIENCE DOCK, SNAKEROOT,
SNAKEWEED, TWICE WRITHEN

Common trade names
None known.

Common forms
Available as a powder, dried or cut root, or tea.

Source
Different folk cultures use different parts of *Polygonum bistorta,* a member of the Buckwheat family (Polygonaceae). Rhizomes and roots are most prized and are gathered in the fall. Leaves are gathered in the spring. Bistort is native to Europe and naturalized in North America.

Chemical components
There have been reports that *P. bistorta* contains phenolic compounds. Aqueous extracts are rich in tannins (Duwiejua et al., 1994). Rhizomes and roots contain starch, gallic acid, phlobaphene, flavonoids, and a trace of emodin, an anthraquinone.

Actions
The pharmacokinetics of this drug have not been studied. Bistort is one of the strongest botanical astringents known. In a study with rats, bistort significantly inhibited acute and chronic phases of aduvant and carrageenan-induced inflammation (Duwiejua et al., 1994). This effect has not been confirmed in human trials.

Reported uses
Extracts of underground plant parts have long been used to stop external and internal bleeding. The herb has been used externally for hemorrhoids, measles, insect bites and snakebites, and small burns or wounds, and as a mouthwash or gargle for canker sores, gum problems, laryngitis, sore throat, and reduction of pulmonary secretions.

Internally, bistort has been used to treat pulmonary and gastric hemorrhage, jaundice, peptic ulcers, ulcerative colitis, dysentery, and irritable bowel syndrome. It has also been used as an anthelmintic, an antidote for certain poisons and as a douche for excessive vaginal discharge or bleeding.

The 1983 British Herbal Pharmacopoeia reports that bistort exerts an anti-inflammatory activity and lists it as useful in treating diarrhea in children.

Dosage

Some sources recommend that 1 teaspoon of the powdered root can be combined with 1 to 1½ cups of boiling water and taken P.O. for diarrhea. More than 3 cups daily is not recommended.

Adverse reactions

- GI irritation
- Liver damage

Interactions

None reported.

Contraindications and precautions

Avoid use in pregnant or breast-feeding patients; effects are unknown.

Special considerations

- Monitor the patient taking bistort for signs and symptoms of GI irritation.
- Monitor liver function studies in patients taking bistort for signs of liver damage.
- Advise the patient not to take bistort internally for more than 3 or 4 weeks at a time.
- Advise the female patient to avoid use of herb during pregnancy or when breast-feeding.

Points of interest

- The rhizome of bistort is rich in starch and has been roasted and eaten as a vegetable.

Analysis

Bistort may have practical value as an astringent for poultices. Its anti-inflammatory and antiarthritic properties appear promising. Overall, bistort has significant anecdotal data but few scientific studies supporting its use. The lack of scientific trials for any of the therapeutic claims should limit bistort use until such clinical trials can define more precisely the role of bistort in modern medicine.

References

British Herbal Pharmacopoeia, Consolidated ed. London: British Herbal Medicine Association, 1983.

Duwiejua, M., et al. "Anti-inflammatory Activity of *Polygonum bistorta, Guaiacum officinale,* and *Hamamelis virginiana* in Rats," *J Pharm Pharmacol* 46:286-90, 1994.

BLACK CATECHU

ACACIA CATECHU, ACACIA DI CACHOU, ACACIE AU
CACHOU, AMARAJA, CAKE CATECHU, CATECHU, CUTCH,
ERH-CH'A, HAI-ERH-CH'A, KADARAM, KATECHU
AKAZIE, KATESU, KHAIR, PEGU KATECHU, WU-TIEH-NI

Common trade names
(Various manufacturers; available in combination) Diarcalm, Élixir
Bonjean, Enterodyne, Hemo Cleen, Katha, Shanti Bori (used in rur-
al Bangladesh as a component of oral contraceptives), Spanish
Tummy Mixture (may contain pale catechu or black catechu as re-
placement product)

Common forms
Available as a dry powder, in a dried extract or liquid for oral use
(0.3 to 2 g), as a tincture, and as a local injection for hemorrhoids.

Source
The crude drug is prepared as a dried extract from the heartwood of
Acacia catechu, a leguminous tree native to Burma and Eastern India
and naturalized in Jamaica. The extract is prepared by boiling heartwood pieces in water, evaporating this mixture to a syrup, and then
cooling to molds. The dried molds are then broken into pieces.

Chemical components
A. catechu contains 20% to 35% catechutannic acid, 2% to 10% aca-
catechin, catechu-red (a flavonoid), quercetin, and gum.

Actions
No pharmacokinetic studies are known. Most animal studies, in
vivo and in vitro, suggest possible physiologic activities but these activities are poorly described. Studies thus far have suggested that the
herb exerts hypoglycemic effects (Singh et al., 1976), hypotensive effects (Sham et al., 1984), possible antileukemic activity (Agrawal
and Agrawal, 1990), and contraceptive activity (Azad Chowdhury et
al., 1984).

Reported uses
A. catechu is claimed to be useful as a topical agent for sore gums
and mouth ulcerations. It is a powerful astringent and is indicated
for the treatment of diarrhea and other GI problems in numerous
countries (not including the United States). This agent has been
commonly used in India as an ointment for indolent ulcers and has
been used in rural Bangladesh as a component of an antifertility pill
(Azad Chowdhury et al., 1984). Other claims include arresting nose-

bleeds and assisting healing in nipple fissures, and as a contraceptive agent. In the late 1800s, chronic gonorrhea was treated with an infusion of catechu.

Dosage
Dried extract can be given in doses of 0.3 to 2 g P.O. or by infusion (tea). The tincture is given in doses of 2.5 to 5 ml of a 1:5 dilution in 45% alcohol.

Adverse reactions
• Aflatoxin contamination (Roy et al., 1988); aflatoxin is a toxic metabolite of *Aspergillus* that is associated with certain cancers.
• Constipation
• Hypotension
⚠ Unstandardized products may contain high amounts of inactive ash and fungal contaminants such as aflatoxin.

Interactions
Antihypertensives: possible worsening of hypotension. Avoid concomitant use.
Captopril: additional hypotensive effect of catechu (Sham et al., 1984). Avoid concomitant use.
Immunosuppressants: increased risk of fungal infection. Avoid concomitant use.
Iron-containing products: may bind with iron products and gelatin and create an insoluble complex.
Opiate analgesics, verapamil: additive effects. Avoid concomitant use.

Contraindication and precautions
Avoid use in pregnant or breast-feeding patients. Products of the catechu family are contraindicated in patients undergoing immunosuppressive therapy. This herb is also known as a dietary carcinogen (Morton, 1992).

Special considerations
• Know that long-term effects of chronic use of the herb are unknown.
• Monitor blood pressure of hypertensive patient taking this drug.
• Know that black catechu is incompatible with iron or zinc sulfate preparations (Pharmaceutical Society of Great Britain, 1979).
• Warn the patient taking opiate analgesics, verapamil, or other agents known to cause significant constipation about additive effects with catechu.
• Warn the patient about the risk of hypoglycemia, especially a diabetic patient.

● Advise the patient that catechu is not a clinically proven antifertility drug and thus should not replace conventional oral contraceptive therapy.

● Advise the female patient to avoid use of herb during pregnancy or when breast-feeding.

Points of interest

● Although *A. catechu* and pale catechu have the name catechu in common, pale catechu is a different plant—*Uncaria gambier*—a member of the Rubiaceae family and used primarily in the dye industry and as a veterinary astringent.

Analysis

Black catechu products were popular in both the United States and abroad during the mid-1800s and early 1900s. The drug is currently used as an antidiarrheal and antifertility agent in some parts of the world. Human clinical trials are lacking, however, and few animal studies have been conducted. Clinical efficacy in chronic diarrhea has not been proven. Acute and chronic toxic effects are also unknown at this time. Although this agent has been used in female patients with cracked nipples, it is unknown whether these patients were breast-feeding at the time. Although pharmacologically interesting, black catechu cannot be recommended for any ailment until more is known about its risks and benefits.

References

Agrawal, S., and Agrawal, S.S. "Preliminary Observations on Leukaemia-Specific Agglutinins from Seeds," *Indian J Med Res* 92:38-42, 1990.

Azad Chowdhury, A.K., et al. "Antifertility Activity of a Traditional Contraceptive Pill Comprising *Acacia catechu, A. arabica,* and *Tragia involuceria*," *Indian J Med Res* 80:372-74, 1984.

Morton, J.F. "Widespread Tannin Intake via Stimulants and Masticatories, Especially Guarana, Kola Nut, Betel Vine, and Accessories," *Basic Life Sci* 59:739-65, 1992. Abstract.

Pharmaceutical Society of Great Britain, Department of Pharmaceutical Sciences, ed. *The Pharmaceutical Codex*, 11th ed. London: The Pharmaceutical Press, 1979.

Roy, A.K., et al. "Aflatoxin Contamination of Some Common Drug Plants," *Appl Environ Microbiol* 54:842-43, 1988.

Sham, J.S.K., et al. "Hypotensive Action of *Acacia catechu*," *Planta Med* 50:177-80, 1984.

Singh, K.N., et al. "Hypoglycaemic Activity of *Acacia catechu, Acacia suma,* and *Albizzia odaratissima* Seed Diets in Normal Albino Rats," *Indian J Med Res* 64:754-57, 1976.

BLACK COHOSH

BLACK SNAKEROOT, BUGBANE, BUGWORT, CIMICIFUGA, RATTLEROOT, RATTLEWEED, SQUAW ROOT

Common trade names

(Various manufacturers; available in combinations) Black Cohosh, CX, Estroven, FC With Dong Quai, Femtrol, GNC Menopause Formula, Remifemin

Common forms

Caplets: 40 mg, 400 mg, 420 mg
Capsules: 25 mg, 525 mg

Source

The crude drug is extracted primarily from the dried rhizomes and roots of *Cimicifuga racemosa (Actaea racemosa)*. Other sources include other *Cimicifuga* species and *Macrotys actae-oides*. These plants are native to Eastern North America.

Chemical components

Several chemical compounds have been extracted from the black cohosh plant, including steroidal terpenes, acteina, cimigoside, and 27-deoxyactein (Berger et al., 1988). Other constituents include tannins, salicylic acid, and an isoflavone, formononetine.

Actions

Physiologic effects of black cohosh include vascular and estrogenic activity. The vascular action is believed to be attributed to acteina, which in animals produces a hypotensive effect through vagal nerve activity (Genazzani and Sorrentino, 1962).

Most research has focused on the plant's estrogenic activity. In studies with rats, active constituents of the plant were found to bind directly to estrogen receptors and suppress the release of leutinizing hormone (Jarry and Harnischfeger, 1985; Jarry et al., 1985; Duker et al., 1991). A commercial extract reduced leutinizing hormone secretion without affecting follicle-stimulating hormone in a group of menopausal women (Duker et al., 1991). (See *Effect of black cohosh on luteinizing hormone,* page 76.) A study of hysterectomy patients failed to show any advantage of using black cohosh over conventional estrogen replacement therapy (Lehmann-Willenbrock and Riedel, 1988).

Reported uses

Black cohosh has been used as an astringent, diuretic, antidiarrheal, and anti-inflammatory agent. It has also been used to treat menopausal complaints.

RESEARCH FINDINGS
Effect of black cohosh on luteinizing hormone

An ethanolic extract of the rhizome of *Cimicifuga racemosa* (Remifemin) was evaluated for estrogenic activity in 55 menopausal women. One group of subjects received 8 mg of extract daily for 8 weeks; a control group of another 55 women received a placebo. At the end of the 8-week treatment period, the secretion levels of luteinizing hormone (LH) and follicle-stimulating hormone (FSH) were decreased in the group receiving the herb, compared with those who received a placebo. However, only LH suppression was statistically significant. This selective effect was interpreted as an example of the extract's estrogenic activity.

The authors reproduced these effects in rats that had their ovaries removed. Results indicate that the difference in hormonal suppression between *Cimicifuga racemosa* and placebo is because FSH secretion is less sensitive to estrogenic feedback inhibition than LH (Duker et al., 1991).

Dosage
Dosages vary and are not standardized. In studies, dosages ranged from 8 to 2,400 mg P.O. daily.

Adverse reactions
- Hypotension
- Nausea
- Vomiting

⚠ Large doses may induce miscarriage because of the herb's estrogenic effects.

Interactions
Antihypertensives: potential for enhanced hypotensive effect. Avoid concomitant use.

Contraindications and precautions
Contraindicated during pregnancy because of increased risk of spontaneous abortion. Use cautiously in patients taking antihypertensive medications because the vascular action of acteina may cause additional hypotension.

Special considerations
- Monitor blood pressure closely in hypertensive patients.
- Warn the pregnant patient that black cohosh, if taken in large doses, may cause spontaneous abortion.

● Advise the patient receiving antihypertensive medications of the potential additive effects of black cohosh.

Points of interest
● This herb has been found to be effective in treating the symptoms of menopause.

Analysis
Animal and human studies on the use of black cohosh are limited. Data from these studies suggest that the herb's hormonal effects may be beneficial in controlling the symptoms associated with menopause. The majority of clinical data regarding this plant comes from German studies that evaluated only a small number of women. Additional well-controlled trials are needed to define the role for black cohosh in estrogen replacement therapy as compared to traditional pharmacotherapy, particularly the use of conjugated estrogen products.

References
Berger, S., et al. "27-Deoxyactein: A New Polycyclic Triterpenoid Glycoside from *Actaea racemosa*," *Planta Med* 54:579-80, 1988.

Duker E., et al. "Effects of Extracts of *Cimicifuga racemosa* on Gonadotropin Release in Menopausal Women and Ovariectomized Rats," *Planta Med* 57:420-24, 1991.

Genazzani, E., and Sorrentino, L. "Vascular Action Of Acteina, Active Constituent of *Actaea racemosa* L," *Nature* 194:544-45, 1962.

Jarry, H., and Harnischfeger, G. "Studies on the Endocrine Effects of the Contents of *Cimicifuga racemosa*: 1. Influence on the Serum Concentration of Pituitary Hormones on Ovariectomized Rats," *Planta Med* 1:46-49, 1985.

Jarry, H., et al. "Studies on the Endocrine Effects of the Contents of *Cimicifuga racemosa*: 2. In Vitro Binding of Compounds to Estrogen Receptors," *Planta Med* 4:316-19, 1985.

Lehmann-Willenbrock, E., and Riedel, H.H. "Clinical and Endocrinologic Studies of the Treatment of Ovarian Insufficiency: Manifestations Following Hysterectomy with Intact Adnexa," *Zentralbl Gynakol* 110:611-18, 1988.

BLACK HAW

CRAMP BARK, NANNYBERRY, SHEEPBERRY, SHONNY, SLOE, STAGBUSH, SWEET HAW

Common trade names
Black Haw, PMS Serene, Utero-Tone

Common forms
Available as a liquid extract or as the root bark. Also available as capsules or tablets in combination with other herbs and extracts.

Source
The bark of the roots of *Viburnum prunifolium*, a deciduous shrub found in the Eastern United States, has traditionally been used for medicinal purposes.

Chemical components
Scopoletin (6-methoxy-7-hydroxy-coumarin) and other coumarins are thought to contribute to the antispasmodic action of the herb. Other constituents of the root bark include salicin, volatile oil, iso-valeric acid, tannin, and resin. A hemimellitate acid derivative, 1-methyl 2,3-dibutyl hemimellitate, has also been identified in aqueous extracts of stem bark; however, this compound has not been shown to exert antispasmodic properties (Jarobe et al., 1969).

Actions
The uterine relaxant properties of black haw and other *Viburnum* species have been studied in animals. In one investigation, extracts prepared from black haw, *V. opulus*, and two other *Viburnum* species caused complete relaxation of uterine tissue in rats. Further chemical analyses of extracts from black haw and *V. opulus* identified at least four constituents that have uterine relaxant properties (Jarobe et al., 1966).

Reported uses
Black haw has been used most commonly as a uterine relaxant and general antispasmodic. Specific indications include prevention of spontaneous abortion and the treatment of dysmenorrhea, uterine pain, chronic diarrhea, and general musculoskeletal spasms. Human clinical trials are looking to verify these claims.

Dosage
Black haw tincture or bark can be used in a tea and taken t.i.d.

Adverse reactions
● GI irritation

Interactions
Anticoagulants: enhanced effects. Avoid concomitant use.

Contraindications and precautions
Contraindicated in patients with allergies to this plant or related plant species. Also contraindicated in pregnant and breast-feeding patients.

Special considerations
● Monitor the patient taking this agent for signs of bleeding and hypersensitivity reactions.

• Advise the patient to consider traditional uterine relaxants before using black haw; controlled studies on this agent have not been conducted in humans.

• Advise the female patient to avoid use during pregnancy or breastfeeding.

Analysis

Available data on pharmacologic effects of black haw are based on animal studies. Although black haw has been used for many years and was formerly included in the United States Dispensatory, human clinical data are lacking. Most important, information on the safety and adverse effects of black haw is not available. Therefore, this agent should be avoided until more is known about its risks and benefits.

References

Jarobe, C.H., et al. "Uterine Relaxant Properties of *Viburnum*," *Nature* 5064:837, 1966.

Jarobe, C.H., et al. "1-methyl 2,3-dibutyl hemimellitate: A Novel Component of *Viburnum prunifolium*," *J Org Chem* 34:4202-03, 1969.

BLACKROOT

BLACK ROOT, BOWMAN ROOT, BRINTON ROOT, CULVER'S PHYSIC, CULVER'S ROOT, HIGH VERONICA, HINI, *LEPTANDRA*, *LEPTANDRA VIRGINICA*, PHYSIC ROOT, QUITEL, TALL SPEED-WELL, *VERONICA*, *VERONICA VIRGINICA*

Common trade names
None known.

Common forms
Available as dried root or tincture.

Source
Blackroot is made from the dried rhizome and roots of *Veronicastrum virginicum*, which grows in Canada and the United States.

Chemical components
Tannic acid, verosterol (a volatile oil), cinnamic and paramethoxycinnamic acids, gum, resin, mannite, and d-mannitol have been isolated from blackroot. Early studies yielded a substance called leptandrin, which was thought to be the active component (Wood and Bache, 1907). However, there are no recent data to support this.

Actions

Blackroot has a bitter, nauseous taste and irritates gastric and intestinal mucosa, primarily because of the herb's tannin content (Millspaugh, 1974). Tannic acid has astringent properties that act locally on the mucosa of the GI tract. Tannic acid also forms insoluble complexes with alkaloids, glycosides, and certain heavy metal ions.

Blackroot has also been shown to have antiulcer and antisecretory effects in the GI tract as a result of an inhibitory action on the gastric enzyme system.

Mannite and d-mannitol are considered to be osmotic diuretics and work by increasing the transport of sodium and water out of the loop of Henle. There are also data to suggest that cinnamic acid exerts some choleretic effect. In animal studies, cinnamic acid injections increased bile acid flow by 50% (Galecka, 1969). Other animal studies confirmed this effect (Das et al., 1976).

Reported uses

Blackroot has been claimed to be useful as an emetic and a cathartic. Because of its purported biliary action within the GI tract, it has been claimed to be beneficial in relieving jaundice and other symptoms related to liver or biliary congestion. Human trials are lacking.

Dosage

Blackroot possesses emetic and cathartic properties at 15 to 40 grains (1 to 2.6 g); however, the usual reported dose is 1 g. Tea may be made by mixing 1 to 2 teaspoon of dried blackroot in cold water, boiling this solution, and then simmering it for 10 minutes. The dosage of this solution is typically 1 cup t.i.d. The tincture has been administered in doses of 1 to 2 ml t.i.d.

Adverse reactions

• Abdominal pain or cramps
• Changes in stool color or odor
• Drowsiness
• Headache
• Nausea
• Vomiting
⚠ Hepatotoxicity following ingestion of large amounts of dried tea leaves (in the range of ½ lb of tea every 3 to 4 days) has been reported (Haddad and Winchester, 1990).

Interactions

None reported.

Contraindications and precautions

Contraindicated in pregnant and breast-feeding patients; effects are unknown. Avoid large amounts of blackroot, especially in patients with existing hepatic disease because of the potential toxic effects of tannic acid on the liver.

Special considerations

• Know that alkaloids such as atropine and scopolamine, glycosides such as digoxin, and products that contain iron may form insoluble complexes with tannins. Advise patients to avoid use of blackroot with these agents.

⚠ Know that use of this herb should be discontinued if abnormal increases in hepatic transaminase levels occur.

• Warn the patient that little to no scientific data exist in humans to support therapeutic uses for this plant.

• Advise the patient to immediately report symptoms of hepatic injury, such as right upper quadrant pain, jaundice, and fever.

• Advise the female patient to avoid use of the herb during pregnancy or when breast-feeding.

Points of interest

• Settlers gathered knowledge of blackroot from Native American Indians. The Delaware Indians referred to the plant as *quitel;* the Missouri and Osage Indians called it *hini* (Lloyd, 1921).

• Early American doctors used blackroot as a cure for bilious fevers (Wood and Bache, 1907).

Analysis

There is little current information on blackroot's therapeutic uses or effectiveness. Human trials have not been performed that support therapeutic claims for blackroot. The lack of clinical trials limits the usefulness of anecdotal or historical data. No therapeutic claim can be supported at this time.

References

Das, P.K., et al. "Pharmacology of Kutkin and Its Two Organic Constituents, Cinnamic Acid and Vanillic Acid." *Indian J Exp Biol* 14:456-58, 1976.

Galecka, H. "Choleretic and Cholagogic Effects of Certain Hydroxy Acids and Their Derivatives in Guinea Pigs," *Acta Pol Pharm* 26:479-84, 1969.

Haddad, L.M., and Winchester, J.F. *Clinical Management of Poisoning and Drug Overdose,* 2nd ed. Philadelphia: W.B. Saunders Co., 1990.

Lloyd, J.B. *Origin and History of All the Pharmacopeial Vegetable Drugs, Chemicals, and Preparations.* 8th and 9th decennial revisions, Vol. I. Cincinnati: The Caxton Press, 1921.

Millspaugh, C.F. *American Medicinal Plants.* New York: Dover Publications, Inc., 1974. Reprint of 1892 edition.

Wood, G.B., and Bache, F. *Dispensatory of the United States of America,* 19th ed. Philadelphia: Lippincott-Raven Pubs., 1907.

BLESSED THISTLE

CARDO SANTO, CHARDON BENIT, HOLY THISTLE,
KARDOBENEDIKTENKRAUT, SPOTTED THISTLE,
St. Benedict thistle

Common trade names
Blessed Thistle Combo, Blessed Thistle Herb

Common forms
Available as 325-mg and 340-mg capsules, 1-oz packets of dried
herb, 1-oz containers of tincture, and tea.

Source
The crude drug is obtained from the leaves and, especially, the flowers
of the blessed thistle, an annual plant found primarily in Asia and
Europe. Blessed thistle, *Cnicus benedictus (Carbenia benedicta, Carduus benedictus),* is a member of the Compositae family and is related
to daisies, asters, and other flowering plants.

Chemical components
The aerial parts of blessed thistle contain the sesquiterpene lactones
cnicin and salonitenolide. Concentration of sesquiterpene lactones
is quite variable in the Compositae family and depends on climate,
season, geographic location, and soil quality at harvest.

Actions
Blessed thistle purportedly exerts effects on the stomach, liver, heart,
blood, mammary glands, and uterus. The pharmacokinetics of
blessed thistle compounds has not been well documented. In vitro
cytotoxicity has been demonstrated for cnicin (Barrero et al., 1997).
    The antibiotic activity of cnicin and other components of blessed
thistle has also been investigated.

Reported uses
This agent is claimed to be useful for several GI and hepatic disorders as well as for memory improvement, stimulation of lactation,
and relief of menstrual symptoms.

Dosage
Various dosages have been suggested, depending on the intended
use and method of administration. However, lack of human trials
makes it difficult to arrive at specific dosage recommendations. In
addition to capsules and tinctures, some sources recommend the
herb as a tea.

Adverse reactions
• Contact dermatitis and possible airborne contact dermatitis due to cross-sensitivity with other members of the Compositae family. (Sesquiterpene lactones are sensitizers.)
• Nausea
• Vomiting

Interactions
Other herbal drugs based on Compositae: possible cross-sensitivity. Avoid concomitant use.

Contraindications and precautions
Contraindicated in pregnant or breast-feeding patients; effects are unknown. Use cautiously in patients with a history of contact dermatitis, especially in relation to other members of the Compositae family.

Special considerations
• Monitor for contact dermatitis in susceptible patients.
• Caution the patient who wishes to consume this herb that little scientific data on therapeutic benefits are available.
• Advise the female patient to avoid use of herb during pregnancy or when breast-feeding.

Points of interest
• According to legend, blessed thistle was a popular folk remedy and tonic used by monks during the Middle Ages. It was also used to treat bubonic plague.
• Germany allows use of this herb in the treatment of dyspepsia and loss of appetite.

Analysis
Many anecdotal claims are made for this agent, but there are no animal or human clinical data to support them. Use with caution in patients with a history of hypersensitivity reactions.

References
Barrero, A.F., et al. "Biomimetic Cyclization of Cnicin to Malacitanolide, a Cytotoxic Eudesmanolide from *Centaurea malacitana,*" *J Nat Prod* 60:1034-35, 1997.

Crellin, J.K., and Philpott, J. *Herbal Medicine Past and Present. A Reference Guide to Medicinal Plants,* Vol. 2. Durham, N.C.: Duke University Press, 1990.

Reynolds, J.E.F., et al., eds. *Martindale, The Extra Pharmacopeia,* 31st ed. London: Royal Pharmaceutical Society of Great Britain, 1996.

Zeller, W., et al. "The Sensitizing Capacity of Compositae plants. VI. Guinea Pig Sensitization Experiments with Ornamental Plants and Weeds Using Different Methods," *Arch Dermatol Res* 277:28-35, 1985.

BLOODROOT

INDIAN PAINT, RED PUCCOON, REDROOT, TETTERWORT

Common trade names
(Available in combination) Lexat, Viadent

Common forms
Available as an ingredient (sanguinarine) in some toothpastes and oral rinses.

Source
The alkaloid sanguinarine is extracted from the rhizome of *Sanguinaria canadensis*, a herbaceous perennial that is native to North America.

Chemical components
Bloodroot contains several pharmacologically active alkaloids, including the isoquinolone derivatives sanguinarine, homochelidonine, sanguidimerine, chelerythrine, and protopine. Other compounds extracted from bloodroot include coptisine, sanguirubine, and berberine.

Actions
Sanguinarine, the most extensively studied agent in bloodroot, is poorly absorbed from the GI tract. It has broad antimicrobial activity as well as anti-inflammatory properties. Minimum inhibitory concentrations of sanguinarine range from 1 to 32 mcg/ml for most species of bacteria that promote dental plaque (Godowski, 1989).

Sanguinarine converts to a negatively charged iminiun ion that permits the compound to bind to plaque (Godowski, 1989). In addition, sanguinarine can induce mild CNS depression and has a papaverine-like action on smooth muscle and cardiac muscle.

Reported uses
Bloodroot was formerly used as an expectorant but, because of toxicity, fell into disuse. Other claims include use as an emetic, a laxative, and a digestive stimulant.

The efficacy of sanguinarine as an antiplaque agent has been well documented in numerous clinical trials (Godowski, 1989; Kopczyk et al., 1991). In contrast, a recent study of periodontal disease treatments showed no significant advantage to using a sanguinarine dentrifice and oral rinse in conjunction with initial periodontal therapy, such as oral hygiene instruction, scaling, and root planing (Cullinan et al., 1997).

Because of its ability to chemically corrode and destroy tissue, bloodroot has been prescribed as a cure for surface cancers, fungal growths, ringworm, and nasal polyps. In humans, it has been tested topically for the treatment of ear and nose carcinomas. Mouthwashes generally contain dilute concentrations of sanguinarine.

Dosage
Tincture: 0.3 to 2 ml t.i.d.
Extract (1:1 in 60% alcohol): 0.06 to 0.3 ml t.i.d.

Adverse reactions
• Eye and mucous membrane irritation and degradation from contact with root dust or components
• Headache
• Nausea
• Potential for hypotension, shock, coma (with excessive doses in animals)
• Vomiting
⚠ The powdered rhizome and juice of bloodroot are potentially destructive to mammalian tissues.

Interactions
Sanguinarine products containing zinc: increased antimicrobial efficacy of sanguinarine (Eisenberg et al., 1991). Avoid concomitant use.

Contraindications and precautions
Avoid use during pregnancy. Use cautiously under medical supervision on abraded or healing tissue.

Special considerations
• Warn the patient against use of bloodroot or its components unless under strict supervision and guidance of his dentist or other primary health care provider.
• Advise the female patient to avoid use of this herb during pregnancy.

Points of interest
• The FDA has classified bloodroot as an herb unsafe for use in foods, beverages, or drugs. However, the herb is used in homeopathic medicine.

Analysis

Most clinical data support using sanguinarine as an ingredient in toothpaste or oral rinses to control dental plaque. However, a study by Cullinan et al. (1997) showed no benefit of sanguinarine when used in combination with routine periodontal care. It also questioned the use of sanguinarine because the agent offers no advantage over routine periodontal care and is potentially dangerous if ingested orally.

Sanguinarine's efficacy in treating topical cancers, fungal infections, and nasal polyps has not been demonstrated in controlled clinical trials; it cannot be recommended without additional studies. Oral ingestion is associated with tissue destruction and, therefore, its use is not recommended use.

References

Cullinan, M.P., et al. "Efficacy of a Dentrifice and Oral Rinse Containing *Sanguinaria* Extract in Conjunction with Initial Periodontal Therapy," *Aust Dent J* 42:47-51, 1997.

Eisenberg, A.D., et al. "Interactions of Sanguinarine and Zinc on Oral Streptococci and Actinomyces Species," *Caries Res* 25:185-90, 1991.

Godowski, K.C. "Antimicrobial Action of Sanguinarine," *J Clin Dent* 1:96-101, 1989.

Kopczyk, R.A., et al. "Clinical and Microbiological Effects of a *Sanguinaria*-Containing Mouth Rinse and Dentrifice with and without Fluoride During Six Months of Use," *J Periodontol* 62:617-22, 1991.

BLUE COHOSH

BLUE GINSENG, CAULOPHYLLUM, SQUAW ROOT, PAPOOSE ROOT, YELLOW GINSENG

Common trade names

Blue Cohosh Root

Common forms

Available as dried powder, tea, tablets, 1-oz and 2-oz tinctures, and 500-mg capsules.

Source

The aerial parts, roots, and rhizomes of *Caulophyllum thalictroides* have been used to extract active ingredients. This herb is found in parts of Eastern United States and Canada. Seeds of this plant are bright blue in color.

Chemical components

Rhizome and root extracts contain the alkaloids methylcytisine (caulophylline), baptofoline, anagyrine, and magnoflorine; the saponins caulosaponin and cauloside D; and resin, gum, citrollol, phosphoric acid, phytosterol, and starch. Hydrolysis of cauloside D yields hederagenin.

Actions
A glycoside component of blue cohosh stimulates smooth muscle in the uterus, small intestine, and coronary vessels in various animals (Ferguson and Edwards, 1954).

Antifertility actions have been documented in animal studies (Chaudrasekhar and Sarma, 1974; Chaudrasekhar and Raa Vishwanath, 1974). Some anti-inflammatory and antimicrobial actions have been reported as well (Benoit et al.,1976, and Anisimov et al., 1972, respectively). Methylcytisine has pharmacologic activity similar to nicotine, causing elevations in blood pressure, serum glucose levels, and peristalsis (Scott and Chen, 1943).

Reported uses
Early claims for this herb include its use as an anticonvulsant, an agent to enhance menstrual flow, an agent to induce labor, an antispasmodic, and an antirheumatic.

Dosage
Dried rhizome or root: 0.3 to 1 g t.i.d.
Liquid extract (1:1 in 70% alcohol): 0.5 to 1 ml t.i.d.

Adverse reactions
- Chest pain
- GI irritation; severe diarrhea, cramping
- Hyperglycemia
- Hypertension
- Mucous membrane irritation following contact with powdered extract

⚠ Poisoning in children after ingestion of the seeds.

Interactions
Antianginals: may interfere with therapy, leading to increased chest pain and discomfort. Avoid concomitant use.
Antihypertensives: may interfere with therapy, leading to increased blood pressure. Avoid concomitant use.
Nicotine replacements: increased effects of nicotine. Avoid concomitant use.

Contraindications and precautions
Contraindicated in pregnant patients because of the herb's potential uterine stimulating effects. Also contraindicated in patients with heart disease.

Special considerations

● Know that the active agent, methylcytisine, is pharmacologically similar to, though much less potent than, nicotine.
● Monitor for signs and symptoms of overdose, which could resemble nicotine poisoning. Initiate gastric lavage or induce emesis and provide appropriate supportive measures.
● Monitor blood pressure and serum glucose level in patients taking this drug.
● Advise the female patient to avoid use during pregnancy.
● Advise patient to keep blue cohosh products out of reach of children. The bright blue seeds are attractive but poisonous.

Analysis

Blue cohosh is an interesting herb that offers encouraging opportunities for investigation as a therapeutic agent for inflammatory disease or as a contraceptive. The potential for toxicity and worsening of the disease requires considerable investigation to assess risks and benefits of the herb before it can be recommended for use.

References

Anisimov, M.M., et al. "The Antimicrobial Activity of the Triterpene Glycosides of *Caulophyllum robustum* Maxim," *Antibiot Khimioter* 17:834, 1972.

Benoit, P.S., et al. "Biochemical and Pharmacological Evaluation of Plants. XIV: Antiinflammatory Evaluation of 163 Species of Plants," *Lloydia* 393:160-71, 1976.

Chaudrasekhar, K., and Raa Vishwanath, C. "Studies on the Effect of Implantation on Rats," *J Reprod Fertil* 38:245-46, 1974.

Chaudrasekhar, K., and Sarma, G.H.R. "Observations on the Effect of the Low and High Doses of Caulophyllum on the Ovaries and the Consequential Changes in the Uterus and Thyroid in Rats," *J Reprod Fertil* 38:236-37, 1974.

Ferguson, H.C., and Edwards, L.D. "A Pharmacological Study of a Crystalline Glycoside of *Caulophyllum thalictroides*," *J Am Pharm Assoc* 43:16-21, 1954.

Scott, C.C., and Chen, K.K. "The Pharmacologic Action of N-methylcytisine," *Therapeutics* 79:334, 1943.

BLUE FLAG

DAGGER FLOWER, DRAGON FLOWER, FLAG LILY, FLEUR-DE-LIS, FLOWER-DE-LUCE, LIVER LILY, POISON FLAG, SNAKE LILY, WATER FLAG, WILD IRIS

Common trade names

Iridin, Irisin

Common forms

Powdered root: 20 grains (1,300 mg)
Solid extract: 10 to 15 grains (650 to 975 mg)

Fluid extract: 0.5 to 1 fluidram (2.5 to 5 ml)
Tincture: 1 to 3 fluidrams (5 to 15 ml)

Source
The rhizome of *Iris versicolor* yields iridin and an oleoresin. *I. versicolor* is a perennial herb found abundantly in swamps and low-lying areas throughout Eastern and Central North America.

Chemical components
The rhizome contains starch, gum, tannin, 25% acrid resinous matter, 0.025% furfural (a volatile oil), 0.002% isophthalic acid, traces of salicylic acid, lauric acid, stearic acid, palmitic acid, and I-triacontanol. Other constituents include iridin, beta-sitosterol, and iriversical. A number of substances contained in the rhizome are still unidentified.

Actions
Little is known about the phytochemical, therapeutic, or toxicologic properties of blue flag and its components. The acute oral toxicity for furfural is 127 mg/kg (Newall et al., 1996). The root is claimed to possess laxative, diuretic, dermatologic, and anti-inflammatory properties. The commercial products Iridin and Irisin are powdered root extracts with diuretic and intestinal stimulant properties.

Reported uses
Blue flag was used by Native Americans as a cathartic and an emetic. It has been called the liver lily because of its purported ability to cure diseases of the liver. Externally, the poulticed root was used as an anti-inflammatory agent on sores and bruises. Powdered root preparations have been used as diuretics and intestinal stimulants.

Dosage
Available data on dosages relate to use of blue flag as a cathartic.
Solid extract, powdered root: 10 to 20 grains.
Fluid extract, tinctures: 0.5 to 3 fluidrams.

Adverse reactions
• Headache
• Mucous membrane irritation (due to furfural component)
⚠ Iridin has caused poisoning in humans and livestock.
⚠ Severe nausea and vomiting can occur following ingestion of fresh root preparations.

Interactions
None reported.

Contraindications and precautions
Contraindicated in pregnant and breast-feeding patients; effects are unknown.

Special considerations
• Advise the patient to avoid taking this drug internally.
• Inform the patient that contact with eyes, nose, or mouth will cause severe irritation.
• Warn the parents to keep all parts of this plant out of the reach of children.
• Advise the female patient to avoid use of herb during pregnancy or when breast-feeding.

Points of interest
• The fresh rhizome emits a slight but peculiar odor and has a pungent, acrid taste.
• The rhizome of *I. versicolor* is an official pharmaceutical ingredient in the United States Pharmacopoeia.
• When not in bloom, blue flag can be easily mistaken for sweet flag (*Acorus calamus*).

Analysis
Blue flag is a known intestinal irritant and may be dangerous in some conditions; therefore, it cannot be recommended for any disease. The fact that little is known about the phytochemical and toxicologic properties of blue flag and its constituents indicates that this herb is best avoided until further information is available.

References
Newall, C.A., et al. *Herbal Medicines: A Guide for Health-Care Professionals,* 1st ed. London: Pharmaceutical Press, 1996.

BOGBEAN
BUCKBEAN, MARSH TREFOIL, WATER SHAMROCK

Common trade names
None known.

Common forms
Available as dried leaf, liquid extract, and tincture.

Source
Bogbean extract is made from the leaves of *Menyanthes trifoliata,* a member of the Gentianaceae family. This plant is native to swamps and marshes of Europe and North America.

Chemical components

Several acids (caffeic, chlorogenic, ferulic, salicylic, vanillic, folic, palmitic), alkaloids (gentianin, gentianidine, choline), and flavonoids (hyperin, kaempferol, quercetin, rutin, trifolioside) are present in bogbean. Other components include a coumarin, scopoletin, iridoids, carotene, and ceryl alcohol.

Actions

Bogbean is claimed to have both bitter and diuretic properties. An in vitro study suggests that compounds isolated from bogbean may be valuable analgesic agents. The isolation of eight compounds from the dried rhizomes of *M. trifoliata* and their inhibition on prostaglandin synthesis was reported. The results demonstrated that two of the eight compounds showed significant inhibition of prostaglandin synthesis, with compounds two to 14 times more potent than aspirin. The other isolated compounds did not have any effect on prostaglandin synthesis (Huang et al., 1995).

Tertiary references suggest that bile-stimulating properties have been described for both caffeic and ferulic acid. Extracts of bogbean have also demonstrated antibactericidal properties (Bishop and MacDonald, 1951).

Reported uses

Bogbean has been reported to be a rheumatic agent, an appetite stimulant, a cathartic laxative, and an agent for fevers, scurvy, or dropsy (edematous state). Human trials evaluating bogbean for safety and efficacy are lacking.

Dosage

Dried leaf: 1 to 2 g in a tea P.O. t.i.d.
Extract (1:1 in 25% alcohol): 1 to 2 ml P.O. t.i.d. with plenty of juice or water at mealtimes.

Adverse reactions

- Bleeding (potential)
- Hemolysis (Giaceri, 1972)
- Nausea
- Vomiting

⚠ Ingestion may result in severe protracted nausea and vomiting.

Interactions

Anticoagulants (heparin, warfarin): may potentiate action of anticoagulants because of coumarin derivative in bogbean. Avoid concomitant use.
Antiplatelets (aspirin, clopidogrel, ticlopidine): may increase risk of bleeding. Avoid concomitant use.

Contraindications and precautions
Contraindicated in pregnant and breast-feeding patients.

Special considerations
• Monitor for signs of bleeding, especially in patients receiving concomitant anticoagulation or antiplatelet therapy.
• Advise the patient to keep fluid extracts away from children because of possible risk of poisoning.
• Advise the patient to report unusual abdominal pain, vomiting, or dizziness. Tell the patient to discontinue the herb if symptoms continue.

Points of interest
• The fruit of *M. trifoliata,* a plant found predominantly in swamps and bogs, resembles a small bean; hence the name "bogbean."
• Small quantities of bogbean are used as a natural food flavoring in Europe.

Analysis
Although animal studies have documented a few therapeutic pharmacologic uses for bogbean, definitive validation from human clinical trials is not available to justify the use of bogbean for any of its therapeutic claims. Questions about safety remain unanswered.

References
Bishop, C.J., and MacDonald, R.E. "A Survey of Higher Plants for Antibacterial Substances," *Botany* 15:231-59, 1951.
Giaceri, G. "Chromatographic Identification of Coumarin Derivatives in *Menyanthes trifoliata,*" *Fitoterapia* 43:134-38, 1972.
Huang, C., et al. "Anti-inflammatory Compounds Isolated from *Menyanthes trifoliata* L.," *Acta Pharm Sinica* 30:621-26, 1995.

BOLDO

BOLDINE, BOLDO-DO-CHILE

Common trade names
Boldo is a minor ingredient in more than 60 preparations used principally in South America and Europe.

Common forms
Available as a tea, a tincture, and an extract.

Source
Boldine, an alkaloid, is the principal constituent of the leaves and bark of the Chilean boldo tree, *Peumus boldus* (*Boldea boldus*). This small evergreen is native to Chile and Peru and is naturalized in the

Mediterranean region. Boldine has also been found in more than a dozen other trees or shrubs in the laurel, magnolia, and monimia families.

Chemical components
At least 17 different alkaloids occur in the leaves and bark of the boldo tree. Dried boldo leaves have a total alkaloid content of 0.25% to 0.5%. Boldine is the principle alkaloid, constituting approximately 0.1% of the dried leaf. The bark is much richer in alkaloids, with boldine accounting for approximately 75% of the total alkaloid content. Other compounds include flavonoids, volatile oils, a coumarin, resin, and tannins.

Actions
Although boldo is a widely used medicinal plant, its physiologic effects and mechanisms of action are not well known. Pharmacokinetic, pharmacodynamic, and physiologic data in humans are lacking. In studies with dogs, boldo was found to exert a diuretic effect, increasing urinary excretion by 50% (Speisky and Cassels, 1994). In other animal studies, boldo has been shown to relax smooth muscle and prolong intestinal transit time, a process mediated at least in part through anticholinergic actions (Gotteland et al., 1995).

Boldine acted as an alpha-adrenergic blocker and calcium antagonist in rats. When administered parenterally, boldine exerts some inhibitory CNS action, possibly mediated by dopamine receptor blockade (Speisky and Cassels, 1994).

Laboratory tests have shown boldine to be a more potent antioxidant than vitamin E. Other laboratory studies have shown that boldine offers in vitro protection of cytochrome P450 enzyme systems from damage due to exposure to peroxidative attack (Kringstein and Cederbaum, 1995). These findings have led to speculation that boldine may have value as a hepatoprotective agent or as a treatment in free radical–mediated disease states. Finally, studies have demonstrated that boldine is not mutagenic or genotoxic (Speisky and Cassels, 1994; Tavares and Takahashi, 1994).

Reported uses
Boldo is one of the most widely used medicinal plants in Chile. Its principal therapeutic claims are for treating digestive and hepatobiliary disorders. Some human clinical trials appear to validate its use in digestive disorders (Gotteland et al., 1995; Borgia et al., 1981). (See *GI effects of boldo*, page 94.)

Boldo-based preparations are also used for headache, earache, head colds, rheumatism, nervousness, weakness, generalized edema, dyspepsia, flatulence, menstrual pain, syphilis, gonorrhea, and gout.

RESEARCH FINDINGS
GI effects of boldo

A recent study attempted to assess the effects of boldo on mouth-to-cecum transit time in healthy human subjects. Twelve volunteers received either 2.5 g of a dry boldo extract or a glucose placebo during two successive 4-day periods. On day 4 of each period, subjects received 20 g of lactulose. The level of hydrogen exhaled was then measured every 15 minutes to detect changes that would reflect mouth-to-cecum transit time. These results indicated that transit time was significantly greater after the administration of boldo than after the placebo.

This study helps explain the mechanism and effectiveness of boldo in the treatment of digestive disorders (Gotteland et al., 1995). Another study examined boldo given with rhubarb, gentian, and cascara in treating GI complaints. Although useful in improving symptoms of appetite loss, flatulence, and itching, boldo and cascara were more effective than other herbal combinations in treating constipation (Borgia et al., 1981), a further testimony of boldo's effectiveness as a cathartic.

Other therapeutic claims include use as a sedative, mild hypnotic, diuretic, laxative, and anthelmintic.

Dosage
Human clinical trials have used 2.5 g of dried boldo extract P.O. daily.

Adverse reactions
• Possible CNS effects, including seizures, disturbed coordination, and exaggerated reflexes

⚠ Although reports are conflicting, boldo volatile oil may be a toxic volatile oil. In large doses, boldo may cause paralysis of motor and sensory nerves and eventually the muscle fibers, causing death due to respiratory arrest. Toxicologic studies in animals, however, seem to reflect favorably on the claimed low toxicity of boldo. In mice and guinea pigs, doses of 500 to 1,000 mg/kg boldine P.O. were needed to produce death; 15 g boldine P.O. was needed to cause death in a 12-kg dog. Death in these cases was due to respiratory depression. Rats showed no signs of toxicity after ingesting up to 3,000 mg/kg of boldine extract P.O. (Speisky and Cassels, 1994).

Interactions
None reported.

Contraindications and precautions

Contraindicated in patients with existing CNS or respiratory system disorders and in pregnant and breast-feeding patients.

Special considerations

• Instruct the patient to keep boldo preparations and plant parts out of the reach of children.
• Advise the patient with existing CNS or respiratory problems to avoid use of boldo products.
• Advise the patient that additional studies need to be conducted before boldo or its components can be recognized for the treatment of any disorder.
• Instruct the patient to avoid ingestion of the boldo volatile oil because its toxicity index is unknown.
• Advise the female patient to avoid use of herb during pregnancy or when breast-feeding.

Points of interest

• Fossilized boldo leaves over 13,000 years old that have imprints of human teeth have been found in Chile. It is not known whether these leaves were used medicinally by ancient Chileans or whether they were chewed simply for their pleasant and refreshing taste (Speisky and Cassels, 1994).
• More than 60 preparations registered in various countries include boldo as an active ingredient, usually as a minor constituent. Most of these products are indicated for digestive or hepatobiliary disorders. Chile currently exports about 800 tons of dried boldo leaves annually, mainly to Argentina, Brazil, Italy, France, and Germany (Speisky and Cassels, 1994).

Analysis

Further studies are needed to clarify the pharmacology, pharmacokinetics, and toxicology of boldo. Recent findings about boldo's antioxidant and hepatoprotective properties warrant additional investigation. Until the safety and efficacy of boldo preparations are established, this herb cannot be recommended for human use.

References

Borgia, M., et al. "Pharmacological Activity of a Herbs Extract. A Controlled Clinical Study," *Curr Ther Res* 29:525-36, 1981.

Gotteland, M., et al. "Effect of a Dry Boldo Extract on Oro-cecal Transit in Healthy Volunteers," *Rev Med Chil* 123:955-60, 1995.

Kringstein, P., and Cederbaum, A.I. "Boldine Prevents Human Liver Microsomal Lipid Peroxidation and Inactivation of Cytochrome P4502E1," *Free Radic Biol Med* 18:559-63, 1995. Abstract.

Speisky, H., and Cassels, B.K. "Boldo and Boldine: An Emerging Case of Natural Drug Development," *Pharmacol Res* 29:1-12, 1994.

Tavares, D.C., and Takahashi, C.S. "Evaluation of the Genotoxic Potential of the Alkaloid Boldine in Mammalian Cell Systems In Vitro and In Vivo," *Mutat Res* 321:139-45,1994. Abstract.

BONESET

AGUEWEED, CROSSWORT, EUPATORIUM, FEVERWORT,
INDIAN SAGE, SWEATING PLANT, THOROUGHWORT,
VEGETABLE ANTIMONY

Common trade names
(Available in combination) Catarrh Mixture

Common forms
Available as a tea, an extract, and a topical cream.

Source
The crude drug is obtained from the dried leaves and flowering tops of the perennial herb *Eupatorium perfoliatum,* which grows throughout much of the United States and parts of Canada.

Chemical components
Boneset contains flavonoids, such as kaempferol, quercetin, astragalin, and rutin; eupatorin, a bitter, crystalline glycoside; terpenoids; triterpenes; sterols; volatile oil; resin; tannin; crystalline wax; inulin; polysaccharides; sugars; and gallic acid.

Actions
Although boneset is an old herbal standby, especially as an antipyretic, comparatively little is known about its pharmacologically active constituents. Animal studies suggest that boneset exhibits immunostimulatory actions on granulocytes and macrophages of sesquiterpene lactones and polysaccharide fractions of *E. perfoliatum* (Wagner et al., 1985).

Several studies attribute diaphoretic and emetic properties to boneset. In addition, weak to moderate anti-inflammatory activity has been documented for some of the flavonoids and for an alcoholic extract of boneset. Although most members of the genus *Eupatorium* contain hepatotoxic pyrrolizidine alkaloids, these have not yet been found in boneset (Smith and Culvenor, 1981).

Reported uses
Despite over 200 years of anecdotal use as an antipyretic, there has never been a human clinical trial reported that established the effectiveness for this use. A study in Germany failed to find any difference between a homeopathic boneset remedy and aspirin for dis-

comfort of the common cold (Gassinger et al., 1981). Other traditional uses have included acute bronchitis, influenza, congestion of the respiratory mucosa, and as a sedative and expectorant.

Dosage

Extract: 10 to 40 drops (2 to 4 g of plant material) mixed in a liquid P.O. daily.
Tea: 2 to 6 teaspoon of crushed dried leaves and flowering tops steeped in 1 cup to 1 pint of boiling water.

Adverse reactions

- Allergic reactions
- Diarrhea
- Possible hepatotoxicity
- Vomiting

Interactions

None reported.

Contraindications and precautions

Contraindicated in pregnant and breast-feeding patients; effects are unknown.

Special considerations

- Monitor liver function studies periodically.
- Advise the patient that insufficient data exist to recommend this herb as a treatment for any disease state, and that many proven anti-inflammatory compounds exist with known risks and benefits.
- Advise the female patient to avoid use of the herb during pregnancy or when breast-feeding.

Points of interest

- It has been suggested that boneset derived its name from an alleged ability to alleviate dengue fever, also known as "breakbone fever."
- Despite its inclusion in the United States Pharmacopeia for almost a century (1820-1916) and the National Formulary for almost 25 years (1926-1950), boneset's use was never advocated by the traditional medical community. More recently, boneset has been included in homeopathic formulations and herbal mixtures marketed in Europe and to practicing herbalists.
- Boneset was used by Native Americans against malaria. (See *Native Americans fought fever with boneset,* page 98.)

Analysis

Medicinal uses of boneset should be discouraged until more is known about its clinical safety and efficacy. However, because many proven remedies already exist for the range of boneset's claimed therapeutic uses, it is unlikely that additional clinical research will be pursued.

References

Gassinger, C.A., et al. "A Controlled Clinical Trial for Treating the Efficacy of the Homeopathic Drug *Eupatorium perfoliatum* D2 in the Treatment of the Common Cold," *Arzneimittelforschung* 31:732-36, 1981.

Smith, L.W., and Culvenor, C.C. "Plant Sources of Hepatotoxic Pyrrolizidine Alkaloids," *J Nat Prod* 44:129-52, 1981.

Wagner, H., et al. "Immunostimulating Polysaccharides (Heteroglycans) of Higher Plants," *Arzneimittelforschung* 35:1069, 1985.

BORAGE

BEEBREAD, COMMON BORAGE, COMMON BUGLOSS, COOL TANKARD, OX'S TONGUE, STARFLOWER

Common trade names
Borage Oil, Borage Power

Common forms
Capsules (softgels): 240 mg, 500 mg, 1,300 mg borage seed oil (oil contains 20% to 26% gamma linolenic acid [GLA]).

Source
Active components of the drug are obtained from the leaves, stems, flowers, and especially the seeds of borage (*Borago officinalis*), a hardy annual that grows in Europe and Eastern United States.

Chemical components
Borage seed contains a mucilage, tannin, and an essential oil. The fatty acid component of the seed oil consists of linoleic acid, GLA, oleic acid, and saturated fatty acids. The oil also contains small amounts of pyrrolizidine alkaloids, notably amabiline, a known hepatotoxin.

Actions

The mucilage component of borage produces an expectorant-like action. The malic acid and potassium nitrate components produce a mild diuretic effect.

GLA from borage seeds may suppress inflammation and joint tissue injury. GLA is rapidly converted to dihomogammalinoleic acid, an immediate precursor of monoenoic prostaglandin E_1, which has potent anti-inflammatory activity (Levanthal et al., 1993).

Borage teas are claimed to have soothing effects. Studies in rats and humans have suggested that borage can calm the CV response to stress. In one study, borage oil reduced systolic blood pressure and heart rate and reportedly improved the ability to perform tasks. This clinical trial used daily doses of 1.3 g for 28 days but involved only 10 individuals. The mechanism of action is unknown (Mills, 1989).

Reported uses

Borage leaves have been part of European herbal medicine for centuries. During medieval times, the leaves and flowers were steeped in wine and taken to dispel melancholy. Borage has also been used to treat colds and bronchitis and is claimed to possess diaphoretic, expectorant, tonic, and anti-inflammatory properties. (See *Treating joint inflammation with borage,* page 100.) More recently, borage has been used to treat rheumatoid arthritis. Most of the claims for this product are based on anti-inflammatory effects seen in animals and in small, uncontrolled or poorly controlled human trials (Leventhal et al., 1993; Karlstad et al., 1993).

Dosage

In clinical trials, dosages ranged from 1.1 to 1.4 g P.O. daily of borage seed oil.

Adverse reactions

⚠ Although no significant adverse effects have been reported, 1 to 2 g of borage seed oil contains potentially toxic amounts (approximately 10 mcg) of unsaturated pyrrolizidine alkaloids, including amabiline.

Interactions

None reported.

Contraindications and precautions

Contraindicated in pregnant and breast-feeding patients; effects are unknown.

Special considerations

• Monitor liver function studies periodically in patients who consume borage.

RESEARCH FINDINGS
Treating joint inflammation with borage

Two clinical trials showed promising results using gamma-linolenic acid (GLA) in borage seed oil in the treatment of joint disorders. A randomized, double-blind, placebo-controlled 24-week trial was conducted using 37 patients who had rheumatoid arthritis and active synovitis.

The treatment group receiving GLA (1.4 g) as borage seed oil daily showed significant reduction of signs and symptoms of disease activity ($P < 0.05$). Thirty-six percent of the subjects experienced fewer tender joints and 28% had fewer swollen joints. The placebo group showed no such improvement. Of note, many of the patients in both groups also received NSAIDs and some received up to 10 mg of prednisone daily. No patients withdrew from GLA treatment (Leventhal et al., 1993).

In an uncontrolled trial, seven healthy patients and seven patients with rheumatoid arthritis received nine capsules of GLA (1.1 g) daily for 12 weeks. All the patients also received NSAIDs alone, prednisone and NSAIDs, or just acetaminophen. Eighty-five percent of the arthritic patients exhibited apparent clinical improvement, possibly as a result of the administration of GLA (Pullman-Mooar et al., 1990).

• Advise the patient with compromised liver function to avoid using borage because of the potential for liver damage.
• Advise the female patient to avoid use of the herb during pregnancy or when breast-feeding.

Points of interest
• Borage oil (starflower oil) is used as an alternative to evening primrose oil as a source of GLA.

Analysis
A few studies in rats and humans suggest that borage has value as an anti-inflammatory agent for rheumatoid arthritis. However, its exact role in therapy as well as questions about its efficacy and safety remain to be resolved. Other claims for this product are largely unsubstantiated.

References
Karlstad, M. D., et al. "Effect of Intravenous Lipid Emulsions Enriched with Gamma-linolenic Acid on Plasma n-6 Fatty Acids and Prostaglandin Biosynthesis After Burn and Endotoxin Injury in Rats," *Crit Care Med* 21:1740-49, 1993.

Leventhal, L. J., et al. "Treatment of Rheumatoid Arthritis with Gamma-linolenic Acid," *Ann Intern Med* 119:867-73, 1993.

Mancuso, P., et al. "Dietary Fish Oil and Fish and Borage Oil Suppress Intrapulmonary Proinflammatory Eicosanoid Biosynthesis and Attenuate Pulmonary Neutrophil Accumulation in Endotoxic Rats," *Crit Care Med* 25:1198-1206, 1997.

Mills, D.E. "Dietary Fatty Acid Supplementation Alters Stress Reactivity and Performance in Man," *J Hum Hypertens* 3:111-16, 1989.

Pullman-Mooar, S., et al. "Alteration of the Cellular Fatty Acid Profile and the Production of Eicosanoids in Human Monocytes by Gamma-linolenic Acid," *Arthritis Rheum* 33:1526-33, 1990.

BROOM

BANNAL, BROOM TOP, GENISTA, GINSTERKRAUT, HOGWEED, IRISH BROOM TOP, SAROTHAMNI HERB, SCOTCH BROOM, SCOTCH BROOM TOP

Common trade names
None known.

Common forms
Available as root, cigarettes, teas, and extracts.

Source
The crude drug is prepared from the twigs and flowers of *Cytisus scoparius* (*Sarothamnus scoparius*). Broom has been naturalized from Europe to the United States and Canada. This plant should not be confused with Spanish broom (*Spartium junceum*), used in trace amounts in foods and cosmetics.

Chemical components
Broom tops (flowers) contain the alkaloid sparteine. The concentration of this alkaloid ranges from 0.01% to 0.22% in floral parts, and up to 1.5% in twigs. Broom also contains the flavone glycosides oxysparteine, scoparoside, spiraeoside, lupanine, genitoside, and isoquercetin. Kaempferol, quercetin derivatives, isoflavones (sarothamnoside), and caffeic-acid derivatives and essential oils (containing phenylethyl alcohol, phenols, and acids) have also been reported. Broom seeds contain phytohemagglutinins, or lectins.

Actions
The metabolism of sparteine has been repeatedly documented in humans. In addition, studies with rodents show that sparteine inhibits sodium and potassium transport across the cell membrane. This action in cardiac cells mimics the actions of type IA antiarrhythmics agents, such as quinidine and procainamide. Sparteine

produces a negative chronotropic effect and possibly a negative inotropic effect (Pugsley et al., 1995; Raschack, 1974).

Sparteine undergoes oxidative metabolism by way of the cytochrome P-450 system in the liver. Cardiac drugs that share the same CYP2D6 pathway have demonstrated the ability to inhibit sparteine metabolism (Belpaire and Bogaert, 1996). All drugs known to share this metabolic pathway have the potential to interfere with the metabolism of sparteine. Sparteine is also a known oxytocic agent.

Another component of broom, scoparoside, possesses diuretic properties.

Reported uses

Medical folklore and homeopathy have endowed broom with antiarrhythmic, cathartic, diuretic, and emetic properties at high doses. Smoking broom cigarettes is reported to cause relaxation and euphoria. However, some researchers argue that these effects are unlikely to occur because of the small quantity of alkaloids taken into the body through smoking of the plant.

Lectins isolated from the seeds of broom have been used as pharmacologic markers (Young et al., 1984). They have also been used to classify red cell polyagglutinability (Bird and Wingham, 1980). Sparteine, like debrisoquin, is used to characterize metabolizers of the oxidative metabolic pathway CYP2D6 in the liver (Belpaire and Bogaert, 1996).

Dosage

No consensus exists.

Adverse reactions

- Arrhythmias
- Fungal pneumonia; increased risk when contaminated broom tops are smoked as cigarettes
- Headache
- Possible mind-altering sensations from smoking plant parts
- Possible spontaneous abortion from effects of sparteine
- Uterine contractions

⚠ Poisoning from overdose is possible. At toxic concentrations, broom may cause a clinical picture similar to nicotine poisoning: shock, tachycardia, mental status changes, vertigo, nausea, and diarrhea.

Interactions

Antihypertensives: possible alteration in effectiveness of some antihypertensive agents. Avoid concomitant use.

Beta blockers, other cardiac drugs, tricyclic antidepressants: possible increase in effects of these drugs, increasing risk of serious arrhythmias, such as ventricular fibrillation, ventricular tachycardia, brady-cardia, and heart block. Avoid concomitant use.

Cardiac pacemakers: possible interference with proper function of pacemaker. Avoid use of broom in patients with cardiac pacemakers.

Contraindications and precautions

Contraindicated in pregnant patients because broom is known to cause spontaneous abortion. Also contraindicated in patients with hypertension or significantly impaired cardiac function because of the potential for arrhythmias and the agent's ability to increase the tone of the vascular system.

Special considerations

• Warn the patient to avoid ingesting or smoking broom preparations because of potentially dangerous effects on the vascular system.
• Caution the patient that broom is a dangerous herb and lacks approval for any therapeutic use.
• Advise the patient not to confuse this plant with Spanish broom (*S. junceum*).
• Warn the female patient to avoid use of the herb during pregnancy.

Points of interest

• Before the use of hops, broom was used to enhance the taste and intoxicating power of beer.
• The FDA considers this plant unsafe for human consumption. The German E Commission, which oversees drug use in Germany, considers broom effective for certain cardiac disorders.

Analysis

Although broom contains interesting and potentially useful therapeutic agents, the potential for harm appears to outweigh any purported benefits. In addition, all of the potential therapeutic applications for broom are supplied by safer and more effective medications. Additional data are needed to determine more completely the risks and benefits of the pharmacologic alkaloids contained in this plant.

References

Belpaire, F.M., and Bogaert, M.G. "Cytochrome P450: Genetic Polymorphism and Drug Interactions," *Acta Clin Belg* 51:254-60, 1996.

Bird, G.W., and Wingham, J. "Lectins for Polyagglutinable Red Cells: *Cytisus scoparius, Spartium junceum* and *Vicia villosa*," *Clin Lab Haematol* 2:21-23, 1980.

Leung, A.Y. *Encyclopedia of Common Natural Ingredients Used in Food, Drugs, and Cosmetics.* New York: Wiley-Interscience, 1980.

Pugsley, M.K., et al. "The Cardiac Electrophysiological Effects of Sparteine and Its Analogue BRB-I-28 in the Rat," *Eur J Pharmacol* 27:319-27, 1995.

Raschack, V.M. "Wirkungen von Spartein und Spartein-derivaten auf Herz and Kreislauf," *Arzneimittelforschung* 24:753, 1974.

Young, N.M., et al. "Structural Differences Between Two Lectins from *Cytisus scoparius*, Both Specific for D-galactose and N-acetyl-D-galactosamine," *Biochem J* 222:41, 1984.

BUCHU

AGATHOSMA, *BAROSMA BETULINA*, BETULINE, BOCCO, *DIOSMA BETULINA*

Common trade names
None known.

Common forms
Available as dried leaves (for infusion) and a tincture.

Source
Active components of buchu are derived from a volatile oil in the leaves of *Barosma betulina* (*Agathosma betulina*) and the related species *B. serratifolia* and *B. crenulata*, low-lying shrubs that grow in South Africa. The leaves are harvested while the plants are flowering or bearing fruit.

Chemical components
The volatile oil of *B. betulina* leaves contains more than 100 chemicals. Those that may be responsible for the pharmacologic properties attributed to the herb include diosphenol (buchu camphor), pulegone, terpene-4-ol, and a number of flavonoids. Mucilage, resin, and coumarins have been reported in other *Barosma* species.

Actions
Little information is available on the action of buchu. In studies with rats, diosmin, a buchu flavonoid, was found to possess anti-inflammatory activity (Farnsworth and Cordell, 1976).

Reported uses
Buchu is claimed to be useful as a diuretic and in the treatment of urogenital tract infections.

Dosage
Infusion: 1 small glass of the infusion (1 oz dried leaves added to 1 pint boiling water)
Tincture: 1 to 2 ml P.O. t.i.d. or q.i.d.

Adverse reactions
• Diarrhea, nausea, vomiting (volatile oil)
• Hepatotoxicity from volatile oil constituent (pulegone)

- Increased menstrual flow (pulegone)
- Nephritis (volatile oil)
- Spontaneous abortion in pregnant females (pulegone)

Interactions
Anticoagulants: possible enhanced effect of the anticoagulants. Avoid concomitant use.

Contraindications and precautions
Contraindicated in pregnant and breast-feeding patients; pulegone has abortifacient activity and increases menstrual flow. Also contraindicated in patients with kidney infection, mild or moderate kidney disease, and compromised liver function because the herb may exacerbate these conditions.

Special considerations
- Monitor liver function in patients using buchu because of the herb's potential for causing liver damage.
- Instruct the patient to avoid ingesting this plant; little is known about the herb, and some components could be toxic.
- Advise the female patient to avoid use of the herb during pregnancy or when breast-feeding.

Points of interest
- Buchu was once included in the U.S. National Formulary as a diuretic and antiseptic. In 1821, it was listed in the British Pharmacopoeia as a medicine for cystitis, urethritis, nephritis, and catarrh of the bladder.
- In Germany, buchu is used as a treatment for kidney and urinary tract infections and as a diuretic. Its use is not endorsed by German health authorities, however, because the herb's purported actions for those uses have not been substantiated.
- The herb is used as a "cooling diuretic" in Ayurvedic medicine (Frawley and Lad, 1986).

Analysis
The effectiveness of buchu has not been demonstrated in clinical trials or animal studies. Together with the potential damaging effects it can cause in the liver, this herb cannot be recommended.

References
Farnsworth, N.R., and Cordell, G.A. "A Review of Some Biologically Active Compounds Isolated from Plants as Reported in the 1974-1975 Literature," *Lloydia* 39:420-55, 1976.

Frawley, D., and Lad, V. *The Yoga of Herbs.* Twin Lakes, Wis.: Lotus Press, 1986.

BUCKTHORN

COMMON BUCKTHORN, EUROPEAN BUCKTHORN, HARTSTHORN, PURGING BUCKTHORN, WAYTHORN

Common trade names
(Various manufacturers; available in combination) Herbal Laxative, Herbalene, Laxysat Mono Abführ-Tee Nr.2, Neo-Cleanse, Neo-Lax

Common forms
Available as a syrup.

Source
The drug is extracted from the berries of the thorny shrub or tree, *Rhamnus cathartica*. Buckthorn is native to Europe and naturalized in parts of the United States and Canada.

Chemical components
Buckthorn berries are believed to contain tannin, albumen, acetic acid, sugar, and an azotized substance composed primarily of glucosides. Rhamnocathartin, a bitter, yellow amorphous substance, is soluble in water and alcohol. Rhamnin, found in the berries of the shrub, is barely soluble in cold water but is soluble in hot alcohol. Rhamnegine breaks down into crystallizable sugar when heated with a dilute mineral acid. Rhamnotannic acid is formed during the separation of rhamnin and is an amorphous, friable, bitter mass soluble in alcohol and insoluble in water.

Actions
Buckthorn is reported to exert powerful cathartic effects. One study with animals found that the herb may be hepatotoxic in mice, possibly resulting from deposits of monoparticulate glycogen in the cytoplasm. Compounds in *R. cathartica* are thought to interfere with glycogen metabolism (Lichtensteiger et al., 1997).

Reported uses
Buckthorn's main use, as a cathartic, has declined drastically because of its violent mechanism of action and severe adverse effects. A powder or decoction of the bark has been used as a gentle astringent or tonic for skin ailments.

Dosage
No consensus exists.

Adverse reactions
- Abdominal pain
- Anxiety

- Decreased respirations
- Dehydration
- Diarrhea
- Nausea
- Trembling
- Vomiting

Interactions
None reported.

Contraindications and precautions
Contraindicated in pregnant or breast-feeding patients; effects are unknown. Use cautiously in patients with GI problems, such as irritable bowel syndrome, peptic ulcer disease, ulcerative colitis, and Crohn's disease because of worsened symptoms.

Special considerations
- Instruct the patient to keep berries and all buckthorn preparations out of reach of children.
- Warn the patient about potential GI problems with this agent. More gentle and predictable laxatives should be recommended, especially for older patients and young children.
- Advise the female patient to avoid use of the herb during pregnancy or when breast-feeding.

Points of interest
- Buckthorn is now primarily used as a dye. The juice of the berries produces a saffron-colored dye; and the bark, a brilliant yellow. The ripened berries of the plant are often mixed with alum, which results in a sap-green color often used for watercoloring.
- Until the 19th century, syrup of buckthorn was the common form. The syrup was prepared by boiling the juice of a buckthorn with pimento, ginger, and sugar. Because of the severity of the resulting drug's actions, use of the herb was discontinued in humans. The herb was given to animals occasionally as a laxative and was mixed with equal parts of castor oil. The discovery of a more gently acting relative, *R. purshiana,* has led to a more limited use of *R. cathartica.*

Analysis
No clinical trials support the medicinal use of *R. cathartica.* Its violent actions and severe adverse effects suggest that the risks of administration outweigh the benefits. Other medications with a lower incidence of adverse effects and more predictable effectiveness should be considered.

References

Lichtensteiger, C.A., et al. "*Rhamnus cathartica* (Buckthorn) Hepatocellular Toxicity in Mice," *Toxicol Pathol* 25:449-52, 1997.

Millspaugh, C.F. *American Medicinal Plants.* New York: Dover Publications, Inc., 1974. Originally published in 1892.

BUGLEWEED

CARPENTER'S HERB, COMMON BUGLE, EGYPTIAN'S HERB, FARASYON MAIY, GYPSY-WEED, GYPSY-WORT, MENTA DE LOBO, MIDDLE COMFREY, PAUL'S BETONY, SICKLEWORT, SU FERASYUNU, WATER BUGLE, WATER HOREHOUND

Common trade names

None known.

Common forms

Available as a dried herb and as a liquid extract and tincture.

Source

Pharmacologically active compounds are extracted from the roots, stems, leaves, and flowers of *Lycopus virginicus* and *L. europaeus*. These members of the Mint family are native to Europe and North America.

Chemical components

Active constituents of *L. europaeus* include lithospermic, chlorogenic, caffeic, ellagic, and rosmarinic acids, and the flavone glycoside luteolin-7-glucoside. Other compounds include amino acids, minerals, sugars, tannin, ursolic acid, and sinapinic acid. *L. virginicus* was found to contain rosmarinic and caffeic acids (Horhammer et al., 1962).

Actions

Certain active compounds in *Lycopus* species have been found to demonstrate complex endocrine effects in animal models, including a dose-related decrease in immunoglobulin G (IgG) antibody activity. The plant has also been shown to inhibit IgG stimulation of adenylate cyclase in human thyroid membranes and thyroid iodine release in mice in vivo. It is unclear why bugleweed extracts interact with thyroid-stimulating hormone (TSH) and IgG antibody activity (Auf'Mkolk et al., 1985).

A study in horses found that oxidized *Lycopus* plant constituents inhibited serum gonadotropin in pregnant mares. These constituents also inhibited human chorionic gonadotropin (HCG) and prolactin in vitro (Brinker, 1990).

Reported uses

Bugleweed is claimed to have astringent and mild narcotic qualities and has been used for years in the symptomatic treatment of Graves' disease. *Lycopus* was compared to *Digitalis* during the 19th century and was found to lower the pulse without accumulating in the system (Millspaugh, 1974). *L. europaeus* has also been used as a remedy for intermittent fever.

Dosage

For antithyroidal and antigonadal effects, 25 to 50 mg/kg parenterally or 200 to 1,000 mg/kg P.O. in animals (Brinker 1990; Winterhoff et al., 1994).

Adverse reactions

None reported in animal studies with *L. europaeus*. However, *L. virginicus* was shown to inhibit testicular growth in rats (Sourgens et al., 1980). Hyperthyroidism has also been reported.

Interactions

Beta-blockers: possible masking of symptoms of hyperthyroidism. Avoid concomitant use.
Thyroid hormone replacement: possible interference with thyroid replacement therapy. Avoid concomitant use.

Contraindications and precautions

Contraindicated in pregnant and breast-feeding patients; effects are unknown. Use with extreme caution in patients with primary or secondary hypopituitarism, pituitary adenoma, primary or secondary hypogonadism, TSH-stimulating tumors, or related disorders. Use cautiously in patients with systolic dysfunction or heart failure.

Special considerations

• Know that this agent suppresses follicle-stimulating hormone (FSH), luteinizing hormone (LH), HCG, and TSH levels. Depending on the patient's hormone levels, concurrent *Lycopus* administration could enhance or antagonize the effects of these hormones.
• Know that this agent has not been evaluated in other thyroid conditions, such as multinodular goiters and subacute thyroiditis.
• Know that *Lycopus* and related species should not be substituted for antithyroid drugs, such as propylthiouracil and methimazole.
• Instruct the patient with a history of osteoporosis to consult with the health care professional before taking this agent.
• Advise the patient receiving oral contraceptives or fertility medications to consult the health care professional before taking bugleweed.

• Advise the female patient to avoid use of the herb during pregnancy or when breast-feeding.

Points of interest
• *L. europaeus* is said to be frequently sold as *L. virginicus.*

Analysis
Knowledge of the physiologic effects of this agent is derived from in vivo and in vitro animal studies using freeze-dried extracts. While the results of animal studies don't necessarily apply to humans, they nevertheless should inspire caution. Although this agent has been shown to inhibit various hormones, such as FSH, TSH, LH, and HCG, the level of inhibition has not been evaluated. It is difficult to determine the place, if any, of bugleweed in the treatment of Graves' disease, but research suggests that these plants should be investigated more thoroughly.

References
Auf'Mkolk, M., et al. "Extracts and Auto-oxidized Constituents of Certain Plants Inhibit the Receptor-Binding and the Biological Activity of Graves' Immunoglobulins," *Endocrinology* 116:1687-93, 1985.

Brinker, F. "Inhibition of Endocrine Function by Botanical Agents," *J Naturopath Med* 1:1-14, 1990.

Horhammer, L., et al. "Studies on the Ingredients of *Lycopus europaeus,*" *Arzneimittelforschung* 12:1-7, 1962.

Kohrle, J., et al. "Iodothyronine Deiodinases: Inhibition by Plant Extracts," *Acta Endocrin.* Suppl. 16:188-92, 1981.

Millspaugh, C.F. *American Medicinal Plants.* New York: Dover Publications, Inc., 1974. Reprint of 1892 edition.

Sourgens, H., et al. "Antihormonal Effects of Plant Extracts on Hypophyseal Hormone in the Rat," *Acta Endocrin* 234:49, 1980.

Winterhoff, H., et al. "Endocrine Effects of *Lycopus europaeus* L. Following Oral Application," *Arzneimittelforschung* 44:41-45, 1994.

BURDOCK

BARDANA, BEGGAR'S BUTTONS, CLOTBUR, COCKLE BUTTONS, CUCKOLD, EDIBLE BURDOCK, FOX'S CLOTE, GOBO, GREAT BUR, GREAT BURDOCK, HAPPY MAJOR, HARDOCK, LAPPA, LOVE LEAVES, PERSONATA, PHILANTHROPIUM, THORNY BURR, WILD GOBO

Common trade names
(Various manufacturers; available in combination) Anthraxiviore, Burdock Root

Common forms
Available as 425-mg and 475-mg capsules, liquid extract, cream for

topical administration, tincture (made from crushed seeds), dried root, and tea.

Source

The crude drug is extracted from the dried root of the great burdock, *Arctium lappa*, or common burdock, *Arctium minus*. The seeds and leaves of burdock plants have also been used in folk medicine. Burdock is a large biennial herb grown in China, Europe, and the United States. The plant can be identified in the spring by the round heads of its purple flowers.

Chemical components

The principal component of burdock root is a carbohydrate, inulin, which can account for up to 50% of the total plant mass. Additional components include tannins, polyphenolic acids, volatile acids, nonhydroxy acids, polyacetylenes, anthroquinone glycosides, and a plant hormone, gamma-guanidino-n-butyric acid. Seeds contain a glycoside, arctiin, and fixed oils, lignans, chlorogenic acid, a germacranolide, and other compounds. Some commercial teas with burdock have been prone to contamination with atropine.

Actions

Burdock is claimed to exert antipyretic, antimicrobial, diuretic, and diaphoretic activities. Uterine stimulation has been reported in in vivo studies. Animal studies have reportedly shown that burdock extracts demonstrate strong hypoglycemic activity (Lappinina and Sisoeva, 1964) and antagonism of platelet activating factor (Iwakami et al., 1992).

Various in vitro and animal studies have found that burdock possesses antimutagenic effects (Dombradi and Foldeak, 1966; Tsujita et al., 1979).

Reported uses

This agent is claimed to be useful for a wide range of ailments, including gout, ulcers, arthritis, rheumatism, sciatica, lumbar pain, hemorrhoids, and skin disorders, such as eczema, acne, psoriasis, and canker sores. Burdock has also been used as a blood purifier. In the Far East, burdock is used to treat cancer, impotence, and sterility. Current studies have reported the use of burdock in the treatment of kidney stones and HIV infection.

Dosage

Burdock is taken internally as a tea or used externally as a compress. The normal dosage of the tea is 1 cup P.O. t.i.d. or q.i.d.

Adverse reactions
● Allergic dermatitis (Rodriguez et al., 1995)
⚠ Poisoning due to atropine contamination of some commercial burdock teas. Signs and symptoms of toxicity include dilated pupils, blurred vision, and rapid pulse. Treatment, if needed, includes physostigmine reversal (Bryson, 1978; Bryson and Rumack, 1978; Rhoads and Anderson, 1985).

Interactions
Insulin, oral antidiabetic agents: possible increase in hypoglycemic effects. Avoid concomitant use.

Contraindications and precautions
Contraindicated during pregnancy, especially early in pregnancy because of the effects of anthraquinone glycosides found in the roots of burdock plants. Also contraindicated in patients with allergies to the drug or related plant species.

Special considerations
● Inform the diabetic patient that burdock may increase the risk of hypoglycemia and that insulin doses and oral hypoglycemic doses may need to be reduced.
● Advise the patient that burdock products may be significantly contaminated with atropine and that toxicity has resulted from this contamination.
● Inform the patient that little scientific data exist to evaluate burdock in humans.
● Warn the female patient to avoid use of the herb during pregnancy or when breast-feeding.

Points of interest
● Burdock root is commonly eaten in Asia; less often in the United States.

Analysis
Animal and in vitro studies suggest that burdock use might offer therapeutic benefits. However, clinical trials are needed to support these claims. In addition, data regarding the safety and efficacy of burdock are lacking.

References
Bryson, P.D. "Burdock Root Tea Poisoning," *JAMA* 240:1586, 1978.
Bryson, P.D., and Rumack, B.H. "Burdock Root Tea Poisoning," *JAMA* 239:2157, 1978.
Dombradi, C.A., and Foldeak, S. "Antitumor Activity of *A. lappa* Extracts," *Tumori* 52:173-75, 1966.

Iwakami, S., et al. "Platelet Activating Factor (PAF) Antagonists Contained in Medicinal Plants: Ligans and Sesquiterpenes," *Chem Pharm Bull* 40:1196, 1992.

Lappinina, L.O., and Sisoeva, T.F. "Investigation of Some Plants to Determine Their Sugar Lowering Action," *Farmatsevt Zh* 19:52-58, 1964.

Rhoads, P.M., and Anderson, R. "Anticholinergic Poisonings Associated with Commercial Burdock Root Tea," *Clin Toxicol* 22:581-84, 1985.

Rodriguez, P., et al. "Allergic Contact Dermatitis Due to Burdock (*Arctium lappa*)," *Contact Dermatitis* 33:134-35, 1995.

Tsujita, J., et al. "Comparison of Protective Activity of Dietary Fiber Against the Toxicities of Various Food Colors in Rats," *Nutr Rep Int* 20:635-42, 1979.

BUTCHER'S BROOM

BOX HOLLY, KNEE HOLLY, PETTIGREE, SWEET BROOM

Common trade names
(Various manufacturers; available in combination) Butcher's Broom Extract 4:1, Butcher's Broom Root, Hemodren Simple, Ruscorectal

Common forms
Capsules: 75 mg, 110 mg, 150 mg, 400 mg, 470 mg, 475 mg
Also available as liquid extract and tea.

Source
Butcher's broom is extracted from the leaves, rhizomes, and roots of *Ruscus aculeatus,* a low-lying evergreen shrub of the Lily family (Liliaceae). It is native to the Mediterranean region but also grows in Southern United States. Butchers in Europe and the Mediterranean at one time used the leaves and twigs of this plant to scrub chopping blocks clean, hence the name *butcher's broom.*

Chemical components
The major active components of butcher's broom are the steroidal saponins, ruscogenin and neoruscogenin. Flavonoids, coumarins, sparteine, tyramine, and glycolic acid have also been isolated.

Actions
In a study of dog veins, the saponins in butcher's broom produced vasoconstriction by directly activating postjunctional $alpha_1$- and $alpha_2$-adrenergic receptors (Marcelon, 1983).

Studies with animals have evaluated the effect of *R. aculeatus* on the diameter of arterioles and venules (Bouskela et al., 1993) and the effect of local changes in temperature on venous responsiveness to *R. aculeatus* (Rubanyi et al., 1984). Clinical trials suggest that a *Ruscus* preparation relieved symptoms of chronic phlebopathy of the lower limbs (Cappelli et al., 1988). (See *Effect of* Ruscus *on pe-*

ripheral venous disorders.) In addition, the extract of this plant possesses anti-inflammatory properties.

Reported uses
Butcher's broom is claimed to be helpful in the treatment of leg edema, varicose veins, peripheral vascular disease, hemorrhoids, and arthritis. It has also been used as a laxative and a diuretic. Human clinical data to support these claims are limited.

Dosage
For venous phlebopathy in the lower limbs, the dosage of butcher's broom tested in humans was 99 mg P.O. daily (in combination with ascorbic acid and hesperidin).

Adverse reactions
None reported.

Interactions
Antihypertensives: possible reduction in effects of alpha-adrenergic blockers, such as prazosin, doxazosin, terazosin; reduced effectiveness of therapy for benign prostatic hyperplasia (BPH). Avoid concomitant use.
MAO inhibitors: possible hypertensive crisis from tyramine in butcher's broom. Avoid use of herb in patients taking MAO inhibitors.

Contraindications and precautions
Contraindicated in pregnant and breast-feeding patients; effects are unknown. Use cautiously in patients with hypertension or BPH or who are receiving alpha-antagonist therapy.

Special considerations
• Advise the patient that more effective agents exist to treat his disease.
• Remind the patient that long-term effects of butcher's broom are still unknown.
• Warn the patient with circulatory disorders that this herb may interfere with other drugs he's taking.
• Advise the female patient to avoid use of the herb during pregnancy or when breast-feeding.

Analysis
Butcher's broom possesses vasoconstrictive properties but clinical data about these effects are limited. One study suggests that butcher's broom is beneficial in patients with chronic venous insufficiency and varicose veins of the lower limbs. However, the study in-

RESEARCH FINDINGS
Effect of *Ruscus* on peripheral venous disorders

A prospective, double-blind, placebo-controlled, cross-over trial evaluated the effectiveness of the RAES combination—*Ruscus aculeatus* (16.5 mg), hesperidin (75 mg), and ascorbic acid (50 mg)—in 40 patients with chronic venous insufficiency and varicose veins of the lower limbs. The study also examined the tolerance of the combination, administered as two capsules P.O. three times daily with meals.

Patients received either RAES or a placebo for two successive periods of 2 months each with a 15-day drug-free period between each session. Ankle diameter, the extent of malleolar edema, and the presence of related symptoms were monitored.

Itching improved significantly during RAES treatment. Cramping, paresthesia, heavy feeling or tension of the legs, and ankle diameter also decreased. All measurements of venous capacity were reduced with RAES. These parameters were either the same or worse in the placebo group, but did not always achieve statistical significance. RAES treatment was well tolerated during the study.

This study demonstrates that RAES reduces venous capacity and may improve symptoms in patients with chronic venous insufficiency and varicose veins of the lower limbs (Cappelli et al., 1988). Additional studies are needed to confirm these findings.

volved only 40 patients and *R. aculeatus* was used in combination with hesperidin and ascorbic acid.

Butcher's broom may be well tolerated, but additional studies are needed to evaluate this agent's effectiveness in treating venous disease and other vascular conditions. There are currently no clinical data to support the use of butcher's broom for treating hemorrhoids or arthritis.

References

Bouskela, E., et al. "Effects of *Ruscus* Extract on the Internal Diameter of Arterioles and Venules of the Hamster Cheek Pouch Microcirculation," *J Cardiovasc Pharmacol* 22:221-24, 1993.

Cappelli, R., et al. "Use of Extract of *Ruscus aculeatus* in Venous Disease in the Lower Limb," *Drugs Exp Clin Res* 14:277-83, 1988.

Marcelon, G., et al. "Effect of *Ruscus aculeatus* on Isolated Canine Cutaneous Veins," *Gen Pharmacol* 14:103, 1983.

Rubanyi, G., et al. "Effect of Temperature on the Responsiveness of Cutaneous Veins to the Extract of *Ruscus aculeatus*," *Gen Pharmacol* 15:431-34, 1984.

BUTTERBUR

EUROPEAN PESTROOT, SWEET COLTSFOOT, WESTERN COLTSFOOT

Common trade names
(Various manufacturers; available in combination) Alzoon, Butterbur Root Extract, Feverfew/Dogwood Supreme, Neurochol, Petaforce, Wild Cherry Supreme

Common forms
Available as 25-mg standardized capsules, *Petasites* extract, and liquid *Petasites* extract (concentration may vary).

Source
Active compounds of butterbur are extracted from the leaves, flowers, stems, and root stock of *Petasites hybridus, P. officinalis,* or *Tussilago petasites.* Some formulas use extract from the leaves and roots of *P. frigidus,* also known as *P. palmatus, T. palmatum,* or western coltsfoot. These plants are low-lying perennial herbs of the Composite family (Compositae).

Chemical components
The active components of *P. hybridus* are believed to be petasin, oxopetasin esters, and isopetasin. Several studies have found petasin, a sesquiterpene ester of petasol and angelic acid, to be the most active component (Weiss, 1988). Isopetasin and oxopetasin esters have been isolated. Other alkaloids isolated from *P. hybridus* include pyrrolizidine alkaloids senecionine, integerrimine, and senkirkine (Luthy et al., 1983), and petasol and isopetasol (Predescu et al., 1980). *P. frigidus* contains petasin and related esters, saponins, resins, and volatile oils, as well as small amounts of pyrrolizidine alkaloids. The latter occur in young leaves but not in the roots, which are more often used in commercial extracts (Moore, 1995).

Actions
Studies with animals have found that *P. hybridus* extracts possess spasmolytic and anti-inflammatory properties. The extracts reduced intestinal ulcerations and blocked gastric damage in rats. The effects were dose-dependent.

Extracts also inhibited peptido-leukotriene biosynthesis in mouse peritoneal macrophages and did not affect prostaglandin synthesis. Proposed mechanisms include inhibition of 5-lipoxygenase or interference with the utilization of calcium ions in leukotriene production (Brune et al., 1993).

In 1953, studies found a cytostatic effect of *Petasites* extract on fertilized sea urchin eggs, leading to the agent being used later as an analgesic for cancer patients (Weiss, 1988). This effect is not substantiated in other available literature.

Reported uses

Butterbur has been used for thousands of years for GI disorders and GI-related pain as well as for asthma, cough, skin diseases, and spasms of the urogenital tract (Brune et al., 1993). Other therapeutic claims include its use as a diuretic, sedative, antiarthritic, and astringent for cosmetic purposes. Butterbur was prescribed in ancient times as an ointment for ulcers and sores (Bianchini and Corbetta, 1977). References have also been made to an analgesic effect of *Petasites* extracts, but this effect may be secondary to the herb's spasmolytic properties.

P. frigidus may be taken as a tea or smoked. It may also be used as a poultice by patients residing in areas where the plant is endemic, including the United States (Moore, 1995).

Dosage

No consensus exists.

Adverse reactions

- Abdominal pain or pressure
- Difficulty in breathing or swallowing
- Difficulty in urinating
- Discoloration of the eyes or skin
- Discoloration of stool
- Severe nausea
- Sustained constipation
- Vomiting

⚠ Carcinogenic and hepatotoxic effects are possible resulting from the presence of pyrrolizidine alkaloids in the plant (Luthy et al., 1983).

Interactions

None reported. However, concomitant use with anticholinergic agents may not be advisable.

Contraindications and precautions

Avoid use of *Petasites* extracts in pregnant or breast-feeding patients; effects are unknown. Also avoid use of the herb in patients with decreased GI or bladder motility because symptoms of these disorders may worsen.

Special considerations

- Discourage the use of butterbur in patients with disorders that might be worsened by any effect on leukotriene synthesis or calcium-modulated smooth-muscle contractility, especially in the

GI tract. Also discourage use in patients with underlying disorders such as asthma that may become dangerous if inadequately treated.
● Monitor for adverse reactions and report any that occur to the health care professional.
● Advise the female patient to avoid use of the herb during pregnancy or when breast-feeding.

Analysis

Despite the use of butterbur extracts for centuries, little information is available to establish safety and efficacy in the prevention or treatment of any diseases in humans. Although studies with animals suggest a possible mechanism of action for reducing smooth-muscle spasms and inflammation, studies in humans are lacking.

Further research may reveal a beneficial effect of the more active components of *Petasites* extracts, but purification and standardization of these extracts would be required before reliable claims could be made. The active components of *Petasites* extract can vary from batch to batch, and potentially hazardous alkaloids have been identified in these plants.

References

Bianchini, F., and Corbetta, F. *Health Plants of the World: Atlas of Medicinal Plants.* New York: Newsweek Books, 1977.

Brune, K., et al. "Gastroprotective Effects by Extracts of *Petasites hybridus*: The Role of Inhibition of Peptido-leukotriene Synthesis," *Planta Med* 59:494-96, 1993.

Luthy, J., et al. "Pyrrolizidine Alkaloids in *Petasites hybridus* and *P. albus. Pharm Acta Helv* 58:98-100, 1983. Abstract.

Moore, M. *Medicinal Plants of the Pacific West.* Santa Fe, N. Mex.: Red Crane Books, 1995.

Predescu, I., et al. "Contributions to the Chromatographic and Spectral Study of *Petasites hybridus* Extract," *Farmacia Bucharest* 28:241-48, 1980.

Weiss, R.F. *Herbal Medicine.* Beaconsfield, England: Beaconsfield Publishers Ltd., 1988.

CACAO TREE
CACAO, CHOCOLATE, COCOA, COCOA BUTTER
(THEOBROMA OIL)

Common trade names
Various commercial products are available as foods, flavorings, or condiments.

Common forms
Available as cocoa powder, butter, syrup, and extracts.

Source
Cocoa is obtained from the seeds of the cacao tree, *Theobroma cacao*. The tree is native to Mexico, but is now cultivated in many tropical areas, especially western Africa. The crude material (cacao tree and cacao beans) is referred to as cacao, and the processed product is called cocoa. Cacao powder is usually alkalized to improve color, flavor and dispersibility in the process that refines the crude material to cocoa powder. Chocolate is prepared by mixing the cacao powder with sugar, flavoring, and extra cocoa butter fat. Milk chocolate includes milk as an ingredient, whereas dark chocolate does not.

Chemical components
Cocoa powder contains many different compounds, including proteins, fats, and alkaloids such as theobromine, caffeine, and tyramine. Cocoa also contains over 300 volatile compounds, including esters, hydrocarbons, lactones, monocarbonyls, pyrazines, pyrroles, and others. The main components responsible for its flavor are aliphatic esters, polyphenols, aromatic carbonyls, pyrazines, diketopiperazines, and theobromine. Cocoa butter primarily contains triglycerides, including oleic, stearic, and palmitic acids. About 75% of the fats are monounsaturated.

Actions
Theobromine and caffeine are both xanthine alkaloids and have similar actions as CNS and cardiac muscle stimulants, diuretics, and smooth muscle relaxants. However, theobromine has the lowest potency of the xanthine alkaloids in exerting these actions, whereas

theophylline is the most potent. Several studies have suggested that a usual dietary portion of chocolate contains psychoactive doses of caffeine and probably theobromine, which may lead to increased well-being, energy, social disposition, and alertness (Mumford et al., 1996).

In vitro studies of polyphenols in chocolate have demonstrated that they have antioxidant activity. Cocoa phenols also inhibit low-density lipoprotein (LDL) oxidation. Results of another in vitro study suggest that the polyphenols in chocolate exert immunoregulatory effects (Sanbongi et al., 1997).

Reported uses

Cocoa extract is an ingredient in alcoholic and nonalcoholic beverages. Cocoa powder and cocoa syrup are used as flavorings in many different foods and pharmaceutical products. Cocoa butter is commonly used as a suppository and an ointment base as well as an emollient and a skin protectant in creams, lotions, lipsticks, and soaps.

Cocoa butter has also been used to treat wrinkles and to prevent stretch marks during pregnancy. No studies have been conducted demonstrating the therapeutic usefulness of any form of cocoa for these indications.

Flavonoids may decrease atherosclerotic plaque formation through inhibition of LDL oxygenation and may reduce thrombosis by inhibiting cyclo-oxygenases. One study demonstrated that intake of some flavonoids may decrease the risk of death from coronary heart disease in elderly men (Hertog et al., 1993).

Dosage

No consensus exists.

Adverse reactions

● Acne
● Allergic reaction
⚠ Ingestion of 1,000 mg or more of theobromine (222 g of dark chocolate) may cause headache, nausea, insomnia, restlessness, excitement, muscle tremor, tachycardia, mild delirium, and extrasystoles. There have also been at least two reports of toxicity in canines; one dog experienced hyperexcitability and seizures, and then collapsed and died after eating 2 lb of chocolate chips. Two other dogs died suddenly 1 hour after consuming 20 to 30 g of dark chocolate (Stidworthy et al., 1997).

Interactions

MAO inhibitors (nardil, parnate, selegiline): potential vasopressor effects. Avoid concurrent use.

Theophylline: possible inhibition of theophylline metabolism. Avoid ingestion of large amounts of cocoa with theophylline.

Contraindications and precautions

Contraindicated in known hypersensitivity. Use cautiously in patients on low-sodium diets and those with irritable bowel syndrome.

Special considerations

• Restrict cocoa intake in patients with inflammatory bowel syndrome.

• Advise the patient with CV disease or special dietary restrictions to minimize consumption of chocolate products, due to the high sodium and high fat content.

• Caution the patient with arrhythmias or significant CV disease not to ingest large quantities of chocolate products because of the risk of xanthine-induced arrhythmia.

• Tell the patient prone to developing acne to avoid use of cosmetics containing cocoa butter.

Analysis

Cocoa is used in many different cosmetic, food, and pharmaceutical products, and it is generally considered to be nontoxic. Although chocolate contains antioxidant flavonoids that may have beneficial CV effects, such flavonoids are also found in other foods. Other flavonoid-containing foods include some fruits and vegetables which probably have a higher nutritional value as well as much less fat. The potential beneficial effects of cocoa flavonoids in CV disease remain to be proven.

References

Hertog, M.G.L., et al. "Dietary Antioxidant Flavonoids and Risk of Coronary Heart Disease: The Zutphen Elderly Study," *Lancet* 342:1007-11, 1993.

Mumford, G.K., et al. "Absorption Rate of Methylxanthines Following Capsules, Cola, and Chocolate," *Eur J Clin Pharmacol* 51:319-25, 1996.

Sanbongi, C., et al. "Polyphenols in Chocolate, Which Have Antioxidant Activity, Modulate Immune Functions in Humans In Vivo," *Cell Immunol* 177:129-36, 1997.

Stidworthy, M.F., et al. "Chocolate Poisoning in Dogs," *Vet Rec* 141:28, 1997.

CALUMBA

COCCULUS PALMATUS, COLUMBO ROOT

Common trade names

(Available in combination) Amaro Maffioli, Appetiser Mixture, Bitteridina, Ducase, Elixir Spark, Padma-Lax, Richelet, Travel-Caps

Common forms

Available as capsules and an elixir that is often prepared without heating as a cold infusion.

Source

The root of the *Jateorrhiza calumba* (*J. palmata*) plant is dried and powdered. The powder changes from green to a brownish black color as it rapidly absorbs moisture from the air and decomposes. The plant is native to Mozambique and Madagascar.

Chemical components

The plant yields columbamine, jateorhizine, palmatine, three yellow crystalline alkaloids, and columbin, a colorless crystalline principle.

Actions

In studies with anesthetized mice, columbin decreased the sleep time of urethane and alpha-chloralose and prolonged sleep time of hexobarbital (Wada et al., 1995).

Reported uses

No human studies have been reported; anecdotal evidence suggests calumba's use as an antidiarrheal and antiflatulence agent.

Dosage

Although 20 to 40 mg/kg/day P.O. for 5 days was given to mice in an animal study, there are no data on human dosages.

Adverse reactions

None reported.

Interactions

None reported.

Contraindications and precautions

Avoid use of the herb in pregnant or breast-feeding patients; effects are unknown.

Special considerations

• Recommend other agents to the patient requiring the herb as an antidiarrheal agent.
• Advise the female patient to avoid use of the herb during pregnancy or when breast-feeding.

Points of interest

• Calumba is native to Mozambique and the forests of eastern Africa, where it is cultivated for use as a flavoring agent and a dye.

Analysis

Because human clinical trials are lacking, this herb cannot be recommended for use. More studies are needed in animals and humans for proven safety and efficacy. Given the safety and efficacy of currently approved antidiarrheal agents, further investigation and development of this agent is of questionable value.

References

Wada, K., et al. "Columbin Isolated from *Calumbae radix* Affects the Sleep Time of Anesthetized Mice," *Biol Pharm Bull* 18:634-36, 1995.

CAPSICUM

BELL PEPPER, CAPSAICIN, CAYENNE PEPPER, CHILI PEPPER, HOT PEPPER, PAPRIKA, PIMIENTO, RED PEPPER, TABASCO PEPPER

Common trade names

Capsin, Cap-Stun, Capzasin, Dolorac, No Pain HP, Pepper Defense, R-Gel, Zostrix (HP)

Common forms

Cream: 0.025%, 0.075%, 0.25%
Gel: 0.025%
Lotion: 0.025%, 0.075%
Self-defense spray: 5%, 10%

Source

Capsaicinoids are derived from the dried fruit of the plants of the Solanaceae family. The two species most commonly used are *Capsicum frutescens* and *C. annum.* Before the actual capsaicin can be isolated, a concentrate called oleoresin capsicum is formed from the peppers. Extraction of capsaicin forms water-insoluble needles (highly alcohol- and fat-soluble). Other species of *Capsicum* used include *C. baccatum, C. chinensis,* and *C. pubescens.* These peppers should not be confused with the plants that give us common black pepper and white pepper (*Piper* species, family Piperaceae).

Chemical components

Capsicum species can contain up to 1.5% of a capsaicinoid oleoresin. The major components of the oleoresin responsible for the plant's pungent appeal are capsaicin, 6,7-dihydrocapsaicin, nordihydrocapsaicin, homodihydrocapsaicin, and homocapsaicin. Many volatile oils, carotenoids (capsanthin, capsorubin, carotene, lutein), proteins, fats, and high amounts of vitamins A and C are present. The amount of vitamin C present may be as much as four to six times that found in an orange. Provitamins E, P, B_1, B_2, and B_3 have also been identified.

Other plant material contains steroidal alkaloidal glycosides (solanine and solasadine) and scopoletin (coumarin). Each chili pepper contains approximately 0.14% capsaicin, with the highest concentrations in the yellowish-red placenta of the fruit and its attachments.

Actions

Although topical capsaicin produces an extremely intense irritation at the contact point, vesicle formation usually does not occur. The initial dose of capsaicin causes profound pain; however, repeated applications cause desensitization, with analgesic and even anti-inflammatory effects. "Heat" sensation is caused by stimulation of specific local afferent nerve fibers. Analgesic effects may be explained by capsaicin-induced neuronal depletion of substance P, believed to be a mediator in the transmission of painful stimuli from the periphery to the spinal cord. The analgesic effect may also result from the methoxyphenol portion of the capsaicin molecule that may interfere with the lipooxygenase and cyclooxygenase pathways.

Capsaicin does not cause blistering or redness because it does not act on the capillaries or other blood vessels. An externally applied 0.1% capsaicin solution inhibits flare formation after intradermal injection of histamine. Areas of skin (control) without pretreatment of capsaicin developed a wheal, flare, and itching. Flare response is believed to be substance P-mediated.

Juices from the fruits have shown antibacterial properties in vitro. I.V. infusion of capsaicin has been reported to stimulate secretion of epinephrine and norepinephrine from the adrenal medulla of rodents.

Reported uses

Traditional claims surrounding use of capsicum include treatment of bowel disorders, chronic laryngitis, and peripheral vascular disease. Various preparations of capsicum have been applied topically as counterirritants and external analgesics. Topical capsaicin preparations are useful for treating pain associated with postherpetic neuralgia (Bernstein et al., 1987), rheumatoid arthritis, osteoarthritis, diabetic neuropathy, postsurgical pain (including postmastectomy and postamputation pain), and other neuropathic pain and complex pain syndromes (Robbins et al., 1998).

Capsaicin has been suggested for refractory pruritus and pruritus associated with renal failure. A small study has suggested nasal inhalation of capsaicin may be beneficial in nonallergic, noninfectious perennial rhinitis. However, poor tolerability is likely to be of issue with larger clinical trials. One study has reported capsaicin's use for urinary urgency. (See *Treating urinary urgency with capsaicin.*)

RESEARCH FINDINGS
Treating urinary urgency with capsaicin

In a study of six patients, an intravesical capsaicin injection was shown to reduce urinary urgency, bladder capacity, and the micturition threshold pressure (Dasgupta and Fowler, 1997). Five "hypersensitive bladder" patients experienced complete resolution or a clinically relevant reduction in urgency, frequency, and pain for up to 16 days posttreatment. The sixth patient had benign prostatic hypertrophy and did not experience symptomatic improvement. All patients reported adverse effects that included a feeling of "warmth" or burning in the urethra after voiding.

The authors suggested that capsaicin induces diuresis through stimulation of the vesicorenal reflex. Increases in urinary concentrations of sodium and potassium were noted together with increased excretion of prostaglandin E_2.

Capsaicin is also increasingly popular as a nonlethal self-defense spray.

Dosage
Because capsaicin is very potent, concentrations of topical preparations range from 0.025% to 0.25%. Preparations are most effective when applied t.i.d. or q.i.d. and have a duration of action of about 4 to 6 hours. Applications given less frequently typically produce less effective substance P depletion and result in incomplete analgesia.

Adverse reactions
Intensity of adverse reactions are dose- and concentration-dependent.
- Blepharospasm, extreme burning pain, lacrimation, conjunctional edema, and hyperemia. (Ocular complications are rare, and usually result from eye rubbing.)
- Burning pain in nose, sneezing, and serous discharge
- GI discomfort (minimized if seeds are removed from the product prior to ingestion)
- Transient bronchoconstriction, cough, and retrosternal discomfort
- Transient skin irritation, itching, stinging, or erythema without vesicular eruption (diminishes with repeated use)

Interactions
Centrally acting adrenergic agents: may reduce efficacy of antihypertensives such as clonidine or methyldopa. Avoid concomitant use.

MAO inhibitors: may promote toxicity (hypertensive crisis) when used together due to catecholamine release. Avoid concomitant use.

Contraindications and precautions
Contraindicated in patients hypersensitive to capsicum or chili pepper products. Also contraindicated in pregnant patients to avoid possible uterine stimulant effects.

Special considerations
• Know that after topical application, relief occurs as early as 3 days, but may take as long as 14 to 28 days, depending on the condition requiring analgesia.
• Be aware that no evidence exists that topical application causes permanent neurologic injury.
• Tell the patient to avoid contact with eyes, mucous membranes, or nonintact skin.
• Inform the patient to flush the exposed area with cool running water for as long as necessary, if incidental contact occurs.
• Caution the patient taking MAO inhibitors or centrally acting adrenergics against use of this herb.
• Advise the female patient to avoid use of the herb during pregnancy or when breast-feeding.

Points of interest
• Over one third of its total vitamin C content remains after a chili pepper has been cooked; vitamin C is lost completely if the pepper is dried.
• Because of its short-term immobilizing effects, capsaicin is used as a humane self-defense spray. The more popular products contain the capsicum oleoresin, which produces immediate blepharospasm, blindness, and incapacitation for up to 30 minutes.
• Peppers are among the most widely consumed spice in the world with an average per-person consumption approaching as much as 50 mg of capsaicin daily in some Southeast Asian countries.

Analysis
Natural capsicum has been used for centuries. Capsaicin, derived from capsicum, has gained widespread popularity in recent years as an agent for several potential therapeutic applications. Commercially available capsaicin preparations have been proven to be effective adjunctive topical analgesics for some pain and pruritic syndromes. Long term effects of topical application appear benign. For some patients, the initial "burning" sensation and the delayed onset of action may be the most undesirable aspect of its use. The ingestion of capsicum over the amount normally available in food is not recommended.

References

Bernstein, J.E., et al. "Total Capsaicin Relieves Chronic Post-herpetic Neuralgia," *J Am Acad Dermatol* 17:93, 1987.

Dasgupta, P., and Fowler, C.J. "Chillies: From Antiquity to Urology," *Br J Urol* 80:845-52, 1997.

Robbins, W.R., et al. "Treatment of Intractable Pain with Topical Large-Dose Capsaicin: Preliminary report," *Anesth Analg* 86:579-83, 1998.

CARAWAY

CARUM CARVI, KUMMEL, KUMMELOL, OLEUM CARI, OLEUM CARVI

Common trade names
(Various manufacturers; available in combination) Ajaka, BPC 1973, Cholosum N, Concentrated Caraway Water, Digestozym, Divinal-Bohnen, Euflat 1, Flatulex, Galloselect N, Gastricard N, Globase, Eevert-Carmin, Lomatol, Majocarmin, Metrophyt-V, Neo-Ballistol, Sanvita Magen, Spasmo Claim, Tirgon

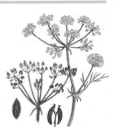

Common forms
Available as caraway oil, 5% volatile oil, caraway water, and caraway seed.

Source
A volatile oil that is distilled from dried ripened seeds of *Carum carvi*, a biennial herb native to Europe and Asia. Caraway water is obtained by soaking 1 oz of bruised seeds in 1 pint of cold water for 6 hours.

Chemical components
Caraway oil is chiefly composed (53% to 63%) of a ketone, carvone, an optical isomer also found in spearmint oil. The oil also contains a terpene, D-limonene.

Actions
Caraway was found to relax the tracheal smooth muscle and increase the resting force (contracture) of ileal smooth muscle in guinea pigs (Reiter and Brandt, 1985). Although this herb has been claimed to have a laxative action, it was not seen in the guinea pigs.

Another study found that caraway oil may inhibit skin tumors in female mice (Schwaireb, 1993). The oil, either applied topically or taken as a dietary supplement, inhibited croton oil-induced skin tumors. This resulted in the disappearance of the tumor and a reduction in the incidence, delay in appearance, retardation, and regression of established papillomas. Topical administration appears to be superior to dietary supplementation in producing these effects (Schwaireb, 1993). Human studies have not been performed to assess the efficacy of caraway oil in preventing toxin-induced skin tumors.

Reported uses

Caraway oil is an aromatic herb and is used in many pharmaceutical preparations as a flavoring agent. It is claimed to be an effective aid for indigestion, flatulence, colic, hiatal hernia, stomach ulcer, constipation, menstrual cramps, bronchitis, and as a gargle for laryngitis.

Ongoing studies are evaluating the role of monoterpenes, found in citrus fruits and caraway-seed oil, in inhibiting carcinogen activation and preventing carcinogen-induced neoplasm (Wattenberg, 1990). D-limonene has been shown to inhibit a tobacco-specific carcinogen when administered immediately before carcinogen challenge, though the extent is unknown.

In a small study evaluating laxative effects of an herbal combination containing caraway, all patients found relief from constipation within the first 2 days. The combination herbal product had no effect on gastric mucosa or ulcer healing rate (Matev et al., 1981). A combination of caraway and peppermint oil was found to decrease or eliminate pain in patients with nonulcer dyspepsia (May et al., 1996).

Dosage

For flatulence, adults dose is 1 to 4 drops of the essential oil in 1 teaspoon water or on a lump of sugar.
For infantile colic, 1 to 3 teaspoons of caraway water.

Adverse reactions

- Diarrhea
- Mucous membrane irritation

Interactions

None reported.

Contraindications and precautions

Contraindicated in patients allergic to caraway oil or its components.

Special considerations

- Monitor for diarrhea and effectiveness of administration.
- Tell the patient that the herb's effectiveness as an antiflatulent or digestant is largely untested and that other available agents have

been widely tested and may be equally as effective or more effective than caraway.

• Advise the patient to check the label carefully to prevent confusion with plain or concentrated caraway water.

Points of interest

• Caraway has been used by many civilizations. Its origin is believed to be with the ancient Arabs, who called the seed *Karawya*. Dioscorides, a Greek physician (A.D. 40 to 90), recommended the oil to be used by "pale-faced girls," possibly due to the agent's claimed stimulant action.

• Caraway oil is used to flavor liqueurs such as aquavit, Kummel, and L'huile de Venus.

• An old superstition states that caraway has the power of retention, preventing the theft of items containing the seed. It was used in love potions to keep lovers from losing interest and straying.

Analysis

Caraway, an established flavoring agent for many pharmaceutical and food products, contains antiflatulent properties. Folklore has produced several therapeutic claims, very few of which can be substantiated with clinical trial data. It might have laxative action and may be used to treat nonulcer dyspepsia. However, studies performed to evaluate the efficacy of caraway in these roles are not definitive. Further human studies are needed to evaluate its effect on neoplasms and whether it possesses anticancer properties.

References

Matev, M., et al. "Use of an Herbal Combination with Laxative Action on Duodenal Peptic Ulcer and Gastroduodenitis Patients with a Concomitant Obstipation Syndrome," *Vutr Boles* 20:48-61, 1981. Abstract.

May, B., et al. "Efficacy of a Fixed Peppermint Oil/Caraway Oil Combination in Non-ulcer Dyspepsia," *Arzneimittelforschung* 46:1149-53, 1996. Abstract.

Reiter, M., and Brandt, W. "Relaxant Effects on Tracheal and Ileal Smooth Muscles of the Guinea Pig." *Arzneimittelforschung* 35:408-14, 1985. Abstract.

Schwaireb, M.H. "Caraway Oil Inhibits Skin Tumors in Female BALB/c Mice," *Nutr Cancer* 19:321-25, 1993.

Wattenberg, L.W. "Inhibition of Carcinogenesis by Naturally Occurring and Synthetic Compounds," *Basic Life Sci* 52:155-66, 1990. Abstract.

CARDAMOM

*Alpinia cardamomum, Amomum cardamon, Amomum
repens, Cardamomi semina, cardamom seeds,
Cardamomum minus, Malabar cardamom, Matonia
cardamom*

Common trade names
None known.

Common forms
Available as dried seeds, whole or powdered.

Source
Cardamom seeds are harvested from the fruits of *Elettaria cardamomum,* a large perennial herb native to southern India. The fruits are gathered before they ripen and split, because seeds from opened fruits are less aromatic. Seeds yield 4% to 6% of a volatile oil.

Chemical components
The volatile oil is primarily composed of 1,8-cineole and alpha-terpinyl acetate (Baruah et al., 1973). Other components include linalyl acetate, linalool, borneol, alpha-terpineol, alpha-pinene, limonene, and myrcene.

Actions
The few studies that report on the pharmacologic action of cardamom are based on in vitro or animal data. Eugenol, a compound found in cardamom and other spices, significantly inhibits tobacco-induced mutagenicity (Sukumaran and Kuttan, 1995). Cardamom oil, given intraperitoneally, was compared with indomethacin for acute carrageenan-induced edema in male rats. Compared with indomethacin, a lower cardamom dose suppressed edema to a lesser extent, whereas a higher dose exerted a more potent anti-inflammatory effect.

In one study, cardamom oil halved the p-benzoquinone-induced writhing in mice, suggesting a possible analgesic effect, and also inhibited the stimulant action of acetylcholine, perhaps explaining its role as an antispasmodic (Al-Zuhair et al., 1996).

Reported uses
Cardamom is a widely used flavoring agent for sweets and coffee and is a standard ingredient in curry. Its medicinal use dates back to ancient times. Herbalists recommended it as an agent to improve digestion and relieve flatulence. When chewed, the seeds have a pleasant taste that may be followed by an increase in saliva and a sensation of warmth in the mouth. The herb has been used for

cough, colds, and bronchitis, and has been recommended as an appetite stimulant in anorexic patients. In addition, cardamom sprinkled on cooked cereal has been reported to help children with celiac disease intolerant to the gluten in grain. Data from human studies cannot be found to support these claims.

Dosage
There are no human studies to support dosing recommendations. Doses listed in other sources are 15 to 30 grains of powder, 1 fluid dram of tincture, or 5 to 30 drops of fluid extract. Seeds are commonly chewed whole, and the powder is often sprinkled on food or included in beverages.

Adverse reactions
• One case of allergic contact dermatitis was reported after a confectioner with chronic hand dermatitis had positive patch test reactions to cardamom and terpenoid compounds (Mobacken and Fregert, 1975).

Interactions
None reported.

Contraindications and precautions
Avoid use of the herb in pregnant or breast-feeding patients; effects are unknown.

Special considerations
• Ingestion of cardamom beyond amounts commonly found in foods is not recommended.
• Inform the patient of the lack of human trials with cardamom. If complaints related to GI dysmotility occur despite use of cardamom, instruct the patient to consult a health care professional.
• Advise the female patient to avoid use of the herb during pregnancy or when breast-feeding.

Analysis
Although cardamom has long been claimed to relieve indigestion and gas, there have been no clinical trials to test this effect and its therapeutic benefit remains unproven. Further study is warranted to evaluate the pharmacologic properties of cardamom, and human data are needed before it can be recommended to treat any medical condition.

References
Al-Zuhair, H., et al. "Pharmacological Studies of Cardamom Oil in Animals," *Pharmacol Res* 34:79-82, 1996.

Baruah, A.K.S., et al. "Chemical Composition of Alleppey Cardamom Oil by Gas Chromatography," *Analyst* 98:168-71, 1973.

Mobacken, H., and Fregert, S. "Allergic Contact Dermatitis from Cardamom," *Contact Dermatitis* 1:175-76, 1975.

Sukumaran, K., and Kuttan, R. "Inhibition of Tobacco-Induced Mutagenesis by Eugenol and Plant Extracts," *Mutat Res* 343:25-30, 1995.

CARLINE THISTLE

ARTEMISIA VULGARIS, *CARLINA VULGARIS*, FELON HERB, MUGWORT, *RADIX CARDOPATIAE*

Common trade names
None known.

Common forms
Available as a liquid or tea.

Source
Active components are obtained from the seeds, fresh roots, and leaves of *Carlina acaulis*.

Chemical components
The plant contains 0.03% to 0.2% volatile oil. The main component is cineole; others include alpha-amyrin, alpha- and beta-pinene, beta-sitosterol, fernenol, quebrachitol, sitosterol, tauremisin, tetracosanol, and thujonestigmasterol. Glycosides include rutinosyl-s quercetin, and 4c-glycosyl flavones, such as orientine, homoorientine, schaftoside, and carlinoside.

Actions
Carline thistle is claimed to be effective as a digestive stimulant, menstruation aid, anthelmintic, antiepileptic, antiseptic, tonic, antispasmodic, colerectic, diaphoretic, diuretic, expectorant, and spasmolytic.

The leaf extract of *Artemisia vulgaris* was found to delay onset of picrotoxin-induced seizures and reduce mortality rates in mice. A plant extract was active against some sarcomas in rats.

Reported uses
Carline thistle is claimed to be effective for cancerous lesions, asthma, bronchitis, cold, dysmenorrhea, fever, gout, epilepsy, chorea, hysteria, rheumatism, gallstones, kidney stones, gastritis, inflammation, rickets, tuberculosis, labor, nervousness, headache, worms, and wounds. Anecdotal human data suggest that the herb is effective in treating pruritus and atopic dermatitis (Tamuki and Muratsu, 1994; Tezhka et al., 1992).

Possible efficacy as a bladder irrigation was suggested by researchers who used *Artemisia vulgaris* as part of an herbal preparation for continuous irrigation of the bladder after prostatic adenotomy. They reported decreased blood loss, bacteremia, and purulent inflammation post-operatively (Davidov et al., 1995).

Dosage
No consensus exists.

Adverse reactions
● Pain, spasms, and possibly seizures (with overdose)

Interactions
None reported.

Contraindications and precautions
Avoid use of the herb in pregnant or breast-feeding patients; effects are unknown.

Special considerations
● Inform the patient that insufficient data exist to recommend use of this herb.
● Advise the female patient to avoid use of the herb during pregnancy or when breast-feeding.

Analysis
Anecdotal reports suggest that carline thistle may be effective for the treatment of pruritic skin lesions and atopic dermatitis. However, safety of the herb or its components are currently not supported by the scientific medical literature. Well-designed and controlled human trials are needed before it can be recommended for any purpose.

References
Davidov, M.I., et al. "Postadenectomy Phytoperfusion of the Bladder," *Urol Nefrol* 5:19-20, 1995.

Tamuki, A., and Muratsu, M. "Clinical Trial of SY Skin Care Series Containing Mugwort Extract," *Skin Res* 36:369-78, 1994. Abstract.

Tezhka, T., et al. "The Clinical Effects of Mugwort Extract on Pruritic Skin Lesions," *Skin Res* 35:303-11, 1992. Abstract.

CASCARA SAGRADA
CALIFORNIAN BUCKTHORN, SACRED BARK

Common trade names
(Various manufacturers; available in combination) Bassoran with Cascara, Bicholax, Cas-Evac, Casvlium, Kondremul with Cascara

Common forms

Available as capsules, bitter and sweet fluid extracts, and as dried bark for teas. Cascara sagrada prepared as a tea isn't popular because of its extremely bitter taste and the availability of standardized pharmaceutical preparations that perform the same functions.

Source

Cascara sagrada is the dried bark of *Rhamnus purshiana*. It should be aged for at least 1 year before use in medicinal preparations, but 3-year-old bark is preferred for pharmaceutical purposes because it will exhibit a milder cathartic activity due to the oxidation of glycosides present in the bark. Cascara sagrada is found along the Pacific Northwest from Canada to California.

Chemical components

Two types of anthracene compounds—emodin glycosides (O-glycosides) and aloinlike C-glycosides—have been reported. The C-glycosides are divided into barbaloin, deoxybarbaloin (chrysaloin), and the cascarosides. Dried, medicinal quality cascara bark yields not less than 7% of total hydroxyanthracene derivatives, calculated as cascaroside A on a dried basis. The cascarosides should make up at least 60% of this total.

Actions

The glycosides found in cascara sagrada are stimulant cathartics that exert their action by increasing the tone of the smooth muscle in the wall of the large intestine and have only minor effects on the small intestine. The drug is transformed by intestinal bacteria into substances that increase peristalsis in the large intestine and help restore intestinal tone.

Reported uses

Cascara sagrada was traditionally used by Native Americans of the Pacific Northwest as a laxative. In 1990, the FDA released the results of its study on OTC products and placed cascara sagrada in category I (safe and effective) as a laxative (Covington et al., 1996). Dried, aged cascara sagrada bark is widely accepted as a mild and effective treatment for chronic constipation (Morton, 1977).

Dosage

Aromatic fluid extract (sweet cascara): 5 ml P.O.
Extract capsules: 300 mg P.O.
Liquid extract (bitter cascara): 1 to 5 ml P.O.

Adverse reactions
- Abdominal pain
- Chronic use or abuse
- Cramping
- Diarrhea
- Discoloration of urine
- Fluid and electrolyte imbalance
- Laxative dependency
- Melanosis coli (darkening pigmentation of colonic mucosa)
- Osteomalacia
- Steatorrhea
- Vitamin and mineral deficiencies
- Vomiting

Interactions
None reported.

Contraindications and precautions
Contraindicated in pregnant and breast-feeding patients because drug crosses the placental barrier, is excreted in breast milk, and increases risk of diarrhea in the breast-fed infant. Although cascara sagrada may be used cautiously during pregnancy, other laxatives (such as bulk-forming or surfactant laxatives) may be preferred.

Special considerations
- Understand that effective bowel regimens for constipation include temporary pharmacotherapy together with sufficient fluid intake and hydration, increasing fiber in the patient's diet, and regular meals and exercise.
- Know that patients with chronic constipation (over 1 week) should be evaluated by a primary health care provider for underlying causes of obstruction.
- Be aware that cascara sagrada appears to be reasonably safe, although the fresher the bark, the higher the risk of adverse reactions.
- Question the patient about laxative use when taking the drug history.
- Inform the patient that the FDA has determined cascara sagrada to be generally safe and effective.
- Advise the female patient to avoid use of the herb during pregnancy or when breast-feeding.
- Remind the patient that cascara sagrada products are only for short term use.

Points of interest
- Cascara sagrada mostly comes from Oregon, Washington, and southern British Columbia. Collections are made during the sum-

mer by peeling off sections of the bark and rolling them into large quills. The bark is then carefully sun dried so that the inner surface is not exposed to the sun and the yellow color is retained. The drug is then processed into its final form.

Analysis
Cascara sagrada is a mild stimulant laxative that has proven to be safe and effective. Although the FDA has approved its use, caution should be used when treating chronic constipation to avoid laxative abuse. Reliable and standardized pharmaceutical forms are preferred because there is no advantage in using the bark as a tea for its medicinal effects. Standardized pharmaceutical products ensure correct dosage and minimize risk of adverse reactions.

References
Covington, T.R., et al., eds. *Handbook of Nonprescription Drugs.* 11th ed. Washington, D.C.: American Pharmaceutical Association, 1996.

Morton, J.F. *Major Medicinal Plants: Botany, Culture and Uses.* Springfield, Ill: Charles C. Thomas Pub., Ltd., 1977.

CASTOR BEAN

AFRICAN COFFEE TREE, BOFAREIRA, CASTOR OIL PLANT, MEXICO WEED, PALMA CHRISTI, TANGANTANGAN OIL PLANT, WONDER TREE, WUNDERBAUM

Common trade names
Alphamul, Aromatic Castor Oil USP 23, Castor Oil Caps USP 23, Emulsoil, Fleet Castor Oil Emulsion, Neoloid, Purge, Ricino Koki, Unisoil

Common forms
Castor oil emulsion: Alphamul 60% (90 ml, 3,780 ml), Emulsoil 95% (63 ml), Fleet Flavored Castor Oil 67% (45 ml, 90 ml), Neoloid 36.4% (118 ml)
Castor oil liquid: 100% (60 ml, 120 ml, 480 ml)
Purge: 95% (30 ml, 60 ml)

Source
Castor oil is obtained by cold-pressing the seeds of *Ricinus communis*, a perennial herb believed to be native to Africa and India.

Chemical components
Castor oil contains 45% to 50% oil. The oil is a mixture of triglycerides, of which 75% to 90% is ricinoleic acid. The poisonous phytotoxins, ricin and ricinine, are present in seed cake and oil.

Actions

Castor oil increases peristalsis and laxative action by stimulating the intramural nerve plexus of the small intestinal musculature. It also promotes fluid and ion accumulation in the colon. Castor oil given orally produces one or more stools 2 to 6 hours after ingestion. Ricin is a poisonous protein that disrupts DNA synthesis and protein metabolism, resulting in cell death.

Reported uses

Castor oil is an official USP product used as a laxative, as a protectant in hair conditioners, and in skin creams for the treatment of rash. Application of the oil to an irritated conjunctiva caused by foreign bodies in the eyes provides soothing relief. Castor oil is frequently used to empty the GI tract of gas and feces before proctoscopy or radiographic studies of the GI tract. Topical application of castor oil has also been claimed to dissolve cysts, growths, or warts, and to soften bunions and corns. The agent is also believed to expel worms if used with anthelmintics. No controlled human trials are available to support these claims.

Dosage

For constipation, 15 to 60 ml castor oil P.O. daily.

Adverse reactions

- Abdominal pain or cramping

Large oral doses:
- Colic
- Nausea
- Severe purgation
- Vomiting

Chronic use:
- Allergic reactions (in persons handling the seeds)
- Fluid and electrolyte loss

⚠ Chewing the seeds may be fatal. Both leaves and seeds are considered poisonous. Ricin and ricinine can cause toxic symptoms, such as irritation of oral cavity and esophagus, abdominal pain, nausea, vomiting, hepatic and renal injury, seizures, and death (Kinamore et al., 1980).

Interactions

None reported.

Contraindications and precautions

Avoid use of the herb in pregnant or breast-feeding patients; effects are unknown. Use cautiously in patients with appendicitis, rectal bleeding, intestinal obstruction, and sensitivity to castor oil.

Special considerations
- Castor oil may be refrigerated to improve palatability.
- Question the patient about laxative use when taking the drug history.
- Instruct the patient to drink plenty of fluids (6 to 8 glasses) daily.
- Warn the patient to use this product for no more than a few days.
- Advise the female patient to avoid use of the herb during pregnancy or when breast-feeding.

Points of interest
- Castor oil flowers develop into spiny capsules containing three seeds (also called "beans"). As they dry, the capsules explode, scattering the seeds.

Analysis
Although castor oil is an official USP product used for its laxative effects, other more gentle and palatable laxatives exist. Standardized forms of this product are available and are recommended over nonstandardized herbal preparations. Other uses claimed for this product have little or no supporting clinical evidence.

References
Kinamore, P.A., et al. "Abrus and Ricinus Ingestion: Management of Three Cases," *Clin Toxicol* 17:401-05, 1980.

CATNIP

CATARIA, CATMINT, CATNEP, CATRUP, CAT'S-PLAY, CATWORT, FIELD BALM, NIP

Common trade names
(Various manufacturers; available in combination) Catnip, Catnip & Fennel, Catnip & Fennel Extract, Catnip Herb, Catnip Mist

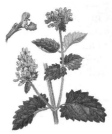

Common forms
Available as capsules (380 mg), liquid, elixir, tincture, and tea.

Source
Obtained from the dried leaves and flowering tops of *Nepeta cataria*, catnip is a common perennial herb found in North America.

Chemical components
The major active ingredients in catnip are volatile oils. The two primary volatile oils are *cis-trans*-nepetalactone and valeric acid. Nepe-

talactone is similar in structure to the sedative ingredient found in valerian root. The seeds also contain linolenic, linoleic, oleic acid, and saturated fatty acids. Other chemicals found in *N. cataria* include acetic acid, buteric acid, citral, dipentene, lifronella, limonene, iridoids, tannins, and terpene.

Actions
N. cataria contains volatile oils that produce sedative effects. An alcoholic extract produced a sedative effect in young chicks. Low to moderate doses caused chicks to sleep, whereas higher doses appeared to have a paradoxical effect (Sherry and Hunter, 1979).

The effect of other drugs on catnip-induced pleasures in cats has been conducted (Hatch, 1972). The psychoactive (hallucinogenic) properties of catnip remain controversial.

Reported uses
The principal anecdotal recommendation for catnip is as a tea for insomnia or restlessness. Despite the lack of human clinical trials, the herb is also said to be useful for the treatment of amenorrhea, anemia, bronchitis, colds, diarrhea, dysmenorrhea, fever, flatulence, headaches, hiccups, hives, indigestion, infantile colic, and toothaches. Catnip has also been used as a stimulant, antispasmodic, diaphoretic, and tonic without scientific data to support these claims. Catnip salve and tea are reported to be folklore remedies for cancer and are believed to have psychoactive and euphoric properties when smoked as a cigarette; mind-altering effects may also occur after accidental ingestion. (See *Psychoactive effects of catnip in a toddler,* page 140.)

Dosage
Human data are lacking.
Tea: pour boiling water on 2 teaspoons of the dried leaves and brew solution for 10 to 15 minutes.
Tincture: 2 to 4 ml P.O. t.i.d.

Adverse reactions
- Headache
- Malaise
- Nausea, vomiting (with large doses)

Interactions
None reported.

Contraindications and precautions
Avoid use of the herb in pregnant or breast-feeding patients; effects are unknown.

RESEARCH FINDINGS
Psychoactive effects of catnip in a toddler

An anecdotal case of altered mental status in a 19-month-old male toddler who ingested catnip tea was reported (Osterhoudt et al., 1997). The toddler consumed an unknown quantity of raisins that had been soaked in the tea. Three hours later, he became restless, cranky, and developed a stomachache. The next day his mother reported that "he looked drugged" and took him to the emergency department. The child's vital signs were as follows: heart rate 199 beats/minute, respiratory rate 28 breaths/minute, blood pressure 131/77 mm Hg, and temperature 99.3° F (37.4° C).

On evaluation, the patient was lethargic but arousable with verbal stimuli. His abdomen was soft with no masses. Cranial nerve function was intact and pain sensation was present. Laboratory values were as follows: leukocytes 7,100/mm^3, hemoglobin 12 g/dl, sodium 135 mEq/L, potassium 4.7 mEq/L, carbon dioxide 18 mmol/L, chloride 99 mEq/L, glucose 98 mg/dl, and BUN 7 mg/dl. Urinalysis and urine toxicology screens were negative. A computed tomography brain scan was unremarkable. The toddler was admitted for observation.

Three hours after admission, he continued to be obtunded and responsive only to physical stimuli. A lumbar puncture was then performed with negative results. Six hours after admission, the toddler had a large bowel movement containing a dozen raisins and some tea leaves. His mental status subsequently improved, and he was discharged the following day. The toddler's symptoms were directly related to his ingestion of catnip and disappeared with the fecal passage of the raisins and tea leaves.

Special considerations
● Ask the patient to reconsider using catnip as a sleep aid because of the lack of scientific data to support this use. Direct such patients to a primary health care provider specializing in sleep disorders.
● Advise the female patient to avoid use of the herb during pregnancy or when breast-feeding.

Points of interest
● *N. cataria* is a perennial herb that is common in Europe and cultivated in the United States. It has an aromatic and mint-like odor.
● Most cat owners buy catnip to use in toys. The scent of the catnip, and not its consumption, is believed to exert the euphoria and sexual stimulation in cats.

Analysis

Although catnip may have sedative effects, human clinical data are lacking. One case report found that catnip altered the mental status of a toddler after he consumed a large amount of raisins soaked in catnip tea. Further studies are needed to evaluate the safety and efficacy of the herb for the claimed therapeutic uses.

References

Hatch, R.C. "Effects of Other Drugs on Catnip-Induced Pleasure Behavior in Cats," *Am J Vet Res* 33:143-55, 1972.

Osterhoudt, K.C., et al. "Catnip and the Alteration of Human Consciousness," *Vet Human Toxicol* 39:373-75, 1997.

Sherry, C.J., and Hunter, P.S. "The Effect of an Ethanolic Extract of Catnip on the Behavior of the Young Chick," *Experientia* 35:237-38, 1979.

CAT'S-CLAW

LIFE-GIVING VINE OF PERU, SAMENTO, UNA DE GATO

Common trade names

(Various manufacturers) Cat's Claw Inner Bark Extract, Vegicaps

Common forms

Tablets, capsules: 25 mg, 150 mg, 175 mg, 300 mg, 350 mg (standard extract); 400 mg, 500 mg, 800 mg, 1 g, 5 g (raw herb)
Also available as teas or tinctures and the cut, dried, or powdered bark, roots, and leaves.

Source

Active components are extracted from the roots, stem bark, and leaves of *Uncaria tomentosa, U. guianensis,* and other species of the woody vine belonging to the Rubiaceae family. The plant is native to the Amazon.

Chemical components

The plant contains oxindole alkaloids, including isopteropodine, pteropodine, isomitraphylline, rhynchophylline, isorynchophylline, and mytraphylline; and indole alkaloidal glucosides, including cadambine, 3-dihydrocadambine, and 3-isodihydrocadambine. Other compounds include quinovic acid glycosides, tannins, proanthocyanidins, polyphenols, catechins (D-catechol), and beta sitosterol.

Actions

Four oxindole alkaloids (isopteropodine, pteropodine, isomitraphylline, and isorynchophylline) have shown immunostimulating properties in vitro, namely increased phagocytotic activity and synthesis of WBCs and enhanced T-helper cell function. Some antitumor activity has also been suggested.

Another alkaloid, rhynchophylline, has been found to inhibit platelet aggregation in rats (Chen et al., 1992), and also to inhibit the sympathetic nervous system, reduce the heart rate, decrease peripheral vasculature resistance, and lower blood pressure (Hemingway and Phillipson, 1974). Mytraphylline, an alkaloid, has weak diuretic properties. The combined effect of these alkaloids appears to be useful in treating CV disorders; however, appropriate studies are lacking.

Another alkaloid, hirsutine, possesses local anesthetic properties and has been shown to inhibit bladder contraction in the guinea pig. High doses of hirsutine inhibited neuromuscular transmission in the rat (Harada and Ozaki, 1976). Both hirsutine and rhynchophylline have shown verapamil-like effects by influencing calcium influx in rabbit aorta strips (Zhang et al., 1987). Other *Uncaria* alkaloids exhibit antiviral activity and antioxidant properties in vitro.

Reported uses

Although claimed to be useful in treating systemic inflammatory diseases (such as arthritis and rheumatism) and inflammatory GI disorders (such as diverticulitis, gastritis, Crohn's disease, dysentery, and ulcerations), human clinical data confirming these uses are lacking.

South American folk medicine has endorsed cat's-claw as a contraceptive. It is anecdotally reported that drinking the tea during a woman's menstrual cycle for 3 consecutive months prevents pregnancy for about 4 years. No scientific support exists for this claim.

Dosage

Usual dosage is 500 to 1,000 mg P.O. t.i.d.

Adverse reactions

• Potential hypotension

Interactions

Antihypertensives: may potentiate effects. Avoid concomitant use.

Contraindications and precautions

Contraindicated in patients undergoing skin grafts and organ transplants, and in those with coagulation disorders or receiving anticoagulants. Avoid use in pregnant or breast-feeding patients; effects are unknown.

Special considerations
● Monitor the patient for signs of bleeding such as petechiae or epistaxis, and for unusual bruising or bleeding gums.
● Recommend another means of contraception if the herb is being used for this purpose.
● Tell the patient to rise slowly from a sitting or lying position to avoid dizziness from possible hypotension.
● Advise the patient to watch for signs of bleeding, especially if anticoagulants are also being taken.
● Advise the female patient to avoid use of the herb during pregnancy or when breast-feeding.

Points of interest
● Clinical trials are evaluating *Uncaria's* ability to fight viruses such as herpes simplex, herpes zoster, and HIV.
● There are about 20 different plants identified as "cat's-claw" in Peru. Botanical verification is required because some species are considered toxic.
● The alkaloid concentration varies seasonally within cat's-claw bark and vines.
● In the 1970s, preliminary research at the Peruvian National Institute of Health demonstrated promising results in treating children with leukemia.
● The plant gets its name from small thorns at the base of the leaf that resemble feline claws.

Analysis
Although cat's-claw may appear to have potential for treating several diseases, more clinical research is required to determine its efficacy and long-term safety. Research is currently being conducted for its potential use in AIDS, leukemia and other cancers, viral infections, allergic respiratory diseases, GI disorders, and osteoarthritis. Studies on cats with leukemia and immunodeficiency virus are also underway.

References
Chen, C.X., et al. "Inhibitory Effect of Rhynchophylline on Platelet Aggregation and Thrombosis," *Chung Kuo Yao Li Hsueh Pao* 13:126-30, 1992.

Harada, M., and Ozaki, Y. "Effect of Indole Alkaloids from *Gardneria* Genus and *Uncaria* Genus on Neuromuscular Transmission in the Rat Limb In Situ," *Chem Pharm Bull* 24:211, 1976.

Hemingway, S.R., and Philipson, J.D. "Alkaloids from South American Species of *Uncaria* (Rubiaceae)," *J Pharm Pharmacol* 26(suppl):113, 1974.

Zhang, W., et al. "Effect of Rhyncophylline on the Contraction of Rabbit Aorta," *Chung Kuo Yao Li Hsueh Pao* 8:425-29, 1987.

CELANDINE

CELANDINE POPPY, COMMON CELANDINE, FELONWORT, GARDEN CELANDINE, GREATER CELANDINE, ROCK POPPY, SWALLOW WORT, TETTER WORT, WART WORT

Common trade names
(Various manufacturers; available in combination) Bloodroot/ Celandine Supreme, Cacau, Celandine Extract, Celandine Tops and Roots, Cytopure, Fennel/Wild Yam Supreme, No. 2040 Headache Remedy, No. 2090 Indigestion Remedy, Venancapsan
Ukrain is available only in Europe as a semisynthetic derivative of celandine alkaloids conjugated with thiophosphoric acid.

Common forms
Available as extracts, tinctures, or teas, and as a prescribed injection in Eastern Europe.

Source
Celandine alkaloids are extracted from the roots and flowering tops of *Chelidonium majus,* a member of the poppy family (Papaveraceae) found commonly in North America, Europe, and Asia. The milky, orange juice from the stems and other parts of the plant has also been used for medicinal purposes. Greater celandine is not related to the plant known as lesser celandine, *Ranunculus ficaria.*

Chemical components
The main alkaloids from the celandine root are chelidonine and coptisine; over 30 isoquinoline alkaloids have been detected as "secondary metabolites." Other compounds include chelidonic acid, chelidoniol, rutin, quercetin, choline, methylamine, histamine, tyramine, other alkaloids, flavonoids, cinnamic acids, and caffeic acid esters.

Actions
Caffeic acid is claimed to have choleretic and antispasmodic activity. Coptisine and caffeoylmalic acid have shown similar spasmolytic activity. Chelidonine has mild central analgesic and strong spasmolytic properties that primarily affect the biliary system.

Extracts of celandine inhibit keratinocyte proliferation, suggesting possible use in the treatment of skin diseases such as warts and psoriasis (Vavreckova et al., 1996). Other researchers found cytotoxic (but not antitumor) activity associated with coptisine chloride and an unidentified alkaloid.

A monograph included with Ukrain referred to a claim that a National Cancer Institute study showed drug action against human cancers. However, Ukrain has *not* been approved by the FDA for use in the United States (Anon., 1997). Ukrain claims to kill cancer cells by inducing apoptosis and inhibiting DNA, RNA, and protein synthesis. Ukrain was found to be toxic to malignant cells at levels that are nonlethal to normal cells. In a study on women with breast cancer, the drug was found to act on malignant cells, making them more recognizable to the immune system, and resulting in their rejection (Brzosko et al., 1996). Ukrain also has immunoregulatory properties.

Reported uses

Celandine has been known to be useful in liver disease, digestive disorders, and eye irritation. The plant sap has been used to remove warts, soften calluses and corns, and loosen bad teeth. Chelidonium alkaloids have been used from the late 1800s in cancer treatment, and in Europe they have also been used to treat colonic polyposis and remove warts, papillomas, condylomas, and nodules. Recently, celandine was found to stimulate the flow of bile and pancreatic enzymes in the treatment of hepatitis, jaundice, gallstones, and biliary inflammation and obstruction. Celandine is also a component of an antiretroviral preparation that may act against the Epstein-Barr and herpes viruses.

Case reports and studies obtained through MEDLINE document Ukrain's success in treating several types and sites of cancer, including breast, colorectal, cervical, testicular, esophageal, urethral, and ovarian; malignant melanoma; optic nerve astrocytoma; and Kaposi's sarcoma in patients with AIDS.

Dosage

Dosage of celandine extract depends on the product and use. Because the alkaloid content varies, it is not always standardized in available products.

Dosage of Ukrain is determined by the patient's immune status. A single dose is 5 to 20 mg per I.V. injection, depending on tumor mass, speed of growth, extent of the disease, and the patient's immune status. In several published studies, Ukrain injections were given every other day.

Adverse reactions

- Dizziness
- Drowsiness
- Fatigue
- Hypotension
- Insomnia
- Nausea
- Polyuria

- Possible embryotoxic effect (animal studies)
- Possible reversible hepatotoxicity
- Restlessness
- Thirst
- Tingling, itching, stabbing pains in tumor area

⚠ The *C. majus* plant must be considered highly toxic. Contact with the sap causes dermatitis, and oral ingestion has been reported to cause abdominal pain, vomiting, diarrhea, fainting, severe stomatitis, gastroenteritis, hemorrhagic gastritis, coma, and even death.

Interactions
Cardiac glycosides (and Ukrain): possible ECG changes. Avoid concomitant use.
Morphine derivatives (and Ukrain): may reduce efficacy. Avoid concomitant use.
Sulfonamides (and Ukrain): may reduce efficacy. Avoid concomitant use.
Sulfonylureas (and Ukrain): may cause hypoglycemia. Avoid concomitant use.

Contraindications and precautions
Contraindicated in children and pregnant or breast-feeding women, and also for prolonged periods (over 2 weeks). Also, herbal supplements or fresh herbs are contraindicated to self-treat serious liver and digestive disorders or other organ systems if disease is suspected.

Avoid direct contact with the fresh plant juices (including the milky sap). Also, avoid use of herb extracts not approved by the FDA for ophthalmic or topical use because blindness, infection, or tissue ulceration may occur.

Special considerations
- Remember that some patients from Europe may receive the herb as a prescription drug.
- Advise the patient that little data exist for use of this plant for any indication.
- Warn the patient that celandine may interact with drugs such as analgesics, antibiotics, and cardiac and antidiabetic agents.
⚠ Warn the patient that oral ingestion has caused major toxicity, even death.

Points of interest
- Ukrain is available by prescription in Europe; however, it is not approved for use in the United States. Products available in the United States are manufactured as herbal nutritional supplements or topical herbal treatments and have not undergone FDA testing. The herb should not be used instead of prescribed medications for

diagnosed ailments or considered equivalent to Ukrain for preventing or treating disease.

Analysis

Although substantial evidence exists that celandine extracts have several pharmacologic effects, there are many reports of harm resulting from plant ingestion. Because of the serious risk of complications of self-treatment of hepatic, GI, and ocular diseases, and the possibility of dermatitis reactions in areas surrounding hyperkeratotic lesions of the skin, the use of celandine supplements and topical agents is not recommended. Alternative, more reliable treatment should be sought from a primary health care provider.

Ukrain might have an important role in the treatment of cancer and other diseases; however, further research is needed before its use in the United States is approved. The drug should not be used for self-treatment or prophylaxis of diseases

References

Anonymous, "UKRAIN Information for Physicians," Nowicky Pharma. Ukrainian Anticancer Institute, Vienna, Austria. Sept. 1, 1997.

Brzosko, W.J., et al. "Influence of Ukrain on Breast Cancer," *Drugs Exp Clin Res* 22:127-33, 1996. Abstract.

Vavreckova, C., et al., "Benzophenanthridine Alkaloids of *Chelidonium majus.* II. Potent Inhibitory Action Against the Growth of Human Keratinocytes," *Planta Med* 62:491-94, 1996.

CELERY

APIUM, CELERY SEED, CELERY SEED OIL, MARSH PARSLEY, SMALLAGE, WILD CELERY

Common trade names

(Available in combination) Cachets Lesourd, Dr. Brown's Cel-Ray, Guaiacum Complex, Herbal Diuretic Complex, Rheumatic Pain, Vegetex

Common forms

Capsules: 450 mg, 505 mg

Source

An oil is obtained by steam distillation of the seeds of *Apium graveolens*, a widely cultivated biennial herb.

Chemical components

Celery is high in minerals, including sodium and chlorine. Celery seed oil contains d-limonene, selinene, and phthalides (3-n-butyl-phthalide, sedanenolide, and sedanonic anhydride).

Actions

Some in vitro studies show that the essential oil has fungicidal, hypoglycemic, and potential anticarcinogenic properties (Hashim et al., 1994). Celery may contain eight anticancer compounds that may detoxify pollutants and cigarette smoke. Two components of celery (3-n-butylphthalide and sedanolide) reduced certain tumors in mice. Another study with rats showed potential cancer reduction; however, human studies are needed to verify these claims.

Reported uses

Celery is used to flavor food, soap, and gum, and is high in fiber and popular with dieters. It is claimed to be useful as a diuretic for bladder and kidney condition; as a sedative, urinary antiseptic, antiarthritic, and spasmolytic; and for nervousness or hysteria. In the Orient, celery is used as a diuretic, digestive aid, antiflatulent, aphrodisiac, and to stimulate menstrual flow; also, the seeds have been used to treat headaches.

In India and Pakistan, celery is used to treat bronchitis, asthma, liver and spleen conditions, rheumatism, hiccups, cough, fever, flatulence, hives, lack of menses, and urine retention or discharge. The seed tincture is used for tension headache, heartburn, toothache, vomiting, hives, and urine retention. In a small clinical trial of hypertensive patients, celery juice was found to lower blood pressure.

Dosage

No consensus exists.

Adverse reactions

- CNS depression (large doses)
- Dermatitis attributed to allergic reactions to volatile oil
- Hypersensitivity reactions (anaphylaxis, angioedema, respiratory complaints, and urticaria)
- Phototoxic bullous lesions (in celery workers; Birmingham et al., 1961)

Interactions

None known.

Contraindications and precautions

Avoid use of celery other than for food purposes in pregnant or breast-feeding patients; effects are unknown.

Special considerations

- Be aware of hypersensitivity reactions when examining agricultural workers who have skin disorders.

• Advise the patient to limit consumption of celery to amounts commonly found in foods.
• Advise the female patient to avoid use of the herb during pregnancy or when breast-feeding.

Points of interest
• Celery tonics and elixirs have been in use since the late 19th century. The ancient Greeks used celery to make wine and served it as an award at athletic games circa 450 B.C.

Analysis
There are several therapeutic claims about celery, but few human trials have been completed. Consumption of quantities beyond that contained in food is not currently recommended.

References
Birmingham, D.J., et al. "Phytotoxic Bullae Among Celery Harvesters," *Arch Dermatol* 83:73, 1961.
Hashim, S., et al. "Modulatory Effects of Essential Oils From Spices on the Formation of DNA Adduct by Aflatoxin B_1 In Vitro," *Nutr Cancer* 21:169-71, 1994.

CENTAURY

BITTER HERB, CENTAUREA, COMMON CENTAURY, EUROPEAN CENTAURY, LESSER CENTAURY, MINOR CENTAURY

Common trade names
None known.

Common forms
Available as the crude herb.

Source
Active components are extracted from the leaves, stems, and flowers of *Centaurium erythraea,* and also *C. umbellatum* and *C. minus.* These are annual or biennial herbs that belong to the Gentian family (Gentianaceae). *C. erythraea* may be referred to as *Erythraea centaurium.*

Chemical components
Centaury contains numerous compounds, including alkaloids (gentianine, gentianidine, and gentioflavine), monoterpenoids (iridoids, gentiopicroside, centapicrin, gentioflavoside, sweroside and swertiamarin), triterpenoids (alpha- and beta-amyrin, erythrodiol, crataegolic acid, oleanolic acid, oleanolic lactone, sitosterol, stigmasterol,

campesterol, brassicasterol, and delta-7 stigmastenol), phenolic acids (protocatechuic, m- and p-hydroxybenzoic acid, vanillic, syringic, beta-coumaric, ferulic, sinapic, and caffeic acids), flavonoids, xanthones (eustomin and demethyleustomin), fatty acids (palmitic and stearic acids), alkanes (nonacosane and heptacosane), and waxes.

Actions
Centaury is claimed to have bitter tonic and sedative properties. Gentiopicrin is known to be an antimalarial agent. The aqueous extract of *C. erythraea* has been shown to have anti-inflammatory activity (Berkan et al., 1991; Mascolo et al., 1987); this anti-inflammatory potency was less than half that of indomethacin.

Two polymethoxylated xanthones, eustomin and demethyleustomin, have shown antioxidant properties (Schimmer and Mauthner, 1996).

Reported uses
Claims for centaury stem from traditional use as a bitter tonic to stimulate appetite. Anecdotal information reports that the agent is used for its astringent properties in cosmetics. Ancient Egyptians used this herb to treat kidney stones.

Dosage
For most uses, 2 to 4 ml of a liquid extract (1:1 in 25% alcohol) or infusion, t.i.d. German sources suggest 1 to 2 g of the crude herb daily.

Adverse reactions
None reported.

Interactions
None reported.

Contraindications and precautions
Avoid use of the herb in pregnant or breast-feeding patients; effects are unknown.

Special considerations
• Inform the patient not to use the herb because little is known about its efficacy.
• Instruct the patient who still wishes to use this herb to avoid chronic use because the long-term effects are not known.
• Advise the female patient to avoid use of the herb during pregnancy or when breast-feeding.

Points of interest
• Centaury is found in trace quantities in vermouth. Usual concentrations are approximately 0.0002% or 2.3 parts per million. Similar quantities occur in some nonalcoholic beverages.

Analysis
Centaury should not be used for any condition because of the lack of safety or efficacy data. There are no human clinical trial data available.

References
Berkan, T., et al. "Anti-inflammatory, Analgesic and Antipyretic Effects of an Aqueous Extract of *Erythraea centaurium*," *Planta Med* 57:34-37, 1991.

Mascolo, N., et al. "Biological Screening of Italian Medicinal Plants for Anti-inflammatory Activity," *Phytother Res* 1:28-31, 1987.

Schimmer, O., and Mauthner, H. "Polymethoxylated Xanthones from the Herb of *Centaurium erythraea* with Strong Antimutagenic Properties in *Salmonella typhimurium*," *Planta Med* 62:561-64, 1996.

CHAMOMILE

COMMON CHAMOMILE, ENGLISH CHAMOMILE, GERMAN CHAMOMILE, HUNGARIAN CHAMOMILE, ROMAN CHAMOMILE, SWEET FALSE CHAMOMILE, TRUE CHAMOMILE, WILD CHAMOMILE

Common trade names
Chamomile Flowers, Chamomile Tea, Chamomile Organic, Chamomilla, Classic Chamomile

Common forms
Available as capsules (354 mg, 360 mg), liquid, tea, and in many cosmetic products.

Source
"True chamomile" refers to the German or Hungarian version of chamomile. Pharmacologically active compounds are extracted from dried flower heads of *Matricaria recututa (M. chamomilla)*. Another type of chamomile is Roman or English chamomile *Chamaemelum nobile (Anthemis nobile)*.

Chemical components
Both kinds of chamomile contain similar compounds. One component of the volatile oil, chamazulene, is formed from natural precursors during steam distillation, and comprises about 0.5% of the flower head. The essential oil mostly consists of alpha-bisabolol, an unsaturated monocyclic sesquiterpene alcohol; other compounds

include angelic and tiglic acid esters, farnesol, nerolidol, germacranolide, amyl and isobutyl alcohols, anthemol, anthemic acid, phenolic and fatty acids, phytosterol, choline, inositol, apigenin, luteolin, quercetin and associated glycosides, coumarins, scopoletin-7-glucoside, umbelliferone, and heniarin.

Actions

The German and Roman chamomiles have similar pharmacologic profiles. In studies with rats, the volatile oil has been found to have anti-inflammatory, antiallergic, antidiuretic, and sedative properties. Some chamomile compounds have been reported to stimulate liver regeneration following oral administration. Others have shown in vitro antitumor activity against human cells. Studies in animals and in vitro models have shown that bisabolol and chamazulene exert anti-inflammatory activity; bisabolol also shows antispasmodic activity. Luteolin and apigenin, two flavonoids in the essential oil, have antispasmodic effects and anti-inflammatory activity similar to indomethacin. Chamomile also exhibits some antibacterial and antifungal activity. Bisabolol has shown antiulcer effects in rats by inhibiting the development of ethanol-, indomethacin-, or stress-induced ulcers (Mann and Staba, 1986). The volatile oil has been reported to lower serum urea concentrations in rabbits.

Reported uses

Chamomile has been used mainly in the treatment of stomach disorders, such as GI spasms, other GI inflammatory conditions, and insomnia because of its purported sedative properties. Other uses include treatment of menstrual disorders, migraine, epidermolysis bullosa, eczema, eye irritation, throat discomfort, and hemorrhoids, and as a topical bacteriostat.

Oral chamomile extract was found to induce a deep sleep in most patients undergoing cardiac catheterization (Mann and Staba, 1986). The extract has also been used as a mouthwash (Fidler et al., 1996).

Dosage

Chamomile is usually taken as a tea, prepared by adding 1 tablespoon (3 g) of the flower head in hot water for 10 to 15 minutes and then taken up to q.i.d. Because of its poor water solubility, only a small amount of the volatile oil is obtained. However, tea preparation extracts the hydrophilic flavonoid components. Long-term consumption of low concentrations of the volatile oil in chamomile tea may have a cumulative therapeutic effect.

Adverse reactions

- Allergic conjunctivitis
- Anaphylaxis

- Contact dermatitis
- Emesis

Interactions
Anticoagulants: may potentiate effects. Avoid concomitant use.
Other medications taken concurrently: potential for decreased absorption of these agents secondary to chamomiles antispasmodic activity in the GI tract. Avoid concomitant use.

Contraindications and precautions
Avoid use in pregnant or breast-feeding patients. Chamomile is believed to be an abortifacient, and some of its components have shown teratogenic effects in several animals (Habersang et al., 1979). Use cautiously in hypersensitivity to the components of the volatile oils or in patients at risk for contact dermatitis.

Special considerations
- Caution the patient with a history of atopy against use of this herb.
⚠ Advise the female patient to avoid use of the herb during pregnancy or when breast-feeding.

Analysis
Chamomile is well known for its purported antispasmodic and anti-inflammatory activities. Limited human data are available to evaluate its clinical effectiveness in treating GI disorders.

References
Fidler, P., et al. "Prospective Evaluations of a Chamomile Mouthwash for Prevention of 5-FU-Induced Oral Mucositis," *Cancer* 77:522-24, 1996.
Habersang, S., et al. "Pharmacological Studies with Compounds of Chamomile. IV. Studies on Toxicity of Alpha-Bisabolol," *Planta Med* 37:115-23, 1979.
Mann, C., and Staba, E.J. "The Chemistry, Pharmacology, and Commercial Formulations of Chamomile," In *Herbs, Spices and Medicinal Plants: Recent Advances in Botany, Horticulture and Pharmacology,* Vol 1. Arizona: Oryx Press, 235-80, 1986.

CHAPARRAL

CREOSOTE BUSH, GREASEWOOD, *HEDIONDILLA*

Common trade names
None known.

Common forms
Available as tablets, capsules, and teas.

Source
Active components are extracted from the leaves of *Larrea tridentata* or *L. divaricata,* a desert-dwelling evergreen shrub native to the southwestern United States and Mexico.

Chemical components
Phenolic compounds isolated from *L. tridentata* include nordihyroguaiaretic acid (NDGA) and the related lignans, nor-isoguaiasin, dihydroguaiaretic acid, partially demethylated dihydroguaiartic acid, and 3'-demethoxyisoguaiasin. Younger plants yield more phenolic compounds than older plants.

Actions
The biologic activity of chaparral is attributed to NDGA, a lipoxygenase inhibitor that was previously used as a food additive to prevent fermentation and decomposition. Despite studies showing NDGA to have an anticancer effect in vitro, earlier research by the National Cancer Institute found no such effect in vivo (Cunningham et al., 1997; Pavani et al., 1994). Some reports suggest that NDGA may stimulate certain malignancies, such as renal cell carcinoma.

NDGA has been shown to inhibit proviral expression, and thus may be able to interrupt the life cycle of the causative organism in HIV infections (Gnabre et al., 1995).

Results from an in vitro study of rat hippocampal neurons suggest that NDGA may play a neuroprotective role in Alzheimer's disease (Goodman et al., 1994).

Reported uses
Chaparral tea is derived from the plant leaves. It was widely used as a remedy by Native Americans for bronchitis, colds, skin disorders, and pain. Human clinical trials are lacking to support the claim of anticancer properties.

Dosage
No consensus exists. Teas are suggested for daily consumption.

Adverse reactions
- Contact dermatitis
- Renal cell carcinoma
- Renal cystic disease

⚠ Hepatotoxicity (cholestatic hepatitis). Jaundice is characterized with markedly increased serum liver function values. Onset occurs within 3 to 52 weeks after ingestion, and symptoms resolved within 1 to 17 weeks after stopping herb in most cases. Some damage, however, progressed to cirrhosis and acute liver failure, requiring transplantation (Sheikh et al., 1997).

Interactions
None reported.

Contraindications and precautions
Use of herb is contraindicated because of numerous reports of serious hepatotoxicity.

Special considerations
⚠ Use of chaparral has been associated with severe irreversible hepatotoxicity, sometimes requiring liver transplantation.
• Monitor the patient who has taken this herb for changes in liver function, jaundice, fatigue, and other signs of hepatotoxicity.
• Caution the patient against use of chaparral because of its strong hepatotoxic property.

Points of interest
• Chaparral is considered to be an unsafe herb and was removed by the FDA from its "generally recognized as safe" list in 1970.
• Anecdotal reports indicate that chaparral tea was used as an anticancer agent from the late 1950s to the 1970s.

Analysis
In vitro studies have yielded conflicting results for the use of NDGA, the active component of chaparral, in treating cancer, AIDS, and Alzheimer's disease. Further in vivo and human clinical studies are needed. Because of its strong association with liver toxicity, use of this herb is not currently recommended.

References
Cunningham, D.C., et al. "Proliferative Responses of Normal Human Mammary and MCF-7 Breast Cancer Cells to Linoleic, Conjugated Linoleic Acid and Eicosanoid Synthesis Inhibitors in Culture," *Anticancer Res* 17:197-203, 1997.

Gnabre, J.N., et al. "Inhibition of Human Immunodeficiency Virus Type 1 Transcription and Replication by DNA Sequence-Selective Plant Lignans," *Proc Natl Acad Sci USA* 92:11239-43, 1995.

Goodman, Y., et al. "Nordihydroguaiaretic Acid Protects Hippocampal Neurons Against Amyloid Beta-Peptide Toxicity, and Attenuated Free Radical and Calcium Accumulation," *Brain Res* 654:171-76, 1994.

Pavani, M., et al. "Inhibition of Tumoral Cell Respiration and Growth by Nordihydroguaiaretic Acid," *Biochem Pharmacol* 48:1935-42, 1994.

Sheikh, N.M., et al. "Chaparral-Associated Hepatotoxicity," *Arch Intern Med* 157:913-19, 1997.

CHASTE TREE

AGNEAU CHASTE, CHASTEBERRY, GATILLIER, HEMP
TREE, KEUSCHBAUM, MONK'S PEPPER

Common trade names
None known.

Common forms
Available as capsules, tinctures, and teas.

Source
Active components are extracted from the dried, ripened fruits and
the root bark of *Vitex agnus-castus.*

Chemical components
Several new luteolin-like flavonoids, iridoid glycosides; aucubin, eu-
rostoside, agnuside, some triterpenoids, and an alkaloid, vitricine,
have been isolated from the root bark. Both free and conjugated
forms of progesterone and hydroxyprogesterone have also been isolated from the leaves and flowers. Testosterone and epitestosterone
were detected in the flower parts. Androstenedione was extracted
from leaves.

    Essential oils contain mono- and sesquiterpenoids; alpha-pinene
and beta-pinene, limonene, cineole, sabinene, castine, eucalyptol,
myrcene, linalool, citronellol, cymene, camphene, carophyllene, farnesene, cardinene, and ledol.

Actions
The herb is claimed to have anti-inflammatory, antiandrogenic,
progesterone-like, and antimicrobial effects. Recently isolated
flavonoids exhibit antineoplastic activity (Hirobe et al., 1997) and
studies with rats have shown a hypoprolactinemic effect (Sliutz et
al., 1993).

Reported uses
Claims for chaste tree include usefulness for several endocrine and
female reproductive tract disorders, including menstrual cycle regulation, uterine bleeding, ovarian insufficiency, aiding lactation, and
combating acne. Human data supporting these claims are sparse. A
German abstract described a study of women with latent hyperprolactinemia in which prolactin secretion was reduced and both the
luteal phase and luteal secretion of progesterone was normalized
(Milewicz et al., 1993). Another report argued against use of the

herb in multiple follicular development because of resulting de-
ranged hormone levels (Cahill et al., 1994).

Dosage
Dosage used in the German study was 20 mg capsules P.O. daily.
Other dosages are usually teas or tinctures.

Adverse reactions
- Abdominal pain
- Cramping
- Diarrhea
- Headache
- Increased menstrual flow
- Pruritus
- Rash

Interactions
None reported.

Contraindications and precautions
Avoid use of the herb in pregnant or breast-feeding patients; effects
are unknown.

Special considerations
- Keep effects of this herb in mind if the patient reports increased
menstrual flow.
- Advise the female patient to avoid use of the herb during pregnancy or when breast-feeding, or if she is planning pregnancy.
- Advise the patient that most information on this herb comes from
foreign studies, which make interpretation of results difficult.

Points of interest
- A German formulation of chaste tree is indicated for menstrual
disorders due to primary or secondary corpus luteum insufficiency,
premenstrual syndrome, mastodynia, inadequate lactation, and
menopausal symptoms.
- Postmarketing surveillance in Germany has determined that the
herb is discontinued due to adverse reactions only 1% of the time.
- Monks were said to have chewed the leaves of this plant to help
them maintain their vow of celibacy.

Analysis
It may be worth investigating chaste tree further in disorders specific to women. The lack of data on long-term safety and clinical efficacy preclude conclusive recommendations.

References

Cahill, D., et al. "Multiple Follicular Development Associated with Herbal Medicine. *Hum Reprod* 9:1469-70, 1994.

Hirobe, C., et al. "Cytotoxic Flavonoids from *Vitex agnus-castus*," *Phytochemistry* 46:521-24, 1997.

Milewicz, A., et al. "*Vitex agnus-castus* Extract in the Treatment of Luteal Phase Defects Due to Latent Hyperprolactinemia. Results of a Randomized Placebo-Controlled Double-Blind Study," *Arzneimittelforschung* 43:752-56, 1993.

Sliutz, G., et al. "*Agnus castus* Extracts Inhibit Prolactin Secretion of Rat Pituitary Cells," *Horm Metab Res* 25:253-55, 1993.

CHAULMOOGRA OIL

CHAULMOGRA OIL, GYNOCARDIA OIL, HYDNOCARPUS OIL

Common trade names
None known.

Common forms
Available as a topical oil, and a salt form of oil for S.C. injection.

Source
Active components are extracted from seeds of *Hydnocarpus wightiana, H. anthelmintica,* and *Taraktogenos kurzii.*

Chemical components
The seeds contain about 50% of the brownish-yellow chaulmoogra oil; the remaining components include chaulmoogric acid, hypnocarpic acid, gorlic acid, and fatty acids (palmitic and oleic acids).

Actions
Chaulmoogra oil has demonstrated efficacy against *Mycobacterium leprae* in laboratory experiments and case reports (Levy, 1975). It has also been listed as an antileprotic agent.

Reported uses
Folk literature and ancient Hindu and Chinese documents suggest that chaulmoogra oil is an effective treatment for leprosy. (See *Chaulmoogra and leprosy.*)

Dosage
No consensus exists. Dosage is derived from quantity of chaulmoogra oil injected S.C.

FOLKLORE
Chaulmoogra and leprosy

Throughout the ages, leprosy has been greatly feared. Lepers would be declared legally dead and have their possessions redistributed; in Norway, lepers were forced to wear cowbells around their necks as they walked to warn oncoming pedestrians.

In the 1920s, an adventurous explorer-botanist, Joseph Rock, set out to locate a plant he had never seen and knew little about (Dobelis, 1996). After hearing stories of leprosy cures involving this rare, exotic plant, Rock traveled the globe searching jungles, swamps, mountains, and valleys of the Far East and India until finally obtaining some seeds in an Indian market.

Investigation revealed that the seeds came from a local tree that grew 50 to 60 feet tall and had leathery leaves and large, white flowers. Rock collected a large quantity of the seeds and was able to naturalize the plant in Hawaii. Approximately 20 years later, the active components in the seeds of the chaulmoogra tree provided the elemental materials for synthesizing the first anti-leprostatic agents.

Adverse reactions
● Calcinosis cutis (forms precipitates under the skin with S.C. injection; Ohtaka, 1992)
● GI irritation (with S.C. injection)

Interactions
None reported.

Contraindications and precautions
Avoid use of the herb in pregnant or breast-feeding patients; effects are unknown.

Special considerations
● If the patient suspects a leprosy diagnosis, inform him that more traditional and acceptable forms of antimicrobial therapy exist, and that he should seek medical advice from a health care provider experienced in the therapy and care of leprosy.
● Advise the patient not to attempt administration of this agent unless under close supervision of a health care provider experienced in therapy and care of leprosy.
● Advise the female patient to avoid use of the herb during pregnancy or when breast-feeding.

Points of interest

• Despite a decrease in the incidence of leprosy worldwide, as of 1991 there were 6 million cases of leprosy requiring treatment (Noordeen, 1991). These cases predominate in Africa, Asia, Latin America, and the Pacific; only a few cases exist in Canada, Europe, and the United States.

• The components of chaulmoogra oil have served as the fundamental structure for synthesis of modern antileprostatic pharmaceutical agents.

Analysis

Chaulmoogra oil should be avoided because more accepted and safer therapies for leprosy exist. Its role in the treatment of any disorder, including leprosy, is yet undetermined.

References

Levy, L. "The Activity of Chaulmoogra Acids against *Mycobacterium leprae*," *Am Rev Resp Dis* 111:703-05, 1975.

Noordeen, S.K. "A Look at World Leprosy," *Lepr Rev* 62:72-86, 1991.

Ohtaka, K. "Patients with Calcinosis Cutis: National Leprosarium Matsuoka Hoyo-En' Aomori' Japan," *Nippon Rai Gakkai Zasshi* 61:98-101, 1992.

CHICKWEED

MOUSE-EAR, SATINFLOWER, STAR CHICKWEED, STARWEED, STITCHWORT, TONGUE GRASS, WHITE BIRD'S-EYE, WINTERWEED

Common trade names

(Various manufacturers) Chickweed

Common forms

Available as the crude herb, capsules, tea bags (caffeine-free), liquid extracts (alcohol-free available), tinctures, ointments, and oils.

Source

Components are extracted from the leaves, stems, and flowers of *Stellaria media*, a member of the Caryophyllaceae family that is native to Europe.

Chemical components

The active components are mainly unknown. Herbal literature lists various components such as saponins, nitrate salts, vitamin C, calcium, iron, coumarin, hydroxycoumarin, flavonoids (rutin), vitamin A, and most of the B-complex vitamins.

Actions
None reported. One in vitro animal study isolated two flavonoid components from the herb that possessed antioxidant activity (Budzianowski et al., 1991).

Reported uses
This widely occurring "weed" is commonly prescribed by herbalists as a remedy for both internal and external inflammatory conditions such as rheumatism and skin disorders (eczema and psoriasis), and for its ability to relieve skin irritation and pruritus. Claims have also been made for chickweed as an antitussive, expectorant, and antipyretic as well as an excess-fat reducer because of its mild diuretic and laxative effect.

The herb has also been used internally as a "blood cleanser," and as a demulcent for soothing sore throats and stomach ulcers. Externally, it has been used as a poultice to help draw out fluid from abscesses or boils, and as an ointment or salve to relieve burns, rashes, and insect stings and bites. Chickweed is claimed to be an excellent emollient for dry, chapped skin, and to promote early healing of wounds and cuts.

Dosage
Capsules: 3 capsules P.O. t.i.d.
Liquid extract: 15 to 30 drops (diluted) P.O., up to t.i.d.
Ointment: applied liberally to affected areas as needed, up to q.i.d.
Tea: several times daily as needed.

Adverse reactions
⚠ Herbal literature reports one case of nitrate toxicity in grazing farm animals and one case of human paralysis resulting from ingestion of excessive amounts of the herb. Both reports are attributed to the herb's nitrate content, and the findings remain controversial.

Interactions
None reported.

Contraindications and precautions
Avoid use of the herb in pregnant or breast-feeding patients; effects are unknown.

Special considerations
• Warn the patient about possible adverse reactions that occur with nitrates (hypotension, headache, syncope).
• Caution the patient against consuming this herb because of the lack of clinical data.

● Advise the female patient to avoid use of this herb during pregnancy or when breast-feeding.

Analysis
Despite widespread claims by herbalists of chickweed's potential value for various ailments, there is insufficient clinical evidence to support these therapeutic qualities.

References
Budzianowski, J., et al. "Studies on Antioxidative Activity of Some C-glycosylflavones," *Pol J Pharmacol* 43:395-401, 1991.

CHICORY

BLUE SAILORS, GARDEN ENDIVE, SUCCORY, WILD SUCCORY

Common trade names
Chicory

Common forms
Available as the crude herb, root (roasted and unroasted), and extracts.

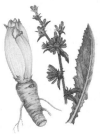

Source
Active components are extracted from the dried roots of *Cichorium intybus*, a biennial or perennial herb native to Europe. The leaves of young plants are used as potherbs, whereas the leaves of older plants can be blanched and eaten like celery. The roots can be boiled and eaten with butter or, more commonly, can be roasted and added to coffee or tea for a bitter taste. The roasted, dried root is also used as a coffee substitute.

Chemical components
The flowers contain cichoriin and the leaves contain chicoric acid (dicaffeoyl tartaric acid), flavonoids, catechol tannins, glycosides, carbohydrates, unsaturated sterols and triterpenoids, and tartaric acid. The roots contain many steam-distillable aromatic compounds. The characteristic aroma of chicory stems from acteophenone. The roots also contain inulin; on roasting, this is converted to oxymethylfurfural, which gives off a coffeelike aroma. Chicory also contains maltol, a taste modifier that intensifies the flavor of sugar.

Actions
Chicory is commonly used as a water-soluble or alcoholic extract. The water-soluble fraction is thought to exhibit sedative effects, and

therefore may antagonize the stimulating effects from coffee and tea. Alcohol extracts are believed to have anti-inflammatory activity (Benoit et al., 1976). Although few data exist regarding chicory use in humans, several animal studies have shown that it reduces cardiac rate by action similar to that of quinidine. This suggests that chicory might be useful in treating arrhythmic disorders.

Reported uses
Chicory is primarily used in herbal lore as a coffee or tea additive because of its ability to antagonize the CNS stimulation brought on by these products. It has also been used as a coffee substitute because of its coffeelike aroma and taste. In folk medicine, chicory root is used as a diuretic and laxative; human data are, however, lacking for this use.

Dosage
Very little information is available.
Crude herb: 3 g P.O. daily.

Adverse reactions
• Contact dermatitis (possibly caused by sesquiterpene lactones; Malten, 1983)

Interactions
None reported.

Contraindications and precautions
No known contraindications. Use cautiously in patients with known cardiac disease because of the agent's potential action on the heart.

Special considerations
• Question the patient about use of the herb when taking the drug history.
• Advise the patient with cardiac disease to avoid this herb or to use it cautiously.

Points of interest
• Chicory has been shown to take up the fungicide quintozene through its roots, which may lead to colonization with certain bacteria in the soil and subsequent contamination of the plant.

Analysis
Chicory has a long history of traditional use. Because of its flavor and aroma, the root has been used as a substitute to coffee or tea. Unlike coffee, chicory may exhibit sedative properties, which may explain its traditional use in offsetting stimulant properties of teas

and coffee. However, these claims remain yet unproven. The plant may have some use as an antiarrhythmic, but further studies are needed. Its use as a laxative is also unclear and should therefore be reserved until human trials are completed.

References

Benoit, P.S., et al. "Biological and Phytochemical Evaluation of Plants. XIV. Anti-inflammatory Evaluation of 163 Species of Plants," *Lloydia* 39:160-71, 1976.
Malten, K.E. "Chicory Dermatitis from September to April," *Contact Dermatitis* 9:232, 1983.

CHINESE RHUBARB

HIMALAYAN RHUBARB, MEDICINAL RHUBARB, RHEI RADIX, RHEI RHIZOMA, RUBARBO, TURKISH RHUBARB

Common trade names
Dahuang Liujingao, Extractum Rhei Liquidum

Common forms
Available as tablets, water- and alcohol-based tinctures, syrups, and extracts.

Source
Active components are derived from the dried root bark of *Rheum palmatum*, a large, perennial herb native to the mountains of Tibet and northwest China.

Chemical components
Chinese rhubarb contains anthraquinones, tannins, and stilbenes. The anthraquinones occur as glycosides and have been identified as chrysophanol, rhein, emodin, and aloe emodin. Other substances include sennosides A, B, and C, and phenolics (such as glucogallin, gallic acid, and catechin).

Actions
The herb's dramatic purgative or laxative effect are attributable to rhein and sennosides. Sennosides act on the large intestine to increase motility after being degraded by microorganisms in the colon. Increased laxative activity appears to correlate with sennoside content. Anthraquinones exhibit a laxative and antimicrobial effect.

Rhubarb extract has been studied in chronic renal failure in the rat (Zhang and El-Nahas, 1996). A recent study found rhubarb to decrease the severity of proteinuria, decrease BUN, and attenuate severity of glomerulosclerosis.

Rhein and emodin inhibit mitochondrial energy production. This may explain the inhibitory effect of rhubarb extracts on renal growth. Hypermetabolism is implicated in initiation of remnant kidney scarring.

In patients with upper GI bleeding, rhubarb has been found to increase blood vessel constriction and promote hemostasis; however, the mechanism of this action is unknown (Dong-hai et al., 1980).

Reported uses

Chinese rhubarb has been used medicinally for centuries as a laxative, an antidiarrheal, and in indigestion, jaundice, GI bleeding, menstrual disorders, conjunctivitis, and traumatic injuries. It has also been used topically for the treatment of burns, scabs, and sores, and as an astringent or styptic to stop bleeding.

The combination of an ACE inhibitor, captopril, and Chinese rhubarb was found to be superior to either agent alone in slowing progression of renal failure (Zhang et al., 1990). Similar results were obtained with rhubarb and other adjuvant drugs. Chinese researchers concluded that such treatments may be used as transitional measures in chronic renal disease before more radical therapies are instituted (Kang et al., 1993).

In patients with GI bleeding, rhubarb was found to help control bleeding, decrease blood loss, reduce need for clotting agents, resolve fever, increase peristalsis of the colon without affecting the stomach or duodenum, and help eliminate extravasated bleeding.

Dosage

For diarrhea, 1 teaspoon P.O. daily of tincture or decoction.
For constipation, ½ to 1 teaspoon P.O. daily of tincture or 1 to 2 teaspoons P.O. daily of decoction.
For upper GI bleeding, 3-g tablets or powder b.i.d. or q.i.d.
When dosing in older children or the elderly over age 65, use lower-strength preparations.

Adverse reactions

• Contact dermatitis (from handling the leaves)
• Discoloration of urine (bright yellow or red)
⚠ Leaves contain poisonous oxalic acid. Consumption causes abdominal pain, burning in mouth and throat, diarrhea, nausea, vomiting, possibly seizures and death with ingestion of large amounts.

Interactions

None reported.

Contraindications and precautions

Contraindicated in pregnant and breast-feeding patients, in children under age 2, and in patients with intestinal problems such as ulcers or colitis. Use of herb for over 2 weeks is contraindicated because it can induce a tolerance in the colon.

Special considerations

• Be aware that most of the literature comes from the Orient, making interpretation of published studies difficult.
• Explain that Chinese rhubarb is not the same as that found in the United States.
• Inform laboratory that the patient's urine will be bright yellow or red in color.
• Advise the patient to take this herb for a short time to avoid problems such as melanosis coli or laxative dependence.
• Caution the patient against preparing Chinese rhubarb formulations at home to avoid the risk of oxalic acid poisoning. Urge the patient to keep this plant out of the reach of children and pets.
• Inform the patient that this herb may color the urine bright yellow or red.
• Advise the female patient to stop taking the herb if pregnancy is being planned or suspected or if breast-feeding is being planned.

Points of interest

• Chinese rhubarb is officially listed in the Chinese Pharmacopia and was mentioned in the Chinese herbal Pen-King (ca. 2700 BC). Rhubarb root is one of the oldest and best known Chinese herbal medicines available. It has also been used in the manufacture of liqueurs and aperitifs.
• Rhubarb species grown in Europe and North America and used for food and medicinal purposes are less potent than Chinese rhubarb.

Analysis

Active medicinal components of Chinese rhubarb suggest its theoretic application as an agent for GI dysmotility. With safety and efficacy data lacking, the herb cannot be recommended for this use.

The use of rhubarb in renal failure and GI bleeding appear intriguing; however, data are from the foreign literature and difficult to interpret. Future studies should focus on these aspects of Chinese rhubarb applications.

References

Dong-hai, J., et al. "Resume of 400 Cases of Acute Upper Digestive Tract Bleeding Treated by Rhubarb Alone," *Pharmacology* 20:128-30, 1980.

Kang, Z., et al. "Observation of Therapeutic Effect in 50 Cases of Chronic Renal Failure Treated with Rhubarb and Adjuvant Drugs," *J Tradit Chin Med* 13:249-52, 1993. Abstract.

Zhang, G., and El Nahas, A.M. "The Effect of Rhubarb Extract on Experimental Renal Fibrosis," *Nephrol Dial Transplant* 11:186-90, 1996.

Zhang, J.H., et al. "Clinical Effects of *Rheum* and Captopril on Preventing
Progression of Chronic Renal Failure," *Chin Med J* 103:788-93, 1990. Abstract.

CHONDROITIN

CAS, CHONDROITIN SULFATE A OR CHONDROITIN-4-
SULFATE, CHONDROITIN-C OR CHONDROITIN-6-SULFATE,
CSS

Common trade names
(Available in combination) 100% CSA, Chondroitin-4 Sulfate,
Purified Chondroitin Sulfate

Common forms
Available as 200-mg and 400-mg capsules and as an injection in
Europe.

Source
Chondroitin is extracted from the cartilage of the bovine trachea.

Chemical components
Chondroitin sulfates are large molecularly sized compounds of glycosaminoglycans (GAGs) and disaccharide polymers composed of
equimolar amounts of D-glucuronic acid, D-acetylgalactosamine,
and sulfates in 30 to 100 disaccharide units.

Purified commercial chondroitin preparations contain combinations of chondroitin-4-sulfate and chondroitin-6-sulfate, which are
negatively charged because of carboxylic and dissociated sulfates.
Structurally, chondroitin sulfates are related to the low-molecular-
weight heparanoid, danaproid sodium.

Actions
Because of their large molecular size, studies have estimated that the
oral absorption of chondroitin sulfates is poor. Chondroitin sulfates
have been shown to control the formation of new cartilage matrix
by stimulating chondrocyte metabolism and synthesis of collagen
and proteoglycan.

Chondroitin sulfates are also reported to inhibit the enzymes human leukocyte elastase and hyaluronidase. High concentrations of
human leukocyte elastase are found in the blood and synovial fluid
of patients with rheumatic disease. Chondroitin sulfates also stimulate the production of highly polymerized hyaluronic acid by synovial cells. Viscosity is subsequently improved and synovial fluid
levels return to normal.

RESEARCH FINDINGS
Chondroitin sulfates and diclofenac in osteoarthritis

A randomized, multicenter, double-blind, 3-month study compared the efficacy of chondroitin sulfates (CS) with that of the NSAID diclofenac sodium (Morreale et al., 1996).

A total of 146 patients with osteoarthritis of the knee were randomized into two groups. During the first month, patients in the NSAID group received diclofenac and placebo t.i.d. During the second and third months, patients received placebo only. Patients in the CS group received CS and placebo t.i.d. during the first month. During the second and third months, patients received CS only. Diclofenac was given for 1 month; CS was given for 3 months. A total of 126 patients completed the study.

At the end of four months, researchers noted a 64.4% decrease in Lequesne Index scores in the group receiving diclofenac as compared with a 29.7% decrease in the group receiving CS. However, mean values for spontaneous pain decreased by 82% for the CS group compared with 36% for the diclofenac group. The difference was statistically significant in favor of CS ($P < 0.01$). There was a reduction in pain on weight-bearing of 53.1% for the CS group compared with a 36.2% reduction in the diclofenac group.

In addition, analgesic consumption was 20% lower in the CS group; consumption was just 5.2% lower in the diclofenac group. The authors concluded that, although NSAID-treated patients showed prompt pain reduction, their symptoms reappeared at the end of the study. In contrast, the CS-treated patients had a slower onset of therapeutic effect, but the effects lasted for up to 3 months following treatment.

Reported uses

Chondroitin is claimed to be useful as a dietary supplement in combination with glucosamine sulfate in osteoarthritis and related disorders. Chondroitin sulfates have been used in ischemic heart disease and hyperlipidemia, as a preservative of corneas for transplantation, and as an adjunct to eye surgery.

Chondroitin sulfates were first evaluated using parenteral administration (Theodosakis, 1997). Other small trials demonstrated improvement in subjective outcomes, such as use of NSAIDs, visual analogue scales for pain, the Lequesne's Index, and patient or physician global assessment. (See *Chondroitin sulfates and diclofenac in osteoarthritis.*)

Dosage

The oral dose is based on the patient's weight; chondroitin is usually given in combination with glucosamine sulfate.

Patients under 120 lb: 1,000 mg glucosamine sulfate plus 800 mg chondroitin sulfates P.O.

Patients between 120 and 200 lb: 1,500 mg glucosamine sulfate plus 1,200 mg chondroitin sulfates P.O.

Patients over 200 lb: 2,000 mg glucosamine sulfate plus 1,600 mg chondroitin sulfates P.O. (Theodosakis, 1997).

The total daily dosage is usually taken with food, in two to four divided doses. Recent studies evaluating chondroitin sulfates alone used doses from 400 mg P.O. b.i.d. or t.i.d., and 1,200 mg P.O. daily as a single dose.

Adverse reactions

• Dyspepsia
• Headache, motor uneasiness, and euphoria were reported with use of chondroitin sulfates (Kerzberg et al., 1987).
• Nausea
• Pain (at injection site with parenteral administration)
⚠ Risk of internal bleeding exists because of the herb's similarity to heparin. Studies in animals found significantly decreased hematocrit, hemoglobin, WBCs, and segmented neutrophils; reduced aggregation in response to adenosine diphosphate and collagen; and significantly decreased platelet count (McNamara et al., 1996). There is no report of bleeding as a result of chondroitin sulfate use in humans.

Interactions

Anticoagulants: may potentiate effects. Avoid concomitant use.

Contraindications and precautions

Avoid use of the herb in pregnant or breast-feeding patients; effects are unknown. Use cautiously in patients with bleeding disorders because of risk of anticoagulation.

Special considerations

• Offer additional support to the patient with osteoarthritis, such as intermittent moist heat application and exercise.
• Instruct the patient to watch for signs of bleeding, especially if he is taking anticoagulants or has a bleeding disorder.
• Advise the female patient to avoid use of the herb during pregnancy or when breast-feeding.

Points of interest

• Public interest in the combined use of chondroitin sulfates and glucosamine sulfate has risen, especially since the publication of a book, *The Arthritis Cure* (Theodosakis, 1997), which claims that the sulfate combination is "the medical miracle that can halt, reverse, and may even cure osteoarthritis."

Analysis

Most data from human trials are flawed in study design, and clinical trial data on the glucosamine sulfate and chondroitin sulfates combination are lacking. Therefore, these data must be interpreted cautiously. Long-term clinical trials with better study design and size are needed.

The Arthritis Foundation cannot currently recommend the use of glucosamine sulfate and chondroitin sulfates for osteoarthritis or other types of arthritis.

References

Kerzberg, E.M., et al. "Combination of Glycosaminoglycans and Acetylsalicylic Acid in Knee Osteoarthrosis," *Scand J Rheumatol* 16:377-80, 1987.

McNamara, P.S., et al. "Hematologic, Hemostatic, and Biochemical Effects in Dogs Receiving an Oral Chondroprotective Agent for Thirty Days," *Am J Vet Res* 57:1390-94, 1996.

Morreale, P., et al. "Comparison of the Anti-inflammatory Efficacy of Chondroitin Sulfate and Diclofenac Sodium in Patients with Knee Osteoarthritis," *J Rheumatol* 23:1385-91, 1996.

Theodosakis, J. *The Arthritis Cure.* New York: St. Martin's Press, 1997.

CINNAMON

BATAVIA CASSIA, BATAVIA CINNAMON, CASSIA, CASSIA LIGNEA, CEYLON CINNAMON, CHINESE CINNAMON, CINNAMOMOM, FALSE CINNAMON, PADANG CASSIA, PANANG CINNAMON, SAIGON CASSIA, SAIGON CINNAMON

Common trade names

None known. Various manufacturers produce the herb for use as a spice for foods.

Common forms

Available as dried bark, dried leaves, powder, and cinnamon oil.

Source

Active components are derived from the dried bark, leaves, and twigs of various species of *Cinnamomum:* Ceylon cinnamon (*C. zeylandicum*), Saigon cinnamon (*C. loureirii*), and others. *C. zeylanium* grows in Sri Lanka, southeastern India, Indonesia, South

America, and the West Indies. Essential oils are removed by steam distillation of the dried bark or leaves.

Chemical components
The main element in the essential oil is cinnamaldehyde. Other components found in smaller amounts include phenols and terpenes (such as eugenol, trans-cinnamic acid, hydroxycinamaldehyde, o-methoxycinnamaldehyde, o-glucoside, and 3-(2-hydroxyphenol)-propanoic acid), cinnamyl alcohol, tannins, mucilage, procyanidins, and coumarins.

Actions
Eugenol has antiseptic and anesthetic properties. Cinnamic aldehyde has shown fungicidal activity in vitro against respiratory tract mycoses such as *Aspergillus niger, A. fuigatis, A. midulans, A. flavus, Candida albicans, C. tropicalis, Histoplasma* and *Cryptococcus neoformans* (Viollon and Chaumont, 1994). O-glucoside and 3-(2-hydroxyphenol)-propanoic acid have reportedly demonstrated gastroprotective activity in rats similar to cimetidine.

Reported uses
Cinnamon oil is widely used in small amounts in toothpaste, mouthwashes, gargles, lotions, liniments, soaps, detergents, and other pharmaceutical products and cosmetics. Claims have been made for cinnamon products as an antidiarrheal, analgesic, and antifungal. In Eastern and Western folk medicine, uses for cinnamon include treating chronic diarrhea, rheumatism, colds, abdominal pain, chest pain, kidney disorders, hypertension, and female disorders.

Dosage
No consensus exists. Most sources cite cinnamon's use as a spice in small quantities only.

Adverse reactions
- Cheilitis
- Facial flushing
- Gingivitis
- Glossitis
- Hypersensitivity reactions, including contact dermatitis, second-degree burns, increased breathing and perspiration, postexcitatory state followed by a period of centralized sedation (drowsiness)
- Increased GI motility
- Increased heart rate
- Perioral dermatitis
- Shortness of breath
- Stomatitis

RESEARCH FINDINGS
Toxic ingestion of cinnamon oil

One case report described acute cinnamon toxicity in a 7-year-old child who had ingested 2 oz of cinnamon oil (Pilapil, 1989). Symptoms of toxicity included a burning sensation in the mouth, chest, and stomach; double vision; dizziness; vomiting; and subsequent collapse.

In the emergency department, the child was drowsy and had warm skin, increased bowel sounds, a pulse of 100/minute, and respiration of 20/minute. The child was given 8 oz of milk for toxicity symptoms, followed 15 minutes later with 15 ml of syrup of ipecac. After the child vomited, activated charcoal (120 ml) was administered.

Symptoms of rectal burning, diarrhea, double vision, and abdominal cramps persisted. GI symptoms and drowsiness lasted for 5 hours, after which the patient was asymptomatic. It is unclear from this report whether persistent GI symptoms resulted from cinnamon ingestion or the use of ipecac and charcoal.

Interactions
None reported.

Contraindications and precautions
Avoid use in pregnant or breast-feeding women over amounts normally found in foods.

Special considerations
• Tell patient that cinnamon should be used only as a spice. Other uses cannot be recommended because of lack of adequate data.
• Advise the patient that cinnamon or its components can cause allergic type reactions, such as skin irritation (including second-degree burns) and mucosal membrane reactions.
• Remind the patient to report unusual signs or symptoms. Cinnamon toxicity involves the GI tract, CNS, and the CV system. (See *Toxic ingestion of cinnamon oil.*)
⚠ Warn parents that children may use cinnamon products as a recreational drug.

Analysis
Human trials evaluating the efficacy of cinnamon for its proposed uses are lacking. Further studies in animals and humans are needed to determine its safety and efficacy.

References

Pilapil, V.R. "Toxic Manifestations of Cinnamon Oil Ingestion In a Child," *Clin Pediatr* 28:276, 1989.

Viollon, C., and Chaumont, J.P. "Antifungal Properties of Essential Oils and Their Main Components upon *Cryptococcus neoformans*," *Mycopathologia* 128:151-53, 1994.

CLARY

CLARY OIL, CLARY SAGE, CLEAR EYE, EYEBRIGHT, MUSCATEL SAGE, ORVALE, SEE BRIGHT, TOUTE-BONNE

Common trade names
None known.

Common forms
Available as an essential oil (5 ml, 10 ml. clear liquid).

Source
The highly aromatic essential oil is steam-distilled from the flowering tops of *Salvia sclarea*, a perennial herb native to southern Europe.

Chemical components
The whole plant contains diterpenes (including sclareol, manool, salvipisone, ferruginol, microstegiol, and candidissiol), sesquiterpenes (caryophyllene oxide, spathulenol), alpha-amaryin, beta-sitosterol, flavonoids (including apigenin, luteolin, and 4-methylapigenin), linalyl acetate, linalool, and pionene.

Actions
The pharmacokinetics of clary's major component, diterpene sclareol, has been studied in vivo using a rat model. When given I.V., sclareol was rapidly cleared by biliary excretion; neither sclareol nor its metabolites were excreted in the urine following I.V. or P.O. administration.

The essential oil of clary produced contracture and inhibition of twitch response to nerve stimulation on skeletal muscle, whereas on smooth muscle it produced contracture with little or no decrease in nerve stimulation (Lis-Balchin and Hart, 1997).

Some diterpenoids and sesquiterpenes extracted from clary have been found to have antimicrobial activity against *Staphylococcus aureus*, *Candida albicans*, and *Proteus mirabilis* (Ulubelen et al., 1994).

Clary is claimed to contain an estrogen-like compound that helps regulate hormonal balance. Its antispasmodic activity is thought to be due to nerol, a component of the essential oil. Although the essential oil has also been studied in humans for effects on the CNS and hematopoietic, immune, and enzyme systems, data are difficult to interpret because they were published in foreign journals.

Reported uses

Claimed to have sedative, euphoric, astringent, anti-inflammatory, and antispasmodic properties, clary is also thought to be useful in treating several ailments including mental fatigue, anxiety, depression, decreased libido, sore throat, digestive and renal problems, premenstrual syndrome, menstrual pain, irregular periods, and menopausal symptoms. It is also used in aromatherapy. The mucilaginous seeds have been used to remove particles of dust from the eyes.

Dosage

For mental fatigue, anxiety, depression, and decreased libido,
Inhalation: apply 2 drops of essential oil to a piece of cloth, then inhale.
Massage: apply 2 to 4 drops of essential oil to 2 teaspoons of carrier oil or lotion.
Baths: add 2 to 10 drops of essential oil to bath water.
For menstrual pain, apply 4 drops of essential oil to a piece of cloth to be used for warm compresses.
For sore throat, hoarseness, laryngitis, add 3 drops of essential oil to a glass of water, then rinse mouth and gargle.

Adverse reactions

• Drowsiness
• Euphoria
• Headache
• Increased menstrual bleeding

Interactions

Alcohol: may potentiate effects. Avoid concomitant use.

Contraindications and precautions

Contraindicated in patients with a history of estrogen-sensitive malignancy because of potential estrogenic effects. Avoid use of the herb in pregnant or breast-feeding patients; effects (other than with food uses) are unknown.

Special considerations

• Monitor the female patient for increased menstrual bleeding or changes in the menstrual cycle.
• Explain that therapeutic effects and safety risks are not well documented.

• Advise the patient to avoid hazardous activities until CNS effects are known.
• Instruct the patient to avoid consumption of other CNS depressants, including alcohol, because of purported sedative effects.
• Warn the patient to report unusual symptoms that occur during herbal therapy to their health care provider.
• Advise the female patient to avoid use of the herb during pregnancy or when breast-feeding.

Points of interest
• In the 16th century, Rhine Valley winemakers added clary to their wines to make the wines more potent.

Analysis
Despite its many claims of therapeutic usefulness, clary has yet to demonstrate clinical efficacy through controlled animal and human trials. This herb cannot be recommended for use until these controlled studies are conducted.

References
Lis-Balchin, M., and Hart, S. "A Preliminary Study of the Effect of Essential Oils on Skeletal and Smooth Muscle In Vitro," *J Ethnopharmacol* 58:183-87, 1997.
Ulubelen, A., et al. "Terpenoids from *Salvia sclarea*," *Phytochemistry* 36: 971-74, 1994.

CLOVES
CARYOPHYLLUM, *EUGENIA AROMATICA*, OIL OF CLOVES, OLEUM CARYOPHYLLI

Common trade names
Dent-Zel-Ite Toothache Relief Drops, Red Cross Toothache Medication

Common forms
Available as drops (85% eugenol), mouthwashes, fluid or oil extracts, and in cigarettes.

Source
Active components are extracted by steam distillation from the dried flower buds of *Syzgium aromaticum* (also known as *Eugenia caryophyllata* or *Caryophyllus aromaticus*), an evergreen tree native to Southeast Asia.

Chemical components

The agent is composed primarily of the phenolic substances eugenol and acetyl eugenol. Eugenol comprises 90% to 95% of the phenolic compounds obtained from the plant and is extracted as a volatile oil. It is chemically known as 2-methoxy-4-(2-propenyl) phenol. Other compounds include a terpene, caryophyllene, and small amounts of alpha-humulene and beta-carophyllene.

Actions

Cloves are reported to have both analgesic and antiseptic activity. The primary mechanism for the analgesic activity of cloves is believed to be inhibition of prostaglandin biosynthesis from cyclooxygenase and lipoxygenase blockade by eugenol (Rasheed et al., 1984). However, other mechanisms may also exist, such as a reduction in pain perception produced by the phenolic activity of eugenol on nociceptors in dental pulp.

The antiseptic activity of cloves is also related to eugenol. Eugenol has been reported to have antimicrobial activity against various bacteria and *Candida albicans*. The antimicrobial activity of eugenol is poorly described, but is thought to be due to a membrane-active antibacterial effect from the phenolic activity of eugenol (Briozzo et al., 1989).

Reported uses

Clove oil has been widely used topically in the treatment of toothache, and has also been added to mouthwashes as an antiseptic. Some in vitro data have confirmed its anti-inflammatory and antimicrobial activity.

Dosage

Depending upon the product being used, doses can vary from 5 to 30 drops for the fluid extract, 1 to 5 drops for the oil extract, and ½ to 1 oz of oral mouth rinses containing clove oil.

Adverse reactions

- Bronchospasm
- Hemoptysis
- Local tissue irritation
- Oral tissue sensitivity
- Pulmonary edema

⚠ Potential damage to viable soft tissue and airway epithelium injury. High-altitude pulmonary edema (accompanied by airway inflammation) has been associated with clove cigarette smoking (Hackett et al., 1985).

Interactions
None reported.

Contraindications and precautions
Avoid the use of topical clove oil because it may cause further damage to dental pulp or supporting periodontium.

Special considerations
• Know that the American Dental Association (ADA) has not accepted clove oil and eugenol as safe and effective nonprescription drugs for toothaches.
• Toothaches or dental pain may signify a more serious problem. Advise the patient to seek professional dental advice regarding such pain. Restrict the application of clove and eugenol to persons trained in its use, such as dentists.
• Question the patient about use of clove cigarettes (if he is a smoker) when taking the patient's history.
• Advise the patient that application of clove oil or eugenol-containing products may cause more damage to viable dental pulp or soft tissue.

Points of interest
• The FDA-appointed advisory review panel on nonprescription drugs has reclassified eugenol to a Category III nonprescription drug (products that have insufficient data available on their use as nonprescription drugs).
• The ADA accepts clove oil and eugenol for professional use only by dentists.
• The German Commission E has approved cloves for use as a local anesthetic and antiseptic.

Analysis
Most clinical data on the use of clove oil or eugenol is obtained from in vitro studies. There are no well-controlled studies in humans evaluating the analgesic and antiseptic properties of clove oil or eugenol. Although data on the effects of clove oil and eugenol on prostaglandin synthesis suggest an analgesic role, further studies are needed.

References
Briozzo, J., et al. "Antimicrobial Activity of Clove Oil Dispersed in a Concentrated Sugar Solution," *J Appl Bacteriol* 66:69-75, 1989.
Hackett, P.H., et al. "Clove Cigarettes and High Altitude Pulmonary Edema," *JAMA* 253:3551-52, 1985. Letter.
Rasheed, A., et al. "Eugenol and Prostaglandin Biosynthesis," *N Engl J Med* 310:50-51, 1984. Letter.

COENZYME Q10
CO-Q10, MITOQUINONE, UBIDECARENONE, UBIQUINONE

Common trade names
Adelir, Co-Q10, Heartcin, Inokiton, Neuquinone, Taidecanone, Ubiquinone, Udekinon

Common forms
Tablets: 25 mg, 50 mg, 100 mg, 200 mg
Capsules: 10 mg, 30 mg, 60 mg, 100 mg

Source
Co-Q10 (2,3 dimethoxy-5 methyl-6-decaprenyl benzoquinone) is an endogenous antioxidant found in small amounts in meats and seafood. Although Co-Q10 is found in all human cells, its highest concentrations occur in the heart, liver, kidneys, and pancreas. It is found naturally in the organs of many mammalian species. The "10" in Co-Q10 designates the number of isoprene units of the molecular side chain, and this is specific for humanoid ubiquinone. Japan retains all of the world's patents for the product and is the major supplier of the world's Co-Q10.

Chemical components
Ubiquinones (redox carriers, electron transport shuttles) are lipid-soluble benzoquinones involved in electron transport in the cell's mitochondria, where they are most concentrated. Co-Q10 is classified as a fat-soluble quinone with characteristics common to many vitamins. It is a unique substance, but resembles niacin in general biosynthetic performance. Chemically, its structure resembles vitamin K.

Actions
Co-Q10 is proven to have antioxidant and membrane-stabilizing properties. It participates in the electron transfer process within the oxidative respiration chain and is a part of oxidative phosphorylation. Co-Q10 prevents the depletion of metabolic substrates required for resynthesis of adenosine triphosphate (ATP). Without Co-Q10, ATP cannot be regenerated through this pathway. Co-Q10 is a powerful intramembrane antioxidant and free radical scavenger, protecting cell membranes and DNA from oxidative damage. Co-Q10 simply protects tissue from ischemic cellular damage.

Reported uses
Ubiquinone is marketed to treat several diseases and disorders, including ischemic heart disease and heart failure. The basis for Co-Q10 use is that patients with significant heart disease (New York

RESEARCH FINDINGS
Co-Q10 in heart failure

In a large, double blind, placebo-controlled study with Co-Q10 (2 mg/kg/day) and conventional treatment, 651 patients with New York Heart Association class III or IV heart failure over 1 year's duration demonstrated a significant reduction in hospitalizations—23% versus 37% (Morisco et al., 1993). Similarly, episodes of pulmonary edema and cardiac asthma were reduced in the study group (20 versus 51, and 97 versus 198, respectively; both P < 0.001) compared with controls.

The authors concluded that the addition of Co-Q10 to conventional therapy significantly reduced hospitalization for decompensated heart failure and the incidence of serious complications in patients with heart failure.

Heart Association [NYHA] class III to IV) have Co-Q10 deficiency relative to normal, healthy individuals (NYHA class I to II). (See *Co-Q10 in heart failure.*)

In patients who received Co-Q10 daily for 5 years, the mean ejection fraction increased after only 6 months, and improved by 87% in the study subjects (Sinatra et al., 1997).

Epidemiologic evidence exists that high vitamin E doses may reduce the risk of coronary artery disease. Coantioxidants such as Co-Q10 may make vitamin E an even more efficient antioxidant for low-density lipoproteins (Vasankari et al., 1997).

Other conditions in which Co-Q10 claims to be useful include angina pectoris, hypertension, doxorubicin cardiotoxicity, arrhythmias, mitral valve prolapse, periodontal disease, immunodeficiency, diabetes, deafness, and Bell's palsy.

Dosage
Dosages used in clinical trials ranged from 50 to 300 mg P.O. daily.

Adverse reactions
- Anorexia
- Diarrhea
- Epigastric discomfort
- Ischemic tissue damage (during intense exercise)
- Mild nausea

Interactions
Oral antidiabetic agents: may theoretically inhibit some Co-Q10 enzymes and thus, inhibit functions of exogenously administered Co-Q10.

Warfarin: Co-Q10 may diminish response to warfarin. Monitor patient.

Contraindications and precautions
Use cautiously in patients who may be allergic to Co-Q10 or its formulation.

Special considerations
• Caution the patient against performing intense exercise during Co-Q10 therapy because damage of ischemic tissue may occur.
• Instruct the patient with heart failure to report changes in his condition to the primary health care provider.

Analysis
Despite its usefulness in the symptomatic treatment of heart failure, Co-Q10 has not been shown to reduce mortality. Comparative trials are needed to evaluate this agent with standard treatments (such as ACE inhibitors, beta blockers, and aspirin) to determine survival rates. Co-Q10 also needs to be further evaluated in the treatment of other diseases before its use can be recommended.

References
Morisco, C., et al. "Effect of coenzyme Q10 Therapy in Patients with Congestive Heart Failure. A Long-Term Multicenter, Randomized Study." *Clin Invest* 71:s134-36, 1993.

Sinatra, S.T., et al. "Coenzyme Q10: A Vital Therapeutic Nutrient for the Heart with Special Application in Congestive Heart Failure," *Conn Med* 65:707-11, 1997.

Vasankari, T.J., et al. "Increased Serum and Low-Density-Lipoprotein Antioxidant Potential After Antioxidant Supplementation in Endurance Athletes," *Am J Clin Nutr* 65:1052-56, 1997.

COFFEE
BEAN JUICE, *COFFEA ARABICA*, CAFÉ, ESPRESSO, JAVA, ROBUSTA COFFEE, SANTOS COFFEE

Common trade names
(Various manufacturers) Maxwell House, Eight O'clock, Bean Company, Folgers

Common forms
Available as whole dried or ground beans, and freeze-dried or spray-dried crystals (instant coffee). Caffeine is widely used in analgesics, stimulants, allergy medicines, cold products and dietary aids.

Source

The fruits of the *Coffea arabica* bush are commonly cultivated for their most popular seeds (referred to as beans after roasting). Grown in semitropical areas, other coffee species are also used (*C. canephora, C. robusta*). The best known coffee-growing areas are Central and South America, Africa, Jamaica, and Hawaii. Freshly picked berries are either sun-dried ("natural" or dry process) or subjected to depulping machines and then dried ("washed" or wet process). The roasting and blending of other beans gives each coffee its characteristic flavor. Before roasting, caffeine is extracted from green (unripened) beans with organic solvents.

Chemical components

Active components include caffeine, trigonelline, chlorogenic acid, galactomanan (carbohydrate) protein, free amino acids, polyamines, tannins, some B vitamins, and trace quantities of niacin. Coffee oil contains fatty acids, stearic acids, sterols, tocopherols, cafestol, cahweol, and lanosterol. Over 100 aromatic compounds have been identified in coffee, including some furan derivatives, pyrazines, pyrroles, oxazoles, and various acids.

Actions

Caffeine, a methylxanthine, is responsible for most of coffee's effects. It binds to adenosine receptors in the brain and acts as a stimulant. The normal elimination half-life of caffeine is 3.5 to 4.5 hours, but can double in pregnancy and last for days in a fetus.

Caffeine increases fatty acid metabolism and basal metabolic rate, and affects metabolism of other drugs. It contains diterpenes that can cause increase in cholesterol, low-density lipoproteins (LDLs), and triglycerides. Changes in heart rate and mild elevations in blood pressure can also occur (Van Dusseldorp, 1989).

Caffeine stimulates gastrin release, adrenocorticotropin hormone, and cortisol, and mildly raises interocular pressure. It also has a weak diuretic effect that may be severe if abused. In patients with detrusor instability, it may cause an increase in detrusor pressor. Chlorogenic acid, found in moderate amounts in coffee, possesses stimulant, diuretic, and choloretic properties.

Retrospective studies have reported a possible link between caffeine and bladder and pancreatic cancer; over half of coffee's mutagenic activity can be attributed to methylglyoxal.

Reported uses

Endurance runners have used coffee to increase fatty acid metabolism and aid exercise tolerance. The effect of coffee on angina patients was to increase exercise tolerance and delay time to angina.

Coffee may act as a bronchodilator and was shown to have a similar effect on pulmonary function tests. However, much larger doses of coffee would be needed to match the bronchodilating potency of traditional agents such as theophylline and aminophylline.

Caffeine was found to help cold sufferers be more alert and lower their general feeling of malaise. Postprandial coffee consumption by elderly patients has been shown to circumvent postprandial hypotension and reduce falls.

In cattle models, coffee was used to lower postpartum complications. It reduced the incidence of diarrhea, normalized temperature, and reduced mortality by 75%.

Dosage
No consensus exists. The lethal dose of caffeine is reported to be 10 g.

Adverse reactions
- Diuresis
- Extrasystole
- Gastroesophageal reflux disease (GERD)
- Glaucoma due to temporary caffeine-induced intraocular pressure
- Headache
- Increased blood pressure
- Insomnia
- Mild delirium and excitation
- Muscle fasciculations (twitches, tremors)
- Nausea
- Possible aggravated CV disease; effects on lipids are controversial
- Possible lowered seizure threshold (in patients with refractory psychiatric disorders receiving electroconvulsive therapy)
- Peptic ulcer disease
- Restlessness
- Tachycardia

Interactions
None reported.

Contraindications and precautions
Avoid use of coffee in pregnant or breast-feeding patients; effects are unknown.

Special considerations
- Consider coffee intake as a cause in patients complaining of insomnia.
- Question the patient about the daily consumption of coffee.
- Monitor the cardiac patient for arrhythmias if coffee is being consumed.

- Remind the patient that chronic consumption of coffee can lead to caffeine withdrawal symptoms when it is abruptly discontinued; "rebound" headaches may occur.
- Advise the patient with hyperlipidemia to minimize consumption of coffee because of adverse effects on lipid profiles.
- Warn the patient against coffee consumption in patients with GERD because coffee may exacerbate the disease.
- Advise the female patient to avoid use of the herb during pregnancy or when breast-feeding.

Points of interest
- Clinical trials dispell the belief that caffeine exacerbates arrhythmias (Graboys et al., 1989) or produces lasting increases in blood pressure (Van Dusseldorp et al., 1989).
- Colombian and Central American coffee seems to be preferred over Brazilian and African varieties by American consumers.
- Coffee charcoal (charred outer portion of beans) is used to treat nonspecific acute diarrhea in Germany.

Analysis
Although coffee is relatively harmless, some patients may be adversely affected by the pharmacologic effects of caffeine. A conservative approach may be to currently limit coffee consumption in patients with hypercholesterolemia, hypertension, or gastric diseases, and in pregnant or breast-feeding patients.

References
Graboys, T.B., et al. "The Effect of Caffeine on Ventricular Ectopic Activity in Patients with Malignant Ventricular Arrhythmia," *Arch Intern Med* 149:637-39, 1989.
Van Dusseldorp, M., et al. "Effect of Decaffeinated Versus Regular Coffee on Blood Pressure," *Hypertension* 14(5):563-69, 1989.

COLA TREE
KOLA NUT, KOLANUT

Common trade names
(Various manufacturers; available in combination) Colloidal Energy Formula, Kola Nut, Starter, Ultra Diet Pep

Common forms
Available as nuts or seeds. Extracts of the seeds are also available in capsules, tablets, and fluid extracts. Cola nut extract is widely used as a flavoring in carbonated soft drinks in the United States.

Source

Cola nitida and *C. acuminata* are evergreen trees native to western Africa, Sri Lanka, and Indonesia. They belong to the Sterculia family (Sterculiaceae), which also includes cacao or chocolate. The active components are extracted from the seeds.

Chemical components

Caffeine is the primary component of cola seeds; other notable components include the alkaloid theobromine, tannins, and phenols.

Actions

Caffeine and theobromine are both methylated xanthines, and are similar in action to theophylline by inhibiting phosphodiesterase, which increases intracellular levels of cAMP. Primary effects are CNS stimulation, cardioacceleration, increased blood pressure, bronchodilation, increased gastric acid secretion (Ibu et al., 1986), and diuresis.

Chewing cola nuts tends to increase salivary pH (Gaye et al., 1990), which may contribute to the reduced incidence of tooth decay observed in habitual users. Cola tannins are reported to be carcinogenic. Other studies have shown an extremely high level of methylating activity that is attributed to nitrosamide or nitrosamine formation in subjects who chewed cola nuts, possibly leading to an increased incidence of oral carcinoma (Atawodi et al., 1995). Cola compounds have also shown antibacterial activity (Ebaba et al., 1991).

Reported uses

Current herbal therapy promotes cola as an antidepressant, antidiarrheal, CNS and cardiac stimulant, diuretic, and aphrodisiac. However, human clinical studies are lacking to support these claims. Traditional uses include treatment of several mood or personality disorders, dyspnea, heart disease, and diarrhea. The most common use has been as a CNS stimulant. Although studies evaluating the CNS and cardiac effects of caffeine have been performed in animals, therapeutic implications for humans have not been established. Anecdotally, the bark has been used to treat wounds, and the root is sometimes chewed to clean teeth and freshen the breath.

Dosage

Fluid extract: 5 to 40 drops (¼ to 2 teaspoons) P.O. up to t.i.d. at meals, with juice or water.
Solid extract: 2 to 8 grains (130 to 520 mg) P.O. per dose.
Decoctions: 1 to 2 teaspoons unextracted powder boiled in 1 cup water for 10 to 15 minutes.
Most commercial preparations are standardized to approximately 10% caffeine content.

Adverse reactions
- Allergic reactions
- Alterations of brain, kidney, liver, and testicular enzyme activity
- Anxiety
- Bradycardia
- Decreased luteinizing hormone release
- Excitation
- Gastric pain (with increased acid secretion)
- Hypertension
- Hypotension
- Nervousness
- Palpitations
- Staining of oral mucosa (bright yellow, when cola nuts chewed)
- Tachycardia

Interactions
Analgesics, antipyretics: may increase the half-life of these agents. Avoid concomitant use.

Contraindications and precautions
Cola nuts or their extracts are contraindicated in pregnant or breast-feeding patients; in those with hypertension, arrhythmias, or gastric ulcer; and in patients at risk of stroke. Also contraindicated in patients allergic to chocolate because cross-sensitivity reactions may occur.

Special considerations
- Know that smokers who also chew cola nuts are at an increased risk of developing oral carcinoma.
- Monitor the cardiac patient for arrhythmias and changes in blood pressure.
- Tell the patient to report changes in mood or behavior.
- Advise the patient with chocolate allergy to avoid this herb.
- Advise the female patient to avoid use of the herb during pregnancy or when breast-feeding.

Points of interest
- Cola nut is considered to be therapeutically useful for mental and physical fatigue according to the German Commission E monograph.

Analysis
The contribution of the cola tree to the Western economy is assured as it is the primary source of caffeine for carbonated soft drinks. Small amounts of cola nut extract are probably harmless, and would be equivalent to a strong cup of coffee or the standard dose of OTC

caffeine products. Other components, whose activities have not been fully investigated, may contribute to as-yet unidentified toxicity.

Although caffeine and theobromine in cola nuts have useful CNS and respiratory system effects, it would be better to select single-ingredient medications that have a standardized dose and known adverse effects. Additional research is required to develop complete adverse effect and toxicity profiles and to identify new antimicrobial activities.

References

Atawodi, S.E., et al. "Nitrosatable Amines and Nitrosamide Formation in Natural Stimulants: *Cola acuminata, C. nitida,* and *Garcinia cola,*" *Food Chem Toxicol* 33:625-30, 1995.

Ebana, R.U., et al. "Microbiological Exploitation of Cardiac Glycosides and Alkaloids from *Garcinia kola, Borreria ocymoides, Kola nitida,* and *Citrus aurantifolia,*" *J Appl Bacteriol* 71:398-401, 1991.

Gaye, F., et al. "Experimental Study of Variations of Salivary pH Affected by Chewing Cola," *Dakar Med* 35:148-55, 1990.

Ibu, J.O., et al. "The Effect of *Cola acuminata* and *Cola nitida* on Gastric Acid Secretion," *Scand J Gastroenterol* 124(Suppl):39-45, 1986.

COLTSFOOT

ASS'S-FOOT, BULLSFOOT, COUGHWORT, FARFARA, FIELDHOVE, FILUIS ANTE PATREM, FOALSWORT, HALLFOOT, HORSE-HOOF, KUANDONG HUA, PAS DÍANE

Common trade names
None known.

Common forms
Available as extract, tincture, syrup, and tea.

Source
Active components are extracted from dried leaves, flowers and, sometimes, roots of *Tussilago farfara,* a low-growing perennial herb that commonly occurs in Europe, England, Canada, and the northern United States.

Chemical components
The plant contains many compounds, including tannins, carotenoids, flavonoids, senkirine, senecionine, tussilagone, a glucoside, phytosteol alcohol, dihydride alcohol, a terpene alcohol, and mucilage.

Actions
The components of *T. farfara* have different pharmacologic effects. Mucilage supplies the demulcent effect of coltsfoot. L-652,469, a re-

cently discovered chemical, acts as a calcium channel blocker and an inhibitor of platelet activation factor, a component in the asthma process, in rabbits and humans (Li et al., 1988). In studies with animals, tussilagone showed a pressor effect similar to that of dopamine but without the tachyphylaxis (Hwang et al., 1987). Other studies have found an anti-inflammatory and gram-negative antibacterial activity.

Senkirkine is thought to cause hepatotoxicity in animals. Urinary bladder papilloma was also observed (Hirono et al., 1976).

Reported uses
Coltsfoot was first used 2,000 years ago in Asia and Europe primarily for asthma, bronchitis, and cough. Although some recommend the herb to be smoked for respiratory relief, heat destroys the mucilage that provides coltsfoot's demulcent effects.

Dosage
Dried herb: 0.6 to 2.9 g P.O. by decoction.
Liquid extract (1:1 in 25% alcohol): 0.6 to 2 ml P.O. t.i.d.
Tincture (1:5 in 45% alcohol): 2 to 8 ml P.O. t.i.d.
Syrup (liquid extract 1:4 in syrup): 2 to 8 ml P.O. t.i.d.
Tea: 1 to 3 teaspoons of dried flowers or leaves in 1 cup of boiling water P.O. t.i.d.

Adverse reactions
- Diarrhea
- Fever
- Increased blood pressure
- Jaundice
- Loss of appetite
- Nausea
- Upper respiratory infection
- Vomiting

Interactions
Antihypertensives: may antagonize hypotensive effects. Avoid concomitant use.

Contraindications and precautions
Avoid use in pregnant or breast-feeding patients; effects are unknown. Use cautiously in patients allergic to other members of the composite family (Compositae), such as chamomile or ragweed, because cross-sensitivity may occur. Also use cautiously in hypertensive patients because of its pressor effect.

Special considerations
• Monitor blood pressure of the patient taking this herb.
• Explain that there are insufficient data regarding coltsfoot's safety and efficacy profiles.
• Assess the patient for jaundice.
• Advise the female patient to avoid use of the herb during pregnancy or when breast-feeding.
• Instruct the patient to report unusual symptoms while taking this or other herbal supplements.
• Tell the patient to avoid coltsfoot if he is allergic to chamomile or ragweed.

Points of interest
• Coltsfoot was once used as a flavoring agent in candy.

Analysis
The little information available about coltsfoot is based on animal research and, therefore, is difficult to extrapolate to humans. Coltsfoot's CV effects and carcinogenic potential, and the risk of an allergic reaction, should be considered before use. Because of the lack of data, the use of coltsfoot cannot currently be recommended. The FDA has classified this herb as of "undefined safety" and Canada has banned its use.

References
Hirono, J., et al. "Carcinogenic Activity of Coltsfoot, *Tussilago farfara*," *Jpn J Cancer Res* 67:125-29, 1976.

Hwang, S., et al. "L-652,469 as a Dual Receptor Antagonist of Platelet Activating Factor and Dihydropyridines from *Tussilago farfara*," *Eur J Pharmacol* 141:269-81, 1987.

Li, Y.P., et al. "Evaluation of Tussilagone: A Cardiovascular-Respiratory Stimulant Isolated from Chinese Herbal Medicine," *Gen Pharmacol* 19:261-63, 1988.

COMFREY

BLACKWORT, BRUISEWORT, KNITBONE, SLIPPERY ROOT

Common trade names
None known.

Common forms
Available as a tea (dried leaf and whole root), blended plant extract also known as "green drink," and a cream.

Source

An oil is extracted from the leaves and roots of *Symphytum officinale*, a member of the Borage family (Boraginaceae). Comfrey is a perennial herb that grows in temperate regions, including western Asia, North America, and Australia.

Chemical components

Comfrey contains a few compounds that show medicinal activity. Mucilage, a mucopolysaccharide of fructose and glucose, is concentrated in the root up to 29%. Allantoin, tannin, pyrrolizidine alkaloids, triterpenoids, asparagine, and a phenolic acid (rosmarinic acid) are also found in the plant.

Actions

Mucilage is reported to possess demulcent properties by forming a protective film, soothing irritation and inflammation. Allantoin is claimed to be a cell-growth stimulator, accounting for the herb's ability to stimulate wound healing. Tannin provides the astringent properties and rosmarinic acid imparts anti-inflammatory properties.

Reported uses

The application of comfrey is limited to claims for healing wounds. Historically, comfrey was used for several internal ailments, such as ulcers of the bowels, stomach, liver, and gallbladder; however, because the alkaloids are converted to toxic metabolites by liver enzymes after being ingested, internal use is no longer recommended.

External application of comfrey products is not considered to be as dangerous as oral administration.

Dosage

The oil from the leaves and root can be incorporated in ointments or as a compress. Although comfrey has been used as a tea, it is not recommended for internal use in the United States or Canada because of its toxicity. Limit external application to 10 days or less.

Adverse reactions

● Carcinogenic potential (caused hepatocellular adenomas and urinary bladder tumors in animals; Hirono et al., 1978)

⚠ Hepatotoxicity: Several studies report on hepatic venoocclusive disease caused by pyrrolizidine alkaloids in the plant (Mattocks, 1980).

Interactions

None reported.

Contraindications and precautions

Internal use of comfrey is contraindicated. Also contraindicated in pregnant or breast-feeding patients and in young children; effects are unknown. Do not use the root for medicinal purposes. Apply the mature leaves externally on intact skin for a limited period of time only.

Special considerations

• Monitor wound appearance and size if the patient is taking this herb to promote healing.
• Assess the patient for signs and symptoms of hepatotoxicity.
• Caution the patient against consumption of the herb.
• Advise the patient to try commercially available antiseptic ointments and creams before attempting to use this herb to promote wound healing.
• Advise the female patient to avoid use of the herb during pregnancy or when breast-feeding.

Analysis

Although comfrey has a long history of therapeutic claims for several ailments, it is potentially hepatotoxic and thus should not be consumed. Anecdotal and reports on animal studies suggest medicinal benefit for wound healing. Commercially available topical antiseptic agents are more likely to be safe and effective.

References

Hirono, I., et al. "Carcinogenic Activity of *Symphytum officinale*," *J Natl Cancer Inst* 61(3):865-69, 1978.
Mattocks, A.R. "Toxic Pyrrolizidine Alkaloids in Comfrey," *Lancet* 11:1136-37, 1980.

CONDURANGO

CONDOR-VINE BARK, CONDURANGO BARK, CONDURANGO BLANCO, EAGLE-VINE BARK, GONOLOBUS CONDURANGO TRIANA, MARSEDENIA CONDURANGO

Common trade names

Conduran, Condurango, Condurango Bark

Common forms

Available as dried or powdered bark, liquid extract, or tincture.

Source

Condurango is the dried bark of *Marsedenia condurango,* a member of the milkweed family (Asclepiedaceae) that is native to Ecuador and other parts of South America.

Chemical components

Condurango contains tannin, small quantities of a strychnine-like alkaloid, caoutchouc, conduragin, condruit, essential oil, phytosterin, resin, sitosterol, and condurangoglycoside (an aglycone). Other components of the bark include vanillin, *p*-coumaric acid, catteic acid, chlorogenic acid, neochlorogenic acid, coumarin, 7-hydroxycoumarin, esculetin, cichorin, and flavonoids.

Actions

Tannic acid has local astringent properties that act on the GI mucosa; it also forms insoluble complexes with some heavy metal ions, alkaloids, and glycosides. Tannic acid has also been shown to have antiulcerogenic and antisecretory effects within the GI tract.

Saponin glycosides, referring to condurangoglycoside, have a bitter taste and are irritating to the mucous membranes. In humans, they are generally nontoxic after oral ingestion; however, they act as potent hemolytics when given I.V. (Budavari, 1996). Coumarin is converted to 7-hydroxycoumarin by the cytochrome P-450 enzyme system (Klaassen, 1996). Although coumarin is considered to be a less active anticoagulant than warfarin, doses of 4 g have been shown to decrease sympathetic nerve activity. The presence of a strychnine-like compound may also contribute to the herb's proposed uses because strychnine (from the dried ripe seed of *Strychnos Nux-vomica*) has been used medicinally as a bitter.

Reported uses

Condurango is mainly used as an astringent, bitter, or appetite stimulator, and promotes functional stomach activity. Its bark is claimed to relax the nerves of the stomach, thus making it suitable for tension- or anxiety-induced indigestion. The herb has also been suggested for use as an analgesic, diuretic, hemostatic, nervine, or tonic.

In the late 1800s, condurango was considered a cure for the early stages of cancers of the breast, epithelium, esophagus, face, lips, neck, pylorus, skin, stomach, and tongue, and also for lymphadenomas. Although human studies are lacking, two glycosides were isolated from condurango bark and found to have antitumor activity against sarcoma-180 and Ehrlich cancers in rats (Hayashi et al., 1980). Natives of South America have used the herb to treat chronic syphilis.

Dosage

Condurango bark: 1 to 4 g P.O.
Tincture: 1 to 2 ml P.O. t.i.d.
Powdered bark: 1 to 2 teaspoonsful mixed with 1 cup boiling water and left to stand for 10 to 15 minutes before consumption.

Adverse reactions
• CNS stimulation (stiff neck and facial muscles, restlessness, excitable reflexes, seizures)
• Visual disturbances, vertigo, sweating, and increased urine output (after ingestion of 12 g of bark)
⚠ Poisoning from conduragin ingestion (bark compound believed to be a violent poison)
⚠ Seizures ending in paralysis (after conduragin ingestion and overdoses of bark itself)

Interactions
None reported, although the potential for drug interactions exists.
Agents using the CYP2A6 enzyme system (carbamazepine, paroxetine, ritonavir, sertraline): altered metabolism of these agents because coumarin also uses this pathway. Avoid concomitant use.
Iron-containing products, alkaloid-related substances (atropine, scopolamine), medicinal glycosides (digoxin): prevention of absorption of these drugs when used with condurango. Avoid concomitant use.

Contraindications and precautions
Contraindicated in patients with preexisting hepatic disorders or disease. Parenteral administration of tannic acid has been used as an experimental hepatotoxin. Also contraindicated in patients with a history of seizures or other disorders of the nervous system and in pregnant or breast-feeding patients.

Use cautiously in patients with preexisting hepatic disease or who are also taking other medications metabolized by the cytochrome P-450 enzyme system.

Special considerations
• Discontinue the herb immediately if an abnormal increase in liver transaminases occurs.
• An abnormal change in the therapeutic levels of other concurrent medications may occur because of competition for metabolism through the cytochrome P-450 enzyme system.
• Advise the patient to report symptoms of hepatic injury (right upper-quadrant pain, jaundice, fever) and other adverse effects immediately.
• Instruct the patient to immediately discontinue the herb if muscle stiffness or rigidity, excitable reflexes, or seizures occur.
• Advise the patient to avoid hazardous activities, such as driving, until tolerance to the herb is known.
• Advise the female patient to avoid use during pregnancy or when breast-feeding.

Analysis

Human studies are lacking. Antitumor activity was reported in rats (Hayashi et al., 1980). Excessive amounts of the herb are not recommended because of the risk for adverse reactions on the liver, interactions with drugs metabolized through the cytochrome P-450 enzyme system, and possible stimulant effects on the CNS.

References

Hayashi, K., et al. "Antitumor Active Glycosides from Condurango Cortex," *Chem Pharm Bull* 28:1954-58, 1980.
Klaassen, C.D. *Casarett and Doull's Toxicology: The Basic Science of Poisons.* 5th ed. New York: McGraw-Hill Book Co., 1996.

CORIANDER

CHINESE PARSLEY, CILANTRO, ORIANDER

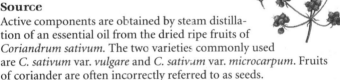

Common trade names
None known.

Common forms
Available as a crude extract of the fruits.

Source
Active components are obtained by steam distillation of an essential oil from the dried ripe fruits of *Coriandrum sativum.* The two varieties commonly used are *C. sativum* var. *vulgare* and *C. sativum* var. *microcarpum.* Fruits of coriander are often incorrectly referred to as seeds.

Chemical components
Fruits contain a volatile oil. Major components of the oil include coriandrol, monoterpene hydrocarbons, alpha pinene, limonene, phellandrene, camphene, terpinene, para cymene, borneol, camphor, geraniol, carvone, and geranyl acetate; anethole, caryophyllene oxide, and elemol. Other components in fruit include oleic, petroselinic and linolenic acids; sitosterols, triacontanol, tricosanol, tricontane, octadecenoic acid, proteins, starch, sugars, coumarins, psoralen, angelicin, scopoletin, and umbeliferone; flavonoid glycosides (quercetin 3-glucuronide, isoquercetin, coriandrinol, rutin); tannins; chlorogenic and caffeic acids.

Generally, the composition of the leaves is similar to the fruit, except that there is less volatile oil and more protein; ascorbic acid is also present in the leaves.

Actions

Coriander has been reported to possess several potentially beneficial pharmacologic effects. These effects have been shown in animal and laboratory models and include cytotoxic and lipolytic activity, hypoglycemic effects, and larvicidal, antifungal, and antibacterial activity.

Coriander oil was observed in vitro to suppress the formation of DNA adducts by acting on microsomal enzymes, and may signal a potential use as an anticarcinogen (Hashim et al., 1994). Aqueous extracts of fresh coriander produced a dose-dependent anti-implantation effect but failed to produce complete infertility in rats (Al-Said et al., 1987).

Reported uses

Coriander is usually used with other ingredients as a flavoring agent. The fruits are used extensively in all types of food dishes. In Oriental cooking, coriander is referred to as Chinese parsley; in Spanish cooking, it is called cilantro. It is also popular as a flavoring agent in beverages, frozen dairy desserts, candy, puddings, gelatins, and relishes. The oil is used in creams, lotions, and perfumes (maximum 0.6%), and sometimes added to tobacco. Coriander is claimed to be effective as an anthelmintic and antiarthritic and in enhancing the functional activity of the stomach.

Dosage

No consensus exists.

Interactions

Hypoglycemic agents: enhanced hypoglycemic effect. Monitor blood glucose levels closely during coriander use.

Adverse reactions

- Allergic reactions to the essential oils
- Fatty infiltration of liver

Contraindications and precautions

Avoid use of the herb in pregnant or breast-feeding patients; effects are unknown.

Special considerations

- Explain that insufficient evidence exists to support a role for coriander for medicinal purpose.
- Advise the patient not to ingest more of this herb than that commonly found in foodstuffs because of potential untoward pharmacologic effects.
- Advise the female patient to avoid use of the herb during pregnancy or when breast-feeding.

Points of interest
• The highest reported levels of coriander in foodstuffs are 0.52% (fruits) in meat products and 0.12% (oil) in alcoholic beverages.

Analysis
Coriander is most appropriately used as a flavoring agent. There are no human data for its effectiveness for other purposes.

References
Al-Said, M.S., et al. "Post-coital Antifertility Activity of the Seeds of *Coriandrum sativum* in Rats," *J Ethnopharmacol* 21:165-73, 1987.

Hashim, S., et al. "Modulatory Effects of Essential Oils from Spices on the Formation of DNA Adduct by Aflatoxin B$_1$ In Vitro," *Nutr Cancer* 21:169-75, 1994.

CORKWOOD
CORKWOOD TREE, PITURI

Common trade names
None known.

Common forms
Available as an extract of the corkwood tree (leaves and stems) in tablets and liquid.

Source
The active ingredients are extracted from the leaves, stems, and root bark of *Duboisia myoporoides*, a member of the Solanaceae family that is native to Australia.

Chemical components
The corkwood tree is a rich source of alkaloids and has been used as a commercial source of scopolamine. The major alkaloids found in young leaves and stems are valtropine and scopolamine; other alkaloids—trigloyl tropine, valeroidine, and hyoscyamine—occur in lesser quantities. Alkaloids extracted from older leaves and stems include scopolamine, valtropine, hyoscyamine, butropine, poroidine, valeroidine, acetyl tropine, noratropine, isoporoidine, apohyoscine, and tropine. The young root and bark of the tree yield tropine, valtropine, hyoscyamine, valeroidine, atropine, scopolamine, and apohyoscine. Similar alkaloids are found in old root and bark samples. Nicotine and nornicotine have also been reported in the leaves (Coulsen and Griffin, 1967, 1968).

Actions
Scopolamine and the other alkaloids found in corkwood are antimuscarinic or muscarinic cholinergic blocking agents, and exhibit a wide range of pharmacologic effects. When taken in therapeutic doses, scopolamine may cause drowsiness and a dream-like state. However, larger doses may result in excitement or restlessness and hallucinations. These antimuscarinic agents may also affect heart rate, reduce gastric and salivary secretions and GI motility, and cause pupillary dilatation and blurred vision due to cycloplegia.

Reported uses
The corkwood tree was principally used as a main source of scopolamine and atropine before the availability of other commercial sources. Scopolamine is commonly used for the prevention of motion-induced nausea and vomiting, and atropine has limited use in treating GI motility disturbances. It has been reported that the corkwood leaves were chewed by native Australians for their stimulant effects and also used in hunting to stun animals. Extracts of the leaves have been used medicinally as a substitute for atropine.

Dosage
No consensus exists. The leaves have been chewed for their stimulant effect.

Adverse reactions
Adverse reactions from corkwood alkaloids are related to their antimuscarinic action. (See *Hyoscine poisoning from corkwood.*)
• Alterations in heart rate
• Blurred vision
• Constipation
• Cycloplegia
• Disorientation
• Drowsiness
• Dry mouth or skin
• Euphoria
• Excitation (in high doses)
• Fatigue
• Hallucinations (in high doses)
• Urine retention

Interactions
Amantadine, beta blockers, digoxin, tricyclic antidepressants and other drugs with anticholinergic or anticholinergic-like effects: enhanced anticholinergic-like effects. Avoid concomitant use.

RESEARCH FINDINGS
Hyoscine poisoning from corkwood

In 1981, four case reports described accidental and occupational exposure to the corkwood tree or leaves, resulting in clinical hyoscine poisoning. During the harvesting of commercially grown trees in Australia, exposure to the dust and leaf particles led to mydriasis and cycloplegia ("cork-eye") in workers. Exposure of several hours resulted in dry mouth, facial flushing, delirium, depression, irrational behavior, or withdrawal. This syndrome has been described as being "corked up" (Pearn, 1981).

Ingestion of a mixture of boiled corkwood leaves and coffee has been shown to cause hallucinations and intoxication-like behavior. Dilated pupils have been noted in children at schools near commercial corkwood tree farms. No specific treatments were described and patients recovered after several hours of nonexposure to corkwood.

Contraindications and precautions

The herb and its products are contraindicated in patients hypersensitive to antimuscarinic agents; in those with glaucoma, CV disease, obstructive GI conditions, myasthenia gravis, obstructive uropathy or renal disease, or other medical conditions that may be exacerbated by antimuscarinic agents; and in pregnant or breast-feeding patients.

Special considerations

• Consider exposure to this agent if the patient manifests pupillary, vision, or behavioral changes.
• Advise the patient already receiving anticholinergic-like agents to avoid taking corkwood because of risk of enhanced anticholinergic effects.
• Caution patient who may be at risk for disease exacerbation or adverse effects from anticholinergic drugs against use of the herb.
• Advise the female patient to avoid use of the herb during pregnancy or when breast-feeding.

Analysis

Although corkwood leaves and stems have been used for medicinal purposes, primarily as an atropine substitute, no clinical studies of the plant have been undertaken. Antimuscarinic toxicity has been reported following occupational or accidental exposure, with absorption though the mucous membranes and upper respiratory tract. Medicinal use of the plant is currently not recommended.

References

Coulsen, J.F., and Griffin, W.J. "The Alkaloids of *Duboisia myoporoides*. I. Aerial Parts," *Planta Med* 15:459-466, 1967.

Coulsen J.F. and Griffin W.J. "The Alkaloids of *Duboisia myoporoides*. II. Roots," *Planta Med* 16:174-81, 1968.

Pearn, J. "Corked Up: Clinical Hyoscine Poisoning with Alkaloids of the Native Corkwood, *Duboisia*," *Med J Aust* 2:422-23, 1981.

COUCHGRASS

DOG GRASS, QUACK GRASS, *TRITICUM*, TWITCHGRASS, WHEAT GRASS

Common trade names
(Various manufacturers; available in combination) Aqua-Rid, Arcocaps, Diuplex

Common forms
Capsules: 380 mg
Tablets: 60 mg

Source
Most medicinal products use the roots of *Agropyron repens*. Couchgrass is commonly found in Europe and has been introduced to the United States.

Chemical components
Couchgrass contains fructose, glucose, mannitol, inositol and triticin, a carbohydrate similar to inulin, and pectin. Other compounds include unspecified cyanogenetic glycosides, tricin and other flavonoids, and saponins. Volatile oils include agropyrene (95%), carvacrol, trans-anethole, carvone, thymol, menthol, menthone, p-cymene and sesquiterpenes, fixed oil, and a vanillin glucoside.

Actions
Couchgrass is believed to induce mild diuretic and sedative effects in rats. Antimicrobial activity has been reported with agropyrene. Very weak anti-inflammatory activity was documented in the carrageenan-induced rat-paw edema model.

Reported uses
Couchgrass has been used as a mild diuretic. Other claimed uses include treatment of urinary tract infections, cystitis, premenstrual syndrome, and arthritis (Reynolds, 1996).

Dosage
Manufacturers of Diuplex suggest 2 to 3 tablets P.O. once or twice daily (360 mg daily).

Adverse reactions
• Contact dermatitis
• Electrolyte depletion

Interactions
None reported.

Contraindications and precautions
Avoid use of the herb in pregnant or breast-feeding patients; effects are unknown. Use cautiously because there is a risk of ergot toxicity because of contamination of the couchgrass' grain with a fungus containing ergot.

Special considerations
• If unprocessed couchgrass is used, discard those with black spores.
• Monitor the patient for signs of ergot poisoning.
• Warn the patient of the potential for ergot poisoning.
• Advise the female patient to avoid use of the herb during pregnancy or when breast-feeding.

Analysis
Information regarding the safety and efficacy of this agent is scant. No clinical trials or published case reports were found.

References
Reynolds, J., ed. *Martindale: The Extra Pharmacopoeia,* 21st ed. London: Royal Pharmaceutical Society of Great Britain, 1996.

COWSLIP

AMERICAN COWSLIP, ARTETYKE, ARTHRITICA, BUCKLES, CREWEL, DRELIP, FAIRY CUP, HERB PETER, KEY OF HEAVEN, KEYFLOWER, MAY BLOB, MAYFLOWER, OUR LADY'S KEYS, PAIGLE, PALSYWORT, PASSWORD, PEAGLE, PETTY MULLEINS, PLUMROCKS

Common trade names
None known.

Common forms
Available as dried flowers and liquid extracts.

Source
Active components are derived from the flowers of *Primula veris,* which is native to the mountains of western North America.

Chemical components
Cowslip contains many compounds, including carbohydrates (galactose, glucose, xylose, and others); flavonoids (apigenin, luteolin, kaempferol, quercetin); phenols (primulaveroside and primveroside); primin, a quinone; saponins; tannins; silicic acid; and a volatile oil identical to mannitol.

Actions
Cowslip is claimed to impart sedative, diuretic, antispasmodic, and expectorant properties. Saponins are not well absorbed orally, but cause GI irritation.

Studies with animals have suggested that saponins in cowslip produce both hypo- and hypertensive effects (Cebo et al., 1976). In vitro studies suggest the saponins inhibit prostaglandin synthetase, imparting a weak anti-inflammatory and analgesic effect (Cebo et al., 1976). Flavonoids may be responsible for anti-inflammatory and antispasmodic activity. Tannins typically exhibit astringent properties.

Reported uses
The claims that cowslip is effective as a sedative-hypnotic to treat insomnia, hysteria, and anxiety associated with restlessness and irritability are based on traditional folklore medicine and animal studies. Human clinical trials are lacking.

Dosage
Dried flowers: 1 to 2 g P.O. as an infusion t.i.d.
Liquid extract (1:1 solution in 25% alcohol): 1 to 2 ml P.O. t.i.d.

Adverse reactions
- Contact dermatitis (Primin is a potential contact allergen.)
- Diarrhea
- Hemolysis
- Hepatotoxicity (possibly due to tannin content)
- Nausea
- Vomiting

⚠ Severe GI irritation (Raw cowslip leaves are thought to cause severe GI symptoms and may compromise heart function.)

Interactions
Antihypertensives: may interfere with therapy. Avoid concomitant use.

Diuretics: may potentiate effects. Avoid concomitant use.
Sedatives: may potentiate effects of other sedative agents. Avoid concomitant use.

Contraindications and precautions
Avoid use of the herb in pregnant or breast-feeding patients; effects are unknown.

Special considerations
• Monitor the patient for allergic reactions, adverse GI effects, and hepatotoxicity.
• Explain that the safety of cowslip has not been established.
• Advise the female patient to avoid use of the herb during pregnancy or when breast-feeding.

Analysis
Little information is available regarding cowslip's chemical and pharmacologic properties. Because safety data are lacking, large doses and prolonged use of cowslip is not recommended.

References
Cebo, B., et al. "Pharmacologic Properties of Saponin Fraction from Polish Crude Drugs," *Herb Pol* 22:154-62, 1976.

CRANBERRY

BOG CRANBERRY, ISOKARPALO (FINLAND), MARSH APPLE, MOUNTAIN CRANBERRY, PIKKUKARPALO (FINLAND), SMALL CRANBERRY

Common trade names
(Various manufacturers; available in combination) Cranberry Power, Cranberry Whole Fruit, Cran Relief, Cran-Tastic

Common forms
Capsules: 475 mg, 500 mg
Juices: usually 10% to 20% pure
Also available as powdered concentrates of varying strengths.

Source
Cranberries are trailing evergreen shrubs that grow in various climates, most notably in acidic bogs, from Tennessee to Alaska. The juice or powdered concentrate of *Vaccinium macrocarpon, V. oxycoccus,* and *V. erythrocarpum* is made from whole berries (fruit); the skins and seeds are then screened out.

Chemical components

Cranberry juice contains many compounds, some of which are considered active. Citric, malic, quinic, and benzoic acids are present. Quinic and benzoic acids break down and form hippuric acid found in urine. Carbohydrates, especially fructose and oligosaccharides, are considered active ingredients for antibacterial activity. Anthocyanin and proanthocyanidins are also found in cranberry. The berries are a minor source of ascorbic acid.

Actions

Studies in mice and humans have demonstrated cranberry's ability to interfere with bacterial adherence to uroepithelial surfaces. In vitro studies using extracts of *Vaccinium* fruits (blueberries and cranberries) have shown possible antitumor activity.

Reported uses

Cranberry has been proposed as a nonantibiotic treatment to prevent urinary tract infections (UTI) and has a 100-year history of being used to prevent recurrent UTI. (See *Cranberry juice and urinary tract infection.*) Mice given cranberry juice as a water supply demonstrated that bacterial adherence was significantly inhibited in urine (Sobota, 1984). Human clinical trials have also been promising.

Although Europeans have proposed cranberry as an anticancer drug, well-designed trials are lacking. Cranberry has been proposed to help urostomy patients with skin irritations from urine. It has also been used in drug overdose cases to help with urinary excretion of phencyclidine.

Dosage

Most studies gave patients between 10 and 16 oz juice P.O. daily or 1 to 2 capsules of concentrate P.O. daily.

Adverse reactions

Cranberry is well tolerated, except for possible diarrhea if excessive quantities are ingested.

Interactions

No significant drug interactions identified. Although not specifically documented, cranberry has the potential to enhance elimination of some drugs normally excreted in urine.

Contraindications and precautions

Use cautiously in patients with benign prostatic hypertrophy and urinary obstruction.

RESEARCH FINDINGS
Cranberry juice and urinary tract infection

Many urinary tract infections (UTI) are caused by enteric flora, and about half are caused by *Escherichia coli*. The bacterium uses surface pili (fimbrie) to attach to carbohydrate structures on the uroepithelial cell lining of the urinary tract. The two most common fimbrie types are a mannose-sensitive type I fimbrie and the P fimbrie.

Extracts of *Vaccinium* fruits have been found to inhibit *E. coli* adhesion (Ofek et al., 1996). Cranberry juice has two chemical components that can affect the ability of the bacteria to adhere to the cell lining. Fructose, found in many fruit juices, inhibits mannose-sensitive type I fimbrie. A large-molecular-weight compound similar to the Tumms-Harefall glycoprotein inhibits P fimbrie. Only blueberries and cranberries of the *Vaccinium* type contain both fructose and the large-molecular-weight compound.

Because approximately 25% of isolates have different adhesion characteristics, future studies that include S-type fimbrie will help clarify cranberry's true role in the treatment of UTI.

The most notable recent clinical trial involved 153 women (Avorn et al., 1994). Patients drank 300 ml of juice daily for 6 months. The placebo drink was similar in taste and color to the actual juice. Results showed the presence of bacteria in the urine in 28% of the placebo group compared with 15% in the cranberry group. Antibiotics were needed for 16 members of the placebo group but only 8 of the cranberry group. Bacteriuria persisted in just 25% of the patients taking cranberry juice compared with almost 100% of the placebo group.

Special considerations
• Counsel the diabetic patient (prone to UTI) to use sugar-free versions, thus minimizing carbohydrate load.
• Advise the patient to drink sufficient fluids to ensure adequate urine flow.
• Remind the patient to notify the primary health care provider if signs of an unresolving UTI (painful urination, urinary bleeding) develop, continue, or worsen.

Points of interest
• The ability of cranberry juice to prevent UTI was noted in 1840 by German scientists who found hippuric acid in the urine of persons consuming the fruit juice. For 100 years, the acidifying and bacteriostatic action of hippuric acid was believed to be caused by anti-

bacterial action. However, during the 1960s, it was found that the hippuric acid concentration was too low to be bacteriostatic and another explanation was pursued.

Analysis

For acute UTI, certain antibiotics remain the mainstay of treatment. However, cranberry juice may be useful as prophylaxis for patients especially prone to UTI, such as diabetics, who are two to three times more prone than nondiabetics. Considering the disadvantages of chronic antibiotic prophylaxis (cost, adverse effects, and promotion of bacterial resistance), consumption of cranberry juice appears to be a safe, inexpensive, and reasonably effective alternative. With future studies, cranberry might be found to be beneficial for patients suffering from conditions of urine retention (such as males with an enlarged prostate or those with spina bifida or diabetes).

References

Avorn, J., et al. "Reduction of Bacteriuria and Pyuria After Ingestion of Cranberry Juice," *JAMA* 271:751-54, 1994.

Ofek, I., et al. "Anti-*Escherichia coli* Adhesion Activity of Cranberry and Blueberry Juices," *Adv Exp Med Biol* 408:179-83, 1996.

Sobota, A.E. "Inhibition of Bacterial Adherence by Cranberry Juice: Potential Use for the Treatment of Urinary Tract Infections," *J Urol* 131:1013-16, 1984.

CREATINE MONOHYDRATE

CREATINE

Common trade names

(Available in combination) Advanced Genetics, Bio-Tech, Champion's Choice, GNC Pro Performance Labs, ISP Nutrition, Joe Weider, Labrada, Metaform, Muscle Tribe, Nature's Best, Universal Nutrition, VitaLife Sport Products

Common forms

Tablets: 2.5 g, 5 g
Powder: 1 teaspoon contains 5 g

Source

Creatine is found in dietary sources such as red meat, milk, and fish. The human body also synthesizes endogenous creatine in the kidney, liver, and pancreas.

Chemical components

Creatine is an amino acid synthesized from the amino acid precursors, arginine and glycine. The highest levels of creatine are found in skeletal muscle, mostly in the form of creatine phosphate. High levels also occur in cardiac and smooth muscle, brain, kidney and spermatozoa; data suggest that creatine amounts in muscle is varied.

Actions

Ingestion of creatine monohydrate increases cellular levels of creatine and creatine phosphate, which maintains high intracellular levels of adenosine triphosphate (ATP), the principal energy source for muscle contraction. As ATP stores become depleted, muscle fatigue ensues. Regeneration of the ATP stores, at a similar rate as ATP hydrolysis, may delay onset of muscle fatigue. The phosphate from creatine phosphate is transferred to adenosine diphosphate, restorating ATP and releasing free creatine. Creatine phosphate also transfers ATP equivalents from within the mitochondria to the cytoplasm, where ATP is needed for cellular metabolism.

Studies of oral absorption of creatine show that it increases the plasma creatine pool. Low doses of creatine monohydrate produced only a moderate rise in plasma creatine, whereas higher doses resulted in a larger increase. Repeated dosing maintained plasma levels. Oral supplementation also significantly increased total creatine content of skeletal muscle, with the greatest changes in those subjects with low initial total creatine content (Harris et al., 1992).

Reported uses

Creatine is used to enhance exercise performance. It has been shown to improve short-term or intermittent, high-intensity exercise performance such as weightlifting and short-distance running. (See *Creatine and muscle strength enhancement,* page 206.)

In a study using a standardized isotonic exercise-resistance measurement, a significant increase in one repetition maximum free weight bench press was observed. Other anaerobic indices, such as weightlifting repetitions and total weightlifting volume, also showed significant improvements (Earnest et al., 1995). The benefit of creatinine in high-intensity performance exercise with repeated bouts of exercise was also demonstrated by Harris and colleagues (Harris et al., 1993).

Dosage

The amount of creatine ingested in a nonvegetarian diet is 2 g daily. The recommended dose to achieve an ergogenic effect is a loading dose of 15 to 20 g daily taken for the first 5 days, then 5 to 10 g daily as a maintenance dose. Other dose recommendations are 5 to 30 g daily or 2 to 4 g as a chronic supplement. Most clinical trials have used a dose of 20 to 25 g daily for 5 days and then measured exercise performance. Because creatine is a low-molecular-weight com-

RESEARCH FINDINGS

Creatine and muscle strength enhancement

A small, double-blind, placebo-controlled study evaluated the effect of creatine supplementation on muscle strength (Greenhaff et al., 1993). Twelve subjects undertook five bouts of 30 maximal voluntary isokinetic contractions of the knee extensor muscle, interspersed with 1-minute recovery periods, before and after 5 days of placebo or oral creatine. Knee extensor muscle torque—measured by an isokinetic dynamometer—plasma ammonia, and blood lactate accumulation were checked during and after every exercise on each treatment.

The highest torque in all patients was recorded during the initial repetition of each of the five exercise bouts and then declined progressively with each exercise bout. The normal decline in peak torque between the first and last bout was about 30%. No differences were found between the peak torque generated during the exercise bouts before and after ingestion of placebo.

Total peak torque was significantly higher in patients taking creatine for both the second and third bouts of exercise compared with corresponding bouts of exercise before creatine supplementation. No differences were noted in blood lactate accumulation; however, plasma ammonia levels were significantly lower after the fourth and fifth bouts of exercise following creatine ingestion. The authors concluded that creatine enhanced muscular strength.

pound and readily excreted by the kidneys, ingestion of doses over 20 g daily is not valuable.

Adverse reactions
• Dehydration
• GI upset (stomach pain, bloating, diarrhea)
• Increased body weight (perhaps due to water rather than increased muscle mass)
• Muscle cramping

Interactions
Caffeine: may reduce or abolish ergogenic effect of creatine. Avoid concomitant use.

Glucose: may increase creatine storage in muscle. Increase in muscle creatine accumulation because of carbohydrate ingestion may result from a stimulatory effect of insulin on muscle creatine transport. Avoid concomitant use.

Contraindications and precautions

Use cautiously in patients with renal disease because creatine is excreted in the urine. Avoid use of creatine in pregnant or breast-feeding patients; effects are unknown.

Special considerations

• Monitor young athletes for overuse or abuse of this agent.
• Know that urinary excretion of creatinine does not indicate declining renal function. It correlates with the increase in muscle creatine storage seen during creatine supplementation, and reflects the increased rate of muscle creatine degradation to creatinine.
• Athletes participating in a resistance-training program may benefit from creatine supplementation because it allows them to complete workouts at a higher level of intensity and strength.
• Creatine is not on the International Olympic Committee Drug list, but some consider it in a gray zone between doping and substances allowed to enhance performance.
• Advise the patient to avoid long-term (over 30 days) use of this agent until effects are known.
• Tell the patient with renal disease to ingest smaller quantities of creatine, if at all.
• Inform the patient to stop the supplementation or take smaller daily amounts if muscle cramping occurs.
• Remind the patient that this agent is useful only for exercise that is of an intense nature and short duration, or when short bursts of strength are necessary (such as weightlifting, sprinting, or ice hockey).
• Advise the parents of athletes who may take this drug about its action, potential adverse effects, and proper use.

Points of interest

• Anecdotally, low-dose supplementation for 30 days results in increased total muscle creatine stores at a much lower rate than aggressive and higher loading doses. Most creatine uptake appears to occur during the first few days. The kidneys readily excrete creatine not retained by tissues. Because the storage and response to creatine is varied, 20% to 30% of patients may not respond to creatine supplementation.
• Even though creatine was discovered nearly 160 years ago, clinical trials in humans studying its effect on exercise performance were not conducted until 1992.
• A single 5-g dose of oral creatine monohydrate is equivalent to the creatine content of about 2.4 lb (1 kg) of uncooked steak.

Analysis

Although studies have shown that creatine supplementation improves high-intensity intermittent exercise performance, its use in enhancing aerobic exercise or endurance exercise performance is unclear and probably insignificant. Improvement in strength is most likely related to an increase in the rate of phosphocreatine resynthesis from creatine stores during recovery between short-duration, high-intensity exercise.

Because the normal creatine content of muscle varies, response to creatine supplementation is also varied. It appears that patients who start with low creatine levels benefit more from supplementation than those with higher baseline creatine levels. However, the long-term safety of creatine is unknown. Until then, use of this agent cannot be recommended.

References

Earnest, C.P., et al. "The Effect of Oral Creatine Monohydrate Ingestion on Anaerobic Power Indices, Muscular Strength, and Body Composition," *Acta Physiol Scand* 153:207-09, 1995.

Greenhaff, P.L., et al. "Influence of Oral Creatine Supplementation of Muscle Torque During Repeated Bouts of Maximal Voluntary Exercise in Man," *Clin Sci* 84:565-71, 1993.

Harris, R.C., et al. "Elevation of Creatine in Resting and Exercised Muscle of Normal Subjects by Creatine Supplementation," *Clin Sci* 83:367-74, 1992.

Harris, R.C., et al. "The Effects of Oral Creatine Supplementation on Running Performance During Maximal Short Term Exercise in Man," *J Physiol* 467:P74, 1993.

CUCUMBER

WILD COWCUMBER

Common trade names

None known.

Common forms

Available as seeds and juice; used as an ingredient in many cosmetics.

Source

Several active components are derived from the seeds and fruits of *Cucumis sativus,* a low-growing annual vegetable native to northern India.

Chemical components

The cucumber plant is composed mainly of water. The seeds and leaves contain compounds that inhibit trypsin and chymotrypsin.

Seeds contain a fatty oil, proteins, cucurbitin (a glycoside), and resin. The raw juice is reported to contain a mild diuretic.

Actions
The cucumber seeds contain cucurbitin and fatty oil, and possess mild diuretic properties in animals. The purported soothing topical effects of the plant are probably due to its water content.

Reported uses
Some sources claim that cucumber is "nature's best diuretic." However, this claim is not based on human clinical trials but on anecdotal evidence (Liener, 1980). Cucumber is high in potassium, and has been used to correct both high and low blood pressure, although without clinical verification. Cucumber has been used in topical products to soothe irritated skin and is included in face-cleansing cosmetics. The seeds are reported to have cooling and anthelmintic properties.

Dosage
As a diuretic agent, 1 to 2 oz of ground seed is steeped in water and then consumed.
As a cosmetic, the juice is extracted and applied topically.

Adverse reactions
None reported, but fluid and electrolyte loss is possible.

Interactions
Diuretics: may potentiate the effects of fluid and electrolyte loss of other diuretic agents. Avoid concomitant use.

Contraindications and precautions
Avoid use of the herb in pregnant or breast-feeding patients; effects are unknown.

Special considerations
• Monitor the patient periodically for serum electrolytes if excessive quantities are being consumed.
• Inform the patient about the lack of clinical data on this plant.
• Advise the patient that proven and safe diuretic agents are available.
• Advise the female patient to avoid use of the herb during pregnancy or when breast-feeding.

Points of interest
• Cucumbers have a long and distinguished history. They originated in northern India, where they were domesticated over 3,000 years

ago. History records a few noteworthy cucumber fanatics, including the Roman emperor Tiberius, who ate some daily; his gardeners were ordered to find ways to grow them out of season. Even Columbus included them in his experimental gardens on Hispaniola (Haiti) during his second voyage in 1494.

Analysis

There are few clinical data to substantiate medicinal or therapeutic claims for cucumber. Standardized, safe, and effective diuretics eliminate the need to use cucumber for this purpose.

References

Liener, I.E. *Toxic Components of Plant Foodstuffs*. London: Academic Press, 1980.

DAFFODIL
DAFFYDOWN-DILLY, FLEUR DE COUCOU, LENT LILY,
NARCISSUS, PORILLON

Common trade names
None known.

Common forms
None known.

Source
Active components are derived from powders or extracts of the
flowers of *Narcissus pseudonarcissus,* of the Narcissus family
(Amaryllidaceae), common in Europe and the United States.

Chemical components
A crystalline alkaloid, narcisssine, has been isolated from daffodil
bulbs and is identical to lycorine, isolated from *Lycoris radiata.* Other
alkaloids (masonin and homolycorin) and a lectin, known as *Narcissus pseudonarcissus* agglutinin (NPA), have also been found in the
bulbs. Crystals of calcium oxalate have been noted in plant sap.

Actions
Daffodil preparations have astringent properties. Narcissine (lycorine)
acts as an emetic. In one study, extracts containing masonin and homolycorin were found to induce delayed hypersensitivity in guinea
pigs. NPA binds to alpha$_2$-macroglobulin and to glycoprotein 120 of
the HIV in vitro. NPA is inhibitory to HIV-1, HIV-2, and cytomegalovirus (CMV) infections in vitro. NPA also inhibits rabies virus at-
tachment to susceptible cells as well as rubella virus multiplication in
vitro (Balzarini et al., 1991).

Reported uses
Historically, preparations made from boiled daffodil bulbs were
used as an emetic. Plasters made from the bulbs were used locally
for wounds, burns, strains, and joint pain. The powdered flowers
have been used as an emetic. Infusions or syrups have been used in
pulmonary congestion.

NPA, the lectin isolated from daffodil bulbs, is used in biochemical research for its ability to bind with glycoconjugates occurring on viruses such as HIV-1 and HIV-2, simian immunodeficiency virus, CMV, rabies, and rubella. NPA has been used to develop novel enzyme-linked immunoassays for quantitation of envelope glycoprotein 120 on HIV (Balzarini et al., 1991).

Dosage
Some sources give 20 grains to 2 drams of powdered flowers, 2 to 3 grains of extract P.O. as an emetic.

Adverse reactions
• Contact dermatitis (Gude et al., 1988)
• Hypersalivation
• Miosis
• Nausea
• Vomiting
⚠ Respiratory or CV collapse
⚠ Narcissine (lycorine) causes eventual collapse and death by paralysis of the CNS. Accidental poisoning by daffodil bulbs has been reported in Switzerland, Germany, Finland, Sweden, the Netherlands, Britain, and the United States.

Interactions
None reported.

Contraindications and precautions
Daffodil flowers and bulbs are poisonous. Ingestion of even small quantities can lead to rapid death. Avoid use of the herb in pregnant or breast-feeding patients; effects are unknown.

Special considerations
• Caution the patient against consumption of any part of this plant.
• Warn the patient to keep plant parts out of reach of children and pets.
• Advise the female patient to avoid use of the herb during pregnancy or when breast-feeding.

Points of interest
• Daffodil bulbs have been mistaken for onions in cases of accidental poisonings.

Analysis
In vitro studies showing the inhibitory effects of a daffodil-derived lectin on HIV and CMV infections indicate potential in biochemical research and in the development of new immunoassays for these

viruses; however, there is insufficient evidence for future therapeutic use. Therapeutic claims are anecdotal and not based on controlled human trials. Daffodil plants are toxic and caution should be used when handling them. This plant is not recommended for internal use.

References

Balzarini, J., et al. "Alpha-(1,3)- and Alpha-(1-6)-mannose Specific Plant Lectins are Markedly Inhibitory to Human Immunodeficiency Virus and Cytomegalovirus Infections In Vitro," *Antimicrob Agents Chemother* 35:410-16, 1991.

Gude, M., et al. "An Investigation of the Irritant and Allergenic Properties of Daffodils (*Narcissus pseudonarcissus* L., Amaryllidaceae). A Review of Daffodil Dermatitis," *Contact Dermatitis* 19:1-10, 1988.

DAISY

BAIRNWORT, BRUISEWORT, COMMON DAISY, DAY'S EYE

Common trade names
None known.

Common forms
None known.

Source
Several chemical compounds are derived from the fresh or dried flowers and leaves of *Bellis perennis*, a common perennial herb.

Chemical components
The flower heads contain saponins, tannin, organic acids, an essential oil, bitter principle, flavones, and mucilage.

Actions
Daisy is claimed to have astringent and anti-inflammatory properties.

Reported uses
The Iroquois Indians used the daisy as a GI aid. It has also been used as an expectorant, astringent, mild analgesic, antidiarrheal, antitussive, and an antispasmotic. When used as an infusion in the home, daisy was reported to treat catarrh, arthritis, rheumatism, liver and kidney disorders, diarrhea, and act as a blood purifier.

The plant also has been reportedly used externally in compresses and bath preparations for the treatment of skin disorders, wounds, and bruises (Launert, 1981).

Dosage
Tincture: 2 to 4 ml t.i.d.
Infusion: 1 teaspoon of dried herb steeped in boiling water for 10 minutes and taken t.i.d.

Adverse reactions
None reported.

Interactions
None reported.

Contraindications and precautions
Avoid use of the herb in pregnant or breast-feeding patients; effects are unknown.

Special considerations
• Although daisy has been used as food in some parts of the world, pharmacologic effects are largely undocumented. Therefore, use with caution.
• Monitor the patient taking this herb for adverse effects.
• Advise the female patient to avoid use of the herb during pregnancy or when breast-feeding.

Analysis
Although the daisy has a long history of anecdotal safety, no clinical data exist to substantiate the claims for medicinal purposes. Moreover, its chemical components have not been well described.

References
Launert, E. *The Hamlyn Guide to Edible and Medicinal Plants of Britain and Northern Europe.* London: Hamlyn Publishing Group Ltd., 1981.

DAMIANA
HERBA DE LA PASTORA, MEXICAN DAMIANA, OLD WOMAN'S BROOM, ROSEMARY

Common trade names
Damiania, Damiana Root

Common forms
Available as a tincture, capsule, powder, or tea.

Source
Damiana comes from the leaves of the Mexican shrub *Turnera diffusa*. It is also found in the southwestern United States and South America. The plant has an aromatic smell and a pleasant taste.

Chemical components

Studies indicate that damiana contains a volatile oil, with an odor similar to chamomile, that primarily consists of 1,8-cineol and pinenes. Additional compounds include thymol, sesquiterpenes, gonzalitosin (a cyanogenic glycoside), a bitter element, resin, tannins, gum, mucilage, starch, and possibly, caffeine.

Actions

The pharmacologic activity of the plant is unknown. No active components have been identified as the basis for damiana's alleged aphrodisiac and hallucinogenic effects.

Reported uses

Damiana has traditionally been used as an aphrodisiac. It was available in the United States in the 1870s as a tincture, and used as an aphrodisiac to "improve the sexual ability of the enfeebled and aged." It is thought to increase pelvic secretions. Some researchers believe that drinking damiana as a tea or smoking the leaves can produce a euphoric and relaxed state, similar to the effects of marijuana (Lowry, 1984). Other reported uses include a mild purgative, diuretic, tonic, and antidepressant.

Dosage

Tincture: up to 2.5 ml P.O. t.i.d.
Powdered herb: 18 g in a 500-ml decoction P.O. (taken as a tea) t.i.d.

Adverse reactions

- Hallucinations
- Irritation of urethral mucosa (May contribute to illusion of "aphrodisiac" effects.)
- Possible liver injury (excessive amounts)

Interactions

None reported.

Contraindications and precautions

Contraindicated in pregnant or breast-feeding patients; effects are unknown.

Special considerations

- Monitor the patient for hepatotoxicity if excessive amounts of the herb are ingested.
- Observe the patient taking damiana who experiences hallucinations; rule out other drugs that may cause similar effects.
- Question the patient about reason for consumption of this herb; suggest available alternative agents and assist him in accessing an

appropriate medical specialist or primary health care professional.
- Advise the female patient to avoid use of the herb during pregnancy or when breast-feeding.
- Advise the patient to avoid hazardous activities until CNS effects of the drug are known.

Analysis
Although damiana is claimed to have aphrodisiac and hallucinogenic effects, evidence to support these claims is lacking. A detailed review of damiana's history indicates that claims of the herb's use stem from a hoax.

References
Lowry, T.P. "Damiana," *J Psychoactive Drugs* 16:267-68, 1984.

DANDELION
LION'S TOOTH, PRIEST'S-CROWN, WILD ENDIVE

Common trade names
(Various manufacturers) Dandelion

Common forms
Available as capsules, extracts, and teas.

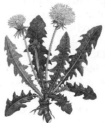

Source
Active components are obtained from the leaves and roots of *Taraxacum officinale* or *T. laevigatum,* common low-growing weeds native to Europe and Asia and naturalized worldwide.

Chemical components
Dandelions contain many compounds, including caffeic, parahydroxyphenylacetic, chlorogenic, linoleic, linolenic, oleic, and palmitic acids; minerals such as potassium, iron, silicon, magnesium, sodium, zinc, manganese, copper, and phosphorus; resins, taraxasterol, taraxacin, taraxacum, taraxerin, taraxerol, and terpenoids; vitamin A, and vitamins B, C, and D. Other compounds include carotenoids (taraxanthin), choline, inulin, pectin, phytosterols, sugars, and triterpenes.

Actions
Taraxacum, a dandelion compound, increases gastric and salivary juice secretions, stimulates the release of bile from the gallbladder and liver, and acts as a mild laxative. In addition, a leaf extract was found to exert a stronger diuretic effect in rats and mice than a root

extract (Racz-Kotilla et al., 1974). An anti-inflammatory effect has also been shown for dandelion root extract in an animal model (Mascolo et al., 1987).

Dandelion is considered a liver and kidney tonic because of its choleretic effects and ability to directly stimulate contraction of the gallbladder, thus releasing stored bile. Results obtained from human and animal studies showed improvement in jaundice, liver conges- tion, gallstones, hepatitis, and bile duct inflammation.

Extracts of dandelion markedly inhibited the growth of cancer cells, perhaps by its resemblance to tumor polysaccharides such as lentinan. Also in the United States, antibodies to active polypeptides in tumor-induced mouse ascites fluid were produced from dandelion.

Reported uses

Dandelion is claimed to possess laxative, diuretic, bile-stimulating, and antirheumatic properties. Herbalists recommend its use for liv- er and gallbladder disorders, cholecystitis, digestive complaints, con- stipation, and when diuresis may be indicated (premenstrual syn- drome, weight loss, heart failure, and hypertension).

Dandelion's milky sap has been used externally for removing corns, calluses, and warts. The plant is one of nine herbal ingredi- ents of a British proprietary preparation that has been used to treat viral hepatitis.

In a small group of patients, dandelion root was used successfully to treat chronic, nonspecific colitis, bringing relief from abdominal pain, constipation, and diarrhea.

Dosage

Dried root: 2 to 8 g P.O. by infusion or decoction t.i.d.
Dried leaf: 4 to 10 g P.O. by infusion t.i.d.
Fluid extract (1:1 in 25% alcohol): 4 to 8 ml P.O. (1 to 2 teaspoon) t.i.d.
Tincture of root (1:5 in 45% alcohol): 5 to 10 ml P.O. t.i.d.
Juice of root: 4 to 8 ml P.O. t.i.d.

Adverse reactions

- Blockage of GI or biliary tract
- Contact dermatitis (in allergic patients)
- Gallbladder inflammation
- Gallstones

Interactions

Antidiabetic agents: may potentiate effects, promoting hypogly- cemia. Avoid concomitant use.
Antihypertensives: possible additive or synergistic hypotensive effect. Avoid concomitant use.

Diuretics: may potentiate fluid and electrolyte losses. Avoid concomitant use.

Contraindications and precautions

Avoid use of the herb in pregnant or breast-feeding patients; effects are unknown.

Special considerations

• Monitor intake and output and serum electrolytes in patients taking dandelion and diuretics concomitantly.
• Monitor serum glucose in diabetic patients taking dandelion. Adjust therapy as needed.
• Instruct the patient taking dandelion with an antihypertensive agent to watch for symptoms of an exaggerated hypotensive effect (orthostatic hypotension, dizziness, syncope); advise him to rise slowly from a sitting or lying position if orthostatic hypotension develops.
• Advise the diabetic patient to monitor glucose more carefully because hypoglycemia may occur.
• Advise the female patient to avoid use of the herb during pregnancy or when breast-feeding.

Points of interest

• Dandelion root is sometimes roasted and used as a coffee substitute. The flowers are used to make wine and schnapps. The plant is also frequently used as a food, mainly in soups and salads.
• Dandelion contains more vitamin A than carrots.

Analysis

Dandelion is a well known herbal remedy and a natural food item. Unfortunately, scientific data are lacking to justify its reported therapeutic uses. The plant has been used in foods for several years without adverse effects. However, it should not be ingested in amounts larger than what is normally present in foods or drinks.

References
Mascolo, N., et al. "Biological Screening of Italian Medicinal Plants for Anti-Inflammatory Activity," *Phytotherapy Res* 1:28-9, 1987.
Racz-Kotilla, E., et al. "The Action of *Taraxacum officinale* Extracts on the Body Weight and Diuresis of Laboratory Animals," *Planta Med* 26(3):212-17, 1974.

DEVIL'S CLAW
GRAPPLE PLANT, WOOD SPIDER

Common trade names
(Various manufacturers; available in combination) Devil's Claw,
Devil's Claw Capsule, Devil's Claw Secondary Root, Devil's Claw
Vegicaps

Common forms
Capsules: 200 mg, 420 mg, 499 mg, 510 mg, 750 mg
Also available as teas or tinctures.

Source
The drug is extracted from the roots and secondary tubers of *Harpagophytum procumbens*, a member of the Pedalia family (Peda-
liaceae).

Chemical components
The major active ingredient in devil's claw is harpagoside. Other
compounds include harpagide, procumbide, stigmasterol, beta sitosterol, fatty acids, aromatic acids, triterpenes, sugars, gum resins,
and flavonoids.

Actions
Harpagoside possesses anti-inflammatory properties. Unlike conventional NSAIDs that alter arachidonic acid metabolism, the herb's
anti-inflammatory effects were not produced by this mechanism in
animals and humans. Harpagoside was found to produce negative
chronotropic and positive inotropic effects by altering the mechanisms that regulate the calcium influx in smooth muscles. Reduced
blood pressure and heart rate, and antiarrhythmic activity have
been reported in animals. In contrast, harpagide possesses negative
chronotropic and inotropic properties.

Reported uses
Devil's claw is claimed to be useful as an antiarthritic, antirheumatic, and appetite stimulant. Despite one finding of an anti-inflammatory effect, other studies have failed to replicate this finding in either
humans or animals (Whitehouse et al., 1983). A study using rats
evaluated the efficacy of the plant in reducing edema of the hind
foot and found no effect on the edema and insignificant alteration
of prostaglandin synthetase activity.

Other therapeutic claims, which lack scientific support, include
treatment of allergies, arteriosclerosis, boils, climacteric problems,
dysmenorrhea, GI disturbances, headaches, heartburn, liver and

kidney disorders, lumbago, malaria, neuralgia, nicotine poisoning, and skin cancer.

Dosage
Dosage of devil's claw tested in humans for decreased eicosanoid production was 2,000 mg P.O. daily (Moussard et al., 1992).

Adverse reactions
None reported.

Interactions
None reported. However, use cautiously in patients also taking antiarrhythmic medications.

Contraindications and precautions
Contraindicated in patients with gastric or duodenal ulcers. Also contraindicated in pregnant patients because it may stimulate uterine contractions; alleged abortive properties of devil's claw remain controversial.

Special considerations
• Monitor heart rate and rhythm of patients taking antiarrhythmics and devil's claw.
• Advise the patient taking the drug for anti-inflammatory effect that many OTC and prescription anti-inflammatory agents exist that have known risks and benefits.
• Tell the female patient taking this agent to report if pregnancy is being planned or is suspected.
• Advise the female patient to avoid use of the herb during pregnancy or when breast-feeding.

Points of interest
• The common name, "devil's claw," comes from the plant's unique fruits, which are covered with hooks to facilitate their spread by animals.

Analysis
Evidence for this agent's anti-inflammatory effect is scanty. Larger and well-designed clinical studies in humans need to be conducted to evaluate its efficacy and safety for treating arthritis. There are no clinical data to support its use for other disorders described. Other anti-inflammatory products (such as NSAIDs) are easily available.

References

Moussard, C., et al. "A Drug in Traditional Medicine, *Harpagophytum procumbens*: No Evidence for NSAID-Like Effect on Whole Blood Eicosanoid Production in Humans," *Prostaglandins Leuco Essent Fatty Acids* 46:283-86, 1992.

Whitehouse, L.W., et al. "Devil's Claw (*Harpagophytum procumbens*): No Evidence for Anti-inflammatory Activity in the Treatment of Arthritic Disease," *Can Med Assoc J* 129:249-51, 1983.

DHEA

DEHYDROEPIANDROSTERONE

Common trade names

(Various manufacturers; available in combination) Born Again's DHEA Eyelift Serum, DHEA Men's Formula, DHEA with Antioxidants 25 mg, DHEA with Bioperine 50 mg

Common forms

Capsules: 5 mg, 25 mg, 50 mg
Tablets (timed-release): 15 mg
Cream: 4 oz (with other vitamins and herbs)

Source

Steroid precursors found in members of the yam family (Dioscoreaceae) have been used to produce dehydroepiandrosterone (DHEA). Most commercially available DHEA is produced in Europe and China.

Chemical components

Besides its occurrence in certain plants, the steroid hormone DHEA is secreted by the zona reticularis of the adrenal glands in primates. Serum levels of DHEA decline dramatically after age 40 in humans.

Actions

Several physiologic effects have been ascribed to DHEA, including its conversion into androgens and estrogens, and its ability to raise serum IGF-1 levels, a mediator of human growth hormone. The degree of androgenic versus estrogenic effect of DHEA appears to depend on the patient's hormonal milieu. In men, DHEA has also been reported to increase levels of several immune cell types (Khorram et al., 1997).

Reported uses

Numerous claims for health benefits with regular DHEA use are being touted in the scientific and lay press. These include immune system enhancement; antidiabetogenic, antineoplastic, and antiatherosclerotic effects; osteoporosis prevention; treatment for certain autoimmune conditions; and a general antiaging effect. One small, uncontrolled study has evaluated DHEA in the treatment of depression. (See *DHEA and depression.*)

Dosage
Of the few human studies available, most used a dose of 50 mg daily. Serum levels of DHEA sulfate should be checked periodically during exogenous replacement, and the dose adjusted to youthlike levels (3,600 ng/ml for men, 3,000 ng/ml for women).

Adverse reactions
- Aggressiveness
- Hirsutism
- Insomnia
- Irritability

Interactions
Although not specifically documented, DHEA may interfere with other exogenous androgen or estrogen hormone therapy.

Contraindications and precautions
Contraindicated in patients with prostate cancer, benign prostatic hypertrophy, or estrogen-responsive tumors (such as those of the breast or uterus) because of DHEA's potential of promoting growth of these tumors. Avoid use of the herb in pregnant or breast-feeding patients; effects are unknown.

Special considerations
⚠ Patients over age 40 should be aggressively screened for hormonally sensitive cancers before taking DHEA.
- Monitor the patient for excessive hair growth.
- Instruct the patient to report mood or behavioral changes.
- Advise the female patient to avoid use of the herb during pregnancy or when breast-feeding.

Analysis
Most claims for DHEA use are based on in vitro and nonprimate studies; moreover, nonprimate mammals do not produce significant amounts of endogenous hormone. Although declining DHEA levels in humans may be assumed to act as a marker for aging and degenerative diseases, inconclusive evidence exists that exogenous DHEA replacement will prevent, or be therapeutic for, such conditions. Long-term safety data for DHEA use in humans are also lacking. Larger and more comprehensive trials are needed to determine a role for this agent.

RESEARCH FINDINGS
DHEA and depression

Results of a small, uncontrolled, open-label study may suggest a role for DHEA in treating depression (Wolkowitz et al., 1997). Six middle-aged patients diagnosed with major depression and low basal plasma DHEA levels were given DHEA 30 to 90 mg daily for 4 weeks. Doses were titrated to mimic plasma levels of DHEA observed in younger patients.

After 4 weeks, depression ratings and memory scores had significantly improved compared with baseline scores. The most notable response came from one patient who was treated with DHEA for 6 months. Depression ratings improved 48% to 72%, and semantic memory performance scores improved 63%. Both measurements returned to pretreatment baselines after treatment was discontinued.

The investigators concluded that larger controlled trials are needed to clarify a role for DHEA in depression.

References

Khorram. O., et al. "Activation of Immune Function by Dehydroepiandrosterone (DHEA) in Age-Advanced Men," *J Gerontol A Biol Sci Med Sci* 52(1):M1-M7, 1997.

Wolkowitz, O.M., et al. "Dehydroepiandrosterone Treatment of Depression," *Biol Psychiatry* 41:311-18, 1997.

DILL

DILL SEED, DILLWEED

Common trade names
Atkinson & Barker's Gripe Mixture, Concentrated Dill Water BPC 1973, Neo, Neo Baby Mixture, Nurse Harvey's Gripe Mixture, Woodwards Gripe Water

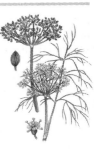

Common forms
Available as dried fruits, distilled or concentrated dill water, or dill oil.

Source
All parts of the plant are used, but most products use the dried ripe fruit, seeds, or flowers of *Anethum graveolens,* a member of the carrot family (Umbelliferae).

Chemical components

Dill plants contain volatile oil (carvone, d-limonene, eugenol, and antheole), flavonoids (including kaempferol, quercetin, and iso-rhamnetin), coumarins, xanthone derivatives, triterpenes, phenolic acids, proteins, fixed oil, myristicin, dillapiole, paraffins, and phellandrene.

Actions

None reported.

Reported uses

Dill is believed to have antiflatulent, aromatic, antispasmodic, lacto-genic, and soporific actions. It is a common ingredient in "gripe water," used to relieve flatulence and colic in infants. It is also used in breast-feeding patients and in cattle to help promote the flow of milk (Morton, 1981). The oil has been used for its antifoaming and antiflatulent action to improve appetite and digestion. The seeds have been used to treat hiccups, stomach pain, halitosis (on chewing), and to strengthen the nails when the hands are soaked in a decoction. There are no controlled human studies available that support these claims. One Bulgarian study concluded that dill oil has weak choleretic effects and should be used with other drugs for benefit (Gruncharov and Tashev, 1973).

Dosage

Dried fruits: 1 to 4 g P.O. t.i.d.
Distilled dill water: 2 to 4 ml P.O. t.i.d.
Concentrated dill water: 0.2 ml P.O. t.i.d.
Dill oil: 0.05 to 2 ml P.O. t.i.d.

Adverse reactions

None reported. Its use as a food additive leads to the belief that few adverse effects exist.

Interactions

None reported.

Contraindications and precautions

Dill weed is contraindicated in patients requiring a low-salt diet because of its high sodium content. Use cautiously in patients with allergies to other spices because dill has allergenic components that have demonstrated cross-sensitivity.

Special considerations

• Periodically monitor serum electrolytes, particularly sodium, in patients taking the herb.

• Explain that the potentially beneficial effects of dill remain un-proven and the safety profile is unknown.

• Recommend that patient first seek medical advice before taking the herb.

• Reinforce the importance of a low-sodium diet in patients who require it.

Points of interest

• The name *dill* is believed to originate from the old Norse word *dil-la* (to lull) because of its sedative and antiflatulent properties. In the Middle Ages, the herb was used by magicians in their potions and magic spells, and was also grown in gardens as a charm against witchcraft and enchantments.

Analysis

Most clinical data on dill weed are from foreign sources or animal models. There are no clinical human data from the United States to support its use for flatulence or colic in infants, or as a stimulant for milk flow, although this appears to be the primary medicinal claim in the herbal literature. More studies are needed to determine the use of dill in children and adults.

References

Gruncharov, V., and Tashev, T. "The Choleretic Effect of Bulgarian Dill Oil in White Rats," *Eksp Med Morfol* 12:155-61, 1973.

Morton, J.F. *Atlas of Medicinal Plants of Middle America: Bahamas to Yucatan.* Springfield, Ill: Charles C. Thomas Publisher, 1981.

DOCK, YELLOW

CHIN CH'IAO MAI, CURLED OR CURLY DOCK, GARDEN PATIENCE, HUALTATA, HUMMAIDH, KIVIRCIK LABADA, NARROW DOCK, NIU SHE T'OU, OSEILLE MARRON (SAUVAGE), SOUR DOCK, SURALE DI BIERDJI, YELLOW DOCK

Common trade names

(Various manufacturers; available in combination) LC Tone, Detox, Rumex Crispus

Common forms

Capsules: 470 mg, 500 mg

Source

A dried extract is prepared from the roots of *Rumex crispus*, a common and troublesome perennial weed that is native to Europe and

Asia. Dock has become naturalized in the United States and now oc-curs along roadsides and in gravelly soils of pastures and meadows.

Chemical components

The primary component of the dried root of *Rumex crispus* is chrysophanic acid; others include rumicin, emodin (oxymethylan-thraquinone), calcium oxalate, oxalic acid, brassidinic acid, tannins, and volatile oils. The stems, leaves, and fruit also contain anthra-quinones and oxalic acid. Loss of activity has occurred if the root is boiled for an extended period of time.

Actions

Rumex species have been studied in vitro and in vivo in animals, and have been found to have both anti-inflammatory and antiviral effects. The anti-itch effect of the leaves of *R. nepalensis* is believed to be caused by the antihistaminic, anticholinergic, and antibrady-kinin properties of the plant (Aggarwal et al., 1986).

A root extract of *R. hastatus* was found to inactivate the herpes simplex virus; antiviral activity against poliovirus and Sindbis virus was unaffected (Taylor et al., 1996). Extracts of the *R. crispus* fruit also showed significant inhibitory activity against HIV reverse tran-scriptase (el-Mekkawy et al., 1995).

An in vitro study of sheep seminal vesicles noted that aqueous and ethanolic extracts of *R. sagittatus* root significantly inhibited cy-clooxygenase activity.

Reported uses

Dock root is said to be an astringent and cathartic. It has been used in syphilis and cutaneous eruptions, particularly of the scrofulous type. Some *Rumex* species were known for curing intermittent fevers, and others have been used in chronic hepatic congestion and dyspepsia. An ointment made by boiling the root in vinegar has been used to treat glandular swellings and various skin diseases such as scabies. Bruising and applying the fresh root is a popular antidote to the rash induced by stinging nettle. Other claimed uses include diuresis and symptomatic treatment of tonsillitis and sore throat.

Dosage

Most in vitro studies reported pharmacologic activity of *Rumex* species in concentrations ranging from 25 to 100 mcg/ml. Doses tested clinically ranged from 2.5 to 5 mg P.O. as a single dose.

Adverse reactions

- Abdominal pain
- Diarrhea
- Hypocalcemia

- Nausea
- Vomiting

⚠ Severe hypocalcemia and metabolic acidosis with resultant death following consumption of excessive quantities. (See *Toxicity of Rumex crispus*, page 228.)

Interactions
None reported.

Contraindications and precautions
Rumex species are contraindicated in pregnant women as a laxative because of the presence of anthraquinones, which have stimulant effects that may lead to miscarriage. Also contraindicated in patients with renal dysfunction or failure, type 1 or 2 diabetes, hepatic disease, and severe electrolyte abnormalities because of the oxalic acid content precipitating in the kidney tubules.

Use cautiously in patients with heart failure, new-onset diabetes, malnutrition, recent thyroid or parathyroid surgery, hypoalbuminemic disease states, or alcoholic disease. Also use with caution in patients also taking drugs known to cause hypocalcemia (such as loop and potassium-sparing diuretics, carbonic anhydrase inhibitors, calcitonin, mithramycin, and phenytoin).

Special considerations
- Monitor serum calcium levels and for signs of hypocalcemia.
- Advise the patient to report sudden onset of nausea, vomiting, or abdominal pain.
- Inform the patient to use very small portions of the herb for culinary purposes, if at all.
- Advise the patient not to use this herb as a replacement for antiviral drugs to treat herpes or HIV.
- Inform the patient with continued allergy or allergic response despite herbal use to notify the health care professional.
- Warn the patient to watch for symptoms of hypocalcemia (fatigue, seizure, muscle spasms, perioral paresthesia, and confusion).
- Instruct the female patient taking the herb to report planned or suspected pregnancy.
- Advise the female patient to avoid use of the herb during pregnancy or when breast-feeding.

Points of interest
- Dock is cultivated in Europe as a vegetable or salad. It is also a popular Himalayan antidote for rash caused by stinging nettles.

RESEARCH FINDINGS

Toxicity of *Rumex crispus*

Although only a few cases of *Rumex* poisonings have been identified in humans, fatal incidents dating back to 1949 have been identified in animals (Panciera et al., 1990). The most recent case in humans involved fatal poisoning due to *Rumex crispus* ingestion (Farr et al., 1989). A 53-year-old patient with insulin-dependent diabetes for 10 years went to the emergency department with symptoms of vomiting and diarrhea after ingesting approximately 500 to 1,000 g of this plant in a sorrel soup.

The patient was dehydrated with moderate metabolic acidosis. Laboratory values were as follows: liver enzymes more than three times the upper limit of normal (AST 8,000 IU/L, ALT 12,000 IU/L); total serum calcium 6.3 mg/dl, with an ionized calcium of 2.3 mg/dl; serum creatinine 5.3 mg/dl (534 mmol/L); BUN 100 mg/dl (18.5 mmol/L); PT ratio 3.14; and fibrinogen 1.2 mg/ml.

The patient lapsed into a coma and exhibited respiratory depression and multiorgan failure. Initially, calcium gluconate was given for the hypocalcemia and sodium bicarbonate for the metabolic acidosis, followed by hemodialysis for the renal insufficiency. Shortly after hemodialysis, the patient experienced arrhythmias that progressed to ventricular fibrillation. The patient died 72 hours after ingesting the plant.

Autopsy revealed birefringent crystals in the kidneys and liver, confirmed later to be calcium oxalate crystals. Other findings included liver necrosis and centrilobular vascular stasis with portal lymphocytic infiltration, necrosis of the proximal and distal convoluted tubules of the kidneys, severe lung edema, and pulmonary congestion. These findings were consistent with *R. crispus* toxicity.

The other family members who had also ingested the plant recovered uneventfully in a few days. The mean lethal dose of oxalic acid in adults is 5 to 30 g. This patient ingested about 6 to 8 g of oxalic acid from the sorrel soup.

Analysis

All clinical data on *Rumex* are from in vitro studies on animals. This herb is best characterized as having mild to moderate antipruritic effects. Although it has been shown to reduce the size of inflammatory wheal reactions, the exact mechanism is unknown. Because of the risk of poisoning in both animals and humans, currently available antihistamine or antiallergy products are recommended instead of the herb.

References

Aggarwal, M., et al. "Effect of *Rumex nepalensis* Extracts on Histamine, Acetylcholine, Carbachol, Bradykinin, and PGs Evoked Skin Reactions in Rabbits," *Ann Allergy* 56:177-82, 1986.

el-Mekkawy S., et al. "Inhibitory Effects of Egyptian Folk Medicines on Human Immunodeficiency Virus (HIV) Reverse Transcriptase," *Chem Pharm Bull (Tokyo)* 43:641-48, 1995. Abstract.

Farr, M., et al. "Fatal Oxalic Acid Poisoning from Sorrel Soup" *Lancet* 23:1524, 1989. Letter.

Panciera, R., et al. "Acute Oxalate Poisoning Attributable to Ingestion of Curly Dock *(Rumex crispus)* in Sheep," *J Am Vet Med Assoc* 196:1981-90, 1990.

Taylor, R.S. et al. "Antiviral Activities of Medicinal Plants of Southern Nepal," *J Ethnopharmacol* 53:97-104, 1996.

DONG QUAI

CHINESE ANGELICA, DRY-KUEI, FP3340010/FP334015/ FT334010, TANG-KUEI, WOMEN'S GINSENG

Common trade names
Dong Kwai, Dong Quai Capsules, Dong Quai Fluid Extract

Common forms
Dong quai tablet (fluid extract): 0.5 g
Raw root: 4.5 g to 30 g (boil or soak in wine)
Also available as injectable forms in foreign countries.

Source
Active components are obtained from the roots of dong quai (*Angelica polymorpha* var. *sinensis*), a fragrant perennial umbelliferous herb native to China, Korea, and Japan.

Chemical components
The volatile oils extracted from the root contain n-butylphthalide, cadinene, safrole, isosafrole, dihydrophthalmic anhydride, carvacrol, succinic acid, nicotinic acid, uracil, ligustilide, vitamin B_{12}, and folinic acid. Coumarin derivatives identified in dong quai include oxypeucedanin, osthole, imperatorin, psoralen, and bergapten. Ferulic acid has also been found.

Actions
Dong quai alters uterine activity in female rabbits. The volatile oil has an inhibitory action on the uterus whereas the nonvolatile and water- and alcohol-soluble components have stimulatory action. In another study, dong quai alone was found not to produce estrogen-like responses in endometrial thickness or vaginal maturation, and also not to be useful in managing postmenopausal symptoms (Hirata et al., 1997).

Studies conducted in rats showed increases in metabolism, oxygen use by the liver, and glutamic acid and cysteine oxidation; these actions may be attributed to vitamin B_{12} and folinic acid that occur in the herb's root.

Dong quai extracts, especially alcoholic extracts, were also found to exert quinidine-type effects, prolong the refractory period, and correct atrial fibrillation in animals. Other studies in rats showed that the plant may prevent atherosclerosis, expand coronary arteries, and increase coronary blood flow. Some coumarins are known to act as vasodilators. Although studies in animals have shown that the volatile oil exerts vasodilatory action to lower blood pressure, the duration of action is short.

Reported uses

Dong quai is recommended by herbalists for many gynecologic disorders, including irregular menstruation, dysmenorrhea, premenstrual syndrome, excessive fetal movement, and chronic pelvic infection. Most claims are based on data from animal studies or small, uncontrolled human trials. The herb has also anecdotally been reported to treat malaria, headache, neuralgia, constipation, toothache, hypertension, herpes zoster, chronic rhinitis, Buerger's disease, Raynaud's disease, hepatitis, hepatocirrhosis, pyogenic infection, ulcerous diseases or abscess, and sepsis.

Dosage

Dosage forms, strengths and extraction forms vary. In the human placebo-controlled study evaluating the estrogenic effects of dong quai on endometrial thickness in postmenopausal woman, 1 g of the root (equivalent to 0.5 mg/kg of ferulic acid) was used.

Adverse reactions

- Bleeding
- Diarrhea
- Fever
- Increased photosensitivity (the psoralens in the herb may cause severe photodermatitis.)

Interactions

Anticoagulants: may potentiate effects. Avoid concomitant use.

Contraindications and precautions

Safrole, a component of the volatile oil, is carcinogenic and not recommended for ingestion. Contraindicated in pregnant or breast-feeding patients because the herb's chemical components may cause fetal harm.

Special considerations
• Monitor the patient for potential bleeding.
• Question the patient about use of this herb and suggest an appropriate specialist to address these health care concerns.
• Warn the patient that some of the herbal components have been shown to increase the risk of some cancers.
• Instruct the patient who becomes photosensitive to use sunblock and to wear adequate clothing and sunglasses.
• Caution the patient against use of this herb for its yet unproven estrogenic effects.
• Advise the female patient to report planned or suspected pregnancy and to avoid use of the herb during pregnancy or when breast-feeding.

Analysis
Despite numerous therapeutic claims for this herb, only a few animal-based studies are available to support them. Dong quai appears to have over 18 different active chemical components, many of which exert widely divergent pharmacologic effects. Some components are carcinogens, while adverse effects of others remain unknown. Extensive testing of individual components is necessary before the herb can be regarded as safe or effective.

References
Hirata, J.D., et al. "Does Donq Quai Have Estrogenic Effects in Postmenopausal Women? A Double-Blind Placebo-Controlled Trial," *Fertil Steril* 68:981-86, 1997.

ECHINACEA

Common trade names
(Various manufacturers; available in combination) Coneflower Extract, Echinacea, Echinacea Angustifolia Herb, Echinacea Fresh Freeze-Dried, Echinacea Glycerite, Echinacea Herb, Echinacea Herbal Comfort Lozenges, Echinacea Purpurea

Common forms
Capsules: 125 mg, 355 mg (85 mg herbal extract powder), 500 mg
Tablets: 335 mg
Also available as hydroalcoholic extracts, fresh-pressed juice, glycerite, lozenges, and tinctures.

Source
Echinacea dietary supplements are obtained from the dried rhizomes and roots of *Echinacea angustifolia* or *E. pallida,* and from the fresh juice of the roots or above-ground parts of *E. purpurea.*

Chemical components
Echinacea contains alkylamides, caffeic acid derivatives, polysaccharides, essential oils, and other constituents, including polyacetylene flavonoids and glycoproteins. The plant also contains three classes of compounds that exhibit nonspecific immunostimulatory activity: alkylamides, chicoric acids and related glycosides, and high-molecular-weight polysaccharides. The concentration of the pharmacologic active constituents varies, depending on the species and plant part used.

Actions
Extract of echinacea stimulates phagocytosis and increases respiratory cellular activity and mobility of leukocytes. No single compo-

nent appears to be responsible for the immunostimulating activity, although the caffeic acid derivatives and high-molecular-weight polysaccharides in echinacea stimulate phagocytosis. The alkylamides in the plant are reported to exert local anesthetic effects and anti-inflammatory activities. Essential oil components produce a tingling sensation on the tongue. Some of those compounds also have insecticidal activity (Jacobson, 1967). Caffeoyl conjugates in the plant stimulate the production of properdin and interferon, and activate adrenal cortex activity. In vitro studies using the fresh-pressed juice of the aerial portion of *E. purpurea* and the aqueous extract of the roots inhibited influenza, herpes infections, and vesicular stomatitis virus.

The extract of echinacea can reduce the growth of *Trichomonas vaginalis* and reduces recurrence of *Candida albicans* infections (Combest and Nemecz, 1997). Intraperitoneal administration of purified arabinogalactan in rats caused activation of macrophages against *Leishmania enrietti*. Arabinogalactan stimulated macrophages to produce tumor necrosis factor, interleukin-1, and interferon beta-2. The lipid soluble compound, 1,8 pentadecadiene exhibits direct antitumor activity (Combest and Nemecz, 1997).

The extract has inhibited edema in rats and inflammation in mice. In vitro studies indicate that the polyphenols from echinacea protect collagen against free radical attack.

Reported uses
Echinacea is claimed to be useful as a wound healing agent for abscesses, burns, eczema, varicose ulcers of the leg and other skin wounds, and as a nonspecific immunostimulant for the supportive treatment of upper respiratory tract infections and urinary tract infections. Two small studies have demonstrated that parenteral administration of purified Echinacin (not available in the United States) may be beneficial as an immunotherapeutic agent in combination with standard chemotherapeutic drugs in the treatment of colorectal or hepatocellular cancer (Lersch et al., 1990, 1992).

Dosage
Expressed juice: 6 to 9 ml P.O. daily.
Capsules containing the powdered herb: equivalent to 900 mg to 1 g P.O. t.i.d.; doses can vary.
Tincture: 0.75 to 1.5 ml (15 to 30 gtt) P.C. two to five times daily. The tincture has been given as 60 gtt P.O t.i.d.
Tea: 2 teaspoon (4 g) of coarsely powdered herb simmered in 1 cup of boiling water for 10 minutes. Avoid this method of administration because some active compounds are water-insoluble.

Adverse reactions
● Adverse effects are uncommon. Allergies may occur in patients allergic to plants belonging to the daisy family. Studies using large dosages in animals demonstrated no toxic effects.

Interactions
None reported.

Contraindications and precautions
Contraindicated in patients with severe illnesses including HIV infection (including AIDS), collagen disease, leukosis, multiple sclerosis, and tuberculosis or other autoimmune diseases. Avoid use of the herb in pregnant or breast-feeding patients; effects are unknown.

Special considerations
⚠ Know that many tinctures contain significant concentrations of alcohol (ranging from 15% to 90%) and may not be suitable for children, alcoholic patients, and patients with liver disease or those taking disulfiram or metronidazole.

⚠ Advise the patient taking the herb for a prolonged time that overstimulation of the immune system and possible immune suppression may occur. Echinacea should not be used longer than 8 weeks; therapy lasting 10 to 14 days is probably sufficient.

● Inform the patient not to delay treatment for an illness that does not resolve after taking this herb.

● Advise the pregnant or breast-feeding patient to avoid use of this herb.

Analysis
Although promising, additional human clinical trial information is needed before a role for echinacea in the treatment or prophylaxis of disease can be defined.

References
Combest, W.L., and Nemecz, G. "Echinacea," *U.S. Pharmacist* October:126-32, 1997.

Jacobson, M. "The Structure of Echinacein, the Insecticidal Component of American Coneflower Roots," *J Org Chem* 32:1646-47, 1967.

Lersch, C., et al. "Stimulation of the Immune Response in Outpatients with Hepatocellular Carcinomas by Low Doses of Cyclophosphamide (LDCY),. *Echinacea purpurea* Extracts (Echinacein), and Thymostimulin," *Arch Gescwulstforsch* 60:379-83, 1990.

Lersch, C., et al. "Nonspecific Immunostimulation with Low Doses of Cyclophosphamide (LDCY), Thymostimulin, and *Echinacea purpurea* Extract (Echinacein) in Patients with Far Advanced Colorectal Cancers. Preliminary Results," *Cancer Invest* 10:343-48, 1992.

ELDERBERRY

ANTELOPE BRUSH (*SAMBUCUS TRIDENTATA*), BLACK
ELDER (*S. NIGRA*), BLUE ELDERBERRY (*S. CAERULEA*),
BORETREE, COMMON ELDER (*S. CANADENSIS*),
DANEWORT (*S. EBULUS*), DWARF ELDER, ELDER,
EUROPEAN ELDER, PIPE TREE, RED ELDERBERRY, RED-
FRUITED ELDER (*S. PUBENS, S. RACEMOSA*), *SAMBUCUS*,
SWEET ELDER

Common trade names
(Various manufacturers) Elderberry Power, Elder Flowers

Common forms
Available as ointments and aqueous solutions of the bark and leaves
as well as oils, ointments, and wine; all are derived from the berries.

Source
Several species of *Sambucus* produce elderberries. Most of the literature refers to *S. nigra* and *S. canadensis,* although other species with
similar chemical components exist. The flowers and berries are used
most often; the inner bark and leaves contain most of the potentially toxic compounds.

Chemical components
The flowers of *S. nigra* contain flavonoid glycosides, a cyanogenic
glycoside (sambunigrine), essential oils, mucilage, tannins, and organic acids. Fruit from the elder (*S. nigra*) contains organic pigments (anthocyanines), amino acids, sugar, rutin, and a substantial
amount of vitamin C (36 mg per 100 g of fruit). The elder leaves
contain 3.5% rutin. The inner bark of the elder also consists of
baldrianic acid. Other species contain additional compounds.

Actions
The elder and several other herbals have traditionally been used for
the treatment of diabetes, although studies in mice indicate that the
agent exerts no effects on glucose control (Swanston-Flatt et al.,
1989). This plant has shown activity against *Salmonella typhi,*
Shigella dysenteriae, and limited activity against *Shigella flexneri*. A
branch tip extract of the red elder (*S. racemosa*) was found to have
strong in vitro antiviral activity against respiratory syncytial virus.
No studies in humans or animals have been reported.

A 1997 study (Yesilada et al., 1997) indicated that *S. nigra* was
somewhat active against the production of inflammatory cytokines
in vitro, giving some merit to folklore suggesting that the plant is effective in the treatment of such inflammatory illnesses as rheuma-

tism, fever, infections, and edema. Elderberries have been reported to have antispasmodic and sedative activities, as well as activities as a diaphoretic, diuretic, and laxative. The herb has been used as a weight-loss agent and an agent to treat colds, "dropsy," kidney disorders, rheumatism, insomnia, and migraines. The cyanogenic glycosides contained in the elder plants release cyanide when hydrolyzed, as when they are chewed; this effect could explain many of the reported actions of this plant.

Reported uses

Elder has been used as an insect repellent, with sprays of the flowers placed in horses' bridles. The powder of the dried elder flowers has been added to water and dabbed on the skin as a mosquito repellent. Clinical support for this use in humans is currently lacking.

Mixed with sage, lemon juice, vinegar and honey, elder has also traditionally been used as a gargle. With peppermint and honey in a hot drink, elder is said to be able to treat a cold, inducing diaphoresis to "sweat out" an illness. Elderberry juice has been used in hair dye and scented ointments. Other reported uses include liver disease, toothache, measles, asthma, burns, cancer, chafing, epilepsy, gout, headache, neuralgia, psoriasis, syphilis, reduction of swelling, and wound healing, although there are no scientific data to support such uses.

Dosage

No consensus exists.

Adverse reactions

• Diarrhea (from berries of the *S. ebulus* and leaves of any species)
• Vomiting (with ingestion of excessive amounts of *S. racemosa* berries)
⚠ Cyanide poisoning from the bark, roots, leaves, and unripe berries of the elder plant. Children making pipes or peashooters from the hollowed shafts of the elder can suffer cyanide poisoning. Ingestion of 60 mg of cyanide has caused death in humans. Emesis and gastric lavage are recommended for known elder plant ingestion. Amyl nitrate, sodium nitrate, and sodium thiosulfate may also be used when cyanide toxicity is suspected.

Interactions

None reported.

Contraindications and precautions

Use elderberry products with caution because of the risk of cyanide toxicity. Berries of the dwarf elder species (*S. ebulus*) are contraindicated. Because all green parts of the elder plant are poisonous, avoid consumption of the leaves and stems. Avoid use of the herb in pregnant and breast-feeding patients.

Special considerations
• Monitor fluid intake and output of patients experiencing GI effects from this herb.
• Be aware that the dwarf elder (*S. ebulus*) is regarded as particularly poisonous. Large doses can cause vertigo, vomiting, and diarrhea (signs of cyanide toxicity).
• Advise the patient that elderberries should never be consumed uncooked because of the risk of cyanide toxicity.
• Advise the female patient to avoid use during pregnancy or when breast-feeding.
⚠ Instruct the patient to keep this plant away from children and pets, and to have the number for the nearest poison control center handy.

Analysis
Use of elderberry products as cathartics isn't recommended because of the risk of cyanide toxicity. Numerous other laxatives and cathartics exist whose safety and efficacy are well established. Safe and effective anti-inflammatory medications are also available for the treatment of rheumatism and other conditions for which elderberries have been used; therefore, elderberry use for these conditions is not recommended. Currently, there appears to be no medicinal use for this herbal product.

References
Swanston-Flatt, S.K., et al. "Glycaemic Effects of Traditional European Plant Treatments for Diabetes. Studies in Normal and Streptozotocin Diabetic Mice," *Diabetes Res* 10:69-73, 1989.
Yesilada, E., et al. "Inhibitory Effects of Turkish Folk Remedies on Inflammatory Cytokines: Interleukin-1$_{alpha}$, Interleukin-1$_{beta}$ and Tumor Necrosis Factor Alpha," *J Ethnopharmacol* 58:59-73, 1997.

ELECAMPANE

AUNEE, ELF DOCK, ELFWORT, HORSEHEAL, SCABWORT, VELVET DOCK, WILD SUNFLOWER

Common trade names
None known.

Common forms
Available as powdered root preparations, fluid extracts, and topical product.

Source

Active ingredients of elecampane are extracted from the dried rhizome and roots of 2- to 3-year-old *Inula helenium* plants.

Chemical components

The main constituents in *I. helenium* are inulin, helenin, volatile oils, and a mixture of sesquiterpene lactones—mainly alantolactone, alantol, and alantic acid.

Actions

Claims for *I. helenium* include antiseptic, bactericidal, diuretic, expectorant, and diaphoretic activities. Anecdotal animal data suggest that the agent exerts relaxant effects on tracheal and ileal smooth muscles (Reiter and Brandt, 1985), and antiparasitic activity against the liver fluke *Clonorchis sinensis* (Rhee et al., 1985). It failed to demonstrate in vitro antiviral activity against the tick-borne encephalitis virus (Fokina et al., 1991). Specific pharmacokinetic and pharmacodynamic data are not available.

Reported uses

I. helenium is claimed to be effective in the treatment of pulmonary disease, bronchitis, asthma, and cough. It is also claimed useful as an antiseptic and a bactericidal agent against *Mycobacterium tuberculosis*, a diuretic, an appetite stimulant, and an agent to treat dyspepsia. Medical data regarding the efficacy of *I. helenium* are largely anecdotal and derived from animal research. Anecdotal human reports suggest possible use as a snake-venom antidote. Large, randomized, placebo-controlled human trials using *I. helenium* have not been conducted.

Dosage

Fresh root: 1 to 2 tablespoon P.O. t.i.d.
Dried root: 2 to 3 g P.O. t.i.d.
Extract: 3 g dried root in 20 ml alcohol and 10 ml water P.O. t.i.d.

Adverse reactions

• Allergic contact dermatitis. Several case reports suggest that the plant is highly allergenic when applied topically. The mechanism is thought to involve degranulation of mast cells. The identified toxin is SL alantolactone.

Interactions

None reported.

Contraindications and precautions

Use cautiously in patients with a history of atopy or in those prone to contact dermatitis.

Special considerations
• Monitor for signs of an allergic reaction in patients prone to hypersensitivity reactions.
• Inform the patient that the allergic reactions may occur when the herb is handled. Advise the patient to take precautions (wear gloves, long sleeves) if handling the agent is likely.
• Advise the patient that there is no approved therapeutic use associated with this agent.

Points of interest
• In France and Switzerland, elecampane root is one of the substances used in the preparation of absinthe, a popular cordial at the turn of the century.

Analysis
Elecampane has been used as a medicinal product for many centuries in Europe and Asia. The presence of volatile oils suggests that the herb might be effective as an expectorant, but the lack of animal or human data limits its usefulness for this condition. Elecampane appears to be safe and well tolerated, but medical supervision is still recommended. Data supporting the use of *I. helenium* suggest some efficacy as an antiseptic and mild GI stimulant; however, the lack of well-designed human trials prevents recommendation for the use of this herb.

References
Fokina, G.I., et al. "Experimental Phytotherapy of Tick-Borne Encephalitis," *Vopr Virusol* 36:18-21, 1991. Abstract.

Reiter, M., and Brandt, W. "Relaxant Effects on Tracheal and Ileal Smooth Muscles of the Guinea Pig," *Arzneimittelforschung* 35:408-14, 1985. Abstract.

Rhee, J.K., et al. "Alterations of *Clonorchis sinensis* EPG by Administration of Herbs in Rabbits," *Am J Chin Med* 13:65-69 1985. Abstract.

EPHEDRA

BRIGHAM TEA, CAO MA HUANG (CHINESE EPHEDRA), DESERT TEA, EPITONIN, HERBA EPHEDRAE, HERBAL, JOINT FIR, MA HUANG, MAHUUANGGEN (ROOT), MEXICAN TEA, MORMON TEA, MUZEI MU HUANG (MONGOLIAN EPHEDRA), NATURAL ECSTACY, POPOTILLO, SEA GRAPE, SQUAW TEA, TEAMSTER'S TEA, YELLOW ASTRINGENT, YELLOW HORSE, ZHONG MA HUANG (INTERMEDIATE EPHEDRA)

Common trade names
(Available in combination) Herbal Fen-Phen, Power Trim, Up Your Gas

Common forms
Available as crude extracts of root and aerial parts, tablets (approximately 7 mg), and teas.

Source
There are many forms of ephedra, the most common being *Ephedra sinica* and *E. nevadensis*. Other forms include *E. trifurca, E. equisetina,* and *E. distachya*. The ephedra species is an evergreen plant with a pinelike odor. Pharmaceutical properties result from components in the seeds and stems.

Chemical components
The primary active ingredient is the alkaloid ephedrine. Not all ephedra species contain ephedrine but of those that do, most contain 0.5% to 2.5% alkaloids. *E. equisetina* contains the most ephedrine, whereas the American species, *E. nevadensis* and *E. trifurca,* lack the agent. Other alkaloids commonly found in ephedra species include methylephedrine, methylpseudoephedrine, pseudoephedrine, norpseudoephedrine (cathine), norephedrine, ephedine, ephedroxane, and pseudoephedroxane. Other compounds include a volatile oil (varies in components depending on source), ephedrans, catechin, gallic acid, tannins, flavonoids, inulin, dextrin, starch, pectin and some common plant acids, sugars, and trace minerals. The root contains ephedradines, feruloylhistamine, moakonine and mahuannins. The woody stems contain alkaloids, which are almost always absent in the fruit and root.

Actions
Most of ephedra's activity stems from the ephedrine component, which produces amphetamine-like actions. Ephedrine acts as a CNS stimulant, produces mydriasis, enhances myocardial contraction and heart rate, causes bronchodilation, decreases GI motility, and stimulates peripheral vasoconstriction with an associated elevation in blood pressure. Pseudoephedrine is similar in adrenergic activity but is less potent than ephedrine. It also possesses stronger diuretic properties than ephedrine. A Chinese abstract reports that the agent can preserve renal function and correct certain electrolyte disorders in rats (Wang and Hikokichi, 1994). *E. altissima* yields several mutagenic N-nitrosamines in vitro. The significance of this finding is unclear.

Reported uses
Ephedra has been used in Chinese medicine for several years for bronchial asthma, coughs, colds, flu, fever, chills, headaches, edema, nasal congestion, and arthralgias. In the West, it is commonly used for its CNS stimulant properties ("natural ecstasy") and as an ap-

petite suppressant ("natural fen-phen"). The use of ephedra faces little debate about its vasoconstrictive properties when used for conditions marked by edematous tissues and congested membranes. Nevertheless, the use of standardized pharmaceuticals containing ephedrine and pseudoephedrine has mostly taken the place of crude ephedra products.

Dosage
American species of ephedra (*E. nevadensis* and *E. trifurca*) are used for teas. Herbalists typically recommend placing ½ oz of dried branches in a pint of boiling water and steeping this mixture for 10 to 20 minutes.

⚠ The FDA prohibits the sale of ephedra in quantities of 8 mg or more per dose, and advises individuals to take less than 8 mg every 6 hours and no more than 24 mg daily. They further advise that ephedra products not be used for more than 7 consecutive days.

Adverse reactions
Some ephedra-related adverse effects appear to be dose-related.
- Anxiety, restlessness
- Confusion
- Constipation (due to tannin content)
- Dizziness
- Exfoliative dermatitis
- Headache
- Insomnia
- Nervousness
- Psychosis
- Urine retention
- Uterine contractions

⚠ Arrhythmias, cardiac arrest
⚠ Myocardial infarction
⚠ Seizure
⚠ Stroke

Interactions
Beta blockers: may enhance sympathomimetic effects on vasculature from unopposed alpha agonist effect, increasing risk of hypertension. Avoid concomitant use.

Ephedra alkaloids, MAO inhibitors: may increase risk of hypertensive crisis. Avoid concomitant use.

Phenothiazines: may block alpha effects of ephedra causing hypotension and tachycardia. Don't use together.

Theophylline: may increase risk of GI and CNS adverse effects. Avoid concomitant use.

Contraindications and precautions

Contraindicated in pregnancy because of the risk of uterine stimulation, and in diabetic patients because of the herb's hyperglycemic effects. Use cautiously in patients with hypertension, preexisting cardiac arrhythmias, angina, other cardiac disease, prostatic enlargement, and in those with a history of cerebrovascular disease.

Special considerations

• Closely monitor younger patients taking ephedra for adverse reactions. Many of the heart attacks, seizures, and strokes reported to the FDA occurred in previously healthy young adults.

⚠ Know that the FDA has found more than 800 cases, including 17 deaths, from adverse reactions associated with ephedrine products.

• Monitor the patient for behavioral or mood changes.

• Recommend standard pharmaceutical formulations of ephedrine and pseudoephedrine for patients with a valid need for these compounds.

• Advise the patient with hypertension, diabetes, cardiac disease, or prostatic enlargement to avoid use of ephedra.

• Advise the diabetic patient to monitor his serum glucose level closely.

• Warn the patient to watch for adverse reactions (especially chest pain, shortness of breath, palpitations, dizziness, or fainting), and advise him to quickly seek medical attention if these occur.

• Advise the patient to take less than 8 mg of the herb every 6 hours and not to exceed 24 mg daily. Also, stress that it is not wise to use the product for over 7 consecutive days.

Points of interest

• The FDA issued warnings against the use of ephedra as an appetite suppressant, and advises that ingestion over the recommended amount may result in heart attack, stroke, seizure, or death. The FDA prohibits the marketing of ephedrine with other CNS stimulants, such as caffeine and yohimbine.

Analysis

Unquestionably, the principal components in some *Ephedra* species can play a valid role in medicine, especially in the treatment of edema and congestion. With standardized formulations of the active constituents available OTC, the ingestion of the herbal product seems to be unwarranted.

References

Wang, G.Z., and Hikokichi, O. "Experimental Study in Treating Chronic Renal Failure with Dry Extract and Tannins of Herbal Ephedra," *Chin J Stomatol* 14:485, 1994.

EUCALYPTUS

FEVERTREE, GUM TREE, TASMANIAN BLUE GUM

Common trade names
Eucalyptamint, Eucalyptus Oil

Common forms
Available as an oil and a lotion.

Source
The drug is extracted from the leaves of the eucalyptus globulus labill plant.

Chemical components
The eucalyptus plant is composed of several chemicals, including eucalyptrin, hyperoside, quercetin, quecitrin, tannins, and associated acids. The primary constituent of the volatile oil is eucalyptol (1,8-cineole).

Actions
Although eucalyptus has been shown in rabbits to possess hypoglycemic activity, its mechanism of action is unknown. Eucalyptus produces a stimulant effect on nasal cold receptors. It is also a counterirritant and causes an increase in cutaneous blood flow (Hong et al., 1991). Eucalyptus has also been shown to exert antimicrobial, antifungal, and anti-inflammatory effects (Egawa et al., 1977; Pattnaik et al., 1996; Santos et al., 1997)

Reported uses
The herb was first used more than 100 years ago for the relief of nasal congestion. When inhaled eucalyptus was evaluated in human patients, the changes in nasal resistance were similar to that of breathing air alone (Burrow et al., 1983).

Dosage
For various uses, typical oral dosages include 0.05 to 0.2 ml (eucalyptol), 0.05 to 0.2 ml (eucalyptus oil), or 2 to 4 g (fluid extract). For topical use, 30 ml oil is mixed with 500 ml water.

Adverse reactions
• CNS, GI, and respiratory reactions may occur even with low doses
• Cyanosis
• Delirium
• Dizziness
• Epigastric burning

- Miosis
- Muscular weakness
- Nausea
- Vomiting
⚠ Seizures

Interactions
None reported.

Contraindications and precautions
Eucalyptus oil is contraindicated in patients receiving hypoglycemic therapy and in pregnant or breast-feeding patients.

Special considerations
- Monitor for adverse reactions, and institute seizure precautions where appropriate.
- Advise the patient that the herb should be diluted before internal or external use.
- Instruct the patient to keep this agent away from children and pets.
- Advise the pregnant or breast-feeding patient to avoid use of the herb.

Analysis
Although eucalyptus is widely consumed, very little clinical data support its claims. Data on the herb's antimicrobial and antifungal effects have not been evaluated in human or animals; therefore, use of eucalyptus cannot be recommended.

References

Burrow, A., et al. "The Effects of Camphor, Eucalyptus, and Menthol Vapors on Nasal Resistance to Airflow and Nasal Sensation," *Acta Otolaryngol* 96:157-61, 1983.

Egawa, H., et al. "Antifungal Substances Found in Leaves of Eucalyptus Species," *Specialia* 15:889-90, 1977.

Hong, C., et al. "Effects of a Topically Applied Counterirritant (Eucalyptamint) on Cutaneous Blood Flow and on the Skin and Muscle Temperature," *Am J Phys Med Rehabil* 70:29-33, 1991.

Pattnaik, S., et al. "Antibacterial and Antifungal Activity of Ten Essential Oils In Vitro," *Microbios* 86:237-46, 1996.

Santos, F., et al. "Mast Cell Involvement in the Rat Paw Oedema Response to 1,8-cineole, the Main Constituent of Eucalyptus and Rosemary Oils," *Eur J Pharmacol* 331:253-58, 1997.

EYEBRIGHT

MEADOW EYEBRIGHT, RED EYEBRIGHT

Common trade names
None known.

Common forms
Available as a lotion or infusion for internal use.

Source
Eyebright comes from *Euphrasia officinalis* (common name, eyebright), and is an annual plant that grows to approximately 1 foot.

Chemical components
Eyebright is composed of carbohydrates, tannins, alkaloids, sterols, phenolic acids, caffeic acids, aucubin, flavonoid glycosides, amino acids, and a volatile fraction.

Actions
None of the plant's constituents exert significant therapeutic effect. Despite the claim that caffeic acid exerts bacteriostatic properties, this effect has not been scientifically documented. A study using extracts of *E. officinalis* in vitro revealed that eyebright exerts a significant cytotoxic effect (Trovato et al., 1996).

Reported uses
Eyebright has been claimed to be useful as a lotion or through internal consumption in the treatment of conjunctivitis and blepharitis. Other reported indications include eye fatigue and styes.

Dosage
For ophthalmic use, soak a pad in an infusion and apply to the eyes as a compress. As an eyewash, 5 to 10 drops of tincture in water. An infusion for oral consumption has been prepared by steeping the plant in boiling water.

Adverse reactions
- Confusion
- Diminished vision
- Headache
- Itching
- Nasal congestion
- Photophobia
- Redness and swelling of the margins of the lids
- Sneezing

• Violent pressure in the eyes with tearing
• Weakness

Interactions
None reported.

Contraindications and precautions
No known contraindications.

Special considerations
• Monitor for adverse reactions, particularly during ophthalmic use.
• Advise the patient that this herb should not be used to treat ophthalmic conditions because of risk of ophthalmic infection.
• Advise the patient to avoid use of the herb because of the risk of cytotoxic effects.
• Instruct the patient to report changes in vision, and eye swelling, redness, or discharge.
• Advise the patient to wear sunglasses and to avoid bright light.

Points of interest
• The plant has been used since the Middle Ages to treat bloodshot or irritated eyes. Its use for this condition evolved because the flowers, which have spots and stripes, resemble bloodshot eyes.

Analysis
No evidence exists that eyebright is effective as an ophthalmic agent. The risk of ophthalmic infection is high with this product because preparations may not be sterile. Thus, eyebright cannot be recommended for use.

References
Trovato, A., et al. "In Vitro Cytotoxic Effect of Some Medicinal Plants Containing Flavonoids." *Boll Chim Farm* 135:263-66,1996.

FALSE UNICORN ROOT

BLAZING STAR, FAIRYWAND, HELONIAS DIOICA, STARWORT

Common trade names
None known.

Common forms
Available as dried roots, chopped for decoction, as a tincture, or as a component of tablets used for menopausal symptoms.

Source
The drug is extracted from the root system of *Chamaelirium luteum* in autumn. The plant is native to North America, is generally harvested from the wild, and is rarely cultivated.

Chemical components
The key constituents of false unicorn root are steroidal saponins and the glycosides chamaelirin and helonin.

Actions
Claims for the pharmacologic activity of *Chamaelirium luteum* include diuretic effects, uterine and ovarian tonic effects, and genitourinary stimulant activities. No scientific data are available to support these claims. The steroidal saponins are claimed to stimulate the uterus, but no supporting evidence exists.

Reported uses
False unicorn root has traditionally been promoted for menstrual and uterine problems. The presence of steroidal saponins in the drug is claimed to be effective as a uterine tonic in amenorrhea and dysmenorrhea, in liver dysfunction, and as a stimulant in genitourinary weakness (Grieve, 1996). No published clinical trials or other clinical evidence is available to support these claims.

Dosage
For menopausal symptoms, 5 to 10 drops of tincture P.O. four to six times daily. Or, if using a decoction, ½ cup P.O. b.i.d.

Adverse reactions
None reported.

Interactions
None reported.

Contraindications and precautions
Avoid use in pregnant patients. Also, avoid use in breast-feeding patients; effects are unknown.

Special considerations
• Know that reported beneficial effects of false unicorn root may take months to appear.

Points of interest
• This herb was listed as a uterine tonic and a diuretic in the *U.S. National Formulary* from 1916 to 1947.

Analysis
There is no documented evidence that false unicorn root is effective for conditions affecting the uterus and ovaries. The lack of animal and human data to support its claims and the unknown risks associated with the agent's use limit its usefulness. This product cannot be recommended at this time because of the lack of clinical trials.

References
Grieve, M. *A Modern Herbal.* New York: Barnes & Noble, Inc., 1996.

FENNEL

ANETH FENOUIL, BITTER FENNEL, CAROSELLA, COMMON FENNEL, FENCHEL, FENOUIL, FENOUILLE, FINOCCHIO, FLORENCE FENNEL, FUNCHO, GARDEN FENNEL, HINOJO, LARGE FENNEL, SWEET FENNEL, WILD FENNEL

Common trade names
Bitter Fennel, Sweet Fennel

Common forms
Volatile oil in water: 2% (Sweet Fennel), 4% (Bitter Fennel)

Source
Fennel is usually obtained from the seeds of *Foeniculum vulgare,* from which is extracted the essential oil. The root of this plant is also considered useful.

Chemical components

The seeds of *F. vulgare* contain 2% to 6% volatile oil, 20% fixed oil (composed of petroselinic acid, oleic acid, and linoleic acid), and high concentrations of tocopherols. Other components of the seeds include flavonoids, umbelliferone, kaempferols, stigmasterol, proteins, sugars, vitamins, and minerals. The herb has a high potassium and calcium content. The volatile oil consists of anethol, fenchone, estragole, limonene, camphene, and alpha-pinene. Other components of the herb include monoterpene hydrocarbons, sabinene, alpha-phellandrene, myrcene, terpinenes, terpinolene, fenchyl alcohol, anisaldehyde, and myristicin apiole.

Actions

Fennel and its volatile oil are reported to have stimulant and antiflatulent properties. Fennel oil with methylparaben has been shown to inhibit the growth of *Salmonella enteriditis* and to a lesser extent *Listeria monocytogenes* (Fyfe et al., 1997). The oil inhibited the twitch response in smooth muscle, and tracheal and ileal muscles in guinea pigs (Lis-Balchin and Hart, 1997). Aqueous fennel extracts increase ciliary function of frog epithelium. An acetone extract of fennel seeds produced an estrogenic effect on the genital organs of male and female rats (Malini et al., 1985).

Reported uses

Despite fennel's claims to increase milk secretion, promote menses, facilitate birth, and increase libido, human data are lacking.

Dosage

For GI complaints, 0.1 to 0.6 ml P.O. daily of the oil, or 5 to 7 g of the fruit daily.

Adverse reactions

- Contact dermatitis
- Nausea
- Photodermatitis
- Seizures
- Tumors (An essential oil component, estragole, has caused tumors in animals.)
- Vomiting

⚠ Pulmonary edema (rare)

⚠ The fennel plant may be mistaken for poison hemlock, which contains the strong narcotic coniine. Ingestion of a small amount of hemlock causes vomiting, paralysis, and death.

Interactions

None reported.

Contraindications and precautions

Use cautiously in patients allergic to other members of the Umbelliferae family, such as celery, carrots, or mugwort. Avoid use in pregnant patients.

Special considerations

• Inform the patient this herb cannot be recommended for any use because of insufficient evidence.
• Remind the patient that the long-term risks of herb's use are not known.
• Advise the patient to avoid sun exposure if photodermatitis occurs.
• Advise the pregnant or breast-feeding patient to avoid use of fennel.
• Inform the patient who may grow this plant to avoid mistakenly retrieving hemlock, which may be fatal if ingested.

Points of interest

• Fennel is used as a flavoring in liquors, baked goods, meat products, snacks, and gravies. The highest concentration of fennel in foods cannot exceed 0.119%. In soaps, lotions, and perfumes, the maximum is 0.4%.

Analysis

Because of a lack of clinical data, fennel cannot be recommended as treatment for any condition.

References

Fyfe, L., et al. "Inhibition of *Listeria monocytogenes* and *Salmonella enteriditis* by Combinations of Plant Oils and Derivatives of Benzoic Acid: The Development of Synergistic Antimicrobial Combinations," *Int J Antimicrob Agents* 9:195-99, 1997.

Lis-Balchin, M., and Hart, S. "A Preliminary Study of the Effect of Essential Oils on Skeletal and Smooth Muscle In Vitro," *J Ethnopharmacol* 58:183-87, 1997.

Malini, T., et al. "The Effects of *Foeniculum vulgare* Mill Seed Extract on the Genital Organs of Male and Female Rats," *Indian J Physiol Pharmacol* 29:21, 1985.

FENUGREEK

BIRD'S-FOOT, GREEK HAYSEED, TRIGONELLA

Common trade names

Fenugreek Seed, Fenu-Thyme

Common forms

Available as a crude drug; extracts in liquid and spray; dried forms; seeds in a dried powder or capsules; and as a poultice.

Source

Fenugreek, or *Trigonella foenum-graecum*, is native to countries on the eastern shores of the Mediterranean. The plant is cultivated in India, Egypt, Morocco and, occasionally, in England. The medicinally active component of fenugreek is found exclusively in the seeds, which are cultivated in sickle-like pods, each containing 10 to 20 brownish seeds.

Chemical components

The seeds contains saponins (diosgenin, tigogenin, gitogenin, trigogenin, yamogenin, neotigogenin, fenugreekine, neogitogenin, smilagenin), alkaloids (trigonelline, gentianine, carpaine, choline), proteins, and amino acids (lysine, tryptophan, 4-hydroxyisoleucine, histadine, and arginine). Other components include coumarin, mucilage fiber, vitamins (including nicotinic acid), minerals, and lipids.

Actions

Hypocholesterolemic activity in rats and dogs has been attributed to the fiber and saponin components of the seeds. Nicotinic acid, in unknown amounts in the seeds, is thought to contribute to lowering cholesterol. Most studies report a reduction of total cholesterol and triglyceride levels; however, the extent of reduction varied.

Fenugreek has been shown to exert hypoglycemic effects in rabbits, rats, and dogs. The saponin fenugreekine has been reported to possess cardiotonic, diuretic, hypoglycemic, antiviral, and antihypertensive properties.

Aqueous and alcoholic extracts of fenugreek have shown a stimulant action on the uterus of guinea pigs, especially during late pregnancy. Aqueous extracts have also been found to increase heart rate and exert anti-inflammatory and diuretic activity in animals (Newall et al., 1996). Fenugreek extracts may decrease calcium oxalate deposition in the kidney (Ahsan et al., 1989).

Reported uses

Fenugreek has traditionally been used to treat constipation, anorexia, dyspepsia, gastritis, and other related GI conditions. Topical formulations have been used for leg ulcers, myalgia, gout, wounds, and lymphadenitis. Additional claims include use as an antidiabetic agent and as a treatment for tuberculosis and cellulitus. These claims await verification from clinical trials.

Dosage

Seeds: 1 to 6 g P.O. t.i.d.
Powdered drug: 50 g to ¼ L of water applied topically.

Adverse reactions
- Bleeding, bruising
- Hypoglycemia

Interactions
Anticoagulants: possible enhanced hypoprothrombinemic effect of the anticoagulants. Avoid concurrent use.
Antidiabetic agents: possible enhanced glucose-lowering effects. May require dosage adjustments during herbal treatment.
Other oral medications administered concurrently: decreased absorption. Because of the high mucilaginous and fiber content of fenugreek seeds, absorption of other oral medications given concurrently may be impaired. Avoid concurrent use.

Contraindications and precautions
Avoid use of the herb in pregnant women because of risk of oxytocic action.

Special considerations
⚠ Monitor coagulation studies and blood glucose in patients at high risk, especially in those who consume excessive quantities of the plant.
- Monitor the patient for signs of bleeding.
- Advise the patient to report if other medications appear to be less effective.
- Instruct the patient to self-monitor blood glucose levels until the hypoglycemic effects of the herb are known.
- Teach the patient the signs, symptoms, and management of hypoglycemia.
- Instruct the patient to report unusual bleeding or bruising.
- Advise the patient taking fenugreek for its effects on glucose and cholesterol levels that other effective, pharmacologic agents with known morbidity and mortality data exist.

Points of interest
- In the United States, fenugreek is categorized by the FDA as "Generally Recommended As Safe" at concentrations below 0.05%.
- The taste and odor of fenugreek resembles maple syrup. In the past, fenugreek was added to liquid medicinals to mask their taste. A child receiving fenugreek tea was noted to have urine that smelled like maple syrup. This symptom mimics one found in a rare hereditary metabolic disorder, branched-chain hyperaminoaciduria, otherwise known as maple syrup urine disease.

Analysis

Although fenugreek may hold promise for use in diabetes or hyper-cholesterolemia, data regarding dosage, efficacy, and safety have not yet been established for humans, or compared with existing pharmacologic agents with proven beneficial effects. Large-scale clinical trials evaluating morbidity and mortality are needed before the herb can be recommended.

References

Ahsan, S.K., et al. "Effect of *Trigonella foenum-graecum* and *Ammi majus* on Calcium Oxalate Urolithiasis in Rats," *J Ethnopharmacol* 26:249, 1989.
Newall, C.A., et al. *Herbal Medicines. A Guide for Health-Care Professionals.* London: The Pharmaceutical Press, 1996.

FEVERFEW

ALTAMISA, BACHELORS' BUTTON, CHAMOMILE GRANDE, FEATHERFEW, FEATHERFOIL, FEBRIFUGE PLANT, MIDSUMMER DAISY, MUTTERKRAUT, NOSEBLEED, SANTA MARIA, WILD CHAMOMILE, WILD QUININE

Common trade names
(Various manufacturers) Feverfew, Feverfew Glyc, Feverfew Power

Common forms
Available as capsules (pure leaf, 380 mg; leaf extract, 250 mg), liquid, and tablets. The leaves are commonly used to make infusions or teas.

Source
Feverfew, a plant from Europe naturalized in the United States and Canada, bears yellow-green leaves and yellow flowers from July to October. The leaves of the plant are usually dried or used fresh in teas and extracts. The most commonly cited botanical name is *Chrysanthemum parthenium*, synonymous with *Tanacetum parthenium. Matricaria parthenium, Leucanthemum parthenium,* and *Pyrethrum parthenium* are also used to refer to the plant.

Chemical components
The leaves and flowering tops of feverfew contain many mono-quiterpenes and sesquiterpenes, as well as sesquiterpene lactones (chrysanthemolide, chrysanthemonin, 10-epi-canin, magnoliolide, and parthenolide), reynosin, santamarin, tanaparthins, and other compounds. Parthenolide may be absent or occur in variable amounts, depending on geographic and other variables.

Actions

The main active ingredients are the sesquiterpene lactones, particularly parthenolide, which inhibits serotonin release by human platelets in vitro. This may be the mechanism of action for the herb's purported efficacy in treating migraines (Groenewegen and Heptinstall, 1990). Parthenolide also inhibits serotonin release (Heptinstall et al., 1992). Extracts of feverfew contain chemicals that inhibit activation of polymorphonuclear leukocytes and the synthesis of leukotrienes and prostaglandins.

Reported uses

Although initial enthusiasm for feverfew had waned, plant preparations are becoming increasingly popular for use in migraine prophylaxis and as an antipyretic. (See *Feverfew and migraine prophylaxis.*) Feverfew is also claimed to be useful for the treatment of psoriasis, toothache, insect bites, rheumatism, asthma, stomach ache, menstrual problems, and threatened miscarriage.

Dosage

For migraine treatment, average dose of 543 mcg P.O. parthenolide daily.
For migraine prophylaxis, 25 mg of freeze-dried leaf extract P.O. daily; 50 mg of leaf P.O. daily with food; or 50 to 200 mg of aerial parts of plant P.O. daily.

Adverse reactions

• Hypersensitivity reactions
• Mouth ulcerations (common with crude drug)
• Post-feverfew syndrome (withdrawal syndrome characterized by moderate to severe pain and joint and muscle stiffness)

Interactions

None reported.

Contraindications and precautions

Contraindicated in pregnant or breast-feeding women.

Special considerations

• Monitor for allergic reaction.
• Monitor for mouth ulcerations. Encourage proper oral hygiene.
• Know that feverfew potency is often based on the parthenolide content in the preparation, which is variable.
• Instruct the patient not to withdraw the herb abruptly, but to taper its use gradually because of risk of post-feverfew syndrome.
• Assure the patient that several other strategies for migraine treatment and prophylaxis exist, and that these should be attempted be-

RESEARCH FINDINGS
Feverfew and migraine prophylaxis

The efficacy of feverfew for migraine prophylaxis has been assessed in a randomized, double-blind, placebo-controlled clinical trial (Murphy, 1988). The study included 76 patients with classic or common migraine headaches for over 2 years, and at least one attack monthly. All other migraine treatments were discontinued before the trial began. After a 1-month, single-blind, placebo run-in period, the patients were randomized to receive one capsule daily of either placebo or feverfew for 4 months. At that time, the patients were crossed over to the other treatment arm of the study. Patients recorded the number, duration, and severity of each migraine attack. Working days missed, nausea, vomiting, and visual or neurologic effects were noted in their diaries.

Of the 76 patients enrolled, 59 patients completed the trial. The number of attacks during feverfew treatment was reduced by 24% compared with placebo. There was no significant difference in the duration of migraine attacks between the herb and placebo. Nausea and vomiting were reduced significantly with feverfew treatment. The number of working days missed with herbal therapy was 68, whereas that for placebo was 76.

At the end of the study but while still blinded to the therapy received, 59% of patients reported that the feverfew treatment period was more effective; only 24% chose placebo. No significant differences between the two treatments was noted in 17% of patients.

When the study population was subdivided into classic and common migraine or patients who had (or had not) used feverfew previously, the results still showed statistically significant reductions in the number and severity of attacks in all subgroups. There were fewer adverse effects with feverfew than placebo, and there was no evidence of feverfew withdrawal. The authors concluded that the herb is safe and effective in the prophylaxis of migraine attacks.

In another trial, patients already using feverfew for the prophylaxis of migraine attacks were randomized to either placebo or the continued use of the herb (Johnson et al., 1985). Patients switched to placebo experienced significant increases in both the severity and frequency of migraine attacks and arthralgias. These symptoms were later identified as post-feverfew syndrome, a withdrawal syndrome of feverfew. The duration of migraine was not altered by feverfew in either trial.

fore taking products with unknown benefits and risks.
• Remind the patient to promptly report unusual symptoms such as mouth sores or skin ulcerations.

Points of interest
• The concentration of parthenolide in the leaves and flowering tops is highest during the summer, before the seeds are set, and drops rapidly thereafter. This may explain the difference in parthenolide levels between brands of feverfew capsules and tablets.
• The Health Protection Branch of the Canadian government has proposed a standard that formulations contain a minimum of 0.2% parthenolide.

Analysis
Although feverfew has been shown to be effective for migraine prophylaxis in at least two clinical trials, further studies are necessary to define better dosage guidelines and specific drug interactions and mechanisms of actions. For patients in whom standard drug therapy has failed, feverfew appears to be the only treatment that can prevent migraine attacks. Although standardized feverfew preparations with dosages based on free parthenolide content have the best experimental support, no consensus on use exists.

References
Groenewegen, W.A., and Heptinstall, S. "A Comparison of the Effects of an Extract of Feverfew and Parthenolide, a Component of Feverfew, on Human Platelet Activity In Vitro," *J Pharm Pharmacol* 43:553-57, 1990.

Heptinstall, S., et al. "Parthenolide Content and Bioactivity of Feverfew (*Tenacetum parthenium* [L.] Schultz-Bip.). Estimation of Commercial and Authenticated Feverfew Products," *J Pharm Pharmacol* 44:391-95, 1992.

Johnson, E.S., et al. "Efficacy of Feverfew as Prophylactic Treatment of Migraine," *BMJ* 291:569-73, 1985.

Murphy, J.J., et al. "Randomised, Double-Blind, Placebo-Controlled Trial of Feverfew in Migraine Prevention," *Lancet* 2:189-92, 1988.

FIGWORT

CARPENTER'S-SQUARE, COMMON FIGWORT, ROSE-NOBLE, SCROFULA PLANT, SQUARE STALK, STINKING CHRISTOPHER, THROATWORT

Common trade names
None known.

Common forms
Available as a tincture, compress, soak, or wash.

Source

Figwort is most commonly derived from *Scrophularia nodosa* and *S. ningpoensis*. Medicinal components are removed from the dried leaves and flowers. The root has also been used, principally in China.

Chemical components

Figwort consists of the amino acids alanine, isoleucine, leucine, lysine, phenylalanine, threonine, tyrosine, and valine. It also contains flavonoids (diosmetin, diosmin, acacetin rhamnoside, iridoids, aucubin, acetylharpagide, harpagide, harpagoside, isoharpagoside, procumbid and catalpol), caffeic acid, cinnamic acid, ferulic acid, sinapic acid, and vanillic acid. Also present are saponins, cardioactive gylcosides, phytosterol, essential fatty acids, and aspargine.

Actions

Figwort appears to possess antibacterial and anti-inflammatory properties, although the mechanism has not been described. Aucubin and catalpol exert cathartic action in rodents (Inouye et al., 1974). Figwort is related to foxglove, which contains digitalis-like glycosides, and contains chemicals that strengthen the force of cardiac contraction and slow the heart rate.

Reported uses

This herb is believed to be useful for eczema, psoriasis, pruritus, and other chronic skin conditions. Additional claims involve the agent's use as an anti-inflammatory, cardiac stimulant, and an agent for GI disorders.

Dosage

Infusion: 2 to 8 g of dried herb P.O.
Liquid extract: 2 to 8 ml P.O.
Tincture: 2 to 4 ml P.O.
Dosage frequency is unknown.

Adverse reactions

- Bradycardia
- Diarrhea
- Heart block
- Nausea
- Vomiting
⚠ Asystole

Interactions

- *Beta blockers, calcium channel blockers, cardiac glycosides:* possible enhancement of cardiac effects of these drugs. Avoid concurrent use.

Contraindications and precautions

Use cautiously in patients with underlying heart disease or in those at risk for arrhythmias. Avoid use in pregnant and breast-feeding women; safety has not been established.

Special considerations

• Monitor heart rate and rhythm.
• Explain that scientific evidence supporting use of the plant is severely lacking.
• Instruct the patient to immediately report changes in heart rate, light-headedness, weakness, or shortness of breath.
• Caution the patient with underlying heart disease or at risk for arrhythmias against use of figwort.
• Advise the pregnant or breast-feeding patient to avoid use of the herb.

Points of interest

• Figwort is not known to be a component of any food.
• The chemical components of figwort resemble those of devil's claw (*Harpagophytum procumbens*).

Analysis

Literature supporting any use of this plant is lacking. The herb should not be used by any patient, especially those with heart disease.

References

Inouye, H., et al. "Purgative Activities of Iridoid Glucosides," *Planta Med* 25:285-88, 1974.

FLAX

FLAXSEED, LINSEED, LINT BELLS, LINUM

Common trade names

Barlean's Flax Oil, Barlean's Vita-Flax, Flaxseed

Common forms

Available as a powder, capsules, softgel capsules (1,000 mg), and an oil.

Source

Flaxseed is the soluble fiber mucilage obtained from the fully developed seed of *Linum usitatissimum* and is sometimes used in poultices.

Chemical components
Flaxseed and linseed oil are rich (30% to 45%) in unsaturated fatty acids, including linolenic, linoleic, and oleic acids. Approximately 3% to 6% of the plant contains soluble fiber mucilage consisting of galactose, arabinose, rhamnose, xylose, galactuonic, and mannuronic acids. Seed chaff and leaves contain cyanogenic glycosides, linamarin, linustatin, and nicolenustatin. Linamarase can potentiate cyanide release from linamarin. The plant also contain 25% protein. Some products contain additional essential fatty acids, fiber, vitamins, and minerals.

Actions
In humans, linolenic acid decreases total cholesterol and low-density-lipoprotein levels. One study in humans noted a decrease in thrombin-mediated platelet aggregation (Bierenbaum et al., 1993). Flaxseed contains lignans, reported to have weak estrogenic, antiestrogenic, and steroidlike activity. Diets high in flaxseed may lower the risk of breast and other hormone-dependent cancers, although this premise awaits clinical confirmation (Thompson et al., 1997). One study determined that linolenic acid supplement, derived from flax, arginine, and yeast RNA, improved weight gain in some patients with HIV (Suttman et al., 1996).

Reported uses
Flax has been used for constipation, functional disorders of the colon resulting from laxative abuse, irritable bowel syndrome, and diverticulitis. It has also been taken internally as a supplement to decrease the risk of hypercholesterolemia and atherosclerosis, despite the lack of clinical trials evaluating its effects on morbidity and mortality. Externally, flax has been made into a poultice and used to treat areas of local inflammation.

Dosage
For all systemic uses, 1 to 2 tablespoons of oil or mature seeds daily in two or three divided doses. Average dose is 1 oz of oil or mature seeds daily.
For topical use, 30 to 50 g of flax meal applied as a hot, moist poultice or compress as needed.

Adverse reactions
- Diarrhea
- Flatulence
- Nausea

⚠ Immature seedpods are especially poisonous. All parts of the plant contain cyanogenic nitrates and glucosides, particularly linamarin. Overdose symptoms include, but are not limited to, shortness of breath, tachypnea, weakness, and unstable gait, progressing to paralysis and seizures.

Interactions
Laxatives, stool softeners: possible increase in laxative actions of flax. Avoid concurrent use.
Oral medications taken concurrently with herb: possible diminished absorption of oral medications. Avoid taking flax and other drugs concurrently.

Contraindications and precautions
Contraindicated in pregnant and breast-feeding women because the herb's hormonal effects may cause teratogenicity or spontaneous abortion. Avoid use in patients with prostate cancer or suspected or actual ileus.

Special considerations
• Monitor for potential toxicity related to oral ingestion of this herb; cyanosis is a symptom of flax toxicity.
• Encourage the patient to drink plenty of fluids to minimize risk of flatulence.
• Instruct the patient to refrigerate flaxseed oil to prevent breakdown of the essential fatty acids.
• Remind the patient that other cholesterol-lowering therapies exist that have been proven to improve survival and lower the risk of cardiac disease; flax has no such clinical support.
• Instruct the patient never to ingest immature seeds and to keep flax away from children and pets.
• Remind the patient that the long-term risks of flax use are not known.
• Tell the patient to report decreased effects of other drugs being taken.

Points of interest
• Flax has been used as a source of fiber for weaving and clothing for more than 10,000 years. Linseed oil, derived from flax, has been used in paints and varnishes and as a waterproofing agent. Flaxseed cakes are used as a food source for cattle. (See *Uses of flax.*)

Analysis
Supplementation of flax as a source of omega-3 fatty acids and its value in the treatment of inflammatory diseases warrants further investigation. Most claims associated with herbal use are unfounded. The potentially toxic components (cyanogenic nitrates) and the potential mutagenic effect of flax require further study to determine its long-term safety and efficacy.

FOLKLORE
Uses of flax

Archeologists have identfied fibers from flax among the remains of prehistoric Scandinavian lake dwellers, who used flax fibers for purposes other than food.

Linsey-woolsey fabrics created from flax were introduced to the United States by Europeans during the Colonial period. For over two centuries, it remained a fundamental fabric for durable American apparel. The production of linen from flax is thought to be no more difficult than that of cotton or wool yarn.

Flax fibers have been used to make fine paper. The seeds, when immersed in water, developed a slimy coating and were then used as a "protectant," similar to how waxes are used currently. Farmers believed in feeding flax to their horses and cows to maintain a "healthy shine on their coat." Because of their slippery nature, there were tales of fatalities from people having fallen into large vats of seeds and drowned. Linseed oil, expressed from flaxseeds, has long been used in paints and varnishes; however, its popularity has declined since the advent of water-based finishes.

Linseed oil is reportedly useful to veterinarians as a topical demulcent, emollient, and laxative. Finally, contemporary herbal texts suggest that the fibers are suitable for baskets and ornamentation (Dobelis, 1986).

References
Bierenbaum, M.L., et al. "Reducing Atherogenic Risk in Hyperlipidemic Humans with Flax Seed Supplementation: A Preliminary Report," *J Am Coll Nutr* 12:501, 1993.

Dobelis, I.N., ed. *Magic and Medicine of Plants.* Pleasantville, N.Y.: The Reader's Digest Association, Inc., 1986.

Suttman, U., et al. "Weight Gain and Increased Concentrations of Receptor Proteins for Tumor Necrosis Factor After Patients with Symptomatic HIV Infection Received Fortified Nutrition Support," *J Am Diet Assoc* 96:565-69, 1996.

Thompson, L.U., et al. "Variability in Anticancer Lignan Levels in Flaxseed," *Nutr Cancer* 27:26-30, 1997.

FUMITORY

EARTH SMOKE, HEDGE FUMITORY, WAX DOLLS

Common trade names
None known.

Common forms
None known.

Source
Fumitory comes from the *Fumaria officinalis* plant, native to Europe and North Africa but also grown in Asia, North America, and Australia. The leaves and flowering aerial parts of the plant are used to produce fumitory.

Chemical components
Fumitory contains many alkaloids, including protopine (also known as fumarine, an isoquinoline derivative), aurotensine, coridaline, cryptopine, stylopine, cryptocavine, sinactine, n-methylsinactine sanquinarine, and bulbocapnine.

Fumitory also contains fumaric acid salts (fumaricine, fumariline, fumaritine), phlobaphene, yellow dye, flavonoids, quercetin and iso-quercetin-related compounds, benzophenanthridines, chlorogenic acids, caffeic and fumaric acids, mucilage, resinous substances, and other compounds.

Actions
In animals, fumitory extracts exhibit antibacterial actions, vasodilating properties, antispasmodic activity on smooth muscle, positive inotropic effects, a moderate hypotensive effect, modulation of bile flow, and inhibition of biliary calculi formation. In addition, the predominant alkaloid, protopine, has antihistaminic and sedative effects at low doses, and stimulatory and convulsive activity at higher doses (Preininger, 1975). Cryptopine and protopine, when isolated, exert negative chronotropic effects in vitro.

Reported uses
Various therapeutic claims have been made for fumitory, including as a treatment for dermatologic eruptions (milk crust, eczema, and scabies), and as a diuretic and a laxative. None of the data supporting these claims have been published in English. Clinical case reports and animal studies have demonstrated the usefulness of fumitory in treating functional diseases of the biliary system (Hentschel et al., 1995). A Russian report noted that injections of fumitory alkaloids were effective in resolving myocardial ischemia and arrhythmias caused by reversible coronary blood flow disorders (Gorbunov et al., 1980).

Dosage
Dried herb: 2 to 4 g P.O. t.i.d., or a tea with 2 to 4 g of the dried herb P.O. t.i.d.
Liquid extract (1:1 in 25% alcohol): 2 to 4 ml P.O. t.i.d.
Tincture (1:5 in 45% alcohol): 1 to 4 ml P.O. t.i.d.

Adverse reactions
- Bradycardia
- Elevated intraocular pressure
- Hypotension
- Sedation

⚠ Seizures (at high or toxic doses)

Interactions
Antihypertensives: possible enhanced hypotensive effect. Avoid concurrent use.

Beta blockers, calcium channel blockers, digoxin, other agents that slow the heart rate: possible bradycardia, heart block, or asystole. Avoid concurrent use.

Contraindications and precautions
Contraindicated in patients with glaucoma, at risk for seizures, and in pregnant or breast-feeding women.

Special considerations
- Monitor intraocular pressure in patients at risk for glaucoma.
- Monitor heart rate and blood pressure
- Monitor the patient prone to seizures. Inform the patient at risk for seizures that although not reported in humans, studies with animals suggest that high doses or prolonged use of this herb or protopine may exacerbate seizure disorders.
- Instruct the patient to report light-headedness, weakness, shortness of breath, or changes in heart rate.
- Advise the pregnant or breast-feeding patient to avoid use of this herb.

Analysis
Fumitory has not been systematically evaluated in humans. Data from studies with animals are limited. Safety and efficacy for any use remain unproven.

References
Gorbunov, N.P., et al. "Pharmacological Correction of Myocardial Ischemia and Arrhythmias in Reversible Coronary Blood Flow Disorders and Experimental Myocardial Infarct in Dogs," *Kardiologiia* 20:84-87, 1980.

Hentschel, C., et al. "*Fumaria officinalis* (fumitory)—Clinical Applications," *Fortschr Med* 113:291-92, 1995.

Preininger, V. "The Pharmacology and Toxicology of the Papaveraceae Alkaloids," in *The Alkaloids XV.* Edited by Manske, R.H.F. London: Academic Press, 1975.

GALANGAL

ALPINIA OFFICINARUM, CHINA ROOT, CHINESE GINGER, COLIC ROOT, EAST INDIAN ROOT, GALANGA, KAEMPFERIA GALANGA, RHIZOMA GALANGAE

Common trade names
None known.

Common forms
None known.

Source
Alpinia consists of the dried root of *Alpinia officinarum*, a native of eastern and southeastern Asia. The plant has been grown in Hainan (Southern China) and coastal areas around Pak-hoi.

Chemical components
The active ingredients of the root are the volatile oil (consisting of cineol, eugenol, sesquiterpenes, and isomerides of cadinene) and resin (containing kaempferide, galangol, galangin, alpinin, and starch).

Actions
The galangal root is thought to contain inhibitors against prostaglandin biosynthesizing enzyme. Traditionally, galangal is used for its carminative, aromatic, and diaphoretic activities.

A. galanga is reported to have antifungal activity and studies in mice show an antitumor effect (Morita and Itokawa, 1988; Qureshi et al., 1992). The chemical component of *A. galanga*, acetoxychavicol acetate, is thought to have antifungal activity (Janssen and Scheffer, 1985).

Reported uses
There is a lack of well-controlled clinical trials in animals or humans. Therapeutic studies have been primarily conducted in animals. It has been used in Saudi medicine as an antirheumatic agent.

Dosage
Usual dose is 1 g P.O.

Adverse reactions
- Diarrhea
- Nausea
- Vomiting

Interactions
None reported.

Contraindications and precautions
Contraindicated in patients if pregnancy is being planned or is suspected, and in those with chronic disease of the GI tract.

Special considerations
- Tell the patient to consult the health care provider before taking this herb.
- Instruct the female patient to report planned or suspected pregnancy.

Points of interest
- Galanga is related to ginger, both botanically and pharmacologically.

Analysis
There is little well-documented evidence that galangal is effective in rheumatic disorders or fungal infections. The lack of animal and human data to support its claims and the potential risks limit its use. The use of galangal in humans cannot be recommended.

References
Janssen, A., and Scheffer, J.J. "Acetoxychavicol Acetate, an Antifungal Component of *Alpinia galanga*," *Planta Med* 51:507, 1985.

Morita, H., and Itokawa, H. "Cytotoxic and Antifungal Diterpenes from the Seeds of *Alpinia galanga*," *Planta Med* 54:117, 1988.

Qureshi, S., et al. "Toxicity Studies on *Alpinia galanga* and *Curucuma longa*," *Planta Med* 58:124, 1992.

GALANTHAMINE

GALANTHAMINE HYDROBROMIDE

Common trade names
Nivalin

Common forms
Tablets (coated): 5 mg, 10 mg
Ampules: 5 mg

Source

Galanthamine is isolated from the bulbs of the common snowdrop, *Galanthus nivalis*. It is also available as a chemical synthetic.

Chemical components

Galanthamine is a water-soluble alkaloid.

Actions

Galanthamine is a selective, competitive acetylcholinesterase inhibitor. The drug inhibits erythrocyte acetycholinase better than brain acetylcholinesterase. It is nearly 100% bioavailable and crosses the blood-brain barrier. In animal models, the agent attenuates drug- and lesion-induced cognitive deficits (Bores et al., 1996). In healthy male volunteers, galanthamine reversed central anticholinergic syndrome induced by I.V. scopolamine (Baraka and Harik, 1977). Preliminary clinical trials of galanthamine with Alzheimer's patients have provided mixed results. In one placebo-controlled trial of 95 patients with mild to moderate Alzheimer's disease, clinical evaluation indicated significantly less deterioration in patients receiving galanthamine after 10 weeks of treatment (Kewitz et al., 1994). In another trial, the agent did not provide any benefit (Dal-Bianco et al., 1991).

Reported uses

Galanthamine has been used to reverse neuromuscular blockade and, in some countries, for myasthenia gravis and post-polio paralysis. Its use in patients with Alzheimer's disease is approved in Austria but not in the United States. Other medications with similar mechanisms of action have been approved in the United States. More well-controlled clinical trials are needed to document the agent's safety and efficacy.

Dosage

For Alzheimer's disease, initially 5 mg t.i.d., then increase dose to 30 to 40 mg daily. Dosage should reduce acetylcholinesterase activity by 35% to 60%.

Adverse reactions

- Abdominal pain
- Agitation
- Diarrhea
- Dizziness
- Light-headedness
- Nausea
- Sleep disturbances
- Vomiting

Interactions

MAO inhibitors: may cause hypertensive crisis. Don't use together.
Organophosphate fertilizers that inhibit acetylcholinesterase: use with
galanthamine may be harmful. Avoid concomitant use.

Contraindications and precautions

Contraindicated in patients with bradycardia, severe hypotonia, recent myocardial infarction, epilepsy, hyperkinesia, Parkinson's disease, diabetic crisis, and obstructions to the respiratory, digestive, or
urinary tract.

Special considerations

• Instruct the patient to seek medical advice before taking this herb.
• Remind the patient that other conventional, accepted treatment
regimens are available.
• Tell the patient to avoid hazardous activities until CNS effects of
the herb are known.
• Inform the patient who may be at risk of organophosphate fertil-
izer exposure to avoid use of this herb.

Points of interest

• A report in 1983 suggested that the common snowdrop was probably the antidote used by Odysseus to counter the effects of Circe's
poisonous drugs in Homer's epic poem "The Odyssey." If this is
true, this was the first recorded use of galanthamine to reverse central anticholinergic intoxication (Plaitakis and Duvoisin, 1983).

Analysis

There appears to be support for the use of galanthamine in Alzheimer's disease. Based on the mechanism of action, its effects and
safety can be predicted. Further studies are needed to define its exact role in treating this disease. Meanwhile, the use of galanthamine
is questionable because similar agents are available.

References

Baraka, A., and Harik, S. "Reversal of Central Anticholinergic Syndrome by
    Galanthamine," *JAMA* 238:2293-94, 1977.
Bores, G.M., et al. "Pharmacological Evaluation of Novel Alzheimer's Disease
    Therapeutics: Acetylcholinesterase Inhibitors Related to Galanthamine," *J
    Pharmacol Exp Ther* 277:728-38, 1996.
Dal-Bianco, P., et al. "Galanthamine Treatment in Alzheimer's Disease," *J
    Neural Transm Suppl* 33:59-63, 1991.
Kewitz, H., et al. "Galanthamine, a Selective Nontoxic Acetylcholinesterase
    Inhibitor Is Significantly Superior Over Placebo in the Treatment of SDAT,"
    Neuropsychopharmacology 10 (Suppl Part 2):130, 1994.
Plaitakis, A., and Duvoisin, R.C. "Homer's Moly Identified as *Galanthus nivalis*
    L.: Physiologic Antidote to Stramonium Poisoning," *Clin Neuropharmacol*
    6:1-5, 1983.

GARLIC

AIL, ALLIUM, CAMPHOR OF THE POOR, DA-SUAN, KNOBLAUNCH, LA-SUAN, NECTAR OF THE GODS, POOR-MAN'S-TREACLE, RUSTIC TREACLE, STINKING ROSE

Common trade names
Garlic, Garlic-Power, Garlique, Kwai, Kyolic, Odorless Garlic Tablets, One a Day Garlic, Sapec

Common forms
Tablets (garlic extract): 100 mg, 320 mg, 400 mg, 600 mg
Tablets (allicin total potential): 2 to 5 mg
Dried powder: 400 to 1,200 mg
Fresh bulb: 2 to 5 g
Also available as an antiseptic oil, fresh extract, powdered, freeze-dried garlic powder, and garlic oil (essential oil).

Source
Garlic, or *Allium sativum,* is one of the most extensively researched and published medicinal plants. The fresh garlic bulb is usually dried, crushed into a powder, and then compressed to produce a tablet. The tablet form is the most commonly used commercial preparation of garlic. However, raw whole cloves have similar effects.

Chemical components
Garlic is made up of more than 23 constituents, including alliin, s-methyl-l-cysteine sulfoxide, various enzymes (alliinase, peroxidase, myrosinase), ajoenes, proteins, lipids, amino acids, phosphorus, potassium, and zinc. Also isolated are minor concentrations of selenium, vitamins A and C, calcium, magnesium, sodium, iron, manganese, and B-complex vitamins. Garlic contains the highest sulfur content of the *Allium* species, of which several sulfur-containing compounds occur in the volatile oil. Alliin, which is enzymatically converted to allicin, gives garlic its characteristic odor when its clove is crushed and ground. Allicin is believed to be the active ingredient.

Actions
Although garlic and its components are being investigated for several uses, the most commonly studied areas are its potential antithrombotic, lipid-lowering, antitumor, and antimicrobial effects. Cholesterol-lowering effects have been well documented in animals and humans. Garlic lowers total serum cholesterol, triglycerides, and low-density lipoprotein (LDL), while increasing high-density lipoprotein (HDL). One study reported a mean reduction of 6% in total serum cholesterol and 11% in LDL (Jain et al., 1993).

Garlic has documented hypoglycemic activity in rabbits; hypotensive properties in animals and humans; and antibacterial, antifungal, larvicidal, insecticidal, amebicidal, and antiviral activities in several in vitro and in vivo models. A component in garlic oil, methylallyltrisulphide, has been linked with inhibition of ADP-induced platelet aggregation (Makheja et al., 1979). An allicin derivative, ajoene, has also been shown to inhibit platelet aggregation. These effects on the platelets, however, are reported to last only a few hours (Boullin, 1981).

In Chinese studies, garlic has been shown to decrease nitrosamine (a type of carcinogen) and nitrite accumulation. Garlic extract was found to significantly prolong survival in mice injected with virulent cancer cells (Pareddy and Rosenberg, 1993). Also, garlic oil has been shown to be beneficial in rodents with GI hypermotility disorders.

Reported uses

There are many claims for garlic's use, from its ability to ward off evil spirits to healing wounds and curing infections. Most, but not all, human trials have documented garlic's ability to improve serum lipid profiles. However, such studies have been small compared with those evaluating other cholesterol-lowering agents and have not evaluated garlic's effect on morbidity and mortality, nor shown greater reductions in cholesterol than other agents (such as the statins—atorvastatin, lovastatin, simvastatin). (See *Garlic as a lipid-lowering agent,* page 270.) In one study, high allicin doses significantly lowered diastolic blood pressure but tended to produce only slightly lower systolic blood pressure (McMahon et al., 1993).

The antimicrobial properties of garlic have been reported anecdotally. Garlic extract has been used on wounds as recently as World War II. Despite reports of inhibited bacterial growth in vitro, its low potency prohibits garlic from becoming a useful clinical agent. This may be true also for garlic's potential as an antifungal agent.

Preliminary pilot studies with AIDS patients suggest that garlic extract may reduce morbidity. It may also be useful in the treatment of asthma, diabetes, inflammation, heavy metal poisoning, constipation, and athlete's foot; however, there is little, if any, evidence to support these claims.

Dosage

It has been suggested that garlic products be standardized to assure the amount of active ingredient (thought to be allicin) in each form. A German product of 600 mg dried garlic powder corresponds to a 1.3% alliin component and a 0.6% allicin release.

For lipid-lowering action, 600 to 900 mg daily; or average of 4 g (fresh garlic) or 8 mg (garlic oil) daily.

RESEARCH FINDINGS
Garlic as a lipid-lowering agent

A few trials have documented the efficacy of garlic to reduce serum lipid levels. One placebo-controlled, randomized trial studied the effects of a commercial brand of garlic tablet (Kwai) on serum cholesterol in 20 patients with documented serum cholesterol levels of 220 mg/dl or higher for 12 weeks (Jain et al., 1993); patients with triglyceride values over 400 mg/dl were excluded from the study.

After 6 weeks, no significant differences in lipid values could be detected. However, after 12 weeks, both serum total cholesterol and serum low-density lipoprotein were significantly lower by 6% and 11% respectively, compared with placebo. Changes in high-density lipoprotein, triglycerides, glucose, blood pressure, and body weight were small and insignificant. Only one patient complained of "increased belching with a garlic taste." A few patients in the placebo group reported minor adverse effects.

More recently, two trials evaluated garlic preparations in outpatients. In one trial, 5 mg b.i.d. of a steam-distilled garlic oil product produced insignificant results in lipoprotein parameters compared with placebo (Berthold et al., 1998). In the other trial, similar results in both the treatment (900 mg/day garlic) and placebo groups were obtained (Isaacsohn et al., 1998). These results warrant the need for further clinical investigation.

Adverse reactions
• Contact dermatitis; other allergic reactions (asthma, rash, anaphylaxis [rare])
• Diaphoresis
• Dizziness
• "Garlic odor"
• Hypothyroidism
• Irritation of mouth, esophagus, and stomach
• Nausea
• Vomiting
⚠ Chronic use or excessive dosages of garlic may lead to decreased hemoglobin production and lysis of RBCs.

Interactions
Anticoagulants: may increase risk of bleeding. Don't use together.
Antiplatelets: may enhance effects of antiplatelet therapy. Monitor patient.

Contraindications and precautions
Contraindicated in patient sensitive to garlic or other members of the Lilaceae family, and in those with GI disorders such as peptic

ulcer or reflux disease. Also contraindicated in pregnant patients because of its oxytocic effects.

Special considerations

• Measure CBCs on patients taking high-dose or long-term garlic.

• Advise the patient that cholesterol-lowering agents are commonly used for hypercholesterolemia because of their proven survival data and ability to lower cholesterol levels more than garlic.

• Instruct the patient to watch for signs of bleeding (bleeding gums, easy bruising, tarry stools, petechiae) if garlic supplements are taken with hemostatic agents.

• Remind the patient to report adverse reactions promptly.

Points of interest

• In Germany, garlic products are a major OTC sales item.

• Fresh and powdered garlic are commonly used as spices. The FDA has given garlic oil, extract, and oleoresin a "Generally Regarded as Safe" status.

• Although commercial preparations are available as "odorless" or "deodorized" forms, their value is questionable because the beneficial properties of garlic appear to lie with the chemical constituents that give garlic its characteristic smell.

Analysis

Garlic is one of the oldest and most revered herbals, with references to its medicinal value dating back thousands of years. Although beneficial effects on the lipid profile have been described, the data are conflicting; mortality data are also unavailable. It is not known if garlic ingestion alone reduces mortality from coronary artery disease; other medications are available that produce greater reductions in cholesterol and have proven survival benefits. If garlic is to be recommended for its cholesterol-lowering action, it should be used as part of a comprehensive cholesterol-lowering program under the direction of a health care professional. Additional indications for garlic, such as hypertension, GI motility disorders, and AIDS, await sufficient clinical evaluation.

References

Berthold, H.K., et al. "Effect of a Garlic Oil Preparation on Serum Lipoproteins and Cholesterol Metabolism. A Randomized Controlled Trial," *JAMA* 279:1900-02, 1998.

Boullin, D.J. "Garlic as a Platelet Inhibitor," *Lancet* 1:776, 1981. Letter.

Isaacsohn, J.L., et al. "Garlic Powder and Plasma Lipids and Lipoproteins. A Multicenter, Randomized, Placebo-Controlled Trial," *JAMA* 158:1189-94, 1998.

Jain, A.K., et al. "Can Garlic Reduce Levels of Serum Lipids? A Controlled Clinical Study," *Am J Med* 94:632, 1993.

Makheja, A.N., et al. "Inhibition of Platelet Aggregation and Thromboxane Synthesis by Onion and Garlic," *Lancet* 1:781, 1979. Letter.

McMahon, F.G., et al. "Can Garlic Lower Blood Pressure? A Pilot Study," *Pharmacotherapy* 13:406, 1993.

Pareddy, S.R., and Rosenberg, J.M. "Does Garlic Have Useful Medicinal Purposes?" *Hospital Pharmacist Report* 8:27, 1993.

GENTIAN

BITTER ROOT, FELTWORT, GALL WEED, GENTIAN, PALE GENTIAN, STEMLESS GENTIAN, YELLOW GENTIAN

Common trade names
Angostura Bitters (a proprietary cocktail flavoring that contains an alcoholic extract of stemless gentian)

Common forms
Available as stemless gentian tea or extract. Other products include compound gentian infusion BP 1993 and concentrated compound gentian infusion BP 1993.

Source
Gentian is extracted from the roots and rhizome of 2- to 5-year-old *Gentiana lutea* L. plants during the summer months. The bitterness of the product is related to the speed with which the plant is dried: slow drying reduces the bitterness. Stemless gentian is extracted from the entire plant of *Gentiana acaulis* L.

Chemical components
Gentian contains several bitter compounds, including gentiopicrin, gentiin, gentiamarin, gentisin (also called gentianin or gentianic acid), gentisic acid, and gentianose.

Actions
Bitter substances ingested before eating have been thought to improve appetite and aid digestion by stimulating the release of gastric juices and bile. Gentian is most often used as part of an alcoholic beverage. It is difficult to separate the effect of gentian and alcohol because, in moderate amounts, alcohol has similar effects (Dombek, 1993).

Reported uses
Bitters, such as gentian, have been used for centuries for mild to moderate digestive disorders, including loss of appetite, irritable bowel syndrome, colic, flatulence, and heartburn.

Increased salivary flow was observed in patients given, among others, an herbal extract combination containing gentian (Borgia et al., 1981). Similar results were noted in another study by the same researchers using patients with mild GI disturbances (including loss of appetite, dyspepsia, and constipation). No adverse effects were noted. However, the therapeutic efficacy of gentian cannot be determined because of incomplete patient information and because gentian was not compared in a single-ingredient product.

Both gentian and stemless gentian are approved for use in foods. Extracts of stemless gentian are used in foods, cosmetics, and some antismoking products (Dombek, 1993). It has been reported to be active against *Plasmodium* malaria and has been used for malarial fevers (Osol, 1973).

Dosage

The dosage is not well documented.

Tea: ½ teaspoon of coarsely powdered gentian root boiled in ½ cup (120 ml) of water for 5 minutes. This mixture is strained, then taken 30 minutes before meals. If this tea is strong and unpalatable, the amount of herb may be reduced. This decoction can be taken up to q.i.d.

Adverse reactions

● Headache
● Nausea, vomiting (with overdose)

Interactions

None reported.

Contraindications and precautions

Contraindicated in patients with severe hypertension and during pregnancy.

Special considerations

● Be aware that brewing a tea is the best way to take the herb.
● Monitor blood pressure in hypertensive patients taking gentian.
● Warn the patient against collecting the herb in the wild (Garnier et al., 1985) because the nonflowering form of *G. lutea* may be difficult to distinguish from the toxic white hellebore.

Points of interest

● Gentian is no longer listed in the United States Pharmacopoeia but is still included in the European pharmacopoeias, including the British Pharmacopoeia.
● The German Commission E has reported that the constituents of gentian stimulate the taste buds and increase release of saliva and gastric secretions. The herb is regarded as a tonic.

• The dye, gentian violet, is a separate chemical entity and is not derived from plants containing gentian.

• Gentian is one of the flavoring agents in the spirit Vermouth.

• The toxic white hellebore (*Veratrum album*) often grows near gentian. One report noted acute veratrum alkaloid poisoning in people who consumed homemade gentian wine accidentally contaminated with veratrum (Garnier et al., 1985).

Analysis

Gentian-containing products have long been used as bitter tonics. Anecdotal reports and evidence from one small clinical trial that used a combination product suggest that a small amount of the herbal extract, usually mixed with alcohol, can act as an appetite stimulant and digestion aid. The other claims for gentian are poorly documented; use of the herb cannot currently be recommended.

References

Borgia, M., et al. "Pharmacological Activity of an Herb Extract: A Controlled Clinical Study," *Curr Ther Res* 29:525-36, 1981.

Garnier, R., et al. "Acute Dietary Poisoning by White Hellebore (*Veratrum album*). Clinical and Analytical Data. A Propos of 5 Cases," *Ann Med Interne* 136:125-28, 1985.

"Gentian," in *The Lawrence Review of Natural Products.* Edited by Dombek, C. St. Louis, Mo.: Facts and Comparisons, 1993.

Osol, A., ed. *The United States Dispensatory,* 27th ed. Philadelphia: Lippincott-Raven Pubs., 1973.

GINGER

ZINGIBER

Common trade names

(Various manufacturers; available in combination) Cayenne Ginger, Gingerall, Ginger Peppermint Combo, Ginger Power, Ginger Trips

Common forms

Root: 530 mg
Extract 250 mg
Liquid, powder, capsules: 100 mg, 465 mg
Tablets (chewable): 67.5 mg
Also available as teas.

Source

Ginger (*Zingiber officinale*) is a perennial that grows in India, Jamaica, and China. The plant produces green-purple flowers that resemble orchids. The rhizome (root) is found underground and is usually the most valued part of the plant.

Chemical components
The root contains both volatile and nonvolatile compounds. The nonvolatile constituents, which include the gingerols and gingerol-like compounds, are thought to be responsible for ginger's flavor and aromatic properties, as well as any pharmacologic activity. The volatile oil contains zingiberol, zingeberene, curcumene, farnesene, bis-abolene, sesquiphellandrene, and several monoterpenes (linalool, borneol, neral, geraniol and others). Other compounds present are zingibain (a proteolytic enzyme), oleoresins, fats, waxes, carbohydrates, vitamins, and minerals.

Actions
Human studies have shown ginger to inhibit platelet aggregation induced by ADP and epinephrine. Ginger extracts have documented anti-inflammatory effects in rodent models. Specific components of ginger produce varying CV effects. Methanolic extracts of ginger have shown positive inotropic effects in a guinea pig model.

Other studies in animals have suggested that components in ginger may be gastroprotective against various chemical insults and stressors. The GI protective action is postulated to be promoted by increased mucosal resistance and potentiation of the defensive mechanism against chemicals or alterations in prostaglandins, providing more protective effects. Additionally, a study of acetone extracts in mice found them to have similar stimulatory effects on GI motility as that seen with metoclopramide and domperidone (Yamahara et al., 1990).

Reported uses
Claims for ginger include, but are not limited to, its use as an antiemetic, GI protectant, anti-inflammatory agent useful for arthritis treatment, a CV stimulant, an antitumor agent, an antioxidant, and also as a therapy for microbial and parasitic infestations.

The antiemetic effects of ginger have been extensively studied in humans for morning, motion, or sea sickness, and for postoperative nausea and vomiting; most provide support for this action, although there are some that do not. (See *Ginger's antiemetic effects,* page 276.) Doses and duration of therapy varied considerably with each study. The antiemetic properties of ginger are likely to result from local effects on the GI tract rather than on the CNS. Increased gastric peristalsis has been shown in animals, but any mechanism in humans is currently considered speculative.

RESEARCH FINDINGS
Ginger's antiemetic effects

Most research on ginger focuses on its use as an antiemetic agent. In a study designed to mimic seasickness by use of a revolving, motor-driven chair, doses of dimenhydrinate (100 mg), ginger root (940 mg), or chickweed herb were given to 36 blindfolded, seasick-prone patients just before their "spin" in the chair (Mowrey and Clayson, 1982). No one in the chickweed or dimenhydrinate group was able to remain in the chair for the full 6 minutes. Patients receiving ginger root tolerated an average of 5.5 minutes in the chair (50% managed the full 6 minutes), whereas those receiving dimenhydrinate or chickweed remained in the chair an average of 3.5 and 1.5 minutes, respectively. Vomiting occurred in three patients in the chickweed group. Although the results of this study are intriguing, the study design has been questioned.

Two trials evaluated the incidence of postoperative nausea and vomiting in patients receiving powdered ginger root, metoclopramide, or placebo. In the first randomized, double-blind study (Bone et al., 1990), 60 women were given ginger 1,000 mg P.O., metoclopramide 10 mg I.V., or placebo 1.5 hours before undergoing major gynecologic surgery. The incidence of nausea and intensity of nausea favored both active treatment groups over placebo. Postoperative administration of "rescue" metoclopramide was significantly less in both active treatment groups. There were no statistically significant differences that favored one active treatment over the other. Use of postoperative analgesia and sedation was similar in all groups.

The second study (Phillips et al., 1993) evaluated powdered ginger root 1,000 mg P.O., metoclopramide 10 mg P.O., and placebo in 120 patients undergoing gynecologic surgery. The results echoed the results of the earlier trial. Both treatment groups showed better results than placebo, and the need for postoperative antiemetics was lower in the group receiving ginger. No differences were noted in the need for postoperative analgesia, recovery time, time until discharge, or adverse effects.

In another study, 250 mg ginger P.O. q.i.d. was given for 4 days to pregnant women with hyperemesis gravidarum. A significant percentage of women preferred ginger versus placebo treatment (Fisher-Rasmussen et al., 1991).

Ginger was found to provide relief from pain and swelling in patients with rheumatoid arthritis, osteoarthritis, or muscular discomfort (Srivastava and Mustafa, 1992). A proposed mechanism is that it inhibited prostaglandin, thromboxane, and leukotriene biosynthesis.

Dosage

Dosage forms and strength vary with each disease state.
As an antiemetic, studies used 500 to 1,000 mg of powdered ginger
P.O., or 1,000 mg of fresh ginger root P.O.

Adverse reactions

• Possible CNS depression or arrhythmias (with overdose)

Interactions

Anticoagulants: may enhance risk of bleeding.

Contraindications and precautions

Contraindicated in pregnant patients; effects are unknown. Use only
under medical supervision in patients receiving anticoagulants because it may affect bleeding time by inhibiting platelet function.

Special considerations

• Advise the female patient to avoid use of ginger during pregnancy.
• Instruct the patient to watch for signs of bleeding when taking
ginger.
• Explain that no consensus exists with respect to dosing and monitoring.

Analysis

Although there are data that support the use of ginger for therapeutic uses in humans, information to the contrary also exists. It is premature to recommend ginger for any use until long-term, controlled, pharmacologic studies of its constituents as an antiemetic,
anti-inflammatory, or gastroprotective agent are obtained.

References

Bone, M., et al. "The Effect of Ginger Root on Post-operative Nausea and
    Vomiting After Major Gynecological Surgery," *Anesthesia* 45:669-71, 1990.
Fisher-Rasmussen, W., et al. "Ginger Treatment of Hyperemesis Gravidarum,"
    Eur J Obstet Gynecol Reprod Biol 38:19-24, 1990.
Mowrey, D.B., and Clayson, D.E. "Motion Sickness, Ginger and Psychophysics,"
    Lancet 1:655-57, 1982.
Phillips, S., et al. *"Zingiber officinale* (Ginger)—An Antiemetic for Day Case
    Surgery," *Anesthesia* 48:715-7, 1993.
Srivastava, K.C., and Mustafa, T. "Ginger (*Zingiber officinale*) in Rheumatism
    and Musculoskeletal Disorders," *Med Hypotheses* 39:342-48, 1992.
Yamahara, J., et al. "GI Motility Enhancing Effects of Ginger and Its Active
    Constituents," *Chem Phar Bull* 38:430-31, 1990.

GINKGO

EGB 761, GBE, GBE 24, GBX, GINKGO BILOBA,
GINKOGINK, LI 1370, ROKAN, SOPHIUM, TANAKAN,
TEBOFORTAN, TEBONIN

Common trade names
(Various manufacturers; available in combination) Bioginkgo 24/6,
Bioginkgo 27/7, Gincosan, Ginexin Remind, Ginkai, Ginkgoba,
Ginkgo Go!, Ginkgold, Ginkgo Phytosome, Ginkgo Power, Ginkoba

Common forms
Available as ginkgo biloba extract in capsules, tablets, and sublingual
sprays (standardized to contain 24% flavone glycosides and 6% ter-
penes) and as concentrated alcoholic extract of fresh leaf.
Tablets, capsules: 30 mg, 40 mg, 60 mg, 120 mg, 260 mg, 420 mg
Sublingual sprays: 15 mg/spray, 40 mg/spray
Ginkgo biloba extract (24% standardized extract) bound to phos-
phatidylcholine is available as 80-mg capsules.

Source
Ginkgo biloba extract is obtained from the leaves of the *Gingko biloba* tree, formerly *Salisburia adiantifolia*. The tree is also known as
the Maidenhair tree and Kew tree. The extract is produced by a complex multistep process that concentrates the active constituents and
removes the potentially toxic ginkgolic acid.

Chemical components
Ginkgo biloba extract is composed of a complex mixture of polar
and nonpolar compounds. The extract contains various flavonol
and flavone glycosides, 20 carbon diterpene lactones (including
ginkgetin, ginkgolic acid, and isoginkgetin), 20-carbon-diterpene
lactone derivatives termed ginkgolides (of which ginkgolide A, B, C,
J, and M have been identified), and a 15-carbon sesquiterpene
termed bilobalide. Other isolated compounds include ascorbic acid,
catechin, iron-based superoxide dismutase, p-hydroxybenzoic acid,
6-hyroxkynurenic acid, protocatechuic acid, shikimic acid, sterols
including sitosterol, and vanillic acid.

Actions
Ginkgo biloba extract produces arterial and venous vasoactive
changes that increase tissue perfusion and cerebral blood flow. The
physiologic effects are attributed to the extract's ability to produce
arterial vasodilation, inhibit arterial spasms, decrease capillary permeability, reduce capillary fragility, decrease blood viscosity, and reduce erythrocyte aggregation. These effects are probably due to

stimulation of prostaglandin biosynthesis or by indirect vasoregulatory effects on catecholamines (Nemecz and Combest, 1997; Princemail et al., 1989). In addition, ginkgo biloba extract acts as an antioxidant (Kobuchi et al., 1997); ginkgolide B is reported to be a potent inhibitor of platelet activating factor (Koltai et al., 1991).

Reported uses
Ginkgo biloba extract has been studied for the treatment of cerebrovascular disease and peripheral vascular insufficiency. (See *Use of ginkgo in dementia,* page 280.) Other studies have evaluated the use of extract or isolated constituents for disorders such as arrhythmias, asthma, impotence secondary to serotonin reuptake inhibitors, premenstrual syndrome, senile macular degeneration, hearing loss, and vestibular disorders.

Ginkgo biloba extract is claimed to improve mental alertness and overall brain function; evidence for this use, however, is unsubstantiated.

Dosage
For dementia syndromes, 120 to 240 mg P.O. daily in two or three divided doses.
For peripheral arterial disease, vertigo, and tinnitus, 120 to 160 mg P.O. daily in two or three divided doses. Doses as high as 320 mg daily have also been studied. Most studies reported a minimum duration of 4 to 6 weeks of therapy is required before positive effects were noted.

Use of crude, dried leaf preparations or extemporaneous preparation of the leaves as a tea are not recommended because of insufficient quantity of active ingredients.

Adverse reactions
• Contact hypersensitivity reactions
• Dermatitis if contact with fruit occurs. The fruit pulp and seed coats contain ginkgolic acid and bilobin, which are structurally related to the urushiols found in poison ivy, mango fruit rind, and cashew nut shells.
• Diarrhea
• Flatulence
• Headache
• Nausea
• Vomiting
⚠ Bleeding (subdural hematoma, hyphema; rare)
⚠ Seizures (with excessive ingestion of ginkgo seeds by children—more than 50 seeds)

RESEARCH FINDINGS
Use of ginkgo in dementia

At least two studies indicate that ginkgo may be beneficial in patients with dementia. A 52-week, multicenter, randomized, double-blind, placebo-controlled trial (LeBars et al., 1997) followed 309 outpatients with mild to severe dementia from Alzheimer's disease or multi-infarct dementia. Patients were randomly given placebo or ginkgo 120 mg daily and assessed according to the Alzheimer's Disease Assessment Scale-Cognitive Subscale (ADAS), the Geriatric Evaluation by Relative's Rating Instrument (GERRI), and the Clinical Global Impression of Change (CGIC). A small but statistically significant treatment difference in favor of gingko was observed, as demonstrated by improved ADAS and GERRI scores. No difference was detected by CGIC tests. The authors concluded that ginkgo improved cognitive and social functioning for 6 to 12 months in many patients.

A similar trial of 216 patients with Alzheimer's disease or multi-infarct dementia demonstrated that ginkgo, at doses of 240 mg daily, improved various symptoms (Kanowski et al., 1996). In this 24-week study, patients were considered to respond if scores in at least two of the three functional tests increased. Other smaller European trials also indicate that ginkgo benefits patients with dementia and other neurologic disorders; however, these studies lack standardized methods of evaluation. Additionally, patients with medical conditions such as cardiac or liver disease, chronic renal failure, and type 1 diabetes were typically excluded from the study. The safety and efficacy of ginkgo biloba extract in these populations, therefore, have not been evaluated.

Interactions
Anticoagulants, antiplatelets: use ginkgo biloba extract with caution due to its effect on platelet activating factor (PAF). Carefully monitor patients taking anticoagulant or antiplatelet medications.

Contraindications and precautions
Contraindicated in patients with a history of allergy to ginkgo preparations, during pregnancy, and in children. Use cautiously in patients taking anticoagulant medications.

Special considerations
• Advise the patient to report unusual bleeding or bruising.
• Instruct the patient to keep seeds out of reach of children because of the potential risk of seizures with ingestion.

• Advise the patient to avoid contact with the fruit pulp or seed coats because of the risk of contact dermatitis. More potent preparations may cause irritation or blistering of skin or mucus membranes if applied externally.

Points of interest

• Standardized ginkgo biloba extract is among the leading prescriptions in Germany and France, but is available only as a dietary supplement in the United States. Ginkgo was the third-best-selling herbal product in health food stores in the United States in 1997.
• Be aware that this agent is considered an "effective substance for the treatment of peripheral arterial occlusive disease," according to the Federal German Drug Law (1996). This same reference reports that ginkgo's effectiveness is similar to pentoxifylline and just as variable.
• Ginkgo was recently approved in Germany for the treatment of dementia.
• Ginkgo biloba extract preparation bound to phosphatidylcholine is claimed to increases the absorption and incorporation of ginkgo into biologic membranes. There is no published support of these claims.
• The seeds are reported to be edible, are sold at Oriental shops, and are normally boiled before consumption to remove toxic components.

Analysis

Ginkgo might be best characterized as being a mild to moderate vasoactive agent. Most of the clinical data are from animal or foreign studies; many of these trials were flawed and used small sample size, lacked objective outcome measurements, had incomplete descriptions of patient characteristics, had inadequate descriptions of the randomization process, and were of short duration. The most convincing preliminary human trial data seem to suggest a role for this agent in dementia and peripheral vascular disease; however, further studies are needed to define its specific role in therapy. Few studies compare ginkgo with standard-of-care treatments. Allergic reactions have been reported primarily with exposure to the whole ginkgo plant or to contact with the fruit pulp. The potential for such reactions with this agent warrants discriminate use in patients with a history of hypersensitivity reactions.

References

Kanowski, S., et al. "Proof of Efficacy of the Ginkgo Biloba Special Extract EGB 761 in Outpatients Suffering from Mild to Moderate Primary Degenerative Dementia of the Alzheimer Type of Multi-Infarct Dementia," *Pharmacopsychiatry* 29:47-56, 1996.

Kobuchi, H., et al. "*Ginkgo biloba* Extract (EGB 761): Inhibitory Effect of Nitric Oxide Production in the Macrophage Cell Line RAW 264.7," *Biochem Pharmacol* 53:897-903, 1997.

Koltai, M., et al. "Platelet Activating Factor (PAF). A Review of Its Effects, Antagonists and Possible Future Clinical Implications (Part I)," *Drugs* 42:9-29, 1991.

LeBars, P.L., et al. "A Placebo-Controlled, Double-Blind Randomized Trial of an Extract of Ginkgo Biloba for Dementia," *JAMA* 278:1327-32, 1997.

Nemecz, G., and Combest, W.L. "Ginkgo Biloba," *US Pharmacist* 22:144-51, September 1997.

Princemail, J., et al. "Superoxide Anion Scavenging Effect and Superoxide Dismutase Activity of *Ginkgo biloba* Extract," *Experientia* 45:708-12, 1989.

GINSENG

AMERICAN GINSENG, ASIATIC GINSENG, CHINESE GINSENG, FIVE-FINGERS, G115, JAPANESE GINSENG, JINTSAM, KOREAN GINSENG, NINJIN, ORIENTAL GINSENG, SCHINSENT, SENG AND SANG, TARTAR ROOT, WESTERN GINSENG

Common trade names
(Various manufacturers; available in combination) Bio Star, Cimexon, Gincosan, Ginsana, Ginsatonic, Neo Ginsana

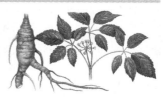

Common forms
No standards exist for ginseng despite availability of chromato-graphic assays for ginsenosides and ginseng polysaccharides.
Capsules: 100 mg, 250 mg, 500 mg
Tea bags: 1,500 mg ginseng root
Extract: 2 oz root extract (in alcohol base)
Root powder: 1 oz, 4 oz
Also available as an oil. Root is available in bulk by the pound.

Source
The most common species is *Panax quinquefolius*, commonly known as American or Western ginseng. Sought after most commonly for its root, other characteristics of the plant ("wild or cultivated") and shapes of the root make it more valuable. Traditionally, ideal plants are at least 6 years of age. *P. ginseng* is known as the Asian, Korean, or Japanese ginseng. The Asian ginseng usually undergoes treatment such as drying or curing before it is sold, whereas the American variety undergoes less manipulation and carries less distinction.

Chemical components

Ginseng is composed primarily of ginsenosides, also known as pan-axosides. Approximately 12 major panaxosides have been isolated, but are found in only minute quantities and are difficult to purify on a large scale. Other components of the plant isolated for pharmacologic effects include a volatile oil, beta-elemine, sterols, flavonoids, peptides, vitamins (B_1, B_2, B_{12}, panthotenic acid, nicotinic acid, and biotin), fats, polyacetylenes, minerals, enzymes, and choline.

Actions

Several pharmacologic effects have been noted that vary with dose and duration of treatment. The panaxosides, found in the root, are thought to be the pharmacologically active agents. Although similar in structure, these compounds sometimes exert opposing pharmacologic effects. For example, ginsenoside Rb-1 has CNS-depressant, anticonvulsant, analgesic, and antipsychotic effects; stress-ulcer preventing action; and acceleration of glycolysis and nuclear RNA synthesis. Ginsenoside Rg-1 has CNS-stimulating, antifatigue, hypertensive, and stress-ulcer aggravating activities. These opposing features form the basis for the theory that ginseng serves to "balance bodily functions."

Another example of these opposing actions is that Rg and Rg-1 enhance cardiac performance, whereas Rb depresses cardiac function. Other ginsenosides have shown antiarrhythmic activity similar to verapamil and amiodarone. Oral ginseng was found to reduce cholesterol and triglycerides, decrease platelet adhesiveness, impair coagulation, and increase fibrinolysis in cholesterol-fed rats. Ginsenosides may reduce stress by acting on the adrenal gland.

Hypoglycemic activity in rodents has been documented, but the mechanism of action has not been proven. (Suzuki and Hikino, 1989). Extracts of ginseng have shown antioxidant activity on human erythrocytes in a laboratory model and prevented the development of morphine-tolerance in rats. Some studies in animals have documented ginseng's anti-inflammatory and antiviral activities, and hepatoprotective effects at low doses (destruction at high doses) in a rat model, whereas others found that tumors in mice were suppressed by components of ginseng (Yun and Choi, 1990).

Reported uses

Ginseng is popularly claimed to minimize or reduce the activity of the thymus gland. Other claims include its use as a sedative, demulcent (soothes irritated or inflamed internal tissues or organs), aphrodisiac, antidepressant, sleep aid, and diuretic. Short-term use of the herb is thought to improve stamina, concentration, healing, stress-resistance (adaptogenic), vigilance, and work efficiency; long-term use is claimed to improve "well-being" in elderly patients with debilitated or degenerative conditions. However, few claims have supporting data from animal studies, and fewer still have data from human studies.

Although studies conducted in humans were mostly small and poorly designed, results suggest that ginseng has several beneficial effects. Improvement in sleep, appetite, emotional lability, and work efficiency in animals and humans indicates the herb's ability to enhance physical and mental performance. Ginseng may also indirectly exhibit corticosteroid-like effects.

Ginseng decreased fasting blood glucose and hemoglobin A_{1C} in both diabetic and nondiabetic patients such that some diabetics were free of insulin therapy for the duration of the study (Sotaniemi et al., 1995). The herb has also been shown to be beneficial in patients with hyperlipidemia, hepatic dysfunction, and impaired cognitive function. (See *Ginseng's effect on cognitive function.*)

Dosage
Dosages vary with the disease state; usually, 0.5 to 2 g dry ginseng root daily or 200 to 600 mg ginseng extract daily, in one or two equal doses.
For improved well-being in debilitated elderly patients, 0.4 to 0.8 g root P.O. daily on a continual basis.

Adverse reactions
- Chest pain
- Diarrhea
- Epistaxis
- Headache
- Hypertension
- Impotence
- Insomnia
- Mastalgia
- Nausea
- Nervousness
- Palpitations
- Pruritus
- Skin eruptions (with ginseng abuse)
- Vaginal bleeding
- Vomiting
- Ginseng abuse syndrome occurs when large doses of the herb are taken concomitantly with other psychomotor stimulants, such as tea and coffee; symptoms include diarrhea, hypertension, restlessness, insomnia, skin eruptions, depression, appetite suppression, euphoria, and edema. The existence of this syndrome is debatable.

RESEARCH FINDINGS
Ginseng's effect on cognitive function

A few studies have been performed to determine ginseng's claim of improved psychomotor performance and cognitive functions.

One randomized, double-blind, placebo-controlled study of 32 healthy male volunteers (age 20 to 24) was performed to evaluate the effect of standardized ginseng extract (Ginsana) on psychomotor performance. Patients were given ginseng 100 mg or placebo b.i.d. for 12 weeks, and evaluated at baseline and at 11 weeks. A favorable effect was shown in attention, logical deduction, and sensory and motor perception within the same individual (acting as his control) at baseline and 11 weeks. However, results were only slightly in favor for ginseng for mathematical reasoning (D'Angelo et al., 1986).

Another randomized, double-blind, placebo-controlled trial evaluated ginseng's effects on cognitive function. The 112 subjects were randomized to receive standardized ginseng or inactive placebo. The primary outcome was the change in score on each cognitive test, evaluated both at baseline and at 8 weeks. Safety was also evaluated by questioning the subjects. Results demonstrate a tendency to faster simple reaction times and better abstract thinking in the ginseng-treated group—the only statistically significant finding (Sorensen and Sonne, 1996).

A third clinical trial evaluated the cognitive effects of a gingko and ginseng combination in healthy volunteers with neurasthenic complaints. This 90-day, double-blind, placebo-controlled, parallel study group involved 64 patients (age 40 to 65) who were randomly assigned to receive 80 mg, 160 mg, 320 mg, or placebo b.i.d., and assessed at baseline and at days 1, 30, and 90. Cognitive outcomes measured were basic memory skills, accuracy and speed of response, and immediate and delayed word and picture recognition. Although well tolerated, the adverse effects most often reported included dizziness, somnolence, and increased frequency of urination. The only significant finding occurred 1 hour after the 320-mg dose, in which cognitive improvement was seen on day 90. A larger dose and shorter dosing interval may be necessary (Wesnes et al., 1997).

One study suffered from a very small sample size. Baseline demographics and characteristics differed significantly between groups in some cases and were not addressed in others. Compliance was only evaluated in one trial; study methods cannot be relied on in some cases because of possible bias in design.

In conclusion, more rigidly controlled human clinical trials are needed before ginseng and its extracts can be recommended for improving cognitive and psychomotor functions.

Interactions

Antidiabetic agents, insulin: use cautiously because of ginseng's hypoglycemic effect.

MAO inhibitors (hypericin, parnate, phenelzine, selegiline, tranylcypromine): adverse reactions include headache, tremors, and mania. Avoid concomitant use.

Contraindications and precautions

Use cautiously in patients with CV disease, hypertension, hypotension, or diabetes, and in those also receiving steroid therapy. Avoid use in pregnant or breast-feeding women; effects are unknown.

Special considerations

• Monitor the patient for signs and symptoms of ginseng abuse syndrome.
• Monitor the diabetic patient for signs and symptoms of hypoglycemia. Advise him to check glucose closely until effects on serum glucose are known.
• Advise the patient not to take ginseng for a prolonged time.
• Tell the patient with preexisting medical conditions to check with his health care professional before taking ginseng.
• Instruct the patient to watch for unusual symptoms (nervousness, insomnia, palpitations, diarrhea) because of risk of ginseng toxicity.
• Advise the pregnant or breast-feeding patient to consult a health care professional before taking ginseng because safety has not been established.

Points of interest

• Ginseng has been given a positive evaluation from the German Commission E.
• It is estimated that about six million people in the United States use ginseng regularly. In oriental cultures, it has been used for its medicinal properties for over 2,000 years.
• Although it was abundant in eastern North America, American ginseng is now considered threatened because of aggressive harvesting of the plant for commercial sales.

Analysis

Public interest in ginseng has increased over the past several years. Although the herb appears to have promising uses, additional human efficacy, toxicity, and interactions data are needed. Ginseng has an interesting and unique pharmacologic profile; however, ingestion of the plant is not without risk despite its use for centuries.

References

D'Angelo, L., et al. "A Double-Blind, Placebo-Controlled Clinical Study on the Effect of a Standardized Ginseng Extract on Psychomotor Performance in Healthy Volunteers," *J Ethnopharmacol* 16:15-22, 1986.

Sorensen, H., and Sonne, J. "A Double-Masked Study of the Effects of Ginseng on Cognitive Functions," *Curr Ther Res* 57:959-68, 1996.

Sotaniemi, E., et al. "Ginseng Therapy in Non-Insulin-Dependent Diabetic Patients," *Diabetes Care* 18:1373-75, 1995.

Suzuki, Y., and Hikino, H. "Mechanisms of Hypoglycemic Activity of Pnaxans A and B, Glycans of *Panax ginseng* Roots: Effects on the Key Enzymes of Glucose Metabolism in the Liver of Mice," *Phytotherapy Res* 3:15-19, 1989.

Wesnes, K.A., et al. "The Cognitive, Subjective, and Physical Effects of a Ginkgo Biloba/Panax Ginseng Combination in Healthy Volunteers with Neurasthenic Complaints," *Psychopharmacol Bull* 33:677-83, 1997.

Yun, T.K., and Choi, S. "A Case-Control Study of Ginseng Intake and Cancer," *Int J Epidemiol* 19:871-76, 1990.

GINSENG, SIBERIAN

ACANTHOPANAX SENTICOSUS, DEVIL'S SHRUB, ELEUTHEROCOCCUS SENTICOSUS, HEDERA SENTICOSA, SHIGOKA, TOUCH-ME-NOT

Common trade names

(Various manufacturers; available in combination) Activex 40 Plus, Gincosan, Ginkovit, Ginseng Complex, Minadex Mix Ginseng, Panax Complex, Siberian Ginseng, Vigoran

Common forms

Available as powders, teas, tinctures, capsules, tablets, and oils.

Source

The drug is extracted from the root and root bark of *Eleutherococcus senticosus,* which belongs to the same family as panax or chinese ginseng (Araliaceae).

Chemical components

Constituents of the root include saponins (termed eleutherosides), which appear to be the active drug and are found in equal concentrations in above-ground parts and roots. The eleutherosides are subgrouped A to G. Other components include essential oil, resin, starch, and vitamin A.

Actions

The saponin portion of Siberian ginseng appears to have affinity for progestin, mineralcorticoid, and glucocorticoid receptors, although not to the extent of panax ginseng. However, unlike panax ginseng, Siberian ginseng binds to estrogen receptors.

When the extract was injected into the peritoneal cavity of mice, a marked hypoglycemic effect was observed (Hikino et al., 1986). Orally administered eleutherococcus was found to decrease plasma glucose levels in rats but had no effect on plasma lactic acid, glucagon, insulin, or liver glycogen levels (Martinez et al., 1984). It is not known if this effect also occurs in humans.

Despite the claim that Siberian ginseng enhances the ability to tolerate stress, ingestion of eleutherococcus was not found to significantly affect the survival of mice under major environmental stress; however, a more aggressive behavior was noted (Lewis et al., 1983).

Reported uses

Siberian ginseng is described as a pungent, bittersweet, warming herb with the purported ability to stimulate the immune and circulatory systems, regulate blood pressure, reduce inflammation, treat insomnia caused by prolonged anxiety, and increase stamina and the ability to cope with stress. Preliminary Russian studies have attempted to verify adaptogenic effects of ginseng in studies of both healthy and nonhealthy patients. These trial results are at best inconsistent, but suggest some favorable effects in certain parameters associated with the patients' ability to withstand stressful conditions.

Studies with animals have indicated no effect on stamina or stress tolerance. In a study involving highly trained distance runners, the herb was found to have no effect on improving exercise tolerance (Dowling et al., 1996). As with other ginseng plants, Siberian ginseng claims to have immunomodulatory actions; it is thought to stimulate macrophages, promote antibody formation, activate complement and increase T-lymphocyte proliferation. An increase in the T-lymphocyte count and an enhancement of the activation state of the T-cells were shown in human patients (Bohn et al., 1987); however, the extent of the proliferation nor the duration of these effects can be determined from this study alone.

Extensive human studies are needed to verify claims of radioprotective or chemotherapeutic effects of Siberian ginseng.

Dosage

No set guidelines exist; however, the most common regimen is 500 to 2,000 mg P.O. daily. Use cautiously because of the lack of uniform content of capsules and substitution with less expensive plants.

Adverse reactions

- Diarrhea
- Difficulty concentrating
- Dizziness
- Euphoria
- Hypertension

- Increased agitation
- Insomnia
- Nervousness
- Skin eruptions
- Vaginal bleeding, estrogenic effects

Interactions

Digoxin: elevated digoxin serum levels. Monitor digoxin use closely.
Hexobarbital: inhibited hexobarbital metabolism. Avoid concomitant use.
Vitamins B_1, B_2, and C: Siberian ginseng may increase excretion of these vitamins. Avoid concomitant use.

Contraindications and precautions

Contraindicated in children and in patients with allergy to ginseng, Siberian ginseng, or ingredients in the preparation.

Special considerations

- Know that most references do not advocate use beyond 3 weeks.
- Be aware that this agent is not uniform in content when packaged and often will be substituted with less expensive plant products.
- Siberian ginseng may be sold as a combination product with panax ginseng. Monitor for adverse effects also associated with panax or Chinese ginseng.
- Advise the patient to report insomnia, nervousness, euphoria, skin eruptions, diarrhea, agitation, or abnormal menstrual bleeding.
- Tell the diabetic patient to closely monitor blood sugar levels and watch for increased effects of antidiabetic medication because of the herb's hypoglycemic effect in animals.
- Advise the patient not to use the herb for longer than 3 weeks.

Analysis

The most prevalent claim for Siberian ginseng is its ability to improve stamina, energy, and exercise performance. This has been proven not to be true. Also, the adaptogenic response, which claims increased resistance to stress, has also been found to be false.

The immunomodulating and radioprotective effects have been studied mostly in animal and foreign trials. Although the data thus far appear promising, particularly for a radioprotective action, larger controlled studies are needed in humans to determine whether the herb not only increases T-cell count and response, but also clinically prevents or hastens recovery from infections.

There are no data to substantiate the other claims for Siberian ginseng. There are no long-term studies either and, thus, its effects over time are not known. Therefore, use of Siberian ginseng beyond 3 weeks is not recommended.

References

Bohn, B., et al. "Flow-Cytometric Studies with *Eleutherococcus senticosus* Extract as an Immunomodulatory Agent," *Arzneimittelforschung* 37:1193-96, 1987.

Dowling, E.A.., et al. "Effect of *Eleutherococcus senticosus* on Submaximal and Maximal Exercise Performance," *Med Sci Sports Exerc* 28:482-89, 1996.

Hikino, H., et al. "Isolation and Hypoglycemic Activity of Eleutherans A, B, C, D, E, F, and G: Glycans of *Eleutherococcus senticosus* Roots," *J Natl Prod* 49:293-97, 1986.

Lewis, W.H., et al. "No Adaptogenic Response of Mice to Ginseng and Eleutherococcus Infusions," *J Ethnopharmacol* 8:209-14, 1983.

Martinez, B., et al. "The Physiological Effects of Aralia, Panax *and Eleutherococcus senticosus* on Exercised Rats," *Jpn J Pharmacol* 35:79-85, 1984.

GLUCOMANNAN

KONJAC, KONJAC MANNAN

Common trade names
Glucomannan

Common forms
Available as powder, capsules, and 600-mg tablets.

Source
The tubers of the plant *Amorphophallus konjac* are typically harvested to yield a chemical called konjac mannan.

Chemical components
Konjac mannan, or glucomannan, is a polysaccharide composed of linked molecules of glucose and mannose. It is purified from konjac flour by chemical treatment with cupric hydroxide and repeated ethanol washings, or by dialysis against water.

Actions
Polysaccharide agents (guar gum, methylcellulose, tragacanth, bran and pectin) such as glucomannan have been shown to delay the absorption of glucose from the bowel (Jenkins et al., 1978). Glucomannan ingestion changes bowel intestinal microbial flora in rodents, although human microbial natural flora may be changed less dramatically (Fujiwara et al., 1991).

Other studies using rodents suggest that the water-soluble form of glucomannan can lower cholesterol, depending on the purity of the herb. A water-insoluble form (referred to as "konnyaku" in Japan) was found not to be able to reduce rat plasma cholesterol (Kiriyama et al., 1969), but it appeared to lower the prevalence of murine lung cancers (Luo, 1992).

Reported uses

Bulk-forming agents such as guar gum (galactomannan, galactose, and mannose), methylcellulose, tragacanth, bran fiber, and pectin are known for their ability to draw water into the lumen of the bowel, promoting hydration of stool and facilitating relief of constipation. Anecdotal reports claim glucomannan to be an effective laxative because of these properties.

Hydrophilic agents have been included as part of weight-loss regimens because of the supposed ability of the agent to produce early satiety and fullness. Glucomannan is becoming a popular component of these weight-loss programs. Clinical trial data supporting the use of glucomannan as a weight-reducing agent are scarce and conflicting, at best. Additional studies are needed in this area.

Studies in healthy human subjects have demonstrated the herb's ability to lower serum cholesterol and glucose. (See *Glucomannan as a cholesterol- and glucose-lowering agent,* page 292.)

Dosage

For lowering cholesterol levels, one study used 3.9 g of glucomannan daily for 4 weeks, stopped for 2 weeks, then resumed treatment again for another 4 weeks; another used 100 ml daily of a 1% solution of glucomannan.

For lowering blood glucose levels, 3.6 to 7.2 g of glucomannan daily was given to diabetic patients for 90 days.

For reducing body weight, an American study used 1.5 g of glucomannan b.i.d. for 8 weeks.

Because of the lack of consistency in trials, no specific dose can be recommended at this time.

Adverse reactions

- Changes in intestinal flora
- Diarrhea, loose stools
- Esophageal and lower GI obstruction
- Flatulence
- Hypoglycemia

⚠ Esophageal perforation as a complication of GI obstruction. Several of these cases required mechanical removal under general anesthesia.

Interactions

Cholesterol-lowering agents: glucomannan may enhance the cholesterol-reducing effects of these agents. Monitor patient.

Oral antidiabetic agents, insulin: may require dosage adjustment during herbal treatment. Monitor patient.

RESEARCH FINDINGS
Glucomannan as a cholesterol- and glucose-lowering agent

Glucomannan has been studied for its ability to lower serum cholesterol and serum glucose. At least two trials have focused on the herb's ability to lower serum glucose.

Glucomannan was given to 13 diabetic patients for 90 days (Doi et al., 1979). After 20 days, serum cholesterol decreased by 11.2% and at 30 days, serum glucose levels declined about 29% (P < 0.025 compared with baseline). Most patients were able to reduce their doses of oral antidiabetic drugs or insulin. Glucomannan was thought to reduce absorption of oral glucose, evidenced by a mean reduction of peak serum glucose values at 30 minutes post-ingestion. The oral glucose tolerance test was also associated with reductions in serum insulin release in patients who received the herb.

The most convincing evidence comes from a larger study of 72 patients with type 2 diabetes. A refined konjac food was given in various forms (powder, noodle, or toast) with normal foods consumed during meals. Diet and activity of the patients remained constant. After 30 and 65 days, fasting blood glucose and 2-hour postprandial glucose values were significantly lower than baseline (P < 0.05 for both). Patients lost an average of 2 kg of body weight during the 65-day study period. Glycosylated hemoglobin fell approximately 15% during this study (P< 0.05). Although low-density lipoprotein and total cholesterol fell slightly, only serum triglyceride values were significantly reduced. High-density lipoprotein values remained unchanged. The researchers concluded that konjac mannan food was useful in the prevention and treatment of hyperglycemia (Huang et al., 1990).

Contraindications and precautions

Avoid use of the herb in pregnant or breast-feeding women; effects are unknown. Use cautiously in patients prone to hypoglycemia or GI dysfunction or obstruction.

Special considerations

• Use glucomannan cautiously in patients prone to gastric obstruction, and in diabetic patients because insulin or oral antidiabetic doses may need to be reduced. Large doses of glucomannan are likely to produce laxative effects, due to its osmotically active properties in the bowel. GI effects may limit tolerance of the herb.

• Stagger administration of other drugs by a few hours; concomitant use may alter absorption of these drugs.

• Monitor the patient for signs of GI or esophageal obstruction (constipation, distended or tense abdomen, loss of appetite, abdominal pain or nausea).

• Monitor the patient for significant changes in bowel habit and periodically check serum electrolytes because of the herb's potential to alter gut flora and act as a laxative.

• Remind the diabetic patient to monitor blood glucose more intensely and consider dosage reductions in insulin or oral antidiabetic agents, if necessary.

• Advise the patient to report if other drugs being used appear to be less effective.

• Inform the patient that long-term effects of this herb are not well known.

Points of interest

• Adverse effects have led to discontinuation of the tablet form of glucomannan in Australia since the mid-1980s.

Analysis

Both animal and human studies support the effectiveness of glucomannan as a cholesterol-lowering agent However, the greater efficacy of modern pharmaceutical agents, such as the statins, forces glucomannan to take a back-seat in the treatment program. Glucomannan may prove to be a valuable adjunct to lipid-lowering therapy; however, larger trials are warranted to adequately describe its adverse effect profile.

Glucomannan's substantial ability to lower blood glucose levels makes it an attractive choice for patients with coexisting hypercholesterolemia and diabetes.

Existing information on its use as a diet aid is conflicting and difficult to interpret.

References

Doi, K., et al. "Treatment of Diabetes with Glucomannan (Konjac Mannan)," *Lancet* 1:987-88, 1979.

Fujiwara, S., et al. "Effect of Konjac Mannan on Intestinal Microbial Metabolism in Mice Bearing Human Flora and in Conventional F344 Rats," *Food Chem Toxicol* 29:601, 1991.

Huang, C.Y., et al. "Effect of Konjac Food on Blood Glucose Level in Patients With Diabetes," *Biomed Environ Sci* 3:123-31, 1990.

Jenkins, D.J., et al. "Dietary Fibres, Fibre Analogues and Glucose Tolerance: Importance of Viscosity," *BMJ* 1:1392, 1978

Kiriyama, S., et al. "Hypocholesterolemic Effect of Polysaccharides and Polysaccharide-Rich Foodstuffs in Cholesterol-Fed Rats," *J Nutr* 97:382, 1969.

Luo, D.Y. "Inhibitory Effect of Refined *Amorphophallus konjac* on MNNG-Induced Lung Cancers in Mice," *Chung Hua Chung Liu Tsa Chih* 14:48, 1992.

GLUCOSAMINE

CHITOSAMINE, GLUCOSAMINE SULFATE, GS

Common trade names
(Various manufacturers; available in combination) Arth-X Plus, Enhanced Glucosamine Sulfate, Flexi-Factors, Glucosamine Complex, Glucosamine Mega, Joint Factors, Nutri-Joint, Ultra Maximum Strength Glucosamine Sulfate

Common forms
Various molecular forms of glucosamine are available, including chlorhydrate, D-glucosamine, hydrochloride, N-acetyl, sulfate, and with potassium chloride added. The preferred form appears to be glucosamine sulfate.
Capsules: 250 mg, 375 mg, 500 mg, 600 mg, 1,000 mg
Tablets: 63 mg, 87 mg, 375 mg, 500 mg, 600 mg, 750 mg

Source
Glucosamine is a natural substance found in mucopolysaccharides, mucoproteins, and chitin. Glucosamine sulfate is synthetically manufactured.

Chemical components
Glucosamine sulfate is the sulfate salt of 2-amino-2-deoxy-D-chitin glucopyranose.

Actions
The administration of glucosamine is believed to stimulate production of cartilage components and allow rebuilding of damaged cartilage (Anon, 1996). Early in vitro studies have found that culture-derived fibroblast increased mucopolysaccharide and collagen synthesis when glucosamine was added (McCarty, 1994).

In vivo and in vitro studies conducted in rats demonstrated glucosamine can severely impair insulin secretion and beta-cell secretory dysfunction similar to that observed in patients with non-insulin-dependent diabetes mellitus (Balkan and Dunning, 1994).

Reported uses
Glucosamine is thought to be useful as an antiarthritic agent in patients with osteoarthritis or other joint disorders. (See *Glucosamine and osteoarthritis.*)

Dosage
The dose used in several clinical trials was 500 mg P.O. t.i.d. Other dosages used were based on patient weight: if weight is below 120 lb

RESEARCH FINDINGS

Glucosamine and osteoarthritis

Early studies in animals reported that oral and parenteral administration of glucosamine retards cartilage degradation and rebuilds damaged cartilage tissue. In early human trials conducted in Europe, some of which were placebo-controlled, glucosamine was given P.O. and by I.M., intra-articular, or I.V. injection for 1 to 3 weeks. All trials demonstrated improvement in pain and range of motion after 1 to 3 weeks, which continued for several weeks after therapy was discontinued. In one study, the investigators used electron microscopic studies and found healthy cartilage with glucosamine, compared with cartilage typical of established osteoarthritis with placebo (Drovanti, 1980).

The three largest randomized, controlled trials to date were carried out by Reichelt (1994) and Drovanti (1980) and colleagues, and Vaz (1982) who evaluated 155, 80, and 40 patients with established osteoarthritis, respectively, for 8 weeks or less. Reichelt's study used a glucosamine dose of 400 mg I.M. twice weekly for 6 weeks compared with placebo; Drovanti's group and Vaz evaluated glucosamine 500 mg P.O. t.i.d. before meals versus placebo or ibuprofen 400 mg P.O. t.i.d. before meals, respectively.

Reichelt and colleagues found significant differences favoring glucosamine over placebo, with lower scores in the Lequesne Index; this improvement was still present 2 weeks after treatment was concluded. In the Drovanti study, symptom scores and joint mobility significantly favored glucosamine over placebo. Vaz reported that the onset of pain relief was more rapid (1 week) with ibuprofen than glucosamine, but at 8 weeks the pain scores were significantly lower with glucosamine than ibuprofen.

Caution must be exercised when interpreting the above results because design flaws may have biased the outcomes, even though this is the best evidence for glucosamine to date. All three trials had a short treatment period and undisclosed blinding techniques; in addition, criteria for selecting the patients and concomitant medications given were not adequately described.

(54 kg), 1,000 mg glucosamine plus 800 mg chondroitin sulfates; between 120 and 200 lb (91 kg), 1,500 mg glucosamine plus 1,200 mg chondroitin sulfates; and if it is above 200 lb, 2,000 mg glucosamine plus 1,600 mg chondroitin sulfates.

Adverse reactions
• Constipation
• Diarrhea

- Drowsiness
- Epigastic pain and discomfort
- Headache
- Heartburn
- Nausea
- Rash

Interactions
None reported.

Contraindications and precautions
No known contraindications. Avoid use in pregnant or breast-feeding women and in children; effects are unknown.

Special considerations
- Monitor glucose levels in diabetic patients.
- Advise the patient that human clinical trials evaluating glucosamine are lacking.
- Suggest other accepted pharmacologic treatment before starting therapy with glucosamine.
- Explain that the long-term effect on beta-cell secretory function in humans is unknown and could be potentially harmful, especially to patients with diabetes or impaired glucose tolerance.

Points of interest
- The Arthritis Foundation does not recommend the use of glucosamine for osteoarthritis or any forms of arthritis because of the lack of efficacy data (Anon, 1996).
- The FDA has not reviewed any studies that confirm claims made for this herb.

Analysis
Although trials have demonstrated that glucosamine sulfate can improve symptoms of osteoarthritis, they all contained major study design flaws and critical problems with data analysis. There are no clinical trials evaluating the use of glucosamine with chondroitin sulfates. Long-term, adequately designed, rigorous, controlled studies are needed before glucosamine's role in the treatment of bone and joint disorders can be determined.

References
Anon. *Glucosamine sulfate treatment. Public information memo #96-05.* Atlanta, GA: Arthritis Foundation. Mar 4, 1996.

Balkan, B., and Dunning, B.E. "Glucosamine Inhibits Glucokinase In Vitro and Produces a Glucose-Specific Impairment of In Vivo Insulin Secretion in Rats," *Diabetes* 43:1173-79, 1994.

Drovanti, A., et al. "Therapeutic Activity of Oral Glucosamine Sulfate in Osteoarthrosis: A Placebo-Controlled Double-Blind Investigation," *Clin Ther* 3:260-72, 1980.

McCarty, M.F. "The Neglect of Glucosamine as Treatment for Osteoarthritis," *Med Hypotheses* 42:323-27, 1994.

Reichelt, A., et al. "Efficacy and Safety of Intramuscular Glucosamine Sulfate in Osteoarthritis of the Knee," *Arzneimittelforschung* 44:75-80, 1994.

Vaz, A.L. "Double-Blind Clinical Evaluation of the Relative Efficacy of Ibuprofen and Glucosamine Sulphate in the Management of Osteoarthrosis of the Knee in Outpatients," *Curr Med Res Opin* 3:145-49, 1982.

GOAT'S RUE

FRENCH HONEYSUCKLE, FRENCH LILAC

Common trade names
Goat's Rue

Common forms
Available as dried leaves.

Source
Goat's rue refers to the dried stalks, leaves, and flowers of *Galega officinalis* of the Leguminosae family (Fabroideae subfamily).

Chemical components
Goat's rue is composed primarily of tannins, bitters, and the alkaloids galegine and paragalegine.

Actions
Goat's rue is reported to have diuretic activity. The galegine alkaloid may reduce plasma glucose levels when administered orally; however, its efficacy as a hypoglycemic agent has not been substantiated in controlled human studies. In 1873, Gillet-Damitte addressed the French Academy and stated that goat's rue increased milk secretion in cows 35% to 50%. The herb's activity as a lactogenic in animals has since been confirmed (Remington et al., 1918). However, its effects on milk production have not been demonstrated in lactating women.

Reported uses
Goat's rue has been claimed to be useful to reduce serum glucose levels in patients with hyperglycemia, and to increase the flow of breast milk in lactating women. The herb has also been used in the management of fever, snakebites, and the plague. Controlled human trials are lacking. The current use of the herb stems from traditional and anecdotal information.

Dosage
Goat's rue fluid extract is prepared by mixing 1 cup of boiling water with 1 teaspoon of the dried leaves; the extract is taken after 10 to 15 minutes P.O. b.i.d.

Adverse reactions
• Headache
• Jitteriness
• Weakness

Interactions
None reported.

Contraindications and precautions
Avoid use of goat's rue extract in infants, children, and pregnant and breast-feeding women, unless approved by a health care professional. Although there are no reports of problems occurring in breast-fed infants, the risk of adverse effects exists.

Special considerations
• Advise the patient to discontinue goat's rue and contact a health care provider if adverse effects occur.
• Inform the patient taking the herb that saliva may be colored yellowish-green.
• Advise the breast-feeding patient to avoid use of this herb.

Points of interest
• Goat's rue is a perennial herb that grows in damp meadows and river banks from Central Europe to Iran. It has been associated with lethal poisonings in sheep grazing on the herb. Clinical signs of animal toxicity include labored breathing, neck edema, frothy nasal discharge, and muscular spasms leading to seizures. Although the mechanism of goat rue's toxicity has not been established, the galegine and paragalegine alkaloids have been implicated (Gresham and Booth, 1991).

Analysis
Clinical data do not support the use of goat's rue as a lactogenic or hypoglycemic agent. Although considered an oral treatment for diabetes before the development of sulfonylureas, the extract was not considered an alternative to insulin (Remington et al., 1918). Because of questionable antihyperglycemic efficacy, the herb is not recommended in diabetes. Similarly, the herb should not be used as a lactogenic in women because the effects on the breast-fed infant are unknown.

References

Gresham, A.C.J., and Booth, K. "Poisoning of Sheep by Goat's Rue," *Vet Rec* 129:197-98, 1991.

Remington, J.P., et al., eds. *The Dispensatory of the United States of America.* 20th ed. Philadelphia: Lippincott-Raven Pubs., 1918.

GOLDENROD

AARON'S ROD, BLUE MOUNTAIN TEA, SWEET GOLDENROD, WOUNDWORT

Common trade names
None known.

Common forms
Available as an aqueous or alcoholic extract.

Source
The active medicinal ingredients are found in the flowers and leaves of the *Solidago virgaurea,* a member of the Asteraceae family. Only one species of goldenrod grows wild in England, but over 130 species are found in the United States. The roots are also valued for their medicinal use.

Chemical components
Chemical compounds identified as having medicinal value include bioflavonoids, saponins, carotenoids, diterpenes, and tannins. The plant also may contain a high concentration of nitrates. The phenolic glycoside, leiocarposide, has also been identified.

Actions
The flavonoids and saponins are used for their diuretic action because they stimulate fluid elimination from the kidneys. The tannins contained in the leaves, stems, and roots are noted for their astringent properties. Anti-inflammatory activity has been studied by several investigators with *Populus tremula* and *Fraxinus excelsior* (combination known as Phytodolor N). Aqueous or alcoholic extracts were tested alone and in combination in models of induced arthritis or edema in the rat paw. Paw edema and arthritic paw volume were reduced by the combinations and agents used alone. Anti-inflammatory activity was demonstrated and also compared to diclofenac (Ghazaly et al., 1992).

Reported uses
Goldenrod has been endorsed by the German E Commission for use as a diuretic, anti-inflammatory, and mild antispasmodic agent. The

herb is widely used in Europe to treat inflammation of the urinary tract, and to prevent the formation or facilitate the elimination of kidney stones (Tyler, 1994). In folklore, the American Indian used goldenrod for treating sore throat and pain. Other uses included stones in the bladder, kidney and intestinal inflammation, and chronic diarrhea. Goldenrod has been used to induce abortion, and an antiseptic lotion and powder have been prepared to treat wounds. Leaves from goldenrod harvested in the Appalachian Mountain region have been used to prepare the blue mountain tea, prescribed for exhaustion and fatigue. The uses for goldenrod are founded on centuries of folklore medicine. No human studies demonstrating the medicinal value of goldenrod have been conducted.

Dosage
A decoction is prepared by mixing 1 to 2 teaspoons (3 to 5 g) of the dried herb with 8 oz water. The mixture is boiled, allowed to stand for 2 minutes, and then strained. Another method uses 30 g of the herb mixed with 300 ml water. One tablespoon of the infusion is ingested t.i.d. or q.i.d.

Adverse reactions
● Respiratory allergy, asthma, hayfever (from extraneous pollens carried by the solidago)
⚠ Emesis, rapid respiration, and death (with ingestion of dried plant)
⚠ Toxicity (emaciation, leg and abdominal edema, GI tract hemorrhage, enlarged spleen—related to parasites, fungus, and rust present in plant)

Interactions
None reported.

Contraindications and precautions
Contraindicated in pregnant women because of the herb's abortive properties.

Special considerations
● The plant is considered to contain high concentrations of nitrates.
● Advise the patient with allergies to avoid use of goldenrod.
● Tell the female patient to immediately report suspected pregnancy.
● Advise the patient to use the herb cautiously as a diuretic or in treating high blood pressure or kidney stones, because its effectiveness has not been proven. Also, tell the patient to consider the effect a delay in seeking medical attention for high blood pressure or kidney pain may have.

• Advise the patient to use the herb with caution for intestinal inflammation or chronic diarrhea.

Points of interest
• In folklore, herbalists used goldenrod to mask the bitterness of other medicines.
• Goldenrod has been popular with herbalists through the centuries for curing stones in the bladder as early as the mid-13th century, and described as an admirable plant for healing wounds.
• Parke-Davis marketed a fluid extract of goldenrod in the 1890s.
• Goldenrod occurs commonly in the United States and may cause an allergic reaction in some individuals. Allergic rhinitis occurring in early spring and fall may be attributed more to ragweed, which blooms at the same time, than to goldenrod (Wunderlin and Lockey, 1988).
• Paradoxically, the herb has been used to treat allergy.

Analysis
There are no human studies documenting the clinical effects of goldenrod. Studies evaluating its diuretic, anti-inflammatory, and cytotoxic effects have been few and performed in vitro or on murine or rat models; toxicity, adverse effects, and contraindications have not been reported. Even though the German E Commission endorsed goldenrod as a diuretic, anti-inflammatory, and antispasmodic agent, scientific evidence of its efficacy in humans is lacking.

References
Ghazaly, M., et al. "Study of the Anti-Inflammatory Activity of *Populus tremula, Solidago virgaurea* and *Fraxinus excelsior*," *Arzneimittelforschung* 42:333-36, 1992.

Tyler, V. *Herbs of Choice: The Therapeutic Use of Phytomedicinals.* New York: Pharmaceutical Products Press, Haworth Press Inc., 1994.

Wunderlin, R.P., and Lockey, R.F. "Questions and Answers," *JAMA* 260:3064-65, 1988.

GOLDENSEAL

EYE BALM, EYE ROOT, GOLDSIEGEL, GROUND RASPBERRY, INDIAN DYE, INDIAN TURMERIC, JAUNDICE ROOT, YELLOW PAINT, YELLOW PUCCOON, YELLOW ROOT

Common trade names
(Also available in combination) Golden Seal Extract, Golden Seal Extract 4:1, Golden Seal Power, Golden Seal Root, Nu Veg Golden Seal Root, Nu Veg Golden Seal Herb

Common forms

Capsules, tablets: 250 mg, 350 mg, 400 mg, 404 mg, 470 mg, 500 mg, 535 mg, 540 mg

Also available as ethanol and water extracts, dried ground root powder, tinctures, and teas.

Source

The rhizome (root stock) of *Hydrastis canadensis* is often used to manufacture the dosage forms. The main chemical components are the alkaloids—hydrastine and berberine. Also present are hydrastinine, canadine, berberastine, candaline, canadaline, chlorogenic acid, carbohydrates, fatty acids, volatile oil, resin, and meconin.

Actions

Goldenseal is claimed to have astringent, anti-inflammatory, oxytocic, antihemorrhagic, and laxative properties. The pharmacologic properties are attributed to berberine or hydrastine, and scientific studies have usually focused on these alkaloids rather than the herb itself.

An alkaloid component of goldenseal was reported to inhibit muscular contractions in rodent smooth muscle, whereas others have shown an oxytocic effect. Goldenseal extracts reduce hyperphagia and polydipsia associated with streptozocin-induced diabetes in mice (Swanston-Flatt et al., 1989).

Berberine was found to decrease the anticoagulant effect of heparin in laboratory tests of heparinated animal and human blood (Preininger, 1975), and to act as a cardiac stimulant (at lower doses), increase coronary perfusion, and inhibit cardiac activity (at higher doses) in animals. Antipyretic activity (greater than aspirin), antimuscarinic, antihistaminic, antitumor, antimicrobial, anthelmintic and hypotensive effects have also been documented for berberine in animal or laboratory models.

Hydrastinine causes vasoconstriction and can produce significant changes in blood pressure.

Reported uses

Claims for goldenseal include, but are not limited to, use for GI disorders, gastritis, peptic ulceration, anorexia, postpartum hemorrhage, dysmenorrhea, eczema, pruritus, tuberculosis, cancer, mouth ulcerations, otorrhoea, tinnitus, and conjunctivitis and as a wound antiseptic, diuretic, laxative, and anti-inflammatory agent. However, there is little, if any, clinical trial data available to support these claims.

Goldenseal was found to be less effective than ergot alkaloids when used for postpartum hemorrhage in humans. Berberine has been shown to shorten the duration of acute *Vibrio cholera* diarrhea and diarrhea caused by some species of *Giardia, Salmonella, Shigella,* and some Enterobactereciae. Clinical studies in patients with hepatic cirrhosis have shown that berberine may correct some laboratory abnormalities and improve biliary secretion and function.

Dosage
Various doses are suggested:
Ethanol and water extract: 250 mg P.O. t.i.d.
Dried rhizome: 0.5 to 1 g t.i.d.

Adverse reactions
- Asystole
- Bradycardia
- CNS depression
- Contact dermatitis
- Diarrhea
- GI cramping and pain
- Heart block
- Leukocytosis
- Mouth ulceration
- Nausea
- Paralysis (with higher doses)
- Paresthesia
- Respiratory depression (with high doses)
- Seizures
- Vomiting

⚠Death may be caused by large alkaloid doses. Symptoms of overdose include GI upset, nervousness, depression, exaggerated reflexes, and seizures that progress to respiratory paralysis and CV collapse.

Interactions
Anticoagulants: may offset the beneficial effects of therapeutic anticoagulants. Avoid concomitant use.
Antihypertensive agents: may interfere or enhance hypotensive effects when taken with goldenseal or its extracts. Don't use together.
Beta blockers, calcium channel blockers, digoxin: may enhance or interfere with the cardiac effects of these drugs. Don't use together.
CNS depressants (alcohol, benzodiazepines): may enhance sedative effects. Avoid use with goldenseal.

Contraindications and precautions
Contraindicated in patients with CV disease, particularly hypertension, heart failure, or arrhythmias, and during pregnancy.

FOLKLORE
History of goldenseal

Goldenseal derives its name from the golden-yellow scars that ultimately appear on the root at the base of the stem. After the stem is broken free, a yellow scar resembling an old-fashioned, gold wax letter seal is left on the root.

Goldenseal has been a popular part of American folklore medicine. The Native Americans were among the first to use the plant. They believed that the root could be used for many diseases, as a paint for their face and skin, as well as a dye for their garments. The plant became so popular to pioneers and settlers that by the early 1900s the country had nearly harvested the plant into extinction. Fearing its demise, the U.S. Department of Agriculture published flyers to promote public interest in the plant.

Formulations of the plant continue to sell for high prices because of a limited supply from farmers able to cultivate crops of *Hydrastis canadensis*.

Special considerations
● Monitor for any unusual symptoms.
● Monitor the patient for signs of vitamin B deficiencies (megaloblastic anemia, peripheral neuropathy, seizures, cheilosis, glossitis, angular stomatitis, seborrheic dermatitis, and infertility).
● Tell the patient to avoid hazardous activities until CNS effects of the agent are known.
● Instruct the patient not to consume the herb because of its potential to cause toxicity.

Points of interest
● Chronic use of the herb has been reported to decrease the absorption of vitamin B and thereby promote its deficiency.
● Tolerance to the herb's pharmacologic effects is thought to develop after only a few weeks of chronic use.
● The berberine alkaloid is also a component of barberry (*Berberis vulgaris*).
● Goldenseal extracts have been a component in sterile eyewashes for many years without supporting evidence for their inclusion. Also, the extracts or their components have been listed in national pharmacopoeias of several countries.
● The herb has been inappropriately used to "mask" the appearance of illicit drugs on urine drug screens in humans and in race horses. This information is false and originates from a fictional literary work that depicts the plant to be useful for hiding opiate ingestion.

• Goldenseal has been used as a dye. The rhizome has a bright yellow color that is popular for staining many fabrics and materials. (See *History of goldenseal.*)

Analysis
The pharmacologic effects of goldenseal have not been adequately studied. Because the risk of toxicity appears excessive for this plant, even some advocacy texts do not support its use for any disorder. Goldenseal and its alkaloids possess some promising pharmacologic properties; additional comprehensive, controlled studies in animals are needed before progressing to human studies.

References
Preininger, V. "The Pharmacology and Toxicology of the Papaveraceae Alkaloids," in *The Alkaloids,* vol 15. Edited by Maske, R.H.F., and Holmes, H.L. New York: Academic Press, 1975.

Swanston-Flatt, S.K., et al. "Evaluation of Traditional Plant Treatments for Diabetes: Studies in Streptozotocin Diabetic Mice," *Acta Diabetol Latina* 26:51-55, 1989.

GOSSYPOL
AMERICAN UPLAND COTTON, COMMON COTTON, COTTON, UPLAND COTTON, WILD COTTON

Common trade names
None known.

Common forms
Available as extracts.

Source
Gossypol is found in seeds, roots, and stems of the cotton plant, *Gossypium hirsutum.* These plants grow in Florida and are cultivated throughout the southern United States. The seeds of the *Gossypium* species vary widely in the quantity of gossypol content.

Chemical components
A polyphenolic binaphthyl dialdehyde (dextro- and levo-rotatory enantiomers), gossypol is the active constituent of cottonseed and other parts of the cotton plant. Cottonseed is also high in protein and low in fat.

Actions
In animal and human sperm cells, gossypol produces visible morphologic damage and reductions in motility, accounting for the

compound's antifertility actions. Gossypol's effects are related to its ability to impair the enzyme, lactate dehydrogenase X, of sperm and sperm-generating cells (Wu, 1989).

Gossypol exerts numerous effects on DNA replication, synthesis, and structural integrity. Tumorogenic potential, common in agents with similar DNA activity, has been reported with gossypin in small studies. Observed disruptions in DNA function in sperm and other cells, combined with gossypol's known inhibition of oxidative phosphorylation, have led researchers to suggest antitumor potential for gossypol. In vitro studies have demonstrated gossypol's inhibitory effect on growth of malignant human cancer cells and growth of cultured human benign prostatic hyperplasia cells (Shidaifat et al., 1997). Derivatives of gossypol have shown antitumor activity against breast tumor epithelial cell lines (Liang et al., 1995).

Laboratory studies suggest that gossypol and a derivative (gossylic iminolactone) have anti-HIV activity; however, this activity is not considered to be due to inhibition of reverse transcriptase (Royer et al., 1995).

Reported uses
Gossypol is claimed to be useful for easing labor and delivery, and for promoting normal menstruation; however, these uses have not been validated.

Studies have shown gossypol to be an effective oral male contraceptive. However, questions regarding the reversibility of these effects have precluded commercial development of this agent. Sperm counts most often return to normal about 3 months after the herb is discontinued, although long-term follow-up of patients have indicated that spermatogenesis may not always return to normal (Wu, 1989).

Other topical formulations have been tested as vaginal spermicides and found to be comparable to other products. Gossypol appears effective in the presence of cervical mucus at low concentrations, and low apparent systemic toxicity (Ratsula et al., 1983).

Dosage
For antifertility use, Chinese studies used 20 mg daily for 60 to 90 days, until the sperm count was reduced to a threshold of 4 million sperm/ml; then, doses of approximately 50 mg weekly are maintained.

Adverse reactions
• Circulatory problems, heart failure
• Diarrhea
• Hair discoloration
• Hypokalemia (due to renal tubular damage)

- Malnutrition
- Rapid muscle fatigue, muscle weakness and paralysis
- Renal toxicity (with high doses)

⚠ Cotton seeds are potentially toxic and may cause death. Domesticated animals have been poisoned from feed containing cotton seeds; postmortem examinations reveal hepatic and pulmonary edema and heart tissue degeneration. Ruminating animals (bovines) appear to be less sensitive to the herb's toxic effects than nonruminants.

Interactions
Other potassium-wasting agents (diuretics): may lead to significant potassium depletion. Don't use together.
Other renal toxins (amphotericin B): may enhance or increase risk of renal toxicity. Avoid concomitant use.

Contraindications and precautions
Avoid use in pregnant or breast-feeding patients; effects are unknown. Use cautiously in patients with renal dysfunction because renal damage may occur.

Special considerations
- Periodically monitor serum creatinine and BUN levels while the herb is being used.
- Monitor serum potassium levels and perform periodic tests of muscle strength in patients taking the herb.
- Explain that other contraception choices are available if the patient wishes to use the herb for this action.
- Warn the patient that permanent infertility may occur with long-term use.

Points of interest
- Gossypol was first identified as an antifertility agent in Chinese epidemiologic studies conducted during the 1950s.
- Processing of commercial cotton seed oil removes the gossypol content of the cotton seeds.
- Gossypol-free cottonseed flour has been suggested as an economic and abundant source of protein, and has been used in baked goods, snacks, and livestock feed.

Analysis
Gossypol has shown promise as an oral contraceptive in males and a vaginal preparation in females. Its systemic use appears daunted by the potential for irreversible sterility. Recent commentaries have suggested the adverse effect profile may be sufficient to disregard use of the product. Further study is needed to determine optimal dosing, route of administration, and incidence of adverse effects. Its

use as a topical vaginal spermicide may be considered, although definitive evidence of safety and efficacy in large human trials is required to establish a role in contraception.

References

Liang, X.S., et al. "Developing Gossypol Derivatives with Enhanced Antitumor Activity," *Invest New Drugs* 13:3:181-86, 1995.

Ratsula, K., et al. "Vaginal Contraception with Gossypol; A Clinical Study," *Contraception* 27:571, 1983

Royer, R.E., et al. "Comparison of the Antiviral Activities of 3-azido-3-deoxythymidine and Gossylic Iminolactone Against Clinical Isolates of HIV-1," *Pharmacol Res* 31:49-52, 1995.

Shidaifat, F., et al. "Gossypol Arrests Human Benign Prostatic Hyperplastic Cell Growth at G_0/G_1 Phase of the Cell Cycle," *Anticancer Res* 17:1003-09, 1997.

Wu, D. "An Overview of the Clinical Pharmacology and Therapeutic Potential of Gossypol as a Male Contraceptive Agent and in Gynaecological Disease," *Drugs* 38:333-41, 1989.

GOTU KOLA

CENTELLA, HYDROCOTYLE, INDIAN PENNYWORT, INDIAN WATER NAVELWORT, TALEPETRAKO, TECA (TITRATED EXTRACT OF *CENTELLA ASIATICA*)

Common trade names
(Various manufacturers; available in combination) Gingko/Gotu Kola Supreme, Gotu Kola Gold Extract, Gotu Kola Herb

Common forms
Capsules: 221 mg, 250 mg, 435 mg, 439 mg, 441 mg
Also available as tinctures and creams.

Source
Centella asiatica is a plant originating from Madagascar. It is also indigenous to India, Sri Lanka, and South Africa.

Chemical components
Gotu kola contains flavonoids (quercetin, kaempferol), various glycosides, terpenoids (asiaticoside, centelloside, madecasoside, brahmoside, brahminoside), madecassol, madecassic acid, asiatic acid, asiaticentoic acid, centellic acid, centoic acid, isothankuniside, fatty acids, amino acids, phytosterols, and tannin. The root region contains 14 different polyacetylenes.

Actions
Most studies have been carried out in animals. Brahmoside and brahminoside showed CNS-depressant effects (decreased motor

activity, increased sleep time, and slightly decreased body temperature) in rats and mice in vivo.

Antifertility activity against human and rat sperm was demonstrated in vitro. Asiaticoside and brahmiroside were believed to be the active constituents; however, spermicidal or spermostatic action could not be shown. Centella extract was found to significantly reduce the fertility of female mice. Centella asiatica was shown to be effective in destroying cultured cancer tumor cells.

Reported uses
Claims for gotu kola include uses as an antipsoriatic, antifertility, antihypertensive, and anticancer agent, and an agent for wound healing, varicose veins, chronic hepatic disorders, rheumatism, and mental fatigue.

A cream formulation of hydrocotyle was shown to be effective in patients with psoriasis (Natarajan et al., 1973). In another study, a hydrocotyle extract was found to be useful for preventing and treating keloids and hypertrophic scars (Bosse et al., 1979); a cortisone-like effect has been proposed for the agent's action. Hydrocotyle has also been used in patients with chronic skin maladies, including cutaneous ulcers, surgical wounds, and gynecologic wounds.

TECA showed significant improvement in symptoms, including edema, in patients with venous insufficiency of the lower limbs (Pointel et al., 1987). Asiaticoside has been shown to improve the general ability and behavioral patterns of mentally retarded patients.

Dosage
Dosages vary with disease state and with the trial cited. Usual doses are 0.6 g of the dried leaf t.i.d. or 450 mg capsule, once daily.

Adverse reactions
- Burning sensation (with topical use)
- Contact dermatitis
- Hypercholesterolemia
- Hyperglycemia
- Pruritus
- Sedation (with large doses)

Interactions
Antidiabetic and cholesterol-lowering agents: high doses of the herb may interfere with the actions of these agents. Don't use together.

Contraindications and precautions
Contraindicated in pregnant and breast-feeding patients. Use cautiously in patients with a history of contact dermatitis.

Special considerations
• Know that two of the active ingredients have been reported to cause CNS depressant effects in animals; monitor the patient for these effects.
• Advise the patient that drowsiness and sedation may occur.
• Tell the patient that a burning sensation may occur when the herb is applied.
• Advise the patient to use another contraceptive method if the herb is being used for this purpose.
• Tell the patient to report planned or suspected pregnancy.
• Instruct the patient not to use the herb continuously for over 6 weeks.

Points of interest
• Historically, Sri Lankans propagated the myth that gotu kola promoted longevity after witnessing elephants chewing on the plant leaves.
• Do not confuse with kola nuts, kola, or cola—an ingredient in Coca-Cola—all of which contain caffeine, unlike gotu kola.

Analysis
Gotu kola appears to be an interesting herb with promise in the areas of wound healing and specific dermatalogic disorders. Additional research in humans is necessary to determine its long-term efficacy and safety profile.

References
Bosse, J.-P., et al. "Clinical Study of a New Antikeloid Agent," *Ann Plast Surg* 3:13-21, 1979.

Natarajan, S., et al. "Effect of Topical Hydrocotyle Asiatica in Psoriasis," *Indian J Dermatol* 18:82-85, 1973.

Pointel, J.P., et al. "Titrated Extract of *Centella asiatica* (TECA) in the Treatment of Venous Insufficiency of the Lower Limbs," *Angiology* 38:46-50, 1987.

GRAPESEED
VITIS COIGNETIAE, VITIS VINIFERA

PINEBARK
MUSKAT, PINUS MARITIMA, PINUS NIGRA

Common trade names
(Various manufacturers; available in combination) Mega Juice, NutraPack, Pycnogenol

Common forms

Available as 25- to 300-mg tablets and capsules.

Source

Grapeseeds are extracted from the seeds of *Vitis vinifera*. Pinebark is extracted from the bark of the European coastal pine *Pinus maritima* or *Pinus nigra*.

Chemical components

The active ingredients in grapeseed and pinebark extracts are flavonoids, or proanthocyanidins (tannins), which are polyphenol oligomers derived from flavan-3-ols and flavan-3,4-diols. Additional active ingredients in grapeseed extract include essential fatty acids and tocopherols. The extract of *V. coignetiae* also contains epsilon-viniferin, oligostilbenes, ampelopsin A, ampelopsin C, ampelopsin F, and combinations of vitisin A and cis-vitisin A.

Actions

Grapeseed proanthocyanidins demonstrate antilipoperoxidant activity and xanthine oxidase inhibition (Covington, 1996). They also inhibit collagenase, elastase, hyaluronidase and beta-hyaluronidase—enzymes responsible for skin turnover. Grapeseed extract from *V. coignetiae* has shown protective effects on rat hepatocytes in vitro; however, ampelopsin C and the combination of vitisin A and cis-vitisin A exhibited hepatotoxic effects. In rat small intestines, grapeseed tannins interfere with mucosal proteins and promote cell regeneration. Grapeseed extract inhibits 5'-nucleotidase activities in snake venoms and rat livers, has therapeutic effects in Ehrlich ascites carcinoma, inhibits growth of *Streptococcus mutans*, and inhibits glucan formation from sucrose. When injected intradermally into rabbits, pinebark proanthocyanidins inhibit degradation of skin connective fibers.

Reported uses

Grapeseed and pinebark extracts are touted as antioxidants to treat circulatory disorders (hypoxia from atherosclerosis, inflammation, and cardiac or cerebral infarction). In European studies, patients with peripheral circulatory disorders given pinebark extract showed improvements in pain, limb heaviness, and swelling. These studies were small, uncontrolled or poorly controlled, and involved a wide range of doses. Additionally, grapeseed extract has been anecdotally reported to be useful for treating inflammatory conditions, varicose veins, and cancer.

Dosage
Tablets, capsules: 25 to 300 mg P.O. daily for up to 3 weeks have been suggested; then maintenance dose of 40 to 80 mg P.O. once daily.

Adverse reactions
None reported.

Interactions
None reported.

Contraindications and precautions
No known contraindications.

Special considerations
• Instruct the patient with a circulatory disorder not to delay seeking medical attention if symptoms worsen (changes in sensation, color, or temperature of extremity).

Points of interest
• Proanthocyanidins were extracted from pinebark in 1951 and marketed under the name Pycnogenol. In 1970, proanthocyanidins were extracted from grapeseeds.

Analysis
Although grapeseed extract is very popular in Europe, there are insufficient clinical data to support the use of grapeseed or pinebark extracts for treatment of any disease for which there is claimed therapeutic benefit. The lack of tolerance and safety data only emphasizes our lack of knowledge of these products. Anecdotally, there are reports that these extracts are effective in circulatory disorders and are well tolerated. Further controlled trials are needed before any recommendations can be made.

References
Covington, T.R., ed. *The Handbook of Nonprescription Drugs.* Washington, D.C.: American Pharmaceutical Association, 1996.

GREEN TEA
MATSU-CHA, TEA

Common trade names
Various manufacturers.

Common forms
Available as teas and capsules.

Source

Green tea is prepared from the steamed and dried leaves of *Camellia sinensis*, a large shrub with evergreen leaves native to eastern Asia. Green tea is different from black tea in that it is produced from leaves that have been withered, rolled, fermented, and dried. Because of the curing process, the properties of the green tea are very similar to that of the fresh leaf.

Chemical components

Green tea contains polyphenols (catechins), tannins, flavonols, and methylxanthines (caffeine, theophylline, theobromine). Commercially prepared green tea extracts are standardized to contain 60% polyphenols and, depending on the method of preparation, the tea may contain 1% to 4% caffeine.

Actions

The chemopreventative effect of green tea is attributed to the polyphenols (epigallocatechin and epigallocatechin-3-gallate); these agents are believed to inhibit cell proliferation and tumor promotion-related activities and have antioxidant actions. Animal models involving rodent lung, esophagus, stomach, intestine, skin, liver, and colon have shown the inhibitory activity of green tea against carcinogens. In vitro studies of green tea polyphenols induced programmed cell death (apoptosis) in human cancer cells (Hibasami et al., 1998; Ahmad et al., 1997).

The caffeine in green tea produces CNS stimulation and the polyphenols inhibit ultraviolet-induced skin carcinogenesis. Green tea has also been suggested as an adjuvant to therapy for AIDS, to prevent drug-resistant mutants, because of its antimutagenic action (McCarty, 1997).

Green tea has also been associated with cholesterol-lowering effects and decreased atherosclerosis (Yang and Koo, 1997). Antibacterial activity has been demonstrated against methicillin-resistant *Staphylococcus aureus* and *Yersinia enterocoltica* in vitro. The fluoride and tannins in green teas are believed to decrease the formation of dental caries.

Reported uses

The Chinese have used green tea leaf and its extracts for thousands of years. Therapeutic claims for this agent include the prevention of cancer, dental caries, hypercholesterolemia, and atherosclerosis. It has been promoted for its diuretic, stimulant, astringent, antibacterial, and radioprotective actions. Studies in animals and in vitro human models have supported the chemopreventative effects and atherosclerosis claims.

Epidemiologic studies in the Asian population have provided additional evidence. Although Japanese patients had a lower risk of cancer with green tea consumption, the difference was not significant (Imai et al., 1997).

Dosage
Epidemiologic studies have suggested possible effects from drinking 6 to 10 cups daily; pharmacokinetic studies indicate that three capsules of green tea extract provide adequate plasma levels.

Adverse reactions
• Allergic reactions (immunoglobulin E-mediated) in patients with green-tea asthma.

Interactions
Doxorubicin: may enhance the antitumor activity of doxorubicin. Monitor patient.
Milk: may inhibit the antioxidant effects of the polyphenol component. Avoid concomitant use.

Contraindications and precautions
No known contraindications. Avoid use in patients with "green tea asthma."

Special considerations
• Because of the risk for serious allergic reactions, avoid use of green and other teas containing epigallocatechin gallate in tea-sensitive individuals.
• Tell the patient that green tea contains caffeine.

Points of interest
• Tea is grown in about 30 countries and, besides water, is the most frequently consumed beverage worldwide. It is considered to be one of the safest beverages because water is boiled in its preparation.
• Tea is generally recognized as safe in the United States.

Analysis
The potential uses of green tea as a preventative for cancer and atherosclerosis have been shown in many animals and suggested by various epidemiologic evaluations, case-control and cohort studies in Asian populations. Although these reports and widespread usage over thousands of years suggest that green tea is relatively safe, further research is necessary in other populations to clarify its impact on cancer risk. More mechanistic, dose-response studies and clinical trials are needed to verify and describe the effects of tea consumption on human carcinogenesis.

References

Ahmad, N., et al. "Green Tea Constituent Epigallocatechin-3-gallate and Induction of Apoptosis and Cell Cycle Arrest in Human Carcinoma Cells," *J Natl Cancer Inst* 89:1881-86, 1997.

Hibasami, H., et al. "Induction of Apoptosis in Human Stomach Cancer Cells by Green Tea Catechins," *Oncol Res* 5:527-29, 1998.

Imai, K., et al. "Cancer-Preventive Effects of Drinking Green Tea Among a Japanese Population," *Prev Med* 26:769-75, 1997.

McCarty, M.F. "Natural Antimutagenic Agents May Prolong Efficacy of Human Immunodeficiency Virus Drug Therapy," *Med Hypotheses* 48:215-20, 1997.

Yang, T.T., and Koo, M.W. "Hypocholesterolemic Effect of Chinese Tea," *Pharmacol Res* 35:505-12, 1997.

GROUND IVY

ALEHOOF, CAT'S-FOOT, CREEPING CHARLIE, *GLECHOMA HEDERACEA*, HAYMAIDS, HEDGEMAIDS

Common trade names

None known.

Common forms

Available as an infusion or tincture of leaves and flowers (aerial parts).

Source

The kidney shaped leaves and purple-blue flowers in whorls of *Glechoma hederacea* is one of the commonest plants grown wild in Great Britain.

Chemical components

Ground ivy contains sesquiterpenes, flavonoids, a volatile oil, a bitter principle (glechomine), saponin, resin, and tannins.

Actions

Ground ivy has not been well studied, thus little is known about its action (Grieve, 1996). It appears to have astringent properties and is claimed to dry secretions and decrease inflammation. It has been used as a diuretic and a decongestant; however, data to support these effects are currently unavailable.

Reported uses

Ground ivy has traditionally and anecdotally been recommended by herbalists to treat disorders of the ear, nose, throat, and digestive system. Its astringent properties have been used to reduce phlegm in sinusitis, bronchitis, hay fever, and allergic rhinitis. Its binding nature has led to its use to treat diarrhea and to dry up watery and mucoid secretions. All the evidence of ground ivy's effectiveness comes from folklore and anecdotal reports; no animal or human trials have been reported.

Dosage
14 to 28 grains prepared as a fluid extract P.O. t.i.d.

Adverse reactions
Appears to be well tolerated; poisoning has occurred in horses who ingest the plant (symptoms include cyanosis, lung congestion, pupil dilation, salivation, and sweating).

Interactions
None reported.

Contraindications and precautions
No known contraindications.

Special considerations
• Explain that little information exists to support a therapeutic use of this herb.
• Suggest other contemporary forms of therapy before starting therapy with this herb.

Points of interest
• Ground ivy is known in parts of England as alehoof because it was used in medieval times to flavor and clarify ale.

Analysis
Ground ivy appears to be a well-tolerated herb often given to children to treat congestive conditions such as sinusitis. Although it may be safe at low doses, animal toxicities have been reported at higher doses; thus, caution must be exercised. Because of the lack of controlled animal or human data, this product cannot be recommended.

References
Grieve, M. *A Modern Herbal.* New York: Barnes & Noble, Inc., 1996.

GUARANA
BRAZILIAN COCOA, GUARANA GUM, GUARANA PASTE, ZOOM

Common trade names
Guarana Plus, Guarana Rush, Happy Motion, Superguarana, Zoom

Common forms

Guarana is a source of caffeine for, and an ingredient of, many soft drinks, including Josta, Dark Dog Lemon, and Guts. Also available in teas, alcoholic extracts, elixirs, capsules, and tablets of varied strength. Guarana is included in the ingredients of several "aphrodisiacs," weight-loss supplements, "energy drinks," vitamin supplements, candies, and chewing gum.

Source

Guarana is a dried paste made from the crushed seeds of *Paullinia cupana* (also known as *P. sorbilis),* a woody vine or shrub native to Brazil and the Amazon basin. This plant is widely cultivated because of its market value as a caffeine source and an ingredient in soft drinks, nutritional supplements, and medicinal products worldwide. It is especially popular in South America, where it has long been used for various disorders.

Chemical components

Caffeine is the active ingredient in guarana. Roasted guarana seeds may have up to 6% caffeine, although one manufacturing process has resulted in soluble guarana containing 10% caffeine. Guarana 800 mg has been reported to contain approximately 30 mg caffeine. The plant may contain tannins (including catechutannic acid, d-catechin, tannic acid, and catechol) and saponins including trace amounts of timbonine, similar to the timbo fish poisons used by Amazonian Indians.

Actions

The effects of guarana are attributed directly to its high caffeine content. The pharmacologic actions of caffeine include CNS stimulation, diuresis, hyperglycemia, cardiac stimulation, coronary and peripheral vasodilation, cerebrovascular vasoconstriction, skeletal muscle stimulation, increased gastric acid secretion, and bronchial smooth muscle relaxation. Although the effects of the saponins and tannins are not completely known, they may also participate in guarana's actions.

Guarana provides increased CNS stimulation over that of tea or coffee, possibly because of the tannin action on caffeine or the effect of fats and saponin on caffeine's absorption (Bempong and Houghton, 1992; Henman, 1982). Antidiarrheal and astringent properties of guarana may also be attributed to the tannins. Catechutannic acid, catechol, and other astringents may relieve diarrhea, but cause constipation in healthy persons.

Recent studies in Brazil showed that guarana decreases thromboxane synthesis in platelets to reverse and inhibit platelet aggregation, effects that may be attributed to the plant's xanthine content.

Reported uses

Guarana has long been used as a CNS stimulant, aphrodisiac, and appetite suppressant; for treatment of diarrhea; and for protection from malaria and dysentery (Henman, 1982). It is currently included in many weight-loss, bodybuilding, and natural vitamin supplements, and smoking cessation products to curb the appetite and provide a feeling of increased energy and mental alertness.

Guarana may be considered similar to coffee, tea, colas, and other caffeine products that are used for the temporary relief of drowsiness and to enhance mental acuity. It may also be used in dermatologic preparations; claims have been made for tannins as protective agents, saponins as as skin softeners, and xanthines as useful agents in reducing dermatitis.

Dosage

Dosage is highly variable and depends on the product and batch. Single doses often contain 200 to 800 mg guarana. Daily intake of guarana should not exceed 3 g P.O. of guarana powder or its equivalent.

A maximum daily caffeine intake of approximately 250 mg (3 to 5 g guarana) has been suggested for nonpregnant adults. Daily dosages of up to 1 g of caffeine have been used without apparent adverse effects, although withdrawal symptoms may occur following discontinuation.

Adverse reactions

Normal consumption:
- Diuresis
- Insomnia

Excessive consumption:
- Agitation
- Anxiety
- Diarrhea
- Headache
- Irritability
- Nausea
- Premature ventricular contractions
- Seizures
- Tachycardia
- Tremors
- Vomiting

⚠ Toxic symptoms (agitation, irritability, tremors, arrhythmias, seizures) can be produced in adults receiving over 1 g caffeine, whereas an acute oral dose of 5 to 10 g caffeine may be lethal.

Withdrawal state (after regular daily consumption):
- Anxiety

- Headache
- Irritability

Interactions

Adenosine: may decrease response. Monitor patient.
Beta-adrenergic agonists: may enhance response. Monitor patient.
Cimetidine, disulfiram, fluoroquinolones, oral contraceptives, phenyl-propanolamine: may increase caffeine serum levels or prolong serum caffeine half-life. Monitor patient.
Iron: absorption may be decreased by coffee and tea if taken within 1 hour of a meal. Avoid concurrent use.
Lithium: caffeine may inhibit clearance of lithium. Monitor patient.
Smoking: enhanced elimination of caffeine and related xanthines.
Theophylline: may cause additive CNS and CV effects. Avoid concomitant use of guarana and other sources of caffeine.

Contraindications and precautions

Guarana and other caffeine-containing products are contraindicated in patients with arrhythmias because high caffeine levels may cause worsening of symptoms and arrhythmias, and inhibit cardioversion with adenosine. Avoid or limit use of caffeine products in pregnant and breast-feeding patients because of an association with low birth weight and caffeine consumption. Avoid, or use with caution, in patients with CV disease, gastric ulcer, chronic headache, or diabetes, and in those currently taking theophylline.

Special considerations

- The caffeine content of any particular guarana product cannot be accurately predicted.
- Caution the pregnant patient against use of the product because it contains caffeine.
- Counsel the patient to reduce guarana use if symptoms resulting from excessive caffeine use occur (tremors, irritability, headache, palpitations).
- Inform the patient that guarana may exacerbate high blood pressure, hiatal hernia, or gastroesophageal reflux disease, and peptic ulcer disease.
- Remind the patients receiving theophylline to avoid guarana because of risk of excessive CNS stimulation.

Points of interest

- Guarana is listed as among those products "Generally Recognized as Safe" by the FDA for use as a food additive. (See *Uses of guarana,* page 320.)
- In 1989 the FDA prohibited the use of caffeine in OTC diet products because of increased agitation, restlessness, tremor and halluci-

FOLKLORE
Uses of guarana

Guarana has been used for stimulant effects similar to coffee and tea; it contains about 3% to 5% of caffeine compared with 2% found in coffee beans and 4% in tea leaves. The plant has been used by many people and various cultures. For example, the French popularized a guarana drink during the early 19th century; others mixed the herb with alcohol to produce a unique beverage. In Central and South America, parts of the guarana plant are used as a fish poison. The Amazon Indians crush the seeds and combine them with cassava flour to make a paste, which is then rolled into sticks and dried. The sticks are later ground on a bone inside the tongue of a large fish (the Pirarucu) or on stone, to generate a powder that could be mixed with water to make a beverage (Henman, 1982).

Guarana is still consumed on a daily basis in many parts of South America. It has emerged as a "natural diet aid" and can be found as a main ingredient in several herbal weight-loss products and soft drinks.

nations reported when caffeine was combined with phenylpropanolamine (DeSimone and Scott, 1995).

• In 1826, the major alkaloid was isolated and named guaranine, which was later shown to be nearly identical to caffeine; theophylline and theobromine were also isolated. Guaranine may still be used in labeling because some reports claim that guaranine is a tetramethylxanthine, whereas caffeine is a trimethylxanthine.

• During processing, small particles of the seed husk of guarana remain in the final product, giving the herb a bitter, chocolate taste.

Analysis

Guarana contains relatively high amounts of caffeine, although it can vary with product and preparation. Although its products are probably as safe as coffee, tea, and colas, caffeine intake should be monitored. Many products contain guarana as an undisclosed ingredient (such as in bodybuilding and weight-loss supplements), and the caffeine content is not always specified. Guarana elixirs contain alcohol, and may contain higher amounts of caffeine than products containing powdered guarana. Caffeine products should be avoided in pregnant and breast-feeding women because caffeine crosses the placenta and is excreted in breast milk.

References

Bempong, D.K., and Houghton, P.J. "Dissolution and Absorption of Caffeine from Guarana," *J Pharm Pharmacol* 44:769-71,1992.

DeSimone, E.M., and Scott, D.M. "Nicotine and Caffeine Abuse," in *Applied Therapeutics: The Clinical Use of Drugs,* 6th ed. Edited by Young, L.Y., and Koda-Kimble, M.A. Vancouver, Wash.: Applied Therapeutics, 1995.

Henman, A.R. "Guarana (*Paullinia cupana* var. *sorbilis*): Ecological and Social Perspectives on an Economic Plant of the Central Amazon Basin," *J Ethnopharmacol* 6:311-38, 1982.

GUM ARABIC

ACACIA, ACACIA ARABICA GUM, ACACIA GUM, ACACIA SENEGAL, ACACIA VER, EGYPTIAN THORN, GUMMAE MIMOSAE, SENEGA

Common trade names
None known.

Common forms
Available as a powder (20 g/package), gum, and syrup (10% gum arabic).

Source
Extracted from the tree *Acacia senegal.* The quality of the gum varies according to the type of gum expression (beetle attack, extreme drought, or tapping) and the growing conditions.

Chemical components
Gum arabic is a complex mixture of calcium, magnesium, and potassium salts of arabic acid. It contains tannin, cyanogenic glycosides, oxidases, peroxidases, and pectinases. It is a heteropolysaccharide composed of D-galactopyranose, D-glucuronic acid, L-arabinose, and L-rhamnose. Acacia powder often contains carbohydrate bases that contain fructose. The gum is soluble in water and insoluble in alcohol, ether, and oils.

Actions
Physiologic mechanisms are poorly described. Purified acacia gum may inhibit the growth and protease activity of suspected periodontal pathogens with marked differences in susceptibility (Clark et al., 1993). Tannins reportedly act as astringents with hemostatic and healing properties; cyanogenic glycosides, oxidases, peroxidases, and pectinases exhibit antimicrobial properties. Gum arabic may also be fermented in the colon, providing a substrate for bacterial nitrogen incorporation and growth. This action increases fecal nitrogen excretion and bacterial masses, while lowering BUN levels.

Reported uses

Two studies evaluated the efficacy of gum arabic in patients with hypercholesterolemia and found no beneficial effect (Haskell et al., 1992; Jensen et al., 1993). Antiplaque and antibacterial effects were noted when gum arabic was used as a chewing gum; lower gingival and plaque scores were reported, implying inhibition of early deposition of plaque.

Gum arabic may also be useful in patients with chronic renal failure on a low-protein diet, because it increases fecal nitrogen content and fecal bacterial mass, and significantly decreases BUN (Bliss et al., 1996). Unsubstantiated claims include treatment of cough, cold, sore throat, diarrhea, dysentery, gonorrhea, burns, sore nipples, inflammations, and nodular leprosy.

Dosage

Dosages vary with the formulation.
For lowering cholesterol: 9.7 to 50 g daily of powdered gum arabic.
For reducing plaque: gum with an unknown quantity of the active ingredient is used.

Adverse reactions

- Bloating
- Contact dermatitis (after exposure to preservative)
- Increased flatulence (dose-dependent effect)
- Increased stool frequency
- ⚠ Nephrotoxicity and hepatotoxicity (with I.V. use)

Interactions

None reported.

Contraindications and precautions

Use cautiously in patients with a history of atopy or those prone to contact dermatitis. Avoid use of the herb in pregnant or breast-feeding patients; effects are unknown.

Special considerations

- Know that this agent is considered a food supplement approved by the FDA and World Health Organization.
- Instruct the patient not to discontinue regular dental care in favor of this herb.

Points of interest

- In 1977, over 11,000 tons of gum arabic was imported to the United States primarily to give body and texture to processed food products.

• This substance is used as an excipient in many OTC and prescription medications to stabilize emulsions and act as a demulcent.

Analysis

Clinical data from studies in hypercholesterolemic patients prove that gum arabic is not an effective agent. Human study data suggest a role for this agent as an antiplaque chewing gum; however, further studies are needed to define its dosage and use in treatment. There are no studies comparing gum arabic with standard care treatments. Although allergic reactions have been reported primarily with exposure to the preservatives, the potential for such reactions warrants discriminate use in hypersensitive individuals.

References

Bliss, D.Z., et al. "Supplementation with Gum Arabic Fiber Increases Fecal Nitrogen Excretion and Lowers Serum Urea Nitrogen Concentration in Chronic Renal Failure Patients Consuming a Low-Protein Diet," *Am J Clin Nutr* 63:392-98, 1996.

Clark, D.T., et al. "The Effects of *Acacia arabica* Gum on the In Vitro Growth and Protease Activities of Periodontopathic Bacteria," *J Clin Periodontol* 20:238-43, 1993.

Haskell, W.L., et al. "Role of Water-Soluble Dietary Fiber in the Management of Elevated Plasma Cholesterol in Healthy Subjects," *Am J Cardiol* 69:433-39, 1992.

Jensen, C.D., et al. "The Effect of Acacia Gum and a Water-Soluble Dietary Fiber Mixture on Blood Lipids in Humans" *J Am Coll Nutr* 12:147-54, 1993.

HAWTHORN

CRATAEGUS EXTRACT, LI 132, MAY, MAYBUSH, WHITETHORN

Common trade names
Cardiplant, Hawthorne Berry, Hawthorne Formula, Hawthorne Heart, Hawthorne Phytosome, Hawthorne Power

Common forms
Available as biologic extracts (4 mg/ml vitexin-2-O-rhamnoside); capsules of berries (510 mg) or leaves (80 mg) standardized to 15 mg oligomeric procyanidines; and extended-release capsules (300 mg of 1.8% vitexin-2-rhamnoside and hyperoside).

Source
Active ingredients are extracted from the berries, flowers, or leaves of *Crataegus* species, commonly *C. laevigata*, *C. monogyna,* or *C. folium*. There are over 300 *Crataegus* species worldwide, and are found in the temperate regions of North America, Asia, and Europe.

Chemical components
Hawthorn is composed primarily of proanthocyanidins and flavonoids (quercetin, hyperoside, vitexin, vitexin-rhamnoside, rutin); other constituents include catechin and epicatechin.

Actions
Studies on animals and in vitro models have suggested CV actions that include dilation of coronary arteries, negative and positive inotropic effects, hypotensive effects, beta-blocking activity, and ACE inhibition. The high bioflavonoid content in some hawthorn species may show antioxidant activity and be cardioprotective in experimental ischemic animal models; the extracts decreased myocardial oxygen consumption and left ventricular work (Lianda et al., 1984). Prophylactic antiarrhythmic potential has also been shown in rabbits administered aconitine. Mild CNS depressant effects have been documented for the hawthorn flower extract.

Reported uses

Claims for hawthorn surround its use in heart failure, paroxysmal tachycardia, hypertension, arteriosclerosis, and Buerger's disease. It may be therapeutically useful in the treatment of New York Heart Association (NYHA) functional class II (mild to moderate) heart failure. Patients with NYHA functional class II heart failure receiving a daily dose of 600 mg of hawthorn extract showed significant clinical improvement over an 8-week period (Schmidt et al., 1994).

Hawthorn, either alone or with coenzyme Q-120, was found to be beneficial and also favor comparably to captopril in patients with heart failure (Tauchert et al., 1994). Other studies have noted the herb's usefulness in patients with stable angina pectoris (Hanak and Bruckel, 1983).

Dosage

A dose of 160 to 900 mg of a standardized extract containing 2.2% flavonoids or 18.75% oligomeric procyanidines P.O. given in two or three doses. The amount of flavonoid (calculated as hyperoside) is 3.5 to 19.8 mg, and that of procyanidins (as epicatechin) is 30 to 168.7 mg.

Adverse reactions

- Fatigue
- Nausea
- Sweating

⚠ Hypotension, arrhythmias, and sedation (with high doses); respiratory failure (in animals)

Interactions

Antihypertensives, nitrates: increased risk of hypotension. Monitor blood pressure closely.
Cardiac glycosides: may potentiate action of the glycoside. Use cautiously.
CNS depressants: may have additive effects. Use cautiously.

Contraindications and precautions

Contraindicated in patients with hypersensitivity to other members of the Rosaceae plant family and in pregnant or breast-feeding patients.

Special considerations

- Monitor patient for adverse CNS effects.
- Instruct the patient to use hawthorn only under medical supervision.
- Advise the patient to avoid hazardous activities until the herb's CNS effects are known.

• Explain that other proven therapies in heart failure should be pursued before taking hawthorn.
• Instruct the patient to seek emergency medical treatment if shortness of breath occurs or if pain occurs in the heart region or spreads to the arm, lower jaw, or upper abdomen.
• Tell the patient who chooses to self-medicate to seek medical advice if symptoms continue for over 6 weeks.

Points of interest
• Germany's Federal Institute for Drugs and Medical Devices approves the use of hawthorn leaf with flower extracts in the treatment of NYHA functional class II heart failure. The extract of berries was not approved because efficacy was not shown.
• Berry preparations are often advertised to the public as a supplement to strengthen and invigorate the heart and circulatory system.

Analysis
Hawthorn has long been used for heart failure in Europe. Several recent foreign studies suggest that it may be effective in treating NYHA functional class II heart failure. Long-term studies using hawthorn that demonstrate prolonged survival are lacking. Future studies should focus on evaluating improvements in NYHA heart failure class, hospital admission rates, quality of life measurements, and whether hawthorn extracts have an effect on mortality.

References
Hanak, T.H., and Bruckel, M.H. "Behandlung Von Leichten Stabilen Formen der Angina Pectoris mit Crataegutt Novo," *Therapiewoche* 33:4331-33, 1983.

Lianda, L., et al. "Studies on Hawthorn and its Active Principle. I. Effect on Myocardial Ischemia and Hemodynamics in Dogs," *J Tradit Chin Med* 4:283-88, 1984.

Schmidt, U., et al. "Efficacy of the Hawthorn *(Crataegus)* Preparation LI 132 in 78 Patients with Chronic Congestive Heart Failure Defined as NYHA Functional Class II," *Phytomedicine* 1:17-24, 1994.

Tauchert, M., et al. "Effectiveness of Hawthorn Extract LI 132 Compared with the ACE Inhibitor Captopril: Multicenter Double-Blind Study with 132 NYHA Stage II," *Munch Med* 136(Suppl):S27-33, 1994.

HELLEBORE, AMERICAN
FALSE HELLEBORE, GREEN HELLEBORE, INDIAN POKE, ITCH-WEED, SWAMP HELLEBORE

Common trade names
Cryptenamine

Common forms
Available as fluid extract, tincture, and powder.

Source
American, or green hellebore, is derived from the dried rhizome and roots of the perennial herb, *Veratrum viride*. Related species include *V. album* (white hellebore), *V. californicum*, *V. officinale* (Cevadilla), and *V. japonicum*.

Chemical components
The main components of the root include several ester glycoalkaloids (pseudojervine, rubijervine, jervine, neogermitrine, cevadine, proto-veratrine, veratridine, and protoveratridine), starch, and resin. The alkaloids are chemically similar to steroids and are considered both medicinally active and toxic. All species contain varying amounts of alkaloids, which explains the varying degrees of action and toxicity.

Actions
The ester alkaloids are responsible for hellebore's physiologic effects, including lowering arterial pressure and heart and respiration rates, and stimulating blood flow into the kidneys, liver, and extremities. The CV response to veratrum alkaloids depends on the agent and dose administered. High doses have paradoxically caused elevated blood pressure (Arena and Drew, 1986).

Veratrum alkaloids are known to have a depolarizing action on nerve membranes, skeletal and visceral muscles, and cardiac tissue. They are believed to increase nerve and muscle excitability, as noted by the adverse effects of increased muscle tone and paresthesia. These agents also produce nausea and emesis; large doses depress respiration and may cause respiratory failure.

Reported uses
Historically, hellebore has been used as an emetic and for pneumonia, peritonitis, neuralgias, epilepsy, and seizures. More recently, veratrum alkaloids have been used in the treatment of hypertension, acute hypertensive crises, hypertensive toxemia of pregnancy, and nephropathies (Arena and Drew, 1986). They have been given parenterally (with success) for managing pulmonary edema resulting from severe acute hypertensive crises. One veratrum alkaloid, germine diacetate, has been used experimentally to treat myasthenia gravis (Anon, 1967).

However, hellebore and the veratrum alkaloids are not currently used because of their narrow therapeutic index and highly toxic nature. Some herbalists may recommend American or green hellebore as a cardiac sedative.

Dosage

For cardiac sedation, 1 to 3 minims fluid extract P.O. every 2 to 3 hours until pulse rate is reduced; or 1 to 2 grains powder P.O.; or 10 to 30 minims tincture P.O. I.V. doses are unknown.

Adverse reactions

- Abdominal pain and distention
- Arrhythmias
- Bradycardia
- Diaphoresis
- Dysgeusia
- Dyspnea
- ECG changes
- Extraocular muscle paralysis
- Hypertension or hypotension
- Increased muscle tone
- Muscular weakness
- Nausea
- Pallor
- Paresthesia
- Respiratory depression
- Salivation
- Seizures
- Sneezing (inhalation)
- Syncope
- Vomiting

⚠ Ingestion of any part of the plant is considered toxic. Signs of overdose are burning throat, impaired vision, abdominal pain, nausea, diarrhea, syncope, shortness of breath, spasms, loss of consciousness, and paralysis. Most cases have not been fatal because of the rapid vomiting that occurs and poor intestinal absorption of the veratrum alkaloids.

Interactions

None reported.

Contraindications and precautions

Contraindicated in patients with hypotension, aortic coarctation, pheochromocytoma, digitalis intoxication, or increased intracranial pressure (unless caused by hypertensive crisis), and during pregnancy.

Special considerations

- American hellebore is considered highly toxic. It has a low therapeutic index that makes it unfavorable for medicinal purposes.

Points of interest

• Veratrine, which once appeared in the Pharmacopoeia (1898) and British Pharmacopoeia Codex, is derived from the plant *V. officinale* (Mexican hellebore) or Sabadilla. It is used as a topical analgesic and a parasiticide. Veratrine contains many of the same alkaloids found in American hellebore in varying amounts.

• Ingestion of the plant *V. californicum,* related to American hellebore, has been associated with causing cyclopia and other related facial deformities in animals.

• Sneezing powders are known to have contained veratrum alkaloids. The powders contained pulverized veratrum album root which, when inhaled, caused many of the same adverse effects seen after ingestion, including nausea, vomiting, diaphoresis, bradycardia, and hypotension (Fogh et al., 1983).

• Veracintine, an alkaloid isolated from *Veratrum album,* and its derivatives have exhibited in vitro cytotoxic effects on leukemia cells.

Analysis

Despite its extensive use in the past for malignant hypertension, hellebore and veratrum alkaloids are no longer preferred for these uses because of their narrow therapeutic index and the emergence of safer and more tolerable agents. The veratrum alkaloids have clear pharmacologic activity; unfortunately, their noxious and toxic adverse effects have limited their use. Because only small amounts of veratrum alkaloid extracts are needed to cause toxic effects, their use is considered extremely dangerous. Hellebore is currently not recommended for medicinal use.

References

Anon. "Veratrum Alkaloids in the Therapy of Myasthenia Gravis," *Can Med Assoc J* 96:1534-35, 1967.

Arena, J.M., and Drew, R.H.,eds. *Poisoning: Toxicology, Symptoms, Treatments,* 5th ed. Springfield, Ill: Charles C. Thomas Publisher, 1986.

Fogh, A., et al. "Veratrum Alkaloids in Sneezing-Powder: A Potential Danger," *J Toxical Clin Toxicol* 20:175-79, 1983.

HELLEBORE, BLACK

BLACK HELLEBORE, CHRISTE HERBE, CHRISTMAS ROSE, EASTER ROSE, MELAMPODE

Common trade names

None known.

Common forms

Available as a fluid or solid extract and powdered root.

Source
The active components are extracted from the dried rhizome and root of the perennial plant, *Helleborus niger*.

Chemical components
The extract may contain hellebrin, an aglycone, and two highly toxic crystalline glycosides—bufadienole helleborin and helleborcin. These glycosides may indicate contamination with other related species. Other components include saponosides, ranunculoside derivatives, resin, fat, and starch. The commercial hellebore roots consist mainly of *H. niger,* and are mostly hellebrin-free. Other related species, especially *H. viridis,* tend to have higher levels of glycosides and aglycones.

Actions
The entire plant is considered poisonous. Extracts of black hellebore are claimed to promote menstrual flow and to have purgative, anthelmintic, and narcotic properties.

    Protoanemonine is thought to cause skin dermatitis, eye irritation, and GI irritations (burning sensation of mouth and throat, abdominal pain, and vomiting). It combines with sulfhydryl groups, which results in subepidermal vesication. Topical application of the freshly bruised plant may cause serious irritation. Early in vitro studies using protoanemonine identified antifungal and cytotoxic properties (Erickson, 1948; Holden et al., 1947).

Reported uses
The plant has been used historically as a purgative and in the treatment of heart failure, intestinal worms, amenorrhea, mental disorders, and anxiety. Other claims for its use include as a diuretic, anesthetic, for the treatment of skin ulcers, and to induce abortion.

    In homeopathy, black hellebore tincture is said to be useful for eclampsia, epilepsy, meningitis, encephalitis, and psychoses. In Europe, black hellebore is used in homeopathy and as adjuvant therapy in the treatment of cancer patients because of its claimed immunostimulatory properties. A recent in vitro study observed increased cytokine production in cells given an extract of black hellebore (Bussing and Schweizer, 1998). To date, there have been no controlled, double-blind, randomized human trials involving black hellebore preparations.

Dosage
For laxative use, 1 to 10 drops fluid extract P.O., 1 to 2 grains solid extract P.O., or 10 to 20 grains powder P.O.

Adverse reactions
- Abdominal pain
- Arrhythmias
- Bradycardia
- Burning sensation of mouth
- Conjunctival irritation
- Dermatitis
- Diarrhea
- Hypotension
- Irregular pulse (with contamination)
- Nasal irritation
- Respiratory failure (with contamination)
- Salivation
- Shortness of breath
- Sneezing
- Vomiting

Interactions
None reported.

Contraindications and precautions
Avoid use of the herb in pregnant or breast-feeding patients; effects are unknown.

Special considerations
- Inform the patient that ingestion of the plant may result in burning of mouth and throat, salivation, vomiting, diarrhea, and abdominal pain.
- Advise the patient that black hellebore is considered to be toxic and therefore should not be consumed.

Points of interest
- *H. niger* blossoms white flowers in the winter, from which it received its name, Christmas rose.
- The name "hellebore" is derived from the Greek *elein* (to injure) and *bora* (food), describing its toxic nature.

Analysis
Besides its use in homeopathy, black hellebore is mainly used as an ornamental garden plant. Though it is being used as a potential immunostimulant, there is currently a lack of controlled human trials to support this claim. Because of its recognized poisonous status and the lack of clinical data to support the medicinal use of black hellebore, it is recommended to avoid products containing components from this plant.

References

Bussing, A., and Schweizer, K. "Effects of Phytopreparation from *Helleborus niger* on Immunocompetent Cells In Vitro," *J Ethnopharmacol* 59:139-46, 1998.

Erickson, R.O. "Protoanemonin as a Mitotic Inhibitor," *Science* 108:533, 1948.

Holden, M., et al. "Range of Antibiotic Activity of Protoanemonin," *Proc Soc Exp Biol Med* 66:54, 1947.

HOPS

Common trade names

(Available in combination) Avena Sativa Compound in Species Sedative Tea, HR 129 Serene, HR 133 Stress, Melatonin with Vitamin B_6, Snuz Plus, Stress Aid

Also available as single-ingredient compounds.

Common forms

Available in herbal tea preparations. Both solid and liquid forms are becoming more popular. There are also anecdotal reports of dried hops being smoked.

Source

Humulus lupulus is a member of the Cannabaceae family (formerly classified within the Moraceae family; the only other genus of Cannabaceae is *Cannabis sativa/indica* also known as marijuana). The hops plant is a perennial, dioecious vine that grows up to 20 feet (6 m). The leaves are trilobed, serrate, and generally opposite. These fruits or flowers grow in conelike leafy bracts at the base of the flower stalk and are generally 2 to 4 inches (5 to 10 cm) long.

Chemical components

More than 330 chemicals have been isolated from the hops plant. They are found in a volatile oil (beta-myrcene, humulene, and linalool) or resin (humulone, lupulone). Other active components include estradiol, colupulone, avermectin, and various alcohols such as xanthohumol and 2-methyl-3-butene-2-ol. Although *Humulus* and *Cannabis* belong to the same family, hops do not contain delta-9-tetrahydrocannabinol as an active constituent.

Actions

The phytoestrogens exert direct estrogenic activity in vitro (Zava et al., 1998). Sedative-hypnotic effects have been shown in mice and humans that are attributed to 2-methyl-3-butene-2-ol (Gerhard et al., 1996; Wohlfart et al., 1983). Colupulone and avermectin both have antibacterial activity. Humulon has been shown to decrease tumor formation and inflammation in mice (Yasukawa et al., 1995).

Colupulone has also been shown to induce hepatic microsomal enzymes whereas xanthohumol inhibits the extramicrosomal hepatic enzyme DGAT in rats, mice, and in vitro (Mannering and Shoeman, 1996).

Reported uses

Historically, hops have been promoted as an analgesic, hypnotic, antispasmotic, anthelmintic, and sedative, and to promote functional activity of the stomach. Anecdotal reports promote the use of hops as a sedative-hypnotic, antidepressant, and for treatment during menopause.

Dosage

No specific dosage is available because hops are often taken either in combination with other herbals or as a tea. However, based upon combination products, the approximate dose of hops may be 2 to 4 mg of the extract.

Adverse reactions

• Anaphylaxis and allergic reactions (predominantly dermatologic manifestations)
• Bronchial irritation and bronchitis (following inhalation)
• Decreased cognitive performance
• Sedation
• Vesicular dermatitis (following direct cutaneous contact with raw plants)

Interactions

CNS depressants (anticholinergics, antihistamines, anxiolytics, antidepressants, antipsychotics, alcohol): may cause additive effects. Use with caution.
Drugs metabolized by the cytochrome P-450 system: may cause decreased plasma levels of these drugs. Avoid concomitant use.
Phenothiazine-type antipsychotics: may cause additive effects on hyperthermia. Avoid concomitant use.

Contraindications and precautions

Contraindicated in patients with estrogen-dependent tumors, such as breast, uterine, or cervical cancer. Use with caution in patients receiving CNS depressants or antipsychotics.

Special considerations

• Know that the herb loses its original activity when stored (only 15% remains after 9 months).
• Warn the patient to avoid hazardous activities until CNS effects of the herb are known.

Points of interest
• Hops are used in the commercial preparation of beer because of the herb's bitter taste and preservative action.

Analysis
In addition to its use in beers, hops have long been used as a sedative-hypnotic. Their use in this case is probably safe when taken infrequently for insomnia, assuming no preexisting conditions or drug therapy exists. Despite its estrogenic activity, the use of hops in menopause is less well founded and thus is not recommended. The lack of specific dose, safety, and efficacy data preclude its recommendation for any use.

References
Gerhard, U., et al. "Vigilance-Decreasing Effects of Two Plant-Derived Sedatives," *Schweiz Rundsch Med Prax* 85:473-81, 1996.

Mannering, G.J., and Shoeman, J.A. "Murine Cytochrome P4503A is Induced by 2-methyl-3-buten-2-ol, 3 methyl-1-pentyn-3-ol (meparfynol), and Tertamyl Alcohol," *Xenobiotica* 26:487-93, 1996.

Wohlfart, R., et al. "The Sedative-Hypnotic Action of Hops. 4. Pharmacology of the Hop Substance 2-methyl-3-buten-2-ol," *Planta Med* 48:120-23, 1983.

Yasukawa, K., et al. "Humulon, a Bitter in the Hop, Inhibits Tumor Promotion by 12-O-tetradecanoylphorbol-13-acetate in Two-Stage Carcinogenesis in Mouse Skin," *Oncology* 52:156-58, 1995.

Zava, D.T., et al. "Estrogen and Progestin Bioactivity of Foods, Herbs, and Spices," *Proc Soc Exp Biol Med* 217:369-78, 1998.

HOREHOUND

COMMON HOREHOUND, HOARHOUND, MARRUBIUM, MARVEL, WHITE HOREHOUND

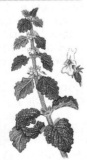

Common trade names
Horehound Herb, Hore Hound Tea

Common forms
Available as capsules of fluid extract (300 mg), lozenges, syrup, tea, powder, and confectionaries.

Source
The extracts are mostly derived from fresh or dried leaves and the flowering tops of *Marrubium vulgare*. This plant, although native to Europe and Asia, has been naturalized to the United States and parts of North America.

Chemical components
The volatile oil marrubiin (a diterpene lactone) is the main bitter component of *M. vulgare;* extracted concentrations range from 0.3% to 1%. Horehound also contains diterpene alcohols, betonicine, tannins, volatile oils, beta-sitosterol (sterol), several flavonoids, waxes, ursolic acid, bitter glycosides, and various sesquiterpene moieties, mucilaginous and resinous substances, and marrubina.

Actions
Horehound is claimed to exert a laxative effect in large doses and a proarrhythmic effect when given in very large doses. In vitro studies with aqueous extracts of horehound have suggested that this herbal extract may antagonize the effects of serotonin (Cahen, 1970). Rabbit studies suggest that the extract can exert a hypoglycemic effect (Roman et al., 1992). Derivatives of marrubiin, but not marrubiin itself, may have minor transient effects on bile secretion.

Reported uses
Anecdotal reports and testimonials claim that horehound is useful as a digestive aid, diuretic, diaphoretic, and expectorant, and for intestinal parasites. Despite its bitter flavor, the herb occurs in several different candies and cough lozenges. The throat-soothing and expectorant properties of horehound have long been popularized by herbalists. There are no human, controlled clinical trials reported that confirm any of these therapeutic claims.

Dosage
For coughs and throat ailments, 10 to 40 drops of extract P.O. in warm water up to t.i.d., 1 to 2 g powder or by infusion P.O. t.i.d., or lozenges P.O. as needed.

Adverse reactions
- Arrhythmias
- Diarrhea
- Hypoglycemia
- Possible spontaneous abortion

Interactions
Agents that enhance or antagonize serotonin release, such as antiarrhythmics, some antidepressants, antiemetics (granisetron, ondansetron), antimigraine agents (ergot alkaloids, sumatriptan): may enhance serotonergic effects. Avoid concomitant use.
Drugs used to lower blood glucose (oral antidiabetic agents, insulin): may augment hypoglycemic effect of drugs. Avoid concomitant administration.

Contraindications and precautions

Contraindicated in pregnant or breast-feeding patients, and in those with diabetes mellitus or arrhythmias.

Special considerations

• Monitor glucose level of diabetic patients.
• Monitor cardiac rate and rhythm.
• Question the patient about the use of this herb and inform him that little information exists regarding safety or effectiveness of this agent.
• Tell the female patient to report planned or suspected pregnancy.
• Inform the diabetic patient that this herb may require dose reductions in insulin or oral antidiabetic agents.

Points of interest

• Although white horehound is listed by the Council of Europe as a natural source of food flavoring, its category (N2) permits that only small quantities can be added to foodstuffs such as liqueurs, candy, and cough drops.
• Black horehound (*Ballota nigra*) may sometimes be found in compounds reported to contain only white horehound (*M. vulgare*).

Analysis

Although horehound has a long history of use as a cough remedy and as a flavoring agent, there is a lack of evidence to promote its use for any other indication. Large doses of horehound should be avoided because adverse effects on cardiac rhythms or blood glucose can occur.

References

Cahen, R. "Pharmacological Spectrum of *Marrubium vulgare*," *CR Soc Biol* 164:1467, 1970.
Roman, R.R., et al. "Hypoglycemic Effect of Plants Used in Mexico as Antidiabetics," *Arch Med Res* 23:59, 1992.

HORSE CHESTNUT

AESCIN, CHESTNUT, ESCINE

Common trade names

Horse Chestnut Extract, Venostasin Retard, Venostat

Common forms

Available as extract using aescin to standardize concentration.

Source

The seeds from *Aesculus hippocastanum,* a member of the Hippo-
castanaceae family, are used to formulate horse chestnut extract—
sometimes known as *Hippocastani semen.* The bark of young
branches should be used; the older bark is poisonous.

Chemical components

Horse chestnut is composed primarily of triterpene glycosides and
the flavonoids (quercetin, kaempferol, astragalin, isoquercetin,
rutin), coumarins (aesculetin, fraxin, scopolin), allantoin, amino
acids, choline, citric acid, and phytosterol. Products are adjusted to
contain triterpene glycosides calculated as aescin (escin).

Actions

Anti-inflammatory actions have been documented for the saponins
(aescin). Aescin reduces transcapillary filtration of water and protein,
and increases venous tone related to increased prostaglandin F_2 alpha
(vasoconstrictor). It stabilizes cholesterol-containing membranes of
lysosomes and limits the release of the enzymes. Usually, the release
of the enzymes is increased in chronic pathologic conditions of the
vein. These enzymes normally breakdown the muco-polysaccharides
in the cell membranes in the capillary walls, but this action is inhibited by aescin (Bombardelli et al., 1996). Aescin has shown notable antiviral activity in vitro toward a strain of influenza virus.

Reported uses

Horse chestnut therapy has been claimed to be effective for the
treatment of varicose veins, diarrhea, fever, phlebitis, hemorrhoids,
and enlargement of the prostate gland. Some data exist to support a
role in venous insufficiency. (See *Horse chestnut and venous insufficiency,* page 338.)

Data also suggest a role in varicose veins. Enzymes responsible for
the metabolism of substances that regulate capillary rigidity and
pore size were found to be reduced in patients with varicose veins
treated with 900 mg horse chestnut extract. These enzymes have
been found to be elevated in varicose vein patients and may play a
role in this disorder (Kreysel et al., 1983).

Dosage

Dosages of 100 to 150 mg P.O. daily of the aescin component, given as
either one or two divided doses, have been clinically tested in humans.

Adverse reactions

- Muscle spasm
- Nausea (with oral use)
- Nephropathy

RESEARCH FINDINGS
Horse chestnut and venous insufficiency

Horse chestnut is claimed to be useful in the treatment of chronic venous insufficiency. Aescin 50 mg b.i.d. was shown to be equivalent to compression stocking therapy in reducing lower leg edema in a 12-week, partially blind, placebo-controlled, parallel study of 240 patients (Diehm et al., 1996).

A second study evaluated 51 postmenopausal female patients who received 100 mg of aescin daily compared with 1,000 mg daily oxerutin (51 patients) daily for 4 weeks, then 500 mg daily for 12 weeks (35 patients). Both groups demonstrated a mean leg volume reduction of about 100 ml, similar to that reported with compression therapy (Rehn et al., 1996).

A smaller study of 20 patients given placebo or 150 mg aescin daily for 6 weeks found that leg volume was significantly reduced in the treatment group and reappeared when the drug was withdrawn. Subjective symptoms of heaviness, tenseness, leg fatigue, and paresthesia improved (Diehm et al., 1992).

• Pruritus, hypersensitivity reactions
• Urticaria
• Vomiting
⚠ Severe bleeding and bruising due to antithrombotic activity of aesculin; shock, hepatotoxicity

Interactions
Anticoagulants, aspirin: increased risk of bleeding because of aesculin, a hydroxycoumarin. Monitor patient.

Contraindications and precautions
Contraindicated in pregnant or breast-feeding patients; effects are unknown. Use cautiously in patients with hypersensitivity to other members of the horse chestnut family and in those with known bleeding disorders.

Special considerations
• Know that the fruit, leaves and older bark are poisonous.
• Monitor liver function tests.
• Inform the patient and health care staff that drug may color urine red.
• Instruct the patient to report unusual bleeding or bruising, yellowing of skin or eyes, fatigue, or fever.
• Advise the patient to use products derived from seeds or bark of young branches only.

• Advise the patient to report changes in effectiveness of other drug therapies.
• Tell the patient to check with the health care provider before taking other prescription or OTC medications that may contain aspirin.

Points of interest
• Germany's Federal Institute for Drugs and Medical Devices recognizes horse chestnut extract as effective in the treatment of chronic venous insufficiency.
• Do not confuse horse chestnut with the buckeye, also called horse chestnut.
• Horse chestnut has been used I.V. in Europe for postoperative edema, presumably for its diuretic activity.

Analysis
Although compression stocking therapy has been the primary treatment option for chronic venous insufficiency, patient compliance is poor. There is currently no allopathic medication indicated for the treatment of venous insufficiency. Thus, a carefully monitored trial of horse chestnut extract may be useful in patients with symptoms associated with this condition.

References
Bombardelli, E., et al. A. "Review: *Aesculus hippocastanum* L," *Fitoterapia* 67:483-511, 1996.

Diehm, C., et al. "Comparison of Leg Compression Stocking and Oral Horse Chestnut Seed Extract in Patients with Chronic Venous Insufficiency," *Lancet* 347:292-94, 1996.

Diehm, C., et al. "Medical Edema Protection—Clinical Benefits in Patients With Deep Vein Incompetence. A Placebo-Controlled, Double-Blind Study," *Vasa* 21:188-92, 1992.

Kreysel, H.W., et al. "A Possible Role of Lysosomal Enzymes in the Pathogenesis of Varicosis and the Reduction in Their Serum Activity by Venostatin," *Vasa* 12:377-82, 1983.

Rehn, D., et al. "Comparative Clinical Efficacy and Tolerability of Oxerutins and Horse Chestnut Extract in Patients With Chronic Venous Insufficiency," *Arzneimittelforschung* 5:483-87, 1996.

HORSERADISH

PEPPERROT

Common trade names
None known.

Common forms
Available as fresh root, powder, or semisolid paste for use as a condiment or spice.

Source

The root of the large leafy perennial, *Armoracia rusticana,* is used to make commercial condiments.

Chemical components

Horseradish contains coumarins (aesculetin, scopoletin, caffeic and hydroxycinnamic acids), ascorbic acid, asparagin, peroxidase enzymes, resin, starch, and sugars. The leaf contains quercetin and kaempferol. The volatile oil contains glucosinolates (mustard oil glycosides), gluconasturtiin, and sinigrin. Isothiocyanate and other compounds are found in the root.

Actions

Horseradish has been used to relieve pain, expel afterbirth, and as an anthelmintic or diuretic; other claimes include antiseptic, circulatory, and digestive stimulant properties. I.V. horseradish peroxidase has caused hypotension in cats (Sjaastad et al., 1984), and the extract has shown anticholinesterase activity (Leiner, 1980).

Reported uses

Horseradish is claimed to be useful for edematous states, certain infections, and inflamed joints.

Dosage

For all uses, 2 to 4 g fresh root P.O. before meals.

Adverse reactions

- Bloody diarrhea, vomiting (with large quantities)
- Hypersensitivity reactions
- Severe mucous membrane irritation

Interactions

Anticholinergics (atropine): may antagonize the effects of the herb. Atropine may be useful in cases of excessive horseradish ingestion.
Cholinergic agents (bethanecol, neostigmine, pyridostigmine): may potentiate parasympathetic effects of these agents. Monitor patient.

Contraindications and precautions

Volatile oil is contraindicated for any use. Avoid use of horseradish in pregnant and breast-feeding patients; effects are unknown. Use with caution in patients with thyroid disease.

Special considerations

- Inform the patient that this plant is poisonous; symptoms in animals include gastritis, hyperstimulation, and excitation progressing to collapse.

● Tell the patient not to grow wild horseradish because it can be confused with pokeweed root, which is considered toxic.

Points of interest
● The FDA consider horseradish to be generally safe. The herb is typically used as a food flavoring in small quantities.
● Horseradish is a common source of peroxidase enzymes.
● Allylisothiocyanate and butylthiocyanate combine with other compounds within the plant when it is destroyed or crushed to produce the characteristic pungent odor.
● Horseradish perioxidase has been used in some chemical tests for blood glucose (Jamnicky et al., 1988) and as a molecular probe in joint disorders (Shiozawa et al., 1983).
● The herb has been used as a taste repellent by mixing it with toxic substances to prevent accidental poisoning of domesticated animals.

Analysis
There is little clinical evidence to support the use of horseradish for any medicinal purposes. Consumption should be limited to quantities normally found in food and food flavorings until more is known about its action and adverse reactions.

References
Jamnicky, B., et al. "Application of Horseradish Peroxidase to Glucose Determination in Body Fluids," *Acta Pharm Jugo* 38:53, 1988.

Leiner, I.E. *Toxic Constituents of Plant Foodstuffs.* New York: Academic Press, 1980.

Shiozawa, S., et al. "Presence of HLA-DR Antigen on Synovial Type A and B Cells: An Immunoelectron Microscopic Study in Rheumatoid Arthritis, Osteoarthritis and Normal Traumatic Joints," *Immunology* 50:587, 1983.

Sjaastad, O.V., et al. "Hypotensive Effects in Cats Caused by Horseradish Peroxidase Mediated by Metabolites of Arachidonic Acid," *J Histochem Cytochem* 32:1328-30, 1984.

HORSETAIL

BOTTLE BRUSH, DUTCH RUSH, PADDOCK PIPES, PEWTERWORT, SCOURING RUSH, SHAVE GRASS

Common trade names
(Available in combination) Goldenrod-Horsetail Compound

Common forms
Available as a liquid extract. Goldenrod-Horsetail Compound is a blend of liquid extracts containing 22.5% goldenrod flowering tips, 22.5% corn silk, 22.5% horsetail, 22.5% pipsissewa leaf, and 10% juniper berry.

Source

Horsetail is obtained from the aerial stems of *Equisetum arvense, Equisetum* species.

Chemical components

Horsetail contains silica and silicic acids, equisetonin (a saponin), flavone glycosides (isoquercitrin, equisetrin, and galuteolin), sterols (beta-sitosterol, campestrol, isofucosterol and cholesterol), trace amounts of alkaloids (nicotine, palustrine and palustrinine), thi-aminase, aconitic acid, and dimethylsulfone.

Actions

The plant has a weak diuretic activity due likely to equisetonin and the flavone glycosides. *E. hyemale* is a more potent diuretic. The herb may act similarly to hydrochlorothiazide; both increase sodium and potassium excretion and increase the urinary pH (Hamon and Awang, 1992). Because *Equisetum* species contain monosilicic acid, which may be a ready source of silicon, horsetail may be useful in strengthening broken bones, connective tissue, and nails.

Reported uses

Horsetail has been used to treat several cancers, fever, gonorrhea, gout, edema, and rheumatism. Other uses include as a styptic, diuretic, urinary tonic, and tissue-strengthening agent in tuberculosis. Horsetail ash has been used for dyspepsia. Its current uses include as a diuretic, and as a silicon supplement for healing broken bones and strengthening connective tissue, teeth, hair, and nails.

Dosage

For acute use, 20 to 40 drops in water P.O. three to five times daily; for chronic use, 20 to 40 drops in water P.O. b.i.d. or t.i.d.

Adverse reactions

- Arrhythmias
- Ataxia
- Fever
- Hypersensitivity reactions
- Muscle weakness
- Seborrheic dermatitis
- Weight loss

Interactions

CNS stimulants: additive effect due to nicotine content of herb. Use cautiously in patients using nicotine replacement aids for smoking cessation.
Diuretics: potentiated effect. Avoid concomitant use.

Contraindications and precautions

Avoid use of large amounts of the herb because nicotine toxicity may occur (muscle weakness, ataxia, weight loss, abnormal heart rate, cold extremities, and fever). Also avoid use of the herb in pregnant or breast-feeding women; effects are unknown.

Special considerations

• Advise the patient to keep the herb out of reach of children and pets.
• Inform the patient that the herb contains nicotine.

Points of interest

• The FDA has classified horsetail as an herb of undefined safety.
• Children have reportedly been poisoned by using the stems as whistles or blowguns.
• Horsetail contains the toxin thiaminase, which inactivates thiamine and causes thiamine deficiency. Irreversible CNS damage may occur in severe thiamine deficiency. In Canada, manufacturers have to prove that their horsetail products are thiaminase-free.

Analysis

Horsetail exerts a weak diuretic activity. Because of its potential toxicity and the availability of safer and more effective diuretic agents, avoid the use of horsetail as a diuretic. Although horsetail is also being marketed as a urinary tonic and a silicon supplement to strengthen hair, bone, nails, and connective tissue, there are no clinical data to support these claims.

References

Hamon, N.W., and Awang, D.V.C. "Horsetail," *Can Pharm J* 125:399-401, 1992.

HYSSOP

Common trade names

None known.

Common forms

Available as commercial or fluid extracts, tinctures, and oils. Fresh or dried flowering tops are used to prepare tea or compress. Narcissus oil is used in fragrances. Narcissus pseudo-narcissus lectin, NPL, (also called narcissus pseudonarcissus agglutinin, NPA) is used in biochemistry.

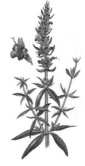

Source
The plant belongs to *Hyssopus officinalis* of family Labiatae.

Chemical components
The herb contains terpenoids (including marrubiin, oleanolic, and ursolic acids), a volatile oil (camphor, pinocamphone, thujone, isopinocamphone, with alpha- and beta-pinene, camphene, alpha-terpinene, linalool, bornylacetate, and others), flavonoids (including diosmin and hesperidiin), hyssopin (a glucoside), tannins, and resin.

Actions
Reported actions include antispasmodic, diaphoretic, antiseptic, hepatic, sedative, stimulant, expectorant, anti-inflammatory, and anti-flatulent; it also has been claimed to promote menstrual flow and to serve as a muscle relaxant. Crude extracts have been shown to inhibit HIV replication in vitro (Kaplan et al., 1990).

Reported uses
Hyssop tea has been used for coughs, colds, bronchitis, asthma, flatulence, indigestion, anxiety, hysteria, and petit mal seizures. Hyssop preparations, especially the volatile oils, have been used externally for cold sores, genital herpes sores, burns, wounds, and skin irritations. Hyssop has been used with white horehound and coltsfoot for coughs and bronchitis; with boneset, elder flower, and peppermint for colds; and with sage as a gargle for sore throats.

Dosage
Tea: infuse 1 to 2 teaspoons dried hyssop in 1 cup of boiling water for 10 to 15 minutes. Drink t.i.d. for cough; gargle t.i.d. for sore throat.
Tincture: 1 to 4 ml t.i.d.

Adverse reactions
• Diarrhea
• Upset stomach

Interactions
None reported.

Contraindications and precautions
Contraindicated in pregnant patients. Use low-strength preparations for elderly patients and in children between ages 2 and 12. Avoid use in children under age 2.

Special considerations
• Do not confuse with giant hyssop, hedge hyssop, prairie hyssop or wild hyssop.
• Instruct the patient to keep out of reach of children and pets.
• Advise the female patient to report planned or suspected pregnancy.
• Advise the patient to use the herb under medical supervision if taken for more than 3 consecutive days.

Points of interest
• The volatile oil is an ingredient in many French liqueurs, specifically Chartreuse and Benedictine. Essential oil is also used in perfume.
• Commercial hyssop is not identical to the Hyssop of the Bible, the latter more commonly identified as *Marjoram* species or the caper plant, *Capparis spinosa*.

Analysis
The presence of volatile oils would suggest that hyssop might be reasonable as an expectorant in the treatment of respiratory disorders (such as cough, bronchitis) and as an antiflatulent in the treatment of digestive disorders (such as bloating, irritable bowel); however, this remains to be proven. Hyssop is generally recognized as safe, but medical supervision is suggested when using it for more than 3 consecutive days. There is no documented evidence that hyssop is effective in its external use in the treatment of burns, wounds and other infections. Even though hyssop extracts have been shown to inhibit HIV in vitro, there is no evidence for the usefulness of hyssop in the treatment of patients with AIDS.

References
Kaplan, K.W., et al. "Inhibition of HIV Replication by *Hyssop officinalis* Extracts," *Antiviral Res* 14:323-37, 1990.

ICELAND MOSS
Cetraria, consumption moss, Iceland lichen,
Lichen islandicus

Common trade names
(Various manufacturers) Iceland Moss

Common forms
Available as throat lozenges, capsules, and creams.

Source
Cetraria islandica, a lichen that grows in the Northern hemisphere, is common in the mountains and heathlands of Iceland. The single-cell, green algae are enclosed in a web of fungal hyphae (root filaments). The lichen may be gathered throughout the year, though it seems to be most abundant between May and September. It should be freed from attached impurities and dried in the sun or shade. The entire plant, or lichen, is used for extraction.

Chemical components
C. islandica is both bitter and mucilaginous. It consists of polysaccharides in the combination of lichenin and isolichenin. Other constituents are lichenic acids, which include fumarprotocetraric, protolichesterinic, and lichesterinic acids. Iceland moss also contains trace amounts of iron and calcium salts and has a high fiber content.

Actions
Protolichesterinic acid from Iceland moss was found to have antibacterial properties against *Mycobacterium tuberculosis, Streptococcus pyogenes,* and *Staphylococcus aureus.* Protolichesterinic acid has further been shown to exhibit antitumor activity against solid-type carcinoma in mice, and potent in vitro inhibiting activity against the DNA polymerase activity of HIV type 1 reverse transcriptase (Ingolfsdottir et al., 1997).

Because of their antibacterial properties, the extracts have been studied for use in pharmaceutical and cosmetic products. The lichen extracts appear to be safe for use as preservatives without interfering with proprietary ingredients (Ingolfsdottir et al., 1985).

Extracts of Iceland moss were recently found to suppress the growth of *Helicobacter pylori*, the organism thought to contribute to the etiology of gastritis and gastric and duodenal ulcer (Ingolfsdottir et al., 1997).

Reported uses

C. islandica has been used in European medicine for the treatment of minor ailments (such as throat irritation and cough), tuberculosis, asthma, and GI disorders such as gastritis. In Iceland, the plant has also been used for symptomatic relief of gastric and duodenal ulcer (Ingolfsdottir et al., 1997). Studies on antitumor and immunostimulating properties of the polysaccharides found comparable carbon clearance assay results as that for the fungal polysaccharide lentinan, which is used clinically in adjuvant cancer therapy in Japan (Ingolfsdottir et al., 1994).

Dosage

Human trials have not yet been performed and, therefore, data regarding safe dosage are unavailable. The decoction can be made by mixing 1 teaspoonful of the shredded moss in 1 cup of cold water, which should then be boiled for 3 minutes and taken P.O. b.i.d. Alternatively, 1 to 2 ml of the tincture P.O. t.i.d.

Adverse reactions

With large doses or prolonged use:
- GI irritation
- Liver toxicity
- Nausea

Interactions

None reported.

Contraindications and precautions

Avoid use of the herb in pregnant or breast-feeding patients; effects are unknown. The bitterness of *Cetraria* is detectable in breast milk.

Special considerations

- Explain that the herb cannot be recommended for any use because of insufficient data.
- Advise the patient to watch for signs of toxicity (abdominal pain, diarrhea, nausea, vomiting, change in color of urine, stool or skin, bleeding).

Points of interest

- Iceland moss has been exported from Iceland and is used abroad to manufacture herbal medicines (particularly in Germany).

Because Iceland is regarded as one of the least polluted countries in the world, the purity of the plants growing in Iceland is desirable. The wild plants are grown organically; fertilizers are not used in the highlands where many of these plants are found.
• Lichens lack roots and derive their energy and nutrients from the surroundings. They are susceptible to contamination by radioactivity and heavy metals. After the Chernobyl accident, the fallout contaminated the lichen in most of Europe; however, the radioactive level in Iceland was almost negligible.

Analysis
Iceland moss derivatives appear to show promise as immunomodulating and anti-tumor agents and may someday find a role in the treatment of *H. pylori*. Further research in human subjects is necessary before any real conclusions can be drawn. Definitive applications and clinical efficacy are not known at this time; however, the lichen extracts appear to be relatively safe in small amounts.

References

Ingolfsdottir, K., et al. "In Vitro Evaluation of the Antimicrobial Activity of Lichen Metabolites as Potential Preservatives," *Antimicrob Agents Chemother* 28:289-92, 1985.

Ingolfsdottir K., et al. "Immunologically Active Polysaccharide From *Cetraria islandica*," *Planta Med* 60:527-31, 1994.

Ingolfsdottir, K., et al. "In Vitro Susceptibility of *Helicobacter pylori* to Protolichesterinic Acid From the Lichen *Cetraria islandica*," *Antimicrob Agents Chemother* 41:215-17, 1997.

INDIGO
COMMON INDIGO, INDIAN INDIGO, QINGDAI

Common trade names
None known.

Common forms
Available as tablets and a blue powder.

Source
Indigo comes from the leaves and branches of a group of plants called *Indigofera*, which consists of many species. Although there are many *Indigofera* species worldwide, only a few exist in the United States (such as *I. tinctoria* and *I. suffruticosa*). *I. tinctoria* is known as the source of natural blue indigo dye, which has been used for hundreds of years.

Chemical components

Leaf fermentation produces the blue indigo dye. The dye comes from a glucoside component of several *Indigofera* species called indican, which is synthesized with different ingredients to produce various coloring agents.

Actions

Studies suggest that *I. tinctoria* may protect against liver damage induced by carbon tetrachloride, whereas other species may have a hepatotoxic effect. Aqueous decoctions with *I. arrecta* have shown a reduction of blood glucose levels in both animals and humans. Studies with *I. arrecta* in mice have shown an increase in plasma insulin levels, and the herb is believed to cause insulin release by stimulation of pancreatic beta-cells.

Indirubin, a minor component of *I. tinctoria*, has been shown to be useful in the treatment of chronic myelocytic leukemia and animal tumors. *I. tinctoria* has been found to significantly increase the survival of rats with cancer (Han, 1994). *I. aspalathoides*, similar to *I. tinctoria*, is believed to have anti-inflammatory activity.

Reported uses

I. arrecta has been reported to treat diabetes; the leaves and plant juice of *I. tinctoria* have been used to treat cancers such as gastric and ovarian. The Chinese have used *Indigofera* as an antipyretic, analgesic, and anti-inflammatory agent, and also for purifying the liver. Other uses of the natural indigo include treating hemorrhoids and scorpion bites, and as an emetic. Indigo is also used with other plants to treat hemorrhagic disease, infantile febrile seizures, mumps, boils, and carbuncles. There are no controlled therapeutic trials supporting these claims; indigo's use is based on anecdotal reports and traditional folklore.

Dosage

No consensus exists.

Adverse reactions

- Dermatitis (with dyes)
- Eye irritation

⚠️Indospicine, a component of *I. spicata*, has teratogenic and hepatotoxic properties, and has also caused cleft palate and embryo death in animals.

Interactions

None reported.

Contraindications and precautions

No known contraindications.

Special considerations

• Tell the patient to keep the herb away from the eyes. Flush with water if contact occurs.
• Advise the female patient to report planned or suspected pregnancy.

Points of interest

• All commercially available natural indigo is prepared synthetically. *I. tinctoria* is believed to be the active ingredient in a well-known, traditional Chinese medicine used for chronic myelocytic leukemia.

Analysis

The many species of the *Indigofera* plant are the common sources of natural blue dye. There is no clinical evidence to substantiate the therapeutic effects of natural indigo, alone or in combination with other ingredients. Because of the lack of clinical trials, this product cannot be recommended at this time.

References

Han, R. "Highlight on the Studies of Anticancer Drugs Derived From Plants in China," *Stem Cells* 12:53-63, 1994.

IRISH MOSS

CARRAGEEN, CARRAGEENAN, CHONDRUS, CHONDRUS EXTRACT, IRISH MOSS EXTRACT

Common trade names

Various manufacturers.

Common forms

Used extensively in small quantities as binders, emulsifiers, or stabilizers in toothpastes, hand lotions, creams, and tablets.

Source

The name Irish moss usually refers to a seaweed, *Chondrus crispus*, or is applied to a mixture of *Chondrus crispus* and *Mastocarpus stellatus*. It can be collected at low tide on the rocky Atlantic coastlines of northwestern Europe and Canada. Carrageenan, a seaweed gum, is processed from *Chondrus crispus* to commercial status through several procedures that can involve cleaning, extraction with sodium hydroxide, filtration and drum rolling, or precipitation with alcohol.

Carrageenan gels are rapidly degraded by acidic environment or heat. Degraded carrageenans lack the "gelling" or viscous properties.

Chemical components
Irish moss contains a large percentage of mucilage, carrageenan, iodine, bromine, iron, and vitamins A and B. Carrageenan is a variable mixture of potassium, sodium, calcium, magnesium, and ammonium sulfate esters of galactose and 3-6 anhydrogalactose copolymers. The three major types of hydrocolloid copolymers are kappa-carrageenan, iota-carrageenan, and lambda carrageenan. Carrageenan readily dissolves in water to form various types of gels with a wide range of characteristics, depending on the type of algae used, manufacturing process, and desired function of the carrageenan.

Actions
Irish moss is reported to have demulcent and emollient properties. Carrageenan extracted from the seaweed is used in the pharmaceutical industry as an emulsifying, suspending, and gelling agent. The gelling fractions are kappa-carrageenan and iota-carrageenan, whereas lambda-carrageenan does not gel. These hydrocolloid properties also make this plant useful to the food industry for various types of jellies.

It has been reported that carrageenan has exhibited numerous pharmacologic effects in vitro and in animals, including lowering cholesterol, limiting food absorption, decreasing gastric secretions, osmotically-active bowel cathartic effects, hypotension, anticoagulant effects, and immunosuppressive activities. Carrageenan has also demonstrated antiproteolytic activity against pepsin and papain in vitro. Interestingly, carrageenan has also been reported to cause GI ulcerations in various animals (Anderson and Soman, 1965). (See *Carageenan and Ebimar,* page 352.)

Reported uses
The herb's actions as a smooth binder have led to its use as a demulcent in ulcers and gastritis. It has also been reported to be valuable for colds, bronchitis, and other respiratory disorders such as tuberculosis. There are no human data to verify these claims. It is used by the pharmaceutical industry as an emulsifying agent for products such as liquid petrolatum and cod liver oil.

When carrageenan is injected into a rodent's paw it produces a consistent inflammatory response. The carrageenan-induced rat paw edema model is a popular and reliable model for testing potential anti-inflammatory compounds.

Carrageenan has also been studied as a carrier for the GI delivery of various drugs. Absorption was enhanced with a carrageenan formulation of doxycycline (Grahnen et al., 1994).

RESEARCH FINDINGS
Carageenan and Ebimar

Carageenan is a sulphated polysaccharide that can be extracted from a seaweed, *Chondrus crispus,* also known as Irish moss. Ebimar (Evans et al., 1965) is a pharmaceutical product derived from carageenan; however, it has a slightly smaller molecular structure than carageenan. Ebimar's reduced viscosity allows it to be more easily administered to patients than carageenan.

Early studies have suggested that sulphated polysaccharides have antiulcer effects. These data led to a comparative trial evaluating Ebimar with aluminum hydroxide gel (antacid) tablets in 35 patients with radiologically-proven gastric or duodenal ulcers. The patients were randomly treated with either 1,000 mg P.O. t.i.d. (chewed and swallowed with meals) and 3,000 mg at bedtime of Ebimar, and 700 mg P.O. t.i.d. (chewed and swallowed with meals) and 2,100 mg at bedtime of aluminum hydroxide gel for the first 3 months, and then crossed over to the alternative treatment every 3 months thereafter. Patients were encouraged to eat dyspepsia-provoking meals and were frequently assessed for symptoms of pain and discomfort, and, radiologic evidence of ulcer healing.

Neither treatment was found to be superior to the other. Although at 5 months, aluminum hydroxide significantly reduced ulcers ($P < 0.05$), this effect was not maintained to the trial's end. Complete ulcer healing between the groups was similar. The investigators concluded that either treatment was beneficial, although Ebimar may cause less constipation. Some patients preferred Ebimar over aluminum hydroxide gel therapy because they claimed that the antacid particles accumulated beneath their dentures, making them uncomfortable.

Dosage

No dosages have been established based on controlled clinical trials. Irish moss is available in some countries in tablet form, but usually is taken as a decoction.

To prepare the decoction, 1 oz of dried plant is added to 1 to 1½ pints of boiling water, simmered gently and strained. It may be sweetened with lemon, cinnamon, or honey and taken b.i.d. or t.i.d. in 1-cup doses.

Adverse reactions
- Bleeding
- Cramping
- Diarrhea

- GI ulcerations (in animals)
- Hypotension
- Infection
- Renal disease (I.V. carrageenan-induced renal lesions in animals)

Interactions

Anticoagulants: may increase the risk of bleeding. Avoid concomitant use.

Antihypertensive agents: may enhance hypotensive effects. Monitor patient.

Other oral drugs: may impair absorption of other drugs. Avoid concomitant use of significant quantities of carrageenan.

Contraindications and precautions

Avoid use of the herb in pregnant or breast-feeding patients; effects are unknown. Contraindicated in patients with active peptic ulcer disease or in those with a history of peptic ulcer disease.

Special considerations

- Monitor blood pressure.
- Monitor the patient for signs of bleeding.
- Tell the patient to avoid dizziness by rising slowly from a sitting or lying position.
- Warn the patient with a history of peptic ulcer disease to avoid use of this agent until its safety and efficacy are known.
- Instruct the patient to watch for signs of bleeding (easy bruising, bleeding gums, tarry stools, epistaxis).
- Explain that carrageenan is considered safe only in small quantities in various foodstuffs and commercial creams and lotions. Oral consumption of larger quantities has not been adequately evaluated.

Points of interest

- Degraded carrageenan is used in preparations for treating peptic ulcers in France.
- Food-grade carrageenan (molecular weight over 50,000 daltons) is thought to be nontoxic because it is not absorbed.
- Carrageenan is used in milk products (chocolate milk, ice cream, sherbets, cottage cheese, evaporated milk, puddings, yogurts, and infant formulas), and to thicken sauces, gravies, jams, and jellies.
- Carrageenan is included in various herbal drinks, weight-loss products, fruit juices, and aloe vera lotions.

Analysis

Although carrageenan (main derivative of Irish moss) is widely used in the pharmaceutical and food industries, therapeutic claims have not been confirmed in controlled clinical human trials. Further study is warranted before Irish moss or its constituents can be recommended for any medical conditions.

References

Anderson, W., and Soman, P.D. "Degraded Carrageenan and Duodenal Ulceration in the Guinea Pig," *Nature* 3:101-2, 1965.

Evans, P.R.C., et al. "Blind Trial of a Degraded Carrageenan and Aluminum Hydroxide Gel in the Treatment of Peptic Ulceration," *Postgrad Med J* 41:48-52, 1965.

Grahnen, A., et al. "Doxycycline Carrageenate—An Improved Formulation Providing More Reliable Absorption and Plasma Concentrations at High Gastric pH than Doxycycline Monohydrate," *Eur J Clin Pharmacol* 46:143-46, 1994.

JABORANDI TREE

ARRUDA BRAVA, ARRUDA DO MATO, INDIAN HEMP, JABORANDI, JAMGUARANDI, JUARANDI, PERNAMBUCO JABORANDI, *PILOCARPUS JABORANDI*

Common trade names
(Various manufacturers; available in combination) Jaborandi, Wonder Gel, X-Tablets

Common forms
The leaves from the jaborandi tree are available as a powder, essential oil, fluid extract, and tincture. Combination products are found as tablets and gels. Pilocarpine is the main active ingredient and is available in many prescription products
Tablets: 5 mg
Ophthalmic solution: 0.25%, 0.5%, 1%, 2%, 3%, 4%, 5%, 6%, 8%, 10%
Ophthalmic gel: 4%
Ocular insert: 20 mcg, 40 mcg

Source
Pilocarpus or jaborandi consists of the leaves of *Pilocarpus jaborandi (Pernambuco jaborandi),* of *P. microphyllus* (Maranham jaborandi), or of *P. pinnatifolius* (Paraguay jaborandi). The plant is native to the northern and northeastern parts of Brazil.

Chemical components
Three alkaloids found in jaborandi are pilocarpine, pilocarpidine, and isopilocarpine. Also reported are jaborine, pilosine, tannic acid, volatile oils (including dipentene), jaboric acid, and pilocarpic acid.

Actions
When applied topically to the eye, pilocarpine stimulates muscarinic receptors; this causes the pupil to constrict and the ciliary body to contract, thus improving the outflow of aqueous humor. Muscarinic alkaloids, when administered orally, stimulate the smooth muscles of the GI tract, increasing motility and tone. The tone and motility of other organs or organ systems (such as ureter, bladder, gallbladder, and biliary ducts) may also be increased. Pilocarpine causes

increased sweating and salivation in humans. It has actions on the CV and respiratory systems (decreases blood pressure, heart rate, and vital capacity). In cats, pilocarpine has been demonstrated to cause cortical stimulation (Brown and Taylor, 1996). Jaborine, a component found in the leaves, may actually be antagonistic to pilocarpine. Tannic acid has local astringent properties that act on the mucosa of the GI tract and has shown antiulcerogenic and antisecretory effects within the GI tract.

Reported uses

Although jaborandi has several reported uses, pilocarpine is usually extracted and employed to stimulate saliva secretion or as a diaphoretic or myotic (Claus, 1956). Pilocarpine is primarily used to treat patients with glaucoma or xerostomia. Other reported uses of the jaborandi plant include treatment of Bright's disease, deafness, diabetes, edema, intestinal atony, jaundice, nausea, nephritis, pleurisy, psoriasis, rheumatism, syphilis, and tonsillitis. A decoction of the leaf, applied locally, has been used as a treatment for baldness.

Dosage

For glaucoma, 1 to 2 drops applied t.i.d. or q.i.d. Refer to package insert for pilocarpine for specific dosing information.
For xerostomia, 15 to 30 mg P.O. daily; 100 mg P.O. is considered to be fatal.

The following daily doses for the leaves has been suggested: powdered leaves, 5 to 60 grains (0.324 to 3.9 g); fluid extract, 10 to 30 drops; tincture, ½ to 1 dram (1.75 to 3 ml).

Adverse reactions

- Bradycardia
- Headache
- Lacrimation
- Nausea
- Salivation
- Sweating
- Visual changes
- Vomiting

⚠ Signs of pilocarpine toxicity include exaggerated muscarinic effects. Extreme cases may lead to severe bronchospasms, hypotension, pulmonary edema, and shock. Treatment consists of atropine administration and general support of the CV and respiratory systems to counteract the effects from pulmonary edema (Brown and Taylor, 1996).

Interactions

Anticholinergic agents (atropine, ipratropium, scopolamine, other belladonna-type alkaloids): effects of these medications may be decreased. Avoid concurrent administration.

Beta blockers: may cause cardiac conduction problems. Monitor patient.

Glycosides, iron-containing compounds, other alkaloids: tannic acid may interact with these agents. Don't use together.

Other prescription products containing pilocarpine, other muscarinic agonists (arecoline, methacholine, muscarine), cholinesterase inhibitors (donepezil, edrophonium, physostigmine): may have an additive effect when used concomitantly. Use cautiously to avoid toxicity.

Contraindications and precautions

Contraindicated in patients with hypersensitivity to pilocarpine, uncontrolled asthma, acute iritis, and angle-closure glaucoma. Avoid use in pregnant or breast-feeding patients. Avoid large doses of jaborandi because hepatic injury may occur, especially in patients with preexisting hepatic disease. Use with caution in patients with significant CV disease, biliary tract or urogenital abnormalities (cholelithiasis, nephrolithiasis), and preexisting cognitive or psychiatric disorders.

Special considerations

• Monitor intraocular pressure in patients at risk for glaucoma.
• Monitor liver transaminases; if these levels increase, the product should be immediately discontinued.
• Know that excessive sweating may lead to dehydration if fluids are not replenished.
• Advise the patient to recognize the toxic symptoms associated with pilocarpine (excessive sweating, lacrimation, salivation, nausea, vomiting, hypotension, and bradycardia); if these occur, tell the patient to discontinue use of the product.
• Instruct the patient to report symptoms of hepatic injury immediately (pain in right upper quadrant, jaundice, fever).
• Warn the patient that pilocarpine may cause visual changes, especially at night, which may impair the ability to drive.
• Advise the pregnant or breast-feeding patient not to use jaborandi.

Analysis

The jaborandi tree is regarded as a source for pilocarpine. Much information exists about the use of pilocarpine for the treatment of glaucoma and xerostomia. However, no human studies are available that support the use of jaborandi leaves for any medicinal purpose. Individuals with glaucoma, xerostomia, or other potentially treatable conditions should seek medical advice before beginning self-medication with jaborandi.

References

Brown, J.H., and Taylor, P. "Muscarinic Receptor Agonists and Antagonists," in *Goodman and Gilman's The Pharmacological Basis of Therapeutics,* 9th ed. Edited by Hardman, J.G. and Limbird, L.E. New York: Mcgraw-Hill Book Co., 1996.

Claus, E.P. *Pharmacognosy,* 3rd ed. Philadelphia: Lea & Febiger, 1956.

JAMAICAN DOGWOOD

FISHFUDDLE, FISH POISON TREE, WEST INDIAN DOGWOOD

Common trade names
(None known for single-ingredient product; available in combination) Willow-Meadowsweet Compound

Common forms
Available as dried preparations of root or bark, tinctures (45% alcohol), fluid extracts (30% to 60% alcohol), and unprocessed bark strips.

Source
Piscidia erythrina grows naturally in West Indies and northern parts of South America; it has been transplanted to Mexico, Texas, and Florida.

Chemical components
Jamaican dogwood contains isoflavones, rotenoids, organic acids, beta-sitosterol, and tannins. Also found are soflavones (erythbigenin, piscidone, piscerythrone, ichthynone, listetin), rotenoids (rotenone, millettone, isomillettone, dehydromillettone, sumatrol) and tartaric acid derivatives (piscidic fukiic, 3'O-methlfukiic acids).

Actions
Isoflavone components, derived as fluid extracts from *P. erythrina* and other plant sources, showed spasmolytic activity in mice (Della-Loggia et al., 1988) and anxiolytic to sedative responses depending on the dose of extract used (Della-Loggia et al., 1981). Antitussive, anti-inflammatory, and antipyretic activities have also been seen in animals.

Reported uses
Jamaican dogwood has been claimed to be a calming agent for patients and for individual parts of the body. Claims include: hypnotic for insomnia; antispasmotic for asthma, whooping cough, renal or intestinal colic; analgesic for toothache, migraines, neuralgias. The

herb also has been used in dysmenorrhea and to help with labor pains. No human trials attesting to the therapeutic benefits of Jamaican dogwood could be found.

Dosage
Doses vary depending on the study cited.
Dried product: 2 to 4 g P.O. daily in divided doses, or 1 teaspoonful in 1 cup of water, simmered for 10 minutes then taken as a tonic.
Tincture: 5 to 15 ml as a daily dose, usually as 2 to 3 ml at a time.
Extract: 1 to 2 drams daily dose, starting with 5 to 20 drops, and increased cautiously.

Doses for analgesic or antispasmodic effect are given three to five times daily; hypnotic doses are given at bedtime.

Adverse reactions
- GI distress
- Nausea
- Sedation
- Symptoms of overdose include diaphoresis, salivation, and tremors. I.V. administration has resulted in toxicity in animals; oral administration appears to have a lower potential for toxicity.

Interactions
CNS depressants (alcohol, benzodiazepines, narcotic analgesics): Jamaican dogwood may potentiate the effects of these agents. Avoid concomitant use.

Contraindications and precautions
Contraindicated in pregnant or breast-feeding patients. Avoid use in patients with CV disease because hypotensive and mild myocardial depression may occur.

Special considerations
- Warn the patient at risk for hypotension or who has CV disease to avoid use of this plant.
- Remind the patient that few, if any, studies have been conducted in humans and that no evidence exists to confirm a therapeutic benefit.
- Tell the patient to avoid hazardous activity until the CNS effects of the herb are known.
- Explain that some constituents of the plant have been shown to have carcinogenic activity.

Points of interest
- Rotene and ichthynone are used by Central and South American fisherman to stun fish, it does not appear to have this effect in mammals.

• Jamaican dogwood is unrelated to the eastern United States plant, the common dogwood, *Cornus florida*.
• The European Council has found Jamaican dogwood not to be suitable for use as a natural food flavoring.

Analysis
Information on Jamaican dogwood is scarce. Consumption of this plant should be avoided until data regarding safety are available.

References
Della-Loggia, R. et al. "Evaluation of the Activity on the Mouse CNS of Several Plant Extracts and a Combination of Them," *Riv Neurol* 51:297-310, 1981
Della-Loggia, R., et al. "Isoflavones as Spasmolytic Principles of *Piscidia erythrina*," *Prog Clin Bio Res* 280:365-68, 1988.

JAMBUL
BLACK PLUM, *EUGENIA CYANOCARPA*, *EUGENIA JAMBOLANA*, JAMBA, JAMBOLÃO, JAMBOOL, JAMBU, JAMBULA, JAMBULON PLUM, JAVA PLUM, SYZYGIUM JAMBOLANUM

Common trade names
None known.

Common forms
Available as a tea or decoctions made from the seeds or dried leaves.

Source
The drug is extracted from the fruits, seeds, and leaves of *Syzygium cuminii,* a 50- to 80-foot tree with edible berries that is native to India and Sri Lanka.

Chemical components
The seeds of *S cuminii* contain gallic acid, ellagic acid, corilagin, 3,6-hexahydroxydiphenoyl-glucose, 3-galloyl glucose, and quercetin.

Actions
Jambul seeds have been claimed to have antihyperglycemic, anti-inflammatory, and antihypertensive effects. In some South American countries, tea made from the leaves are used by diabetics for antihyperglycemic effect (Teixera et al., 1990). However, a recent study found no effect on postprandial blood glucose of jambul seed tea when compared with water in normal rats and rats with streptozotocin-induced diabetes mellitus (Teixera et al., 1997).

The anti-inflammatory effects of jambul seed extract have been evaluated. Jambul seed extract was found to significantly reduce paw edema, although less effectively than phenylbutazone (Chaudhuri et al., 1990). An extract of jambul seeds was found to have neuropsychopharmacologic effects in mice; the animals became quieter and less active, with less spontaneous mobility. Loss of motor coordination and tone, decreased body temperature, and antagonism of amphetamine toxicity were also noted (Chakraborty et al., 1986).

Reported uses
Jambul seeds and extracts are thought to be useful in treating diarrhea and dysentery, and in reducing blood sugar. Although the seeds have some anti-inflammatory and antipyretic properties, the extent of these properties has yet to be defined. Evidence for the therapeutic properties of jambul is anecdotal.

Dosage
No consensus exists. In most cases, tea is prepared from the seeds or leaves of the tree.

Adverse reactions
None reported.

Interactions
CNS depressants: may alter behavior. Avoid concomitant use.

Contraindications and precautions
No specific contraindications. Avoid use in patients with sensitivity to this plant or related species, and in pregnant or breast-feeding patients.

Special considerations
• Monitor the patient for changes in blood pressure or blood glucose.
• Tell the patient to report changes in behavior or coordination.

Points of interest
• A related species, *S. jambos*, has also been used for treating diabetes.

Analysis
Although jambul has been reported to be effective for several medical conditions (diabetes, diarrhea, dysentery), there is little clinical evidence of its efficacy. Some studies have found extracts of jambul seeds and leaves to have anti-inflammatory, antipyretic, and neuropsychopharmacologic effects in animals. Further study on the active constituents of the seeds and leaves is needed to determine the true pharmacologic properties of this plant.

References

Chakraborty, D., et al. "A Neuropsychopharmacologic Study of *Syzygium cuminii*," *Planta Med* 2:139-43, 1986.

Chaudhuri, A.K., et al. "Anti-inflammatory and Related Actions of *Syzygium cuminii* Seed Extract," *Phytotherapy Res* 4:5-10, 1990.

Teixeria, C.C., et al. "Effect of Tea Prepared From the Leaves of *Syzygium jambos* on Glucose Tolerance in Nondiabetic Patients," *Diabetes Care* 13:907-8. 1990.

Teixeria, C.C., et al. "The Effect of *Syzygium cumini* (L.) Seeds on Post-Prandial Blood Glucose Levels in Nondiabetic Rats and Rats with Streptozotocin-Induced Diabetes Mellitus," *J Ethnopharmacol* 56:209-13, 1997.

JIMSONWEED

ANGEL'S TRUMPET, ANGEL TULIP, APPLE-OF-PERU, DEVIL WEED, DEVIL'S-APPLE, DEVIL'S TRUMPET, ESTRAMONIO, GREEN DRAGON, GYPSYWEED, INFERNO, JAMESTOWN WEED, LOCO SEEDS, LOCOWEED, MAD APPLE, MOON WEED, STRAMOINE, STECHAPFEL, STINKWEED, THORN APPLE, TOLGUACHA, TRUMPET LILY, ZOMBIE'S CUCUMBER

Common trade names

None known.

Common forms

Available as an oral and a rectal form. It is also smoked in cigarettes or burnt in powders, and the fumes inhaled.

Source

All parts of *Datura stramonium*, especially the seeds, are toxic. Parts that are used include leaves, flowering tops, roots, and, sometimes, the seeds. The plant occurs in fields, roadside ditches, and refuse sites.

Chemical components

The leaves and seeds contain tropane alkaloids consisting of atropine, hyoscyamine, hyoscine, and scopolamine. The seeds also contain fatty acids (including oleic, linoleic, palmitic, stearic, and lignoceric) and unsaponifiable matter (sitosterol and malic acid proteins). Other plant constituents include flavonoids with anolides, coumarins, and tannins. Although all plant parts are toxic, constituents with the most anticholinergic effects occur in the seeds. Other isolated compounds include datugen, datugenin, total ash, potassium nitrate, and acid-insoluble ash.

Actions

Toxicity is caused by the pharmacologic activity of the tropane alkaloids, which are similar to those found in deadly nightshade (*Atropa belladonna*). These alkaloids are potent central and peripheral cholinergic-blocking agents. Symptoms usually occur within 30 to 60 minutes after ingestion, and may continue for 24 to 48 hours and longer because of delayed GI motility (Ellenhorn, 1997). Ingestion of *D. stramonium* manifests as classic atropine toxicity.

Reported uses

There have been more reports of human than animal poisonings. Case reports in the literature abound of anticholinergic syndrome secondary to seeds being intentionally ingested for the hallucinogenic effect. About 50 to 100 seeds may cause severe intoxication or death. Jimsonweed has been used for several disorders including asthma, whooping cough, muscle spasm, and Parkinsonian symptoms. Being similar in action to belladonna or atropine, this herb may potentially be used as an antispasmodic or mydriatic (Clause, 1961). It also relaxes muscles of the GI, bronchial, and urinary tracts, and reduces digestive and mucous secretions.

Dosage

The dosage was formerly listed as 75 mg (Clause, 1961). It should be noted that the estimated lethal doses of atropine and scopolamine in adults are about 10 mg and over 2 to 4 mg, respectively (Ellenhorn, 1997).

Adverse reactions

• Ataxia, incoordination, psychomotor agitation, extrapyramidal reactions
• Blurred vision
• Changes in mental status (confusion, disorientation, loss of short-term memory, visual and auditory hallucinations, psychosis)
• Decreased bowel sounds
• Difficulty swallowing and speaking
• Dilated pupils
• Dry, hot, flushed skin
• Dry mucous membranes
• Elevated body temperature (related to the inability to sweat)
• Hypertension or hypotension
• Photophobia
• Sinus tachycardia
• Thirst
• Urine retention
⚠Coma, seizures, respiratory failure, CV collapse, and death (with ingestion of plant)

Interactions
Other anticholinergic agents: may exert additive effect. Avoid concomitant use.

Phenothiazines, levodopa, antihistamines, amantadine, thiazides, tricyclic antidepressants, quinidine, disopyramide, procainamide, other agents that interact with atropine and hyoscyamine: may adversely affect the CV system functioning. Avoid concomitant use.

Contraindications and precautions
Contraindicated in pregnant or breast-feeding women and in patients with angle-closure glaucoma, tachycardia, thyrotoxicosis, obstructive disease of the GI tract, obstructive uropathy, or myasthenia gravis.

Special considerations
• Monitor the patient for signs of anticholinergic toxicity (such as change in mental status, incoordination, tachycardia, or hyperthermia).
• Instruct the patient to avoid consumption of the herb.

Points of interest
• Overdose and treatment of the anticholinergic syndrome involves symptomatic and supportive care. Monitoring parameters include heart rate, blood pressure, pulse, mental status, ECG, and respiration rate. Gastric lavage, activated charcoal, or induction of emesis may be helpful. Physostigmine is a potential but controversial treatment.

⚠ *D. stramonium* is toxic at more than small doses, and is also subject to legal restrictions in most countries. It is an illegal drug for nonprescription use in the United States.

Analysis
D. stramonium has a narrow therapeutic window and has not shown promise over current treatments for respiratory, antispasmodic, or mydriatic purposes. The lack of clinical data for this herb and the numerous reports of toxicity warrant discouragement from the use of this herb. It is also considered an illegal drug for nonprescription use.

References
Clause, E.P. *Pharmacognosy,* 4th ed. Philadelphia: Lea & Febiger, 1961.
Ellenhorn, M.J. *Ellenhorn's Medical Toxicology—Diagnosis and Treatment of Human Poisoning,* 2nd ed. Baltimore: Williams & Wilkins Co., 1997.

JOJOBA
DEERNUT, GOATNUT, PIGNUT

Common trade names
Various manufacturers; jojoba is an ingredient in cosmetics and hair treatments.

Common forms
Available as crude wax (jojoba oil), hydrogenated jojoba wax, jojoba butter, and wax beads.

Source
Jojoba oil is obtained from *Simmondsia cainesis* and *S. californica* seeds by expression or solvent extraction.

Chemical components
The highly stable jojoba oil (also referred to as liquid wax) contains long-chain polycarbon esters of fatty acids and alcohols (eicosenoic, docosenoic, oleic and palmitoleic acids, ecosenol, docosenol), simmondsin, small quantities of campesterol, stigmasterol and sitosterol, vitamin E, B vitamins, silicon, chromium, copper, zinc, and iodine.

Actions
Jojoba oil is considered to have emollient properties that soothe chapped skin, psoriasis, and sunburn; relieve dry scalp; remove embedded sebum to help scalp disorders such as dandruff and hair loss; and reduce the acidity of the scalp. An atherogenic diet containing 2% jojoba oil lowered cholesterol in rabbits (Clarke and Yermanos, 1981). Antioxidant activity is most likely related to the alpha-tocopherol content in jojoba (Mallet et al., 1994).

Reported uses
Jojoba has been claimed to be effective in promoting hair growth and relieving skin problems. Its primary applications are to treat chapped skin, dry scalp, dandruff, psoriasis, and dry skin. Jojoba wax beads are used as an exfoliating agent in facial scrubs, skin conditioners, and soaps. Jojoba is also used as a replacement for petrolatum in creams, ointments, lotions, and lipsticks. Other claims include treatment of acne vulgaris, skin abrasions, hair loss, athlete's foot, eczema, pimples, warts, cuts, mouth sores, seborrhea, and wrinkles. Although little clinical evidence is available to support these claims, most applications appear to be based on theory and a long history of anecdotal use.

Adverse reactions
• Contact dermatitis (with topical use)
⚠ Ingestion of *S. chinesis* seeds has lead to toxicity in humans.

Interactions
None reported.

Special considerations
• Advise the patient that jojoba oil is for topical use only.

Points of interest
• Apache and American Southwest Indians and immigrants from Israel have been using jojoba oil to treat superficial conditions for many years.
• It has been suggested that jojoba would function well as an industrial lubricant because of its ability to maintain stability at high temperatures.

Analysis
Jojoba has been used for many years by Native Americans to promote hair growth and relieve skin problems. There have been numerous claims made regarding its effectiveness to treat skin and scalp disorders, but no studies have been done to prove its effectiveness. However, a long history of anecdotal use suggests that the oil is relatively safe if used topically.

References
Clarke, J.A., and Yermanos, D.M. "Effects of Ingestion of Jojoba Oil on Blood Cholesterol and Lipoprotein Patterns in New Zealand White Rabbits," *Biochem Biophys Res Commun* 102:4:1409, 1981.
Mallet, J.F., et al. "Antioxidant Activity of Plant Leaves in Relation to Their Alpha-Tocopherol Content," *Food Chem Toxicol* 49:1:61, 1994.

JUNIPER

A'RA'R A'DI, ARDIC, BACCAL JUNIPER, COMMON JUNIPER, DWARF, GEMENER, GENIEVRE, GROUND JUNIPER, HACKMATACK, HARVEST, HORSE SAVIN, JUNIPER MISTLETOE, *JUNIPERI FRUCTUS*, YOSHU-NEZU, ZIMBRO

Common trade names
(Available in combination) Cold-Plus, Cornsilk Buchu Formula, Formula 600 Plus for Men, Naturalvite, PMS Aid, Regeneration Softgels, SKB

Common forms
Available as capsules, tablets, oral liquid, and essential oil.

Source
The dried ripe fruit of the plant, *Juniperus communis* (family Cupressaccae), also known as female cones or berries, are used for medicinal purposes. The heartwood and tops are used to a lesser extent.

Chemical components
This plant contains volatile oil, juniperin, resin, proteins, formic and malic acids. The volatile oils or essential oils comprise 0.8% to 3% of the cones and consist of piene, sabinene, mycrene and sesquiterpenes. The active constituent responsible for the diuretic action, terpinen-4-ol, varies in concentration. Composition of the volatile oils depends on the season when the plant is harvested.

Actions
The plant's berries have shown significant hypoglycemic effect when given to normoglycemic and diabetic animals (Swanston-Flatt et al., 1990); other observations included weight gain, increased peripheral glucose consumption, and potentiation of glucose-induced insulin release (Sanchez de Medina et al., 1994).

Moderate anti-inflammatory activity was shown in vitro by *J. communis* (Tunon et al., 1995). *Juniper* species also appear to have mild antimicrobial activity. Extracts from bark, sapwood, and leaf had antimicrobial activity similar to that of streptomycin (Clark et al., 1990). Ash from branches and needles is a good source of dietary calcium and iron, and a moderate source of magnesium.

Reported uses
J. communis has been used traditionally in the treatment of kidney infections; a decoction of the branch with berries is still used in some parts of the world (Ritch-Krc et al., 1996). This plant was considered an adjuvant to diuretics in the relief of dropsy due to tubular kidney obstruction. A preparation of fresh berry juice diluted with water has been recommended to be an effective diuretic for children. Although this plant is listed under the therapeutic category of diuretics, there have been no studies to confirm this property. Native Americans used bruised inner bark of *Juniper* to relieve the odor of putrid smelling wounds. Because of its antiflatulent properties, the oil has been used for flatulence and colic.

Dosage
Dosages vary among the few clinical studies reported.
For hypoglycemic activity, in vivo doses ranged between 250 to 500 mg/kg every 24 hours.

For anti-inflammatory activity, in vitro studies used 0.2 mg/ml.
For antimicrobial activity, in vitro studies used 20 mg/ml.
For flatulence and colic, 0.05 to 0.2 ml of juniper oil.

Adverse reactions
• Burning, redness, and sometimes vesicles (with topical use)
• Diarrhea (with large amounts)
• Irritation of the urinary tract, especially kidneys
⚠ *Juniper sabina,* a closely related species, has been used as an abortifacient, but this is poorly substantiated. This plant and others in the *Juniper* class are considered poisonous plants, causing mostly diarrhea and urinary tract irritation.

Interactions
None reported.

Contraindications and precautions
Contraindicated during pregnancy and in patients with renal disease. Use with caution in elderly and diabetic patients, and in those with known contact dermatitis or hypersensitivity reactions. Do not apply to open wounds or skin abrasions.

Special considerations
• Advise the patient to report signs of significant diarrhea or urinary burning.
• Advise the patient that more potent preparations may cause irritation or blistering of skin or mucus membranes if applied externally.
• Inform the patient that this agent should not be used as a replacement for currently available diuretics.

Points of interest
• This agent is still used among the Carrier people of British Columbia. *J. communis* is always used fresh because of its abundant availability.

Analysis
Most clinical data are from in vitro animal studies. The traditional use of this plant as a diuretic and antimicrobial for kidney infections has not been clinically documented. Although evidence suggests activity similar to that of streptomycin, studies in humans are necessary. The hypoglycemic effect of the plant appears promising; however, controlled studies in humans are needed before this agent can be used as an oral antidiabetic agent. This product cannot be recommended for use at this time. Further studies regarding clinical use and dosage are required to determine its therapeutic use.

References

Clark, A.M., et al. "Antimicrobial Properties of Heartwood, Bark/Sapwood and Leaves of *Juniperus* Species," *Phytother Res* 4:15-19, 1990.

Ritch-Krc, E.M., et al. "Carrier Herbal Medicine; Traditional and Contemporary Plant Use," *J Ethnopharmacol* 52:85-94, 1996.

Sanchez de Medina, F., et al. "Hypoglycemic Activity of Juniper Berries," *Planta Med* 60:197-200, 1994.

Swanston-Flatt, S., et al. "Traditional Plant Treatments for Diabetes. Studies in Normal and Streptozotocin Diabetic Mice," *Diabetologia* 33:462-64, 1990.

Tunon, N H., et al. "Evaluation of Anti-inflammatory Activity of Some Swedish Medicinal Plants. Inhibition of Prostaglandin Biosynthesis and PAF-Induced Exocytosis," *J Ethnopharmacol* 48:61-76, 1995.

KARAYA GUM

Bassora tragacanth, Indian tragacanth, kadaya, kadira, karaya gum, katila, kullo, mucara, *Sterculia*, sterculia gum

Common trade names
None known.

Common forms
Karaya gum powder is used to form gels or pastes for bases in food, cosmetics, and pharmaceuticals.

Source
Karaya gum is the dried exudate of *Sterculia urens* and other *Sterculia* species. Native to India and Pakistan, this softwood tree grows to a height of approximately 30 feet. All parts of the tree exude a soft gum when injured. The gum is obtained by defacing the trunk, allowing the gum to seep out and be collected, washed, and dried.

Chemical components
Karaya gum is a high-molecular-weight complex polysaccharide that is composed of residues containing galacturonic acid, beta-D-galactose, glucuronic acid, and L-rhamnose. Because the gum is partially acetylated, it may release acetic acid upon degradation. Trimethylamine has also been identified in hydrolysis products.

Karaya gum contains 12% to 14% moisture and less than 1% acid-insoluble ash. The quality of karaya gum depends on how carefully impurities have been removed. Food-grade gum is usually a white to pinkish gray powder with a slight vinegar odor, whereas pharmaceutical grades may be almost translucent.

Actions
Karaya gum is essentially inert and not associated with significant pharmacologic activity. It is not digested or absorbed systemically. After contact with water, coarse particles in the gum swell, forming a discontinuous type of mucilage that exerts a laxative effect in the bowel. Although preliminary studies suggest that other gums of this type may normalize blood sugar and plasma lipid levels, karaya has not been investigated in this regard.

Reported uses

Karaya gum is used primarily in the pharmaceutical industry as a bulk laxative, and in the food industry as a stabilizer, binder, and emulsifier in products, such as frozen desserts, cheese spreads, whipped cream, meringue powders, and bread and doughnut mixes (Anderson, 1989).

The demulcent properties of the gum make it useful as an ingredient in lozenges to relieve sore throat. The bark has long been used as an astringent. A protective coating of karaya gum applied to dentures has been shown to reduce bacterial adhesion by 98%. In addition, karaya gum is used as a denture adhesive in which the finely powdered gum is dusted onto the dental plate and swells when it touches the moist surface of the gums. This gives a comfortable and tight fit to the plate. Karaya gum was also used in a clinical study of a new delivery system for administering salicylic acid in a skin patch to treat verruca vulgaris (warts). The patch achieved a cure rate of 69% compared with 35% for placebo controls. This treatment was considered safe, effective, and nonirritating (Bart, 1989).

Dosage

Dosage is expressed as a percentage of the karaya gum incorporated into the final product.

Adverse reactions

Karaya gum is generally recognized as safe for internal consumption. Widespread experience with the product throughout the United States and Europe has not been associated with any significant adverse experiences.

Potential problems associated with mucilaginous substances include abdominal pain, diarrhea, and gastroesophageal or esophageal obstruction.

Interactions

None reported.

Contraindications and precautions

Avoid use in pregnant or breast-feeding patients; effects are unknown. Use cautiously, and in modest amounts, in patients prone to gastric outlet obstruction.

Special considerations

• Advise the patient with diabetes to watch for signs and symptoms of hypoglycemia because large quantities of this product may lower glucose levels.
• Instruct the patient to take other medications at least 2 hours before or after ingesting karaya gum.

• Advise the female patient to avoid use of karaya gum products during pregnancy or when breast-feeding.

Points of interest
• The use of karaya gum became widespread during the early 1900s, when it began to supplant tragacanth gum for many uses.

Analysis
Karaya gum has long been used as a bulk ingredient and emulsifying agent in the food and pharmaceutical industries. The gum appears to lack significant pharmacologic activity or toxicity. Clinical use as a bulk laxative appears safe and may be effective, but large controlled clinical studies are unavailable.

References
Anderson, D.M. "Evidence for the Safety of Gum Karaya (*Sterculia* spp.) as a Food Additive," *Food Addit Contam* 6:189, 1989.

Bart, B.J. "Salicylic Acid in Karaya Gum Patch as a Treatment for Verruca Vulgaris," *J Am Acad Dermatol* 20:74-76, 1989.

KAVA

AVA, AWA, KAVA-KAVA, KAWA, KEW, SAKAU, TONGA, YAGONA

Common trade names
Aigin, Antares, Ardeydystin, Cefkava, Kavasedon, Kavasporal, Kavatino, Laitan, Mosaro, Nervonocton N, Potter's Antigian Tablets, Viocava

Common forms
Prepared as a drink from pulverized roots, tablets, capsules, or extract.

Source
Kava comes from the dried rhizome and root of *Piper methysticum,* a member of the black pepper family (Piperaceae). Kava is a large shrub with broad, heart-shaped leaves, and is native to many South Pacific islands.

Chemical components
Pharmacologic activity is attributed to the kavapyrones that occur in the root. Biologically active components are obtained from chemical substitution of the basic pyrone structure. Alpha-pyrone components include yangonin, desmethoxyyangonin, 5,6-dehydromethysticin, 11-methoxyyangonin, and 11-methoxy-nor-yangonin. Methysticin,

kawain, dihydromethysticin, and dihydrokawain are active components from the 5,6-dyhydro-alpha-pyrone structure. Pipermethystine is an alkaloid isolated from the plant leaves of kava.

Actions

More than one mode of action is involved. There is an unquantified synergism among kava components. Components of the root may cause local anesthetic activity that is similar to cocaine but lasts longer than benzocaine. Kava induced a mephenesin-like muscular relaxation in animals, but was found to lack curare-like activity. The limbic system is inhibited by kavapyrones, an effect associated with suppression of emotional excitability and mood enhancement.

In human studies, kava produced mild euphoria with no effects on thoughts and memory. The neuropharmacologic effects of kava include analgesia, sedation, and hyporeflexia. Kava can impair gait and cause pupil dilation. Some pyrones show fungistatic properties against several fungi, including some that are pathogenic to humans.

Reported uses

Kava has been shown to be useful in attenuating spinal seizures and also to have antipsychotic properties. Therapeutic trials have shown a degree of seizure control in epileptic patients, suggesting involvement of the gamma-aminobutyric acid (GABA) receptors. Kava extract has also been studied for anxiety disorders. In a study of patients with anxiety of nonpsychotic origin, kava showed improved scores on the Hamilton Anxiety Scale (Volz et al., 1997). Other medicinal claims of kava include treatment of depression, insomnia, asthma, pain, rheumatism, venereal disease, muscle spasms, and promotion of wound healing.

Dosage

Dosage is usually based on the kavapyrone content, which varies with preparation. Most studies in humans used 70 to 240 mg kavapyrone daily. One study used 90 to 110 mg dried kava extract t.i.d. for the treatment of anxiety (Volz et al., 1997). Doses of freshly prepared kava beverages average 400 to 900 g weekly.

Adverse reactions

- Changes in motor reflexes and judgement
- Visual disturbances

Chronic, heavy use:
- Decreased platelet and lymphocyte count
- Dopamine antagonism
- Dry, flaking discolored skin; reddened eyes (may be related to cholesterol metabolism) (Norton et al., 1994)

• Increased patellar reflexes, shortness of breath, and pulmonary hypertension
• Reduced plasma proteins, urea, and bilirubin levels
• Weight loss

Interactions

Alcohol: increased kava toxicity. Avoid concomitant use.
Alprazolam: may cause coma (Almeida et al., 1996). Avoid concomitant use.
Benzodiazepines, other CNS depressants: additive sedative effects. Avoid concomitant use.
Levodopa: increased Parkinsonian symptoms. Avoid concomitant use.
Pentobarbitol: may cause additive effects. Avoid concomitant use.

Contraindications and precautions

Avoid use of this herb in pregnant or breast-feeding patients, and in children under age 12; effects are unknown. Use cautiously in patients with renal disease, thrombocytopenia, or neutropenia. Avoid concomitant use with psychotropic agents.

Special considerations

• Inform the patient that significant adverse reactions may occur with long term use of kava.
• Tell the patient to avoid alcohol and other CNS depressants because they enhance the herb's sedative and toxic effects.
• Inform the patient that absorption of kava may be enhanced if taken with food.
• Advise the female patient to avoid taking this herb during pregnancy or when breast-feeding.

Points of interest

• Kava, although a depressant, is nonfermented, nonalcoholic, nonopioid and nonhallucinogenic and does not appear to cause physiologic dependence. However, the potential risk for psychological dependence still exists.
• Kava is commonly employed in the South Pacific as a ceremonial beverage. (See *Social significance of kava drinking.*)

Analysis

Kava has been used or studied most frequently for the treatment of anxiety, stress, and restlessness. These uses are supported by limited evidence from a few small clinical trials. In studies of kava as an antianxiety agent, adverse reactions were minimal. However, significant adverse reactions are reported with chronic heavy use. Other therapeutic claims are poorly documented. Additional trials are

FOLKLORE
Social significance of kava drinking

Kava-kava is often enjoyed as a social drink in the South Pacific islands because it induces a pleasant sense of tranquility, sociability, and euphoria. In earlier times, native island women would chew the leaves and rootstalks of the plant into a pulpy mass, spit the contents into a bowl, mix it with water, coconut milk, or other fruit juices, and finally strain the mixture. This cocktail was then consumed at weddings, births, funerals, and other ceremonial rites of passage, similar to how alcohol is consumed in Western society. The plant is now ground and pulverized instead of being chewed. However, this modern version of the kava cocktail may lack the potency of the earlier version, because chewing is thought to enhance emulsification of the active ingredients in the plant (Dobelis, 1986).

needed to establish dosing regimens, drug interactions, therapeutic benefits, and adverse effects.

References

Almeida, J.C., et al. "Coma from the Health Food Store: Interaction Between Kava and Alprazolam," *Ann Intern Med* 125:940, 1996.

Dobelis, I.N. *Magic and Medicine of Plants.* Pleasantville, N.Y: Reader's Digest Association, Inc., 1986.

Norton, S.A., et al. "Kava Dermopathy," *J Am Acad Dermatol* 31:89-97, 1994.

Volz, H.P., et al. "Kava-kava Extract WS-1490 versus Placebo in Anxiety Disorders-A Randomized Placebo Controlled 25-week Outpatient Trial," *Pharmacopsychiatry* 30:1-5,1997.

KELP

BROWN ALGAE, HORSETAIL, *LAMINARIA*, SEA GIRDLES, SEAWEED, SUGAR WRACK, TANGLEWEED

Common trade names
(Various manufacturers) Kelp, Kelp Norwegian

Common forms
Capsules: 380 mcg, 640 mg, 660 mg
Tablets: 150 mcg, 225 mcg
Also available as an aqueous extract or powder.

Source
Active components are derived from the fronds of the marine brown algae (*Laminaria digitata, L. japonica, L. saccharina,* and

Macrocystis pyrifera) that grow along the northern Atlantic and Pacific coasts.

Chemical components

Kelp contains fucoidans, 1-3 beta glucans, algin, laminarin (a polysaccharide found in both soluble and insoluble forms in the plants), laminine, and histamine. Algin is a high-molecular-weight polysaccharide. Kelp is thought to be rich in vitamins, minerals, and iodine.

Actions

Kelp may have some antitumor effects. It was found to protect female mice from the tumorigenic effects of a known carcinogen, and a kelp extract reduced DNA changes induced by several known carcinogens in *Salmonella typhimurium* bacteria (Okai et al., 1993). Neither study, however, provided conclusive evidence that kelp protects against carcinogenic substances. Sulfated laminarin has demonstrated antilipemic, anticoagulant, and antiviral properties (Kathan, 1965).

Reported uses

Kelp is claimed to have antiobesity, antihypertensive, antitumor, anticoagulant, abortifacient, and antirheumatic actions. It was used in Japanese folk medicine for its alleged hypotensive attributes. The rate of breast cancer was found to be low in Japanese patients receiving a high dietary intake of kelp (Teas, 1983). Kelp is also a high-quality source of natural iodine.

Dosage

Dosage is one tablet or capsule daily, providing 500 to 650 mg of ground kelp. This quantity of kelp will provide approximately 250 mcg of elemental iodine (about 150% of the RDA).

Adverse reactions

• Abnormal erythropoiesis
• Acneiform eruptions
• Autoimmune thrombocytopenia
• Bleeding
• Hypotension
⚠ Arsenic poisoning (with contaminated kelp) (Walkin and Douglas, 1975)

Interactions

Anticoagulants: possible increased risk of bleeding complications in patients with coagulation or platelet defects or in those taking aspirin or warfarin concurrently. Avoid concomitant use.

Antihypertensives: potential hypotensive effects; syncope or dizziness may occur. Avoid concomitant use.

Contraindications and precautions
Use cautiously in pregnant patients because of cervical and placental effects associated with topical administration. *Laminaria* "tents," used as natural stents to dilate the cervix during delivery, have been associated with intrauterine fetal death (Agress and Benedetti, 1981).

Special considerations
• Check for arsenic poisoning in the patient who consumes large quantities of kelp on a daily basis.
• Advise the patient prone to cardiac failure or hypotension, such as a patient taking an antihypertensive medication, not to use this agent because of its potential hypotensive effects.
• Advise the female patient to avoid use of kelp products during pregnancy or when breast-feeding.
• Tell the patient on anticoagulant therapy to notify his health care provider if signs and symptoms of bleeding occur (bruises, bleeding gums, or blood in the stool).

Points of interest
• Although natural stents or kelp "tents" have been used to maintain cervical dilatation, contamination of these tents have led to infectious complications and curtailed their use.

Analysis
Based on existing data, kelp cannot be recommended for prevention of cancer. There are no data evaluating the action of kelp and anticoagulants.

References
Agress, R.L., and Benedetti, T.J. "Intrauterine Fetal Death During Cervical Ripening with *Laminaria*," *Am J Obstet Gynecol* 141:587, 1981.

Kathan, R.H. "Kelp Extracts as Antiviral Substances," *Ann N Y Acad Sci* 130: 390-97, 1965.

Okai, Y., et al. "Identification of Heterogenous Antimutagenic Activities in the Extract of Edible Brown Seaweeds, *Laminaria japonica* (Makonbu) and *Undaria pinnatifida* (Wakame) by the Umu Gene Expression System in *Salmonella typhimurium*," *Mutat Res* 303: 63-70, 1993.

Teas, J. "The Dietary Intake of *Laminaria*, a Brown Seaweed, and Breast Cancer Prevention," *Nutr Cancer* 4: 217-22, 1983.

Walkin, O., and Douglas, D.E. "Health Food Supplements Prepared From Kelp—A Source of Elevated Urinary Arsenic," *Clin Toxicol* 8:325-31, 1975.

KELPWARE

BLACK-TANG, BLADDER FUCUS, BLADDER-WRACK,
BLASEN-TANG, QUERCUS MARINA, SEA WRACK,
SEA-OAK, SEETANG

Common trade names
Kelp, Kelp Combination Tabs, Kelp/Lecithin/B6, Kelp Natural
Iodine, Pacific Kelp

Common forms
Available as a dried plant, soft extract prepared with 45% alcohol,
liquid extract, tablets, and softgel formulation with lecithin and B_6.

Source
Fucus vesiculosus (family Fucaceae) is a brown-green seaweed that
grows on rocky areas along the northern coasts of the Atlantic and
Pacific oceans.

Chemical components
The plant is dried with periodic turning to avoid growth of fungus
and development of a putrid odor. The active constituents are prepared from the dried thallus of the plant, which contains algin, iodine, bromine, mannite, and varying amounts of cadmium and
lead. The plant also contains fucoidan, a sulfated polysaccharide.

Actions
F. vesiculosus has been studied mainly in vitro. The anticoagulant effects of fucoidan were found to prolong the activated partial thromboplastin time up to twofold (Dhrig et al., 1997). Kelpware also
showed increased expression of platelet membrane activation markers that may play a role in thromboembolic events in patients with a
malignancy and in those undergoing percutaneous transluminal
coronary angioplasty.

Kelpware has demonstrated antibacterial action against *Escherichia coli* and *Neisseria meningitidis* in vitro, and antifungal action
against *Candida guilliermondii* and *Candida krusei* (Criado and
Ferreiros, 1983, 1984).

Reported uses
The early literature reports use of kelpware for obesity. It has been
used in humans to reduce dietary fat content in patients with morbid obesity. The seaweed was also used for the treatment of exoph-
thalmic and simple goiter because of its iodine content, and reported to be beneficial in patients under age 30. Kelpware has also been
claimed to be useful in menstrual irregularities such as menorrha-

gia, inflammatory disease of the bladder, desquamative nephritis, and fatty degeneration of the heart.

Dosage
For obesity, mix 16 g bruised plant with 1 pint of water; then administer 2 fluid oz P.O. t.i.d.
Alcoholic soft extract: 200 mg to 600 mg P.O.
Alcoholic liquid extract: 4 to 8 ml P.O. before meals.
Tablets: 3 tablets (3.75 grains) taken initially P.O. daily, then increased gradually up to 24 tablets P.O. daily.

Adverse reactions
• Hyperglycemia
• Increased serum creatinine (suggested to be nephrotoxic) (See *Kelpware and nephrotoxicity,* page 380.)
• Polydipsia
• Polyuria

Interactions
Aspirin, anticoagulants: possible additive effects. Monitor patient.

Contraindications and precautions
Contraindicated in pregnant or breast-feeding patients; effects are unknown. Also contraindicated in patients with known malignancies, diabetes, renal dysfunction, severe hepatic disease, heart failure, and recent myocardial infarction; in the elderly; and in those taking drugs known to cause nephrotoxicity. Use cautiously in patients receiving thyroid hormone replacement therapy, lithium, amiodarone, and anticoagulants.

Special considerations
• Monitor serum laboratory results, including creatinine, glucose, PTT and PT/INR.
• Advise the female patient to avoid use during pregnancy and breast-feeding because effects are unknown.
• Advise parents to avoid using kelpware in children because effects are unknown.
• Caution the diabetic patient against use of kelpware.
• Warn the patient that kelpware use may result in signs and symptoms of toxicity from cadmium, lead, arsenic, or bromide.
• Tell the patient to report signs of bleeding, increased thirst, or changes in urinary frequency or volume.
• Inform the patient that kelpware may contain iodine.

RESEARCH FINDINGS
Kelpware and nephrotoxicity

Fucus vesiculosus was once thought to be harmless. However, a recent report of questionable nephrotoxicity has appeared in the literature. An 18-year-old female taking 1,200 mg P.O. t.i.d. of a product containing *F. vesiculosis* for weight loss presented with polyuria, polydypsia, and faintness.

Laboratory values revealed a significantly increased serum creatinine, and urinalysis revealed glucosuria (500 mg/dl), proteinuria, and leucocyturia. Renal biopsy showed moderate interstitial fibrosis, widespread tubular degeneration, and diffuse lymphomonocytic infiltrate. The glomeruli showed scarce and focal mesangial proliferation. Tested samples of the tablets revealed 21.3 mg/kg arsenic, 0.3 ppm cadmium, 0.06 ppm mercury, and 4 ppm chromium. The arsenic content was believed to have contributed to the nephrotoxicity. The patient experienced a complete recovery 1 year after the onset of symptoms (Conz et al., 1998).

Points of interest

• *F. vesiculosus* has been reported to accumulate cadmium and lead in various plant parts, probably from the heavy metal content of sea water.

• Several *Fucus* species along the French coastline are used to make kelpware tablets. The amount of iodine present in kelpware depends on the plant's origin; *Fucus digitatus* contains seven to eight times more iodine than *F. vesiculosus*.

Analysis

Although *F. vesiculosus* appears to possess anticoagulant activity, it cannot be recommended because of the lack of in vivo studies. Most experience with this plant's use is in Europe. The use of kelpware in obesity has received criticism and is generally excluded for morbid obesity.

References

Conz, P.A., et al. "*Fucus vesiculosus: A* Nephrotoxic Alga?" *Nephrol Dial Transplant* 13:526-27, 1998.

Criado, M.T., and Ferreiros, C.M. "Selective Interaction of *Fucus vesiculosus* Lectin-like Mucopolysaccaride with Several *Candida* Species," *Annales de Microbiologie* 134:149-54, 1983. Abstract.

Criado, M.T., and Ferreiros, C.M. "Toxicity of an Algal Mucopolysaccharide for *Escherichia coli* and *Neisseria meningitidis* Strains," *Rev Esp Fisiol* 40:227-30, 1984. Abstract.

Dhrig, J., et al. "Anticoagulant Fucoidan Fractions from *Fucus vesiculosus* Induce Platelet Activation in Vitro," *Thromb Res* 85:479-91, 1997.

KHAT
CAT, CHAT, GAD, KAHT, KAT, MIRAA, TSCHUT

Common trade names
None known.

Common forms
Available as raw leaves.

Source
The raw leaves and tender twigs of *Catha edulis* are harvested for khat. The tree, a member of the staff tree family (Celastraceae), grows to 80 feet and is native to East Africa and the highlands of the Arabian peninsula.

Chemical components
Leaves of khat contain the alkaloids cathinone and cathine. Cathinone is structurally related to amphetamine and, although it is a more powerful stimulant than cathine, it degrades rapidly in the presence of oxygen. Cathine has been identified as norpseudoephedrine. Other similar alkaloids (cathinine, cathidine, eduline, ephedrine), phenylpropyl, phenylpentenylamines, and tannins have also been identified. Fresh leaves contain the most cathinone.

Actions
Cathinone is a sympathomimetic agent with potent CNS stimulating properties. Based on data obtained from animal and human studies, cathinone is considered to be a naturally occurring amphetamine analogue. Khat chewing causes elevated blood pressure, anorexia, vasoconstriction, increased heart rate, pupil dilation, and other amphetamine-like effects. CNS effects range from mild stimulation to euphoria to mania. Psychic dependence, tolerance, and addiction have also occurred.

Blood glucose levels were reduced in animals, but not in humans (Elmi, 1983). An anti-inflammatory effect has been demonstrated in rats for a khat flavonoid. Cathinone suppresses serum testosterone, decreases sperm count and motility, and promotes degeneration of testicular tissue in animals (Islam et al., 1990).

Reported uses
Khat is claimed to be beneficial for treating obesity, depression, and ulcers. It is used in East Africa and the Arabian peninsula as a stimulant to offset fatigue and as an anorexiant.

Dosage

Usually, 100 to 200 g of raw leaf are chewed at a time. The leaves have a sweet taste and cause dryness of the mouth and oropharynx, usually leading to the consumption of large amounts of fluids.

Adverse reactions

- Bilateral optic atrophy (possible idiosyncratic reaction)
- Cardiac problems (arrhythmias, hypertension, tachycardia)
- Cerebral hemorrhage
- Decreased libido (in men)
- Euphoria
- GI problems (stomatitis, esophagitis, gastritis, constipation)
- Hepatotoxicity
- Hyperactivity, aggressiveness, mania, psychoses, hallucinations (with overdose)
- Hyperthermia, sweating
- Low sperm counts, reduced sperm motility (animal and human studies)
- Migraine
- Periodontal disease, oral cancers
- Pulmonary edema, myocardial arrest
- Pupil dilation, decreased intraocular pressure
- Reduced appetite
- Reduced performance on perceptual-visual memory and decision speed tests (with chronic use)

Interactions

Antihypertensives, antiarrhythmics, beta blockers, decongestants, MAO inhibitors, other sympathomimetics: may cause similar interactions as with amphetamines. Avoid concomitant use.

Contraindications and precautions

Contraindicated in patients with CV or renal disease and hypertension. Avoid use of the herb in pregnant or breast-feeding patients because cathinone is a suspected teratogen.

Special considerations

- Monitor the patient for psychological dependence to khat. Depression and sedation may be signs of khat withdrawal. Physical dependence and addiction to khat appears unlikely.
- Warn the patient against chewing khat leaves or products because of the herb's deleterious effects on nutrition and GI function and its association with oral cancer.
- Inform the elderly patient that adverse reactions are likely to occur.
- Advise the female patient to avoid use of the herb during pregnancy or when breast-feeding.

Points of interest
• Khat is consumed in daily social gatherings and is deeply rooted in cultural tradition, especially among Yemen men.
• Khat chewing has become a popular form of drug abuse in East Africa. The "red" type of khat is thought to be superior to the "white" type, which contains less cathinone.
• The sympathetic effects of khat may be described as greater than those of caffeine but less than those of amphetamine.

Analysis
Khat is chewed in Africa and Arabia for stimulation, euphoria, and appetite suppression. Many reports of adverse consequences of overuse and abuse exist in the literature. Symptoms of addiction, tolerance, and psychological dependence are less strong with khat than with amphetamines. Khat and its active ingredient, cathinone, have few, if any, appropriate medical uses.

References
Elmi, A.S. "The Chewing of Khat in Somalia," *J Ethnopharmacol* 8:163-76, 1983.
Islam, M.W., et al. "An Evaluation of the Male Reproductive Toxicity of Cathinone," *Toxicology* 603:223-34, 1990.

KHELLA

AMMI, BISHOP'S WEED, KHELLIN, VISNAGA, VISNAGIN

Common trade names
Khella

Common forms
Available as capsules, tablets, teas, and injectables.

Source
Active components are obtained from fruits and seeds of *Ammi visnaga,* a member of the carrot family (Umbelliferae) that is native to Egypt and other Middle Eastern areas.

Chemical components
Khella contains furanochromones, khellin, visnagin, khellol, and pyranocoumarins. Other compounds include flavonoids (quercetin, kaempferol, isorhamnetin), essential oils (camphor, terpineol, terpinen, linalool oxides), fixed oils, psoralens (methoxypsoralen), and protein.

Actions

Khellin and visnagin act as spasmolytic and vasodilatory agents on the muscles of the bronchi, GI tract, biliary tract, urogenital system, and coronary arteries, similar in action to calcium channel blockers.

When linked with an oxygen atom, khella formed a new compound called cromolyn sodium, formulations of which are used in the preventive treatment of asthma in children, as well as for hay fever, allergic reactions, and bronchospasm.

The photobiological activity of visnagin and khellin against yeasts, bacteria, viruses, and fungi is being studied. In ultraviolet light, these compounds appear to affect cell division and alter DNA. Although still preliminary, research has shown antimutagenicity and antimicrobial activity in plant populations (Jansen et al., 1995; Borges et al., 1998). Furochromones from khella have shown anticonvulsant activity equivalent or superior to phenobarbital (Ragab et al., 1997).

Reported uses

Khella is claimed to be effective in treating cramplike conditions of the GI tract, biliary tract colic, and painful menstruation. Traditionally, it has been used with hawthorn extracts to treat anginal symptoms. Although early research appeared to yield impressive results in relieving anginal symptoms (Osher et al., 1951), other studies have indicated that higher dosages of khella produce intolerable adverse reactions.

Khella may help prevent asthma attacks but does not relieve an ongoing episode. It has been used to prevent bronchial asthma attacks and allergic reactions, and has been used I.V. to treat anaphylactic reactions (Lowe et al., 1994). Extracts of khella have been used to treat psoriasis, and topical khellin with ultraviolet light irradiation has shown effectiveness in treating vitiligo (Jansen et al., 1995). However, topically applied khellin also increases the carcinogenic effects of both ultraviolet light and sunlight (Borges et al., 1998).

Some components of khella may act favorably on total cholesterol levels, protein levels, and atherosclerotic changes in blood vessels, as evidenced by a study in which oral khella increased high-density lipoprotein-cholesterol levels without affecting total cholesterol or triglyceride levels (Harvengt and Desanger, 1983).

Dosage

Average daily doses of 20 mg of khellin have been recommended. *For treatment of angina,* 30 to 300 mg has been used. Sources are typically standardized to a 12% khellin content.

Adverse reactions
- Allergic reactions (itching)
- Sleeplessness
- Weak phototoxic activity has been demonstrated

⚠ Skin malignancies (with topical use in patients predisposed to skin cancer)

With prolonged use or overdose:
- Constipation
- Elevated liver transaminases
- Headache
- Lack of appetite
- Nausea
- Vertigo
- Vomiting

Interactions
Anticoagulants: possible additive effect. Avoid concomitant use.
Calcium channel blockers, other antihypertensives: may potentiate hypotensive effects. Avoid concomitant use.

Contraindications and precautions
Avoid use of the herb in pregnant or breast-feeding patients; effects are unknown. Use cautiously in patients with hepatic disease.

Special considerations
- Periodically monitor liver function tests.
- Recommend that the patient pursue a physician-supervised cardiac workup if khella is being taken as an antianginal.
- Inform the patient that concurrent use of khella may dramatically enhance hypotensive effects of antihypertensive agents.
- Tell the patient on anticoagulant therapy to watch for signs of bleeding (bruises, bleeding gums, or blood in the stool) and to report them to his health care provider.
- Advise the female patient to avoid use of the herb during pregnancy or when breast-feeding.

Analysis
Khella appears to be a strong vasodilator, exerting activity similar to the calcium channel blocking agents. It may be valuable in preventing bronchial and allergic reactions and is being studied for other disorders. However, until adequate human clinical trials are conducted, khella should not be used without the supervision of a health care professional.

References

Borges, M.L., et al. "Photophysical Properties and Photobiological Activity of the Furanochromes Visnagin and Khellin," *Photochem Photobiol* 67:184-91, 1998.

Harvengt, C., and Desanger, J.P. "HDL Cholesterol Increase in Normolipaemic Subjects on Khellin: A Pilot Study," *Int J Clin Pharmacol Res* 3:363, 1983.

Jansen, T., et al. "Provocation of Porphyria Cutanea Tarda by KUVA-therapy of Vitiligo," *Acta Derm Venereol* 75:232-33, 1995.

Lowe, W., et al. "A Khellin-like 7,7'glycerol-bridged Bischromone with Anti-Anaphylactic Activity," *Arch Pharm (Weinheim)* 327:255-59, 1994.

Osher, H.L., et al. "Khellin in the Treatment of Angina Pectoris," *N Engl J Med* 244:315-21, 1951.

Ragab, F.A., et al. "Synthesis and Anticonvulsant Activity of New Thiazolidinone and Thioxoimidazolidinone Derivatives Derived from Furochromones." *Pharmazie (Cairo University, Egypt)* 52:926-29, 1997.

L

LADY'S MANTLE

ALCHEMILLA, BEAR'S FOOT, DEWCUP, LEONTOPODIUM,
LION'S-FOOT, NINE HOOKS, STELLARIA

Common trade names
(Various manufacturers) Lady's Mantle

Common forms
Available as compounded extracts and teas.

Source
The drug is extracted from the roots, leaves,
and flowers of *Alchemilla mollis, A. vulgaris* and
others. The plant is native to Europe but naturalized
to the northeastern United States and Canada.

Chemical components
The major active ingredients are elligitannins and quercetin, a
flavonoid. A glycoside and salicylic acid have also been isolated.

Actions
A water extract of *A. xantochlora* showed antioxidative activity,
whereas an ethanol extract did not (Filipek, 1992). Flavonoid extracts of *A. vulgaris* inhibited the action of several proteolytic enzymes (elastase, trypsin, and alpha-chymotrypsin), suggesting that
it may protect conjunctive and elastic tissues that are detrimentally
affected by proteolytic enzymes (Jonadet et al., 1986). *A. vulgaris* did
not affect the plasma glucose and insulin levels in normal and streptozotocin diabetic mice (Swanson-Flatt et al., 1990).

Reported uses
Lady's mantle is claimed to be useful as an astringent and an aid to
blood clotting. It has been applied topically to wounds to stop bleeding and to promote healing. Lady's mantle is used in women to reduce menstrual bleeding, alleviate menstrual cramps, and regulate
the menstrual cycle. In addition, it has been suggested to be effective
in treating diarrhea because of its tannin content. No controlled trials in humans could be found to verify these claims.

Dosage

Various doses are used for the reported indications. An "infusion" or tea can be prepared from steeping 1 cup boiling water over 2 teaspoons of the dried herb. The tea and tincture (2 to 4 ml) are taken P.O. t.i.d.

Adverse reactions

• Potential for liver damage (related to tannin component)

Interactions

None reported.

Contraindications and precautions

Contraindicated during pregnancy because the herb may stimulate uterine muscle. Avoid use in breast-feeding patients because effects are unknown.

Special considerations

• Periodically monitor liver function tests.
• Advise the female patient to avoid use of the herb during pregnancy or when breast-feeding.
• Warn the patient that very little information is available about this herb.
• Tell the patient to report weakness, fatigue, or jaundice.

Points of interest

• The genus name, *Alchemilla*, is derived from the word alchemy because this herb was believed to bring about miraculous cures. This plant has also been associated with the Virgin Mary because the lobes of the leaves resemble the scalloped edges of a mantle.
• Lady's mantle is also used as an ingredient in herbal cleansing creams and other cosmetics.

Analysis

There are no clinical data to support therapeutic claims for lady's mantle. Data from one animal study suggest that lady's mantle does not affect blood glucose or insulin concentrations. However, it may have antioxidative properties and inhibit some proteolytic enzymes. Human clinical trials are needed to determine the safety and efficacy profiles of this herb.

References

Filipek, J. "Effect of *Alchemilla xantochlora* Water Extract on Lipid Peroxidation and Superoxide Anion Scavenging Activity," *Pharmazie* 47:717-18, 1992.

Jonadet, M., et al. "Flavonoids Extracted from *Ribes nigrum* L. and *Alchemilla vulgaris* L.: 1. In vitro Inhibitory Activities on Elastase, Trypsin and Chymotrypsin. 2. Angioprotective Activities Compared In Vivo," *J Pharmacol* 17:21-27, 1986.

Swanson-Flatt, S.K., et al. "Traditional Plant Treatments for Diabetes. Studies in Normal and Streptozotocin Diabetic Mice," *Diabetologia* 33:462-64, 1990.

LADY'S SLIPPER, YELLOW

AMERICAN VALERIAN, MOCCASIN FLOWER, NERVEROOT, NOAH'S ARK, WHIPPOORWILL'S SHOE, YELLOW INDIAN SHOE

Common trade names
None known.

Common forms
Available as liquid extract, powdered root, dried rhizome, teas, and tinctures. Often used in combination products with other herbal ingredients, such as valerian root.

Source
Active compounds are derived from the rhizome and root of the orchid, *Cypripedium pubescens,* or *C. calceolus.* Other species include *C. parviflorum* and are generally sparsely located in forests of North America and Europe.

Chemical components
The rhizome of *Cypropedium* contains cypripedin, a complex resinoid. Other components include glycosides, resins, quinones, and tannic and gallic acids.

Actions
None reported.

Reported uses
Lady's slipper tea has been used for headaches and nervousness. The powdered root mixed in sugar water has been used as a sedative, mild hypnotic, and antispasmodic. Other claims include epilepsy, hysteria, low fever, nervous depression associated with stomach disorders, and neuralgia.

Dosage
Dried rhizome and root: 2 to 4 g P.O. t.i.d.
Liquid extract (1:1 water and 45% alcohol): 2 to 4 ml P.O. t.i.d.

Adverse reactions
- Contact dermatitis (quinone components)
- Giddiness
- Headache
- Mental excitement leading to hallucinations
- Restlessness

Interactions
Dopamine agonists, similar agents: possible increased hallucinogenic effect. Avoid concomitant use.

Contraindications and precautions
Contraindicated in patients with a history of plant allergies because quinone components may cause contact dermatitis. Also contraindicated in patients susceptible to headaches or mental illness unless under medical supervision. Avoid use of the herb in pregnant or breast-feeding patients; effects are unknown.

Special considerations
- Monitor the patient for psychotic behavior or headaches.
- Warn the patient that there are few clinical data to support therapeutic uses of this herb.
- Tell the patient not to drive or perform activities that require alertness until CNS effects of the herb are known.
- Advise the female patient to avoid use of the herb during pregnancy or when breast-feeding.

Points of interest
- Native American healers used the root of *C. acaule* mixed into a solution for use in a variety of illnesses, including flu and hysteria (Sanchez et al., 1996).
- The herb may be found in combination herb products with Valerian root (*Valerian officinalis*), used for sedative and calming effects.

Analysis
Lady's slipper has not been adequately studied in animal or human models. Pending extensive testing for pharmacologic action, it cannot be recommended for any therapeutic use.

References
Sanchez, T.R., et al. "The Delivery of Culturally Sensitive Health Care to Native Americans," *J Holistic Nurs* 14:295-307, 1996.

LAVENDER

ASPIC, ECHTER LAVENDEL, ENGLISH LAVENDER (*LAVEN-DULA ANGUSTIFOLIA*), ESPLIEG, FRENCH LAVENDER, GARDEN LAVENDER, LAVANDA, LAVANDE COMMUN, LAVANDIN, NARDO, SPANISH LAVENDER (*L. STOECHAS*), SPIGO, SPIKE LAVENDER, TRUE LAVENDER

Common trade names
Lavender, Lavender Flowers

Common forms
Available as oils, flowers, and leaves.

Source
The flowering tops and stalks of *Lavandula officinalis* and other *Lavandula* species (*L. latifolia, L. angustifolia, L. stoechas*) are widely used for their active components. Native to the Mediterranean, lavenders are cultivated widely in American gardens for their color and fragrance. (Lavandin is a hybrid of spike lavender and true lavender.)

Chemical components
Lavender consists of essential oils, mainly monoterpenes. More than 100 compounds are identified in the oil, principally linaloyl acetate, linalool, and tannins; other compounds include ocimene, cineola, camphor, coumarins, flavonoids, phytosterols, pinene, limonene, caproic acid, and perillyl alcohol. Lavender oil, spike lavender oil, and lavadin oil are volatile oils that contain varying amounts of similar compounds.

Actions
Lavender was found to causes CNS depressant effects, anticonvulsant activity, and potentiation of sedative effects of chloral hydrate in rats. Spike lavender oil has been reported to exert a spasmolytic effect on animal smooth muscle, and *L. stoechas* caused hypoglycemia in normoglycemic rats.

Lavender oil fed to rats was found to cause regression of mammary tumors. The active ingredient has been suggested to be perillyl alcohol. The National Cancer Institute is examining this agent in phase II clinical trials in patients with advanced cancers of the breast, ovaries, and prostate (Ziegler, 1996).

In vitro studies report promising results of topical lavender use to eradicate methicillin-resistant *Staphylococcus aureus* and vancomycin-resistant *Enterococcus faecium* (Nelson, 1997). However, no clinical trials are available to confirm these results.

Reported uses

Lavender is regarded by herbalists as a sedative to treat insomnia and restlessness. Other claims include its use in upper abdominal discomfort associated with nervousness, as an appetite stimulant, and to treat migraines and neuralgia. Lavender has also been used as an astringent to treat minor cuts, bruises, and burns, and for pain associated with strained muscles. It has been used as an indoor scent to induce a calming effect.

Dosage

Lavender tea: 1 to 2 teaspoons in 150 ml of hot water; steep for approximately 10 minutes.
Oil (internal): 1 to 4 drops of oil on a sugar cube.
Astringent (external): 20 to 100 g of lavender added to 7.7 gallons (20 L) of water to avoid too strong a scent.

Adverse reactions

With ingestion of large doses (based on narcotic-like potential):
• Constipation
• Contact dermatitis
• CNS and respiratory depression
• Euphoria, mental dullness and confusion, drowsiness
• Headache
• Miosis
• Nausea
• Vomiting

Interactions

CNS sedatives (alcohol, benzodiazepines, narcotics): may potentiate sedative effects. Avoid concomitant use.

Contraindications and precautions

Contraindicated in pregnant or breast-feeding patients and in those taking sedative agents.
⚠ Lavender oil should be considered potentially poisonous. No more than 2 drops of the volatile oil should be consumed. Large doses are reported to exert "narcotic-like" effects.

Special considerations

• Monitor the patient using lavender and other sedatives for signs of excessive sedation or "narcotic-like" symptoms.
• Suggest techniques other than drug therapy (such as behavior modification, light therapy, regular bedtime) to combat insomnia.
• Advise the female patient to avoid use of the herb during pregnancy or when breast-feeding.

• Inform the patient suffering from insomnia that other sedative or hypnotic agents with known risks and benefits are available.

Points of interest
• Lavender has been used in small concentrations to flavor food, but it is cultivated mainly for use as a perfume, potpourri, or in decorations.
• France is a major producer of lavender products.

Analysis
Lavender has been used in traditional medicine for centuries. Unfortunately, there is inadequate clinical evidence for its efficacy in any disease or condition. Controlled studies are necessary before the use of lavender can be recommended.

References
Nelson, R.R.S. "In-Vitro Activities of Five Plant Essential Oils Against Methacillin-Resistant *Staphylococcus aureus* and Vancomycin-Resistant *Enterococcus faecium*," *J Antimicrob Chemother* 40:305-06, 1997.
Ziegler, J. "Raloxifene, Retinoids, and Lavender "Me Too" Tamoxifen Alternatives," *J Natl Cancer Inst* 88:1100-02, 1996.

LICORICE

Chinese licorice, licorice root, Persian licorice, Russian licorice, Spanish licorice, sweet root

Common trade names
(Various manufacturers; available in combination) Full Potency Licorice Root Vegicaps, Licorice ATC Concentrate, Licorice and Garlic, Licorice Root Extract, Licorice Root Tea, Natural Arthro-Rx, Solaray Licorice Root, Tea with Mint, Tummy Soother

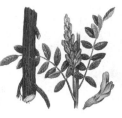

Common forms
Capsules: 100 to 520 mg licorice root
Tablets: licorice root 7 mg and pure concentrated garlic 333 mg
Liquid extracts: licorice extract, deglycyrrhizinized licorice extract
Also available in herbal teas, tobacco products, chewing gums, throat lozenges, and candy.

Source
Most medicinal products use the roots and dried rhizomes of *Glycyrrhiza glabra,* a perennial herb or low-growing shrub. Spanish

licorice is the most common variety and is derived from *G. glabra var typica*. Licorice plants are native to the Mediterranean but are widely cultivated in the United States, Russia, Spain, Turkey, Greece, India, Italy, Iran, and Iraq.

Chemical components

The rhizomes and roots contain 5% to 9% glycyrrhizin (glycyrrhizic acid), a glycoside that is 50 times sweeter than sugar. Hydrolysis of glycyrrhizin yields glycyrrhetic acid, which is not sweet. Other compounds include ammonia, oleane triterpenoids, and glucose, mannose, and sucrose. Aqueous extracts of licorice contain 10% to 20% glycyrrhizin.

Actions

Glycyrrhizin is hydrolyzed by intestinal flora to the pharmacologically active form, glycyrrhetic acid. The main effect of licorice is to potentiate, rather than mimic, endogenous steroids (Davis and Morris, 1991).

Studies in animals suggest that glycyrrhizin and glycyrrhetic acid have mild anti-inflammatory effects. Glycyrrhizin may stimulate gastric mucous synthesis through effects on prostaglandins, which may explain the ulcer healing properties. (See *Licorice-derived products for peptic ulcer disease.*)

Anecdotally, licorice has very effective demulcent (soothing) and expectorant properties, as well as mild laxative and antispasmodic effects. A Chinese licorice preparation called "Zhigancao" has been found to have antiarrhythmic effects, including prolongation of PR and QT intervals. Glycyrrhizin may also lower cholesterol and triglyceride levels, and exert immunosuppressive, antihepatotoxic, and antianemic effects.

Reported uses

Because of its anecdotal use for gastric irritation, licorice derivatives have been studied for antipeptic action. It was evaluated as a treatment for Addison's disease and was found to enhance mineralocorticoid activity, but could not mimic it when adrenal activity was absent.

Glycyrrhizic acid has been used as a shampoo to reduce sebum secretion from the scalp and for eczema, mouth ulcers, and cold sores.

In the United States, glycyrrhizin is used mainly as a flavoring and sweetening agent for bitter drugs, and in tobacco products, chewing gums, candies, beverages, and toothpastes. It is also added to some cough and cold preparations for its expectorant and demulcent (soothing) effects.

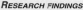

RESEARCH FINDINGS
Licorice-derived products for peptic ulcer disease

Although studies from Europe in the 1940s and 1950s suggested that licorice derivatives could be used to treat peptic ulcers, adverse reactions ranged from headaches and edema to heart failure.

Interest in these agents was revived in the 1960s with the advent of carbenoxolone, a semisynthetic ester of glycyrrhetic acid. This was the first agent derived from traditional medicine to show efficacy against peptic ulcer. Ulcer-healing was demonstrated in 50% to 70% of patients (Marks, 1980). However, other studies failed to show that carbenoxolone or deglycyrrhizinized licorice was superior to cimetidine (Bardhan et al., 1978; LaBrooy et al., 1979; Maxton et al., 1990).

Dosage
For peptic ulcer, 200 to 600 mg P.O. of glycyrrhizin daily for no more than 4 to 6 weeks, according to the German Commission E.

The following tea is believed to provide glycyrrhizin in the middle of this dosage range: 1 teaspoon (2 to 4 g) of crude licorice to ½ cup (120 ml) of boiling water, simmered for 5 minutes. Cool, strain, and take P.O. t.i.d. after food.

Adverse reactions
• Mineralocorticoid effects ("pseudoprimary aldosteronism": headache, lethargy, sodium and water retention, hypokalemia, hypertension)
• Muscle weakness (with hypokalemia)
• Rhabdomyolysis
⚠ Heart failure, cardiac arrest (with overdose)

Interactions
Antihypertensive agents, diuretics: may exacerbate hypokalemic effects of some diuretics. Avoid concomitant use.
Corticosteroids (including topicals): may potentiate effects. Use together cautiously.
Digoxin: may induce hypokalemia and place patient at risk for digoxin toxicity. Avoid concomitant use.
Loratadine, procainamide, quinidine, terfenadine, other agents that may prolong QT interval: may prolong the QT interval and be potentially additive. Use together cautiously.

Spironolactone: may block ulcer healing and aldosterone-like effects of licorice. Avoid concomitant use.

Contraindications and precautions

Contraindicated in patients with hypertension, arrhythmias, and CV, renal, or hepatic disease. Avoid use of the herb in pregnant or breast-feeding patients; effects are unknown. Use cautiously in the elderly under medical supervision.

Special considerations

● Monitor the patient receiving diuretics for hypokalemia.
● Know that a single large dose of licorice is less likely to cause toxicity than prolonged intake of smaller amounts.
⚠ Licorice poisoning may be insidious in nature. Monitor for pseudoprimary hyperaldosteronism causing mineralocorticoid-like effects (headache, lethargy, sodium and water retention, heart failure). Monitor for electrolyte disturbances (potassium, calcium, and sodium) and hypertension, alkalosis, and ECG abnormalities.
● Warn the patient of the dangers of excessive and chronic licorice intake, including fluid retention and electrolyte abnormalities.
● Advise the patient of potential drug interactions.

Points of interest

● Licorice has been used medicinally since Roman times and is popular in Chinese herbal medicine.
● Most "licorice candy" sold in the United States is flavored with anise oil and does not actually contain licorice.

Analysis

Although licorice derivatives have been extensively studied for use against peptic ulcer disease, such products have not performed better than H_2-antagonists and may be less well tolerated. Glycyrrhetic acid may play a role in increasing the topical action of low-potency steroids while minimizing systemic effects; however, this research is still preliminary. Licorice should be taken cautiously because chronic high doses can be very toxic.

References

Bardhan, K.D., et al. "Clinical Trial of Deglycyrrhizinised Licorice in Gastric Ulcer," *Gut* 19:779-82, 1978.

Davis, E.A., and Morris, D.J. "Medicinal Uses of Licorice Through the Millennia: The Good and Plenty of It," *Mol Cell Endocrinol* 78:1-6, 1991.

LaBrooy, S.J., et al. "Controlled Comparison of Cimetidine and Carbenoxolone Sodium in Gastric Ulcer," *BMJ* 1:1308-09, 1979.

Marks, I.N. "Current Therapy in Peptic Ulcer," *Drugs* 20:283-99, 1980.

Maxton, D.G., et al. "Controlled Trial of Pyrogastrone and Cimetidine in the Treatment of Reflux Oesophagitis," *Gut* 31:351-54, 1990.

LILY OF THE VALLEY

CONVALLARIA, JACOB'S LADDER, LADDER-TO-HEAVEN,
LILY CONSTANCY, LILY CONVALLE, MALE LILY, MAY LILY,
MUGUET, OUR-LADY'S-TEARS

Common trade names
None known.

Common forms
Available as extracts.

Source
Active components are derived from leaves, roots, and flowers of
Convallaria majalis, a low-growing perennial herb native to Europe
and naturalized throughout North America.

Chemical components
The entire plant contains cardiac glycosides (convallatoxol, conval-
lotoxin, convallarin, convallamarin, locundjosid, and convallosid—
which transforms into convallatoxin when dried), volatile oil, saponins, asparagin, resin, rutin, chelidonic acid, calcium oxalate, choline, carotene, and wax.

Actions
Tea made from this herb is claimed to have pyrogenic, diuretic,
sedative, and emetic actions. Cardiac effects stem from plant glycosides thought to be less toxic than those of foxglove (digitalis)
(McGuigan, 1984). The plant was also believed to exert hypoglycemic effects, but studies in diabetic mice have shown this to be
false (Swanston-Flatt et al., 1990).

Reported uses
The plant was traditionally used as an antidote to poison gas, a cardiotonic agent, and for treating valvular heart disease. Russian
herbalists have also reported its use as an antiepileptic. The roots
have been used in an ointment to help heal burn wounds and prevent them from scarring. In Germany, the flowers are mixed with
raisins and made into wine.

Dosage
No consensus exists.

Adverse reactions
- Abdominal pain and cramping
- Arrhythmias

- Burning pain in the mouth and throat
- Cold, clammy skin
- Coma
- Dermatitis (leaves)
- Diarrhea
- Dilated pupils
- Dizziness
- Excessive salivation
- Hallucinations
- Headache
- Heart failure
- Hyperkalemia
- Nausea
- Paralysis
- Urinary urgency
- Vomiting

⚠ Death. The entire plant is toxic, causing digitalis-like symptoms. Ingestion of the water in which the cut flowers have been placed can also be toxic. Treatment includes emesis and gastric lavage, followed by activated charcoal, sorbitol cathartic, and supportive care. Perform cardiac monitoring and restore normal sinus rhythm, if necessary, with atropine. Additional effects of plant ingestion may include other rhythm disturbances and hyperkalemia. Treatment is similar to that for digoxin toxicity.

Interactions
Beta blockers, calcium channel blockers: may increase the risk of heart block or bradycardia. Avoid concomitant use.
Digoxin: possible additive effects. Avoid concomitant use.

Contraindications and precautions
All parts of the plant are contraindicated.

Special considerations
- Be aware that lily of the valley has been used in folk medicine as a digitalis substitute. However, it should never be used for any cardiac condition because of its potential for toxicity and lack of accurate dosage information.

Points of interest
- The FDA considers lily of the valley an unsafe and poisonous plant.
- The essential oils of the highly aromatic flowers have been used in perfumes and cosmetics.

Analysis

Existing digoxin and digitalis preparations are available for treating heart failure and other cardiac conditions. There is little use for a highly toxic, insufficiently studied herbal product that might have a similar therapeutic action.

References

McGuigan, M.A. "Plants—Cardiac Glycosides," *Clin Toxic Rev* 6:1-2, 1984.

Swanston-Flatt, S.K., et al. "Traditional Plant Treatments for Diabetes: Studies in Normal and Streptozotocin Diabetic Mice," *Diabetologia* 33:462-64, 1990.

LOBELIA

ASTHMA WEED, BLADDERPOD, CARDINAL FLOWER, EYEBRIGHT, GAGROOT, GREAT LOBELIA, INDIAN PINK, INDIAN TOBACCO, PUKEWEED, RAPUNTIUM INFLATUM, VOMITWORT

Common trade names

(Various manufacturers) Bantron Tablets, Lobelia Capsules, Lobelia Extract, Lobeline Lozenges, Lobidram Computabs

Common forms

Capsules: 395 mg
Tablets: 2 mg
Lozenges: 1 mg
Also available as an extract.

Source

The crude drug is primarily extracted from the dried leaves and tops of *Lobelia inflata,* native to moist woodlands in eastern North America. Other species include *L. berlandieri, L.cardinalis, L. inflata,* and *L. siphilitica.*

Chemical components

Lobelia species contain at least 14 different piperidine alkaloids. The primary alkaloid occurring in most species is lobeline; however, *L. cardinalis* has lobinaline as its primary alkaloid. The emetic alkaloids, lobelanine and lobelanidine, are also found. Lobeline is similar to nicotine, both structurally and pharmacologically.

Actions

Although similar, lobeline is less potent than nicotine. It acts on nicotine receptors in the body and readily crosses both the blood barrier and the placenta. Depending upon the receptor site, lobeline produces several pharmacologic responses. It causes a release of epinephrine and norepinephrine, producing positive inotropic and chronotropic effects on the myocardium, and increases both systolic and diastolic blood pressure.

At low doses, lobeline stimulates respiration, and at large doses it produces a curare-like effect. When administered at toxic doses, lobeline depresses respiration by inhibiting the respiratory centers in the brainstem and causing paralysis of the respiratory muscles (Damaj et al., 1997).

Lobeline increases gastric acid secretion and GI tone and motility. It is well-absorbed from mucous membranes of the mouth, GI tract, and respiratory system. It is metabolized mostly by the liver, kidney, and lungs and is rapidly eliminated by the kidneys (Westfall and Meldrum, 1986).

Reported uses
Lobelia is claimed to be useful as a spasmolytic, antiasthmatic, and emetic. Early settlers smoked lobelia to treat asthma, bronchitis, and other respiratory ailments. Some data suggest that lobelia may be useful as a smoking deterrent because of its nicotine-like effects (Rapp and Olen, 1955).

Dosage
As a smoking deterrent, 0.5 to 2 mg P.O. has been used in tablets or lozenges. The usual dose is 2 mg P.O. after each meal with ½ glass of water for no more than 6 weeks. Doses as high as 8 mg P.O. have been used but caused significant GI distress. Lobeline doses exceeding 20 mg P.O. daily are considered toxic.

Adverse reactions
- Coughing
- Decreased heart rate
- Diaphoresis
- Dizziness
- Epigastric pain
- Fluid retention
- Increased blood pressure
- Nausea, vomiting (in higher doses)
- Palpitations
- Respiratory depression (at high doses) or stimulation (at low doses)
- Seizures
- Severe heartburn
- Tremors

⚠ Although less potent than nicotine, all *Lobelia* species should be considered dangerous. Death has occurred from respiratory depression and paralysis of the respiratory muscles. Symptoms of lobeline overdose include sinus arrhythmia, tachycardia, extrasystoles, partial bundle branch block, profound diaphoresis, hypotension, muscular twitching, seizures, hypothermia, and coma.

Interactions
Nicotine therapy: may potentiate adverse effects of lobeline. Avoid concomitant use.

Contraindications and precautions
Contraindicated in children and pregnant or breast-feeding patients. Use cautiously in patients with hepatic or renal impairment.

Special considerations
• Urge the patient to stop smoking if lobeline is being used to avoid additive effects of nicotine and increased risk of adverse reactions.
• Suggest smoking cessation programs, counseling, behavior modification, nicotine replacement, and other pharmacotherapy to help quit smoking.
• Advise the female patient to avoid use of the herb during pregnancy or when breast-feeding.
• Monitor the patient closely for adverse reactions.
• Warn the patient to avoid use of lobeline for over 6 weeks because of the lack of data on chronic use.

Points of interest
• The FDA advisory review panel on OTC drugs has classified lobeline as having insufficient data available regarding its efficacy as an OTC drug.

Analysis
Because of its similarity to nicotine, lobeline has been used as a smoking deterrent. However, long-term data are not available and clinical trials have not been conclusive. Other safe and effective smoking deterrents are recommended in patients wishing to stop smoking. The risk of serious adverse effects appears to be higher with lobeline than other clinically proven treatments and, therefore, its use as an herbal smoking cessation treatment is not recommended.

References
Damaj, M.I., et al. "Pharmacology of Lobeline, a Nicotine Receptor Ligand," *J Pharmacol Exp Ther* 282:410-19, 1997.

Rapp, G.W., and Olen, A.A. "A Critical Evaluation of a Lobeline-Based Smoking Deterrent," *Am J Med Sci* 230:9-14, 1955.

Westfall, T.C., and Meldrum, M.J. "Ganglionic Blocking Agents," in Craig, C.R., and Stizel, R.E. *Modern Pharmacology,* 2nd ed. Boston: Little, Brown and Company, 1986.

LOVAGE
AETHEROLEUM LEVISTICI, ANGELICA LEVISTICUM,
HIPPOSELINUM LEVISTICUM, MAGGI PLANT,
SEA PARSLEY, SMELLAGE

Common trade names
None known.

Common forms
Available as an herbal tea and essential oil.

Source
Active components are obtained from the roots
and seeds of *Levisticum officinale* and *L. radix*.
These plants are found in southern Europe and
have been naturalized to the United States.

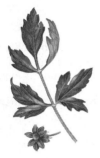

Chemical components
Lovage root contains essential oil that is primarily composed of
phthalide lactones, giving it a characteristic aromatic, spicy odor
(Gijbels et al., 1982). Other compounds include coumarins, terpenoids, and volatile acids.

Actions
When given parenterally in animals, lovage oils cause weak diuresis,
presumably due to mild irritation of renal tubules. It exerts spasmolytic and sedative effects in rodents and has been reported to
stimulate salivation and gastric secretion.

Reported uses
Lovage has been used mainly by herbalists as a diuretic for patients
with pedal edema. It is approved in Germany for irrigation therapy
in urinary tract inflammation and for the prevention of renal
stones.

    The herb is claimed to be useful for gastric discomfort (such as
flatulence), as a spasmolytic and sedative, to dissolve phlegm in the
respiratory tract, and to induce menstruation.

Dosage
Tea: pour 1 cup (150 ml) boiling water into 1.5 to 3 g of finely cut
root of *L. radix* and drain after 15 minutes. Daily dosage is 4 to 8 g
P.O.

Adverse reactions
• Photodermatosis (due to furocoumarin compounds in leaves)

Interactions
Anticoagulants: may potentiate effects. Avoid concomitant use.

Contraindications and precautions
Avoid use of the herb in pregnant or breast-feeding patients; effects are unknown. Use cautiously in patients with a history of plant allergies.

Special considerations
● Monitor serum electrolytes, BUN, and creatinine values periodically during herbal therapy.
● Tell the patient taking lovage for its diuretic effect that pedal edema may indicate heart failure or other potentially dangerous conditions. Advise him to undergo a complete medical examination to rule out the need for aggressive medical treatment.
● Advise the patient that other forms of proven diuretics are available.

Points of interest
● Lovage oil is used as a fragrance in various cosmetics, lotions, and soaps.

Analysis
Although there is some evidence of therapeutic use of lovage in animals, human clinical trials and efficacy and safety data are lacking. Therefore, this herb cannot be recommended at this time.

References
Gijbels, M.J.M., et al. "Phthalides in the Essential Oil From Roots of *Levisticum officinale*," *Planta Med* 44:207-11, 1982.

LUNGWORT
JERUSALEM COWSLIP, JERUSALEM SAGE, LUNG MOSS, LUNGS OF OAK, SPOTTED COMFREY

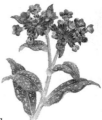

Common trade names
(Available in combination) Lungwort Compound (formerly Bleeders Blend)

Common forms
Available as tablets and extracts.

Source
The drug is obtained from leaves of *Pulmonaria officinalis*, a member of the Borage family.

Chemical components

Lungwort leaves contain allantoin, flavonoids (quercetin and kaempferol), tannins, mucilage, ascorbic acid, saponins, potassium and iron salts, silicic acid, vitamin C, and an anticoagulant glycopeptide.

Actions

Lungwort is claimed to have anti-irritant, expectorant, antitussive, astringent, emollient, and anti-inflammatory actions. Astringent and anti-inflammatory actions are likely attributed to tannins and flavonoids. When applied topically to wounds, tannins cause precipitation of proteins in the surrounding fluids to form a protective coating.

The nondialyzable fraction of the ammonia extract of lungwort contains a glycopeptide that possesses anticoagulant activity in animals (Byshevskii et al., 1990). Lungwort's antitussive activity may be attributed to its mucilage content. The emollient action may be produced by allantoin. The chemical basis for the plant's expectorant action has not been proven.

Reported uses

Lungwort has been used to treat several pulmonary disorders, such as bronchitis, coughs, hoarseness, and influenza. In race horses, lungwort is thought to have a strengthening effect on the animal's lungs to enhance performance; the same effect is thought to occur in humans with tuberculosis. Although these effects could be due to the plant's silica content, there are no data to support these claims. Lungwort has also been claimed to be valuable as an astringent; in diarrhea, GI bleeding, hemorrhoids, and excessive menstruation; and topically to promote wound healing.

Dosage

Tincture: 1 to 4 ml P.O. t.i.d.
Infusion: 1 to 2 teaspoons of dried herb steeped in boiling water P.O. t.i.d.

Adverse reactions

- Contact dermatitis
- GI irritation
- Possible prolonged bleeding time

Interactions

Anticoagulants: may potentiate effects of warfarin. Avoid concomitant use.

Contraindications and precautions

Avoid use of the herb in pregnant or breast-feeding patients; effects are unknown. Also avoid use in patients on anticoagulant therapy. Use cautiously in patients with a history of GI bleeding, thrombocytopenia, or hypersensitivity.

Special considerations

• Monitor PT and INR, and watch for signs of increased bleeding time.
• Inform the patient that insufficient data exist to support a therapeutic use for this agent.
• Advise the patient with respiratory problems (such as asthma, bronchitis, emphysema) to pursue conventional medical therapy.

Points of interest

• Historically, lungwort has been used to treat pulmonary ailments because the spotted leaves resemble the surface of a lung.

Analysis

The chemical basis for lungwort's pulmonary effects is poorly understood. It may be effective as an astringent because of its tannin content. Because there are no human studies to support the safety and efficacy of lungwort, its use cannot be recommended.

References

Byshevskii, A., et al. "Nature, Properties and the Mechanism of the Effect of Blood Coagulation of the Preparation Obtained from *Pulmonaria officinalis*," *Gematol Transfuziol* 35:6-9, 1990.

MADDER
DYER'S-MADDER, GARANCE, KRAPP, MADDER ROOT, ROBBIA

Common trade names
(Available in combination) Nephrubin, Rubia Teep, Rubicin, Uralyt

Common forms
Available as dried root and fluid extract.

Source
The herb consists of the dried roots of *Rubia tinctorum*. The plant is native to parts of the Mediterranean, Europe, and Asia, and is naturalized to parts of North America.

Chemical components
Madder root contains anthraquinone derivatives (ruberythric acid, alizarin, and purpurin), glycosides (including alizarinprimeveroside and lucidinprimeveroside, which is converted to lucidin), an iridoid (asperuloside), resin, and calcium.

Actions
Madder is claimed to have antispasmodic, diuretic, and urinary-stone-inhibiting properties. *R. tinctorum* has been shown to bind the DNA of murine liver, kidney, duodenum, and colonic tissues (Poginsky et al., 1991).

Reported uses
Madder was traditionally used for amenorrhea, jaundice, sciatica, and paralysis. Its use in herbal medicine currently is to treat calcium-containing kidney and bladder stones. Stone formation in rats and rabbits has reportedly been inhibited by dietary intake of fresh madder root. In a rabbit model, administration of anthraquinone derivatives from *R. tinctorum* was found to reduce the rate of bladder calculi formation (Berg et al., 1976).

Dosage
The German Commission E reports a dosage of 30 mg hydroxyanthracene derivatives, calculated as ruberythric acid. Other sources

suggest 20 drops of the fluid extract or 1 capsule (from dried root tincture) t.i.d. for up to 2 months.

Adverse reactions
• Red color of bone, milk, perspiration, saliva, tears, or urine
⚠ Intestinal and liver tumors were induced in rats (Blomeke et al., 1992). However, no effect was shown when fresh madder root was added to the diet of rabbits (Ino et al., 1995).

Interactions
None reported.

Contraindications and precautions
Contraindicated in pregnant or breast-feeding patients because of lucidin's mutagenic and carcinogenic potential.

Special considerations
• Warn the patient about the dangers associated with lucidin, especially if treatment is prolonged.
• Instruct the female patient to report planned or suspected pregnancy.
• Advise the female patient to avoid use of the herb during pregnancy or when breast-feeding.
• Advise the patient wearing contact lenses that madder consumption may stain the lenses.

Points of interest
• Madder was formerly cultivated for its red dye (alizarin), obtained from the roots. Cloth dyed with madder has been found on Egyptian mummies. The red trousers of French soldiers and Turkish fezzes were formerly colored with madder. The production of synthetic alizarin ceased the demand for the natural product. Alizarin colors bone red and was used as a histologic stain in the 1800s to trace bone development and bone cell function.

Analysis
Because of a lack of documented human efficacy and the potential for genotoxicity, the use of madder is strongly discouraged.

References
Berg, W., et al. "Influence of Anthraquinones on the Formation of Urinary Calculi in Experimental Animals," *Urologe [A]* 15:188-91, 1976. Abstract, author's translation.

Blomeke, B., et al. "Formation of Genotoxic Metabolites from Anthraquinone Glycosides Present in *Rubia tinctorum* L.," *Mutat Res* 265:263-72, 1992. Abstract.

Ino, N., et al. "Acute and Subacute Toxicity Tests of Madder Root, Natural Colorant Extracted from Madder (*Rubia tinctorum*), in (C57BL/6 X C3H) F1 Mice," *Toxicol Ind Health* 11:449-58, 1995. Abstract.

Poginsky, B, et al. "Evaluation of DNA-Binding Activity of Hydroxyanthraquinones Occurring in *Rubia tinctorum* L.," *Carcinogenesis* 12:1265-71, 1991. Abstract.

MALE FERN

BEAR'S PAW, ERKEK EGRELTI, HELECHO MACHO, KNOTTY BRAKE, SHIELD FERN, SWEET BRAKE, WURMFARN

Common trade names
Aspidium Oleoresin, Bontanifuge, Extractum Filicis, Extractum Filicis Aethereum, Extractum Filicis Maris Tenue, Male Fern Oleoresin, Paraway Plus

Common forms
Extract: 1.5% to 22% filicin
Male fern extract draught: 4 g of male fern extract
Also available as single or combination product capsules.

Source
The drug is prepared from the dried rhizomes (runners) and roots of *Dryopteris filix-mas,* a perennial fern that grows in Europe, Asia, North America, South America, and northern Africa. Fresh rhizomes are treated with ether to yield the active components. When stored, the rhizomes lose pharmacologic activity in about 6 months.

Chemical components
The active components consist of ether-soluble derivatives of phloroglucinol. Filicic and flavaspidic acids are mainly responsible for the plant's pharmacologic activity, and are inactivated in an alkaline environment. Other compounds include volatile oils, tannin, albaspidin, and desaspidin. Filicin is the collective name given to the mixture of ether-soluble substances obtained in the drug assay and extract. An ethereal extract of European plant material contains approximately 25% filicin, whereas Indian plant material contains about 30%.

Actions
Male fern is well known for its anthelmintic action. (See *Efficacy of male fern extracts against tapeworms.*) Several in vivo trials have been conducted in humans describing successful expulsion of *Taenia solium* (pork tapeworm), *T. saginata* (beef tapeworm), and

RESEARCH FINDINGS

Efficacy of male fern extracts against tapeworms

Two studies evaluated the efficacy of male fern extract in patients who did not respond to other anthelmintics. The eradication cure rate of pork and beef tapeworm was studied in 100 patients ages 5 to 68; the appearance of scoleces (tapeworm heads and mouth parts) in feces after treatment signalled successful therapy. Adults received 6 to 7 g of male fern ethereal extract and children were given 0.25 to 0.50 g for each year of age; the maximum dose was 7 g. The drug was administered by duodenal intubation. Based on the appearance of scoleces, the cure rate achieved was 97%. Three patients in this study experienced adverse effects (nausea and vomiting), but no one experienced intolerance to the extract (Alteric, 1969).

In another study, the effect of male fern against fish tapeworm was tested against three prescribed agents (Laparin, Antiphen, and pumpkin seeds) for tapeworm infestations (Palva, 1963). Although clinical efficacy (expulsion of tapeworms) occurred in all treatment groups, the clinical cure rate (no microscopic evidence of ova in feces) for *Extractum filicis,* Laparin, Antiphen, and pumpkin seeds was 95%, 35%, 52%, and 0%, respectively. The author felt that re-infection could not be a cause of finding ova in stools during follow-up examination and attributed the poor results to inferior anthelmintic activity for these substances (except male fern).

Another study (Mello et al., 1978) examined the efficacy of male fern ethereal extract in 29 patients ages 12 to 60 who had not previously responded to other anthelmintic therapy. The patients received the extract orally, preceded by a hypertonic magnesium sulfate solution. Three cases revealed *Taenia solium* and 26 cases revealed *T. saginata*. The total cure rate was 86%; the cure rates from specific groups were not provided.

Diphyllobothrium latum (fish tapeworm) following treatment with the plant extracts. In the 1950s and 1960s, mepacrine (quinacrine), dichlorophen, and niclosamide were commonly used to expel tapeworms. Male fern is thought to have fewer adverse effects than these agents and is thought to achieve a better cure rate when given by duodenal tube.

Dryopteris phlorophenone derivatives were recently studied in vitro and in vivo for antitumor activity against the Epstein-Barr virus antigen. Among the 33 phlorophenone derivatives tested, aspidin and desaspidin were found to be most active in vitro and showed significant antitumor activity in the mouse. The percentage of induced papillomas per mouse decreased by 50% after 10 to 20 weeks of topical therapy, and papilloma production was also reduced (Kapadia et al., 1996).

Reported uses

Male fern is known as a remedy for intestinal tapeworms. The patient typically received a light diet (to starve the worm) and a laxative the evening before treatment. Upon rising and before eating, the patient was given male fern and another laxative.

Dosage

Adults (fasting state): 3 to 6 ml P.O.
Children up to age 2: up to 2 ml P.O. in divided doses.
Children over age 2: 0.25 to 0.5 ml P.O. per year of age; maximum, 4 ml P.O. in divided doses.

Male fern draught may be given by duodenal tube in a dose of 50 ml to limit GI intolerance. Treatment may need to be repeated. Seven to ten days should elapse between treatments. Male fern may be given as capsules but is considered more effective as a draught.

Adverse reactions

- Abdominal cramps (severe)
- Diarrhea
- Headache
- Hyperbilirubinemia (in animals and humans), albuminuria, dyspnea
- Nausea
- Vomiting

⚠ Optic neuritis, respiratory failure, seizures, cardiac failure, coma, and death have occurred with severe poisoning. Treatment consists of administering a saline cathartic, followed by demulcent fluids, but avoiding fats and oils. Benzodiazepines and ventilatory assistance may be needed for seizures and respiration failure, respectively.

Interactions

Antacids: inactivate the herb. Avoid taking male fern within 1 to 2 hours of taking an antacid.
Fats, oils (such as castor oil): may increase absorption and increase risk of toxicity. Avoid concomitant use.
Proton pump inhibitors (lansoprazole, omeprazole) and other alkaline agents: inactivation of male fern. Avoid concomitant use.

Contraindications and precautions

Contraindicated in the elderly, infants, debilitated patients, or during pregnancy. Also contraindicated in patients with anemia; GI ulceration; or cardiac, hepatic, or renal impairment. Use cautiously in patients receiving medications known to affect bilirubin conjugation or increase liver enzymes such as HMG CoA reductase inhibitors.

Special considerations

• Know that hepatocellular damage has occurred in animals with doses of 500 mg/kg of crude extractum filicis. Liver function test abnormalities and pathologic changes were completely reversible within several days of receiving the initial dose (Valtonen and Takki, 1968).

• Monitor for alterations in liver function tests.

• Tell the patient to take the herb on an empty stomach.

• Advise the female patient to avoid use of the herb during pregnancy or when breast-feeding.

Points of interest

• The Foods Standards Committee of London, England, has recommended that male fern not be used in foods as a flavoring agent.

• Male fern was used by the ancients and was mentioned as an anthelmintic by Galen, Dioscorides, Theophrastus, and Pliny.

Analysis

Male fern has shown promise in treating human tapeworms. However, clinical evidence is sparse, and it is not clear whether the plant exerts sole action or is helped by adjuncts, such as a low-residue diet and laxatives. It would be interesting to compare this plant against praziquantel to determine equivalent efficacy, especially in patients who cannot tolerate praziquantel or niclosamide. The current anthelmintics for tapeworms are much safer compared to male fern. Herbal therapy may be considered if current anthelmintic therapy fails, with thorough consideration of the contraindications and adverse reactions beforehand.

References

Alterio, D.L. "Treatment of Taeniasis with Ether Extract of Male Fern Administered by Duodenal Intubation," *Trop Dis Bull* 66:831, 1969.

Kapadia, G.J., et al. "Anti-Tumor Promoting Activity of *Dryopteris* Phlorophenone Derivatives," *Cancer Lett* 105:161-65, 1996.

Mello, E.B.F., et al. "Oral Treatment of Human Taeniasis by Ethereal Extract of Male Fern (Aspidium) Preceded by the Administration of Hypertonic Solution of Magnesium Sulfate," *Abl Bakt Hyg I Orig A* 248:384-87, 1978. Abstract.

Palva, I.P. "The Effectiveness of Certain Drugs in the Expulsion of Fish Tapeworm," *Ann Med Intern Fenn* 52:89-92, 1963.

Valtonen, E.J., and Takki, S. "Acute Hepatocellular Damage Caused by Oleoresin of the Male Fern in the Rat: An Electron Microscope Study," *Acta Pharmacol Toxicol (Copenh)* 26:169-76, 1968.

MALLOW

BLUE MALLOW, CHEESEFLOWER, CHEESEWEED, FIELD
MALLOW, FLEURS DE MAUVE, HIGH MALLOW, *MALVA
PARVIFLORA*, MALVE, ZIGBLI

Common trade names
Malvedrin, Malveol

Common forms
Available as dried herb and fluid extract.

Source
The drug is obtained from the dried leaves and flowers of *Malva
sylvestris*, a member of the Mallow family (Malvaceae), and is related to the cultivated hibiscus.

Chemical components
Mallow contains flavonol glycosides, mucilage (when hydrolyzed
yields arabinose, glucose, rhamnose, galactose, and galacturonic
acid), anthocyanin (about half is malvin), tannins, and leukocyanins.

Actions
The mucilage contained in the leaves and flowers is responsible for
the herb's emollient and demulcent properties. The plant is also said
to have astringent and expectorant actions.

Reported uses
Mallow preparations are used for irritations of the oral and pharyngeal mucosa, irritative cough, bronchitis, laryngitis, tonsillitis, and
hoarseness, and as a mild astringent. Mallow is also used topically to
reduce swelling and allergic cutaneous irritation, eliminate toxins,
and relieve the pain of skin abrasions and insect stings. The leaves
have been used as a laxative and for gut irritation. Mallow preparations have sometimes been given to children to ease teething pains.
Mallow has been used with yarrow (*Achillea* species) as a douche for
vaginal irritation.

Dosage
The suggested dose is 5 g daily of the chopped, dried herb or by oral
infusion.

Adverse reactions
None reported in humans. Some *Malva* species have been linked to
muscle trembling in cattle.

Interactions
None reported.

Contraindications and precautions
Avoid use of the herb in pregnant or breast-feeding patients; effects are unknown.

Special considerations
- Do not confuse this herb with the similar-sounding marshmallow (*Althaea officinalis*).
- Advise the patient that human clinical trial data are lacking.
- Advise the female patient to avoid use of the herb during pregnancy or when breast-feeding.

Points of interest
- Young mallow leaves and shoots have been eaten since the 8th century B.C. The traditional importance of the herb is captured in the Spanish adage, "A kitchen garden and mallow, sufficient medicines for a home."
- In recent years, mallow's mucilage and anthocyanin components have been analyzed for structural and molecular properties (Farina et al., 1995; Gonda et al., 1990; Tomoda et al., 1989).

Analysis
There are no clinical data to support the use of mallow for any indication. Because of the tannin components, it may reasonably be used as a topical astringent. However, long-term or heavy use should be avoided.

References
Farina, A., et al. "HPTLC and Reflectance Mode Densitometry of Anthocyanins in *Malva silvestris* L.: A Comparison with Gradient-Elution Reversed-Phase HPLC," *J Pharm Biomed Anal* 14:203-11, 1995. Abstract.

Gonda, R., et al. "Structure and Anticomplementary Activity of an Acidic Polysaccharide from the Leaves of *Malva sylvestris* var. *mauritiana*," *Carbohydr Res* 198:323-29, 1990. Abstract.

Tomoda, M., et al. "Plant Mucilages. XLII. An Anticomplementary Mucilage from the Leaves of *Malva sylvestris* var. *mauritiana*." *Chem Pharm Bull (Tokyo)* 37:3029-32, 1989. Abstract.

MARIGOLD

CALENDULA, GARDEN MARIGOLD, POT MARIGOLD

Common trade names
None known.

Common forms
Available as an ointment of 5% flower extract, infusion, or mouthwash.

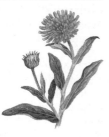

Source
Components are extracted from the small, bright yellow-orange flower heads of *Calendula officinalis*. The shoots and leaves also have been investigated for potentially active compounds. *C. officinalis* is an annual herb native to southern Europe and the eastern Mediterranean, and is naturalized in many parts of the United States and Canada.

Chemical components
Compounds isolated from *C. officinalis* include triterpenoids, oleanic acid glycosides, lutein, carotenoid pigment, sterols, and fatty acids.

Actions
The anti-inflammatory activity of marigold has been demonstrated in mice (Akihisa et al., 1996; Zitterl-Eglseer et al., 1997) and the triterpenoids, primarily faradiol monoester, is thought to be the active component. The unesterfied faradiol equals indomethacin in activity.

Marigold extracts appeared to show antiviral activity against HIV type 1, rhinovirus, and vesicular stomatitis virus (De Tommasi et al., 1991; Kalvatchev et al., 1997).

The healing effect of an ointment containing 5% calendula extract was shown in a rat model. Surgically induced wounds treated with the ointment demonstrated marked physiological regeneration and epithelialization (Klouchek-Popova et al., 1982).

Dietary lutein derived from marigold extract increased tumor latency, suppressed mammary tumor growth, and enhanced lymphocyte proliferation in mice given tumor cell infusions (Chew et al., 1996).

Reported uses
Therapeutic claims for marigold extract include skin healing and antiseptic activities. Ointments have been suggested for leg ulcers, varicose veins, and bedsores. Advocates recommend oral infusions

to aid in digestion and promote bile production. Mouthwashes containing marigold extract have been promoted for gum healing after tooth extraction.

Calendula oil has been used for skin treatments during aromatherapy. The herbal agent has also been promoted for soothing skin inflammations, chapped lips, and cracked nipples from breast-feeding.

Dosage
Ointment: apply topically.
Tincture, tea: 1 to 4 ml P.O. t.i.d.

Adverse reactions
Allergic reactions have been reported with other members of the Compositae family of plants.

Interactions
None reported.

Contraindications and precautions
Avoid use of the herb in pregnant or breast-feeding patients; effects are unknown.

Special considerations
• Do not confuse *C. officinalis* with other ornamental marigolds, such as *Tagetes patula* (French marigold), *T. erecta* (African marigold), and *T. minuta* (Inca marigold). These plants are known for their ability to repel insects and soil nematodes and are often included in vegetable gardens.
• Inform the patient of the risk of allergic reactions.
• Advise the female patient to avoid use of the herb during pregnancy or when breast-feeding.

Points of interest
• Because the plant continuously flowers from May to October, it was given the name Calendula because it was always in bloom on the first day of the month.
• Calendula is believed to have originated in Egypt, where it was valued as a rejuvenating herb.
• During the American Civil War, field doctors are believed to have used marigold leaves on open wounds.

Analysis
Marigold has been used for centuries for its healing effects without documented problems. Although animal models have supported its

healing and anti-inflammatory effects, human studies are lacking. Further research is needed to confirm the other claims for the use of marigold.

References

Akihisa, T., et al. "Triterpene Alcohols from the Flowers of Compositae and their Anti-Inflammatory Effects," *Phytochemistry* 43:1255-60, 1996.

Chew, B.P., et al. "Effects of Lutein from Marigold Extract on Immunity and Growth of Mammary Tumors in Mice," *Anticancer Res* 16:3689-94, 1996.

De Tommasi, N., et al. "Structure and In Vitro Antiviral Activity of Triterpenoid Saponins from *Calendula arvensis*," *Planta Med* 57:250-53, 1991.

Kalvatchev, Z., et al. "Different Effects of Phorbol Ester Derivatives on Human Immunodeficiency Virus 1 Replication in Lymphocytic and Monocytic Human Cells," *Acta Virol* 41:289-92, 1997.

Klouchek-Popova, E., et al. "Influence of the Physiological Regeneration and Epithelialization Using Fractions Isolated from *Calendula officinalis*," *Acta Physiol Pharmacol Bulg* 8:63-67, 1982.

Zitterl-Eglseer, K., et al. "Anti-Oedematous Activities of the Main Triterpendiol Esters of Marigold (*Calendula officinalis* L.), *J Ethnopharmacol* 57:139-44, 1997.

MARJORAM

COMMON MARJORAM, KNOTTED MARJORAM, OLEUM MAJORANAE (OIL), OREGANO, SWEET MARJORAM, WILD MARJORAM

Common trade names
(Various manufacturers) Marjoram, Sweet Marjoram Essential Oil

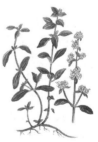

Common forms
Available as dried or powdered leaves and as a tea.

Source
Products identified as marjoram are generally composed of the dried leaves and flowering tops of *Origanum majorana* L., a member of the Mint family (Labiatae). The name wild marjoram is generally a synonym for *O. vulgare*, one of the species more commonly referred to as oregano. Essential oils identified as "Oil of Marjoram" or "Wild Marjoram Oil" have been obtained from thyme (*Thymus mastichina*) and other species.

Chemical components
The essential oil of wild *O. majorana* plants contains the phenolic terpene isomers carvacrol and thymol. Other compounds include triacontane, sitosterol, oleanolic and ursolic acids, rosmarinic acid,

flavonoids, hydroquinone, tannins, and phenolic glycosides (arbutin and methylarbutin).

Actions

An aqueous extract of *O. compactum* inhibited responses to acetylcholine, histamine, serotonin, and nicotine, increasing calcium concentrations and electrical stimulation in smooth muscle from rat and guinea pig ileum and duodenum. These effects were attributed to thymol and carvacrol present in the plants (Van Den Broucke and Lemli, 1980). Marjoram was found to exert some antiviral activity, possibly due to tannins in the plants. Hydroquinone exerted dose-dependent cytotoxic activity on cultured rat hepatoma cells (Assaf et al., 1987). Thymol has been shown to have bactericidal action against several oral bacteria; it is included in some antiseptic mouthwashes and in Cervitec, a varnish used in dentistry. There are several reports of antibacterial, antifungal, and antiviral effects of thymol, carvacrol, and essential oils of the Labiatae.

Reported uses

The dried leaves and flowering tops of the marjoram plant are used mainly in cooking. Marjoram is among the many plants that have been labeled as oregano, but it generally has a milder flavor than the other species. Medicinally, it has been used as an antidote for snakebite and for treating muscle and joint pain, bruises, nausea, infant colic, cough, headache, insomnia, motion sickness, menstrual cramps, amenorrhea, conjunctivitis, and certain cancers. *O. majorana* and *O. vulgare* have been used to stimulate digestion and prevent flatulence (Van Den Broucke and Lemli, 1980).

Dosage

Tea: steep 1 to 2 teaspoons of dried leaves and flower tops for 10 minutes in 1 cup of boiling water; no more than 3 cups should be taken P.O. daily. Alternatively, three doses of ½ to 1 teaspoon of the tincture P.O. daily.

Adverse reactions

⚠ Although no suspected cases of harm from marjoram consumption have been reported, several preparations of essential oil warn against internal use. Thymol and hydroquinone may be toxic.

Interactions

None reported.

Contraindications and precautions

Use in pregnant women should be limited to normal amounts used for cooking because of slight risk of uterine contractions with herbal overdoses. Use cautiously in infants or children because safety of the herb has not been evaluated for this age group.

Special considerations
• Know that the content of thymol, carvacrol, hydroquinone, and other active components varies among plants (and thus in products), and that the volatile oil content may decrease with age.
• Reduce dosage or discontinue the herb if nausea, vomiting, or diarrhea occurs.
• Instruct the patient to notify his health care professional of nausea or diarrhea lasting for more than a few days because these symptoms may indicate serious disease or cause electrolyte imbalance if left untreated.
• Advise the patient to avoid using the volatile oil.
• Tell the patient not to exceed consumption of marjoram in an amount greater than that commonly found in foods.

Points of interest
• Early Greeks believed that marjoram was cultivated by Aphrodite, the goddess of love. The herb is still included in love potions and placed in hope chests or under women's pillows to ensure happy marriages.
• The FDA regards marjoram as "Generally Regarded as Safe."

Analysis
The antispasmodic effect of the extracts may account for its use to treat nausea, colic, and menstrual cramps. Because marjoram is recognized as a safe food additive, moderate consumption in foods or teas is unlikely to cause harm and may be beneficial for these conditions. Although antibacterial, antiviral, and antifungal activity of thymol and carvacrol have been shown in vitro, their concentration is variable; therefore, marjoram should not be relied upon to treat or prevent infections. Its use as a toothache remedy may be related to the antimicrobial activity of thymol on oral bacteria. However, suspected oral infections should be treated with conventional medications.

There is little clinical evidence to support most of the therapeutic claims made for marjoram. Use of marjoram products should be restricted to oral intake or topical use on the skin if desired. Application of marjoram to open wounds or rashes, and especially the eye, should be discouraged.

References
Assaf, M.H., et al. "Preliminary Study of Phenolic Glycosides from *Origanum majorana*; Quantitative Estimation of Arbutin; Cytotoxic Activity Of Hydroquinone," *Planta Med* 53:343-45, 1987.
Van Den Broucke, C.O., and Lemli, J.A. "Antispasmodic Activity of *Origanum compactum*," *Planta Med* 38:317-31, 1980.

MARSHMALLOW

ALTHAEA ROOT, ALTHEA, MORTIFICATION ROOT,
SWEETWEED

Common trade names
None known.

Common forms
Available as whole dried root, dried leaves or
flowers, capsules containing powdered root, and
extracts.

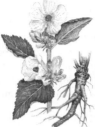

Source
The crude drug is obtained from the dried roots
of *Althaea officinalis,* a perennial herb native to Europe and
naturalized to the United States. Flowers and leaves may also be
used.

Chemical components
Marshmallow root contains starch, mucilage, pectin, and sugar, plus
asparagine, flavonoids, phenolic acids, and calcium oxalate. The
leaves and flowers also contain mucilage, a substance that swells in
water and develops a gel-like consistency. Althea-mucilage O, a rep-
resentative mucous polysaccharide isolated from marshmallow root,
contains rhamnose, galactose, and glucuronic acid. Althea-mucilage
OL is a similar acidic polysaccharide that occurs in the leaves. The
root has also been found to contain scopoletin, quercetin, kaempferol, chlorogenic acid, caffeic acid, and *p*-coumaric acids.

Actions
Althea-mucilage O and OL have been shown to exert a hypoglycemic effect in nondiabetic mice (Tomoda et al., 1987); however, these
effects have not been studied in humans. Antibacterial activity has
also been shown in vitro (Recio et al., 1989).

Although polysaccharides from other plant sources such as tragacanth have been used as bulk-forming laxative products, the laxative
effects of marshmallow mucilages have not been evaluated. Plant
mucilages are commonly used as pharmaceutical vehicles, usually as
suspending agents or viscosity-increasing agents.

Reported uses
Marshmallow has been used as a cough suppressant and to soothe
irritated throats. It is also thought to be useful for intestinal conditions, such as constipation, gastritis, peptic ulcer, and irritable bowel
syndrome. Applied topically, marshmallow purportedly soothes inflamed skin and helps heal minor abrasions.

Dosage

Root: 6 g P.O. daily in crude form or in formulations.
Leaf: 5 g P.O. daily.

Adverse reactions

None reported.

Interactions

Insulin, sulfonylureas: may enhance hypoglycemic effects. Avoid concomitant use.
Other drugs: delayed absorption of other medications when concomitantly administered. Stagger administration of these agents.

Contraindications and precautions

Avoid use of the herb in pregnant or breast-feeding patients; effects are unknown.

Special considerations

• Monitor the diabetic patient for hypoglycemic effects.
• Advise the female patient to avoid use of the herb during pregnancy or when breast-feeding.

Analysis

Marshmallow cannot be recommend for any condition or disease because of the lack of data. Mucilaginous substances may be useful as pharmaceutical agents, but this warrants additional investigation. Consumption of marshmallow in quantities other than that used in foods is not recommended.

References

Recio, M.C., et al. "Antimicrobial Activity of Selected Plants Employed in the Spanish Mediterranean Area, Part II," *Phytother Res* 3:77-80, 1989.
Tomoda, M., et al. "Hypoglycemic Activity of Twenty Plant Mucilages and Three Modified Products," *Planta Med* 53:8-12, 1987.

MAYAPPLE

DEVIL'S-APPLE, HOG APPLE, INDIAN APPLE,
MANDRAKE, UMBRELLA PLANT, WILD LEMON

Common trade names

Condylox, Podocon-25, Podofilm, Warix, Wartec

Common forms

Available as dried rhizome, prescription-only resinous extract (0.5 % podophyllotoxin in alcohol), and concentrated tincture (5%

to 25% solution in alcohol or compound benzoin tincture). A component of mayapple is available commercially in various synthetic anticancer medications.

Source

Active components are derived from rhizome extracts; the USP powdered mixture of resins from *Podophyllum peltatum* is obtained by percolation of the plant with alcohol and precipitation with acidified water. Mayapple is a perennial herb that grows wild in the forests of North America and should not be confused with *Mandragora officinarum,* also known as "mandrake," which is native to the Mediterranean and has different physiologic actions.

Chemical components

Mayapple contains a neutral crystalline substance, podophyllotoxins, amorphous resin, picropodophyllin, quercetin, starch, sugar, fat, and yellow coloring matter. The dried rhizomes and roots of podophyllum peltatum yields some resin. The resin contains aryltetralin lignans calculated as podophyllotoxin. The "podophyllum" resin extract (incorrectly named podophyllin) contains at least 16 physiologically active compounds, including podophyllotoxin, picropodophyllin (the cis isomer of podophyllotoxin), alpha- and beta-pelotins, and quercetin.

Actions

A small quantity of the dried root powder produces a powerful cathartic effect. The resin is a potent spindle poison that blocks mitosis in metaphase, an effect it shares with the vinca alkaloids.

Reported uses

The fruits are the only edible portion of this plant, and can be consumed in drinks, marmalades, and jellies. Mayapple is thought to be useful for treating liver congestion and as an emetic, stimulant, and counterirritant. It has also been used as a powerful cathartic. Antitumor effects are well documented, and mayapple compounds have been incorporated into various synthetic anticancer drugs to treat testicular and ovarian germ cell cancers, lymphomas, small-cell lung cancers, and acute myelogenous and lymphoblastic leukemia.

The concentrated tincture is claimed to be useful for treating warts. The resinous black extract is available by prescription only to topically treat anogenital warts and plantar warts. The Centers for Disease Control and Prevention (CDC) recommends this as an alternative regimen to cryotherapy for external genital or perianal warts, vaginal warts, and urethral meatus warts.

Dosage

Powdered root: 10 to 30 grains.

Tincture: 1 to 10 drops once or twice daily.

5% to 25% solution in alcohol or compound benzoin tincture: apply once weekly on wart and leave for 1 to 6 hours, then wash off. If application is unsuccessful after 4 weeks, consider alternative therapy.

Resin: apply to warts b.i.d. for 3 successive days; repeat at weekly intervals for up to 5 weeks. Treat a small number of warts at one time; do not wash off.

Adverse reactions

- Abdominal pain
- Apnea
- CNS effects (acute psychotic reactions, ataxia, coma, confusion, dizziness, hallucinations, hypotonia, seizures, and stupor) that may take 10 to 15 days to resolve (Dobb et al., 1984).
- Decreased reflexes
- Diarrhea
- EEG changes (persist for several days)
- Hepatotoxicity
- Irritation of skin, eyes, and mucous membranes (resin)
- Leukopenia
- Muscle weakness
- Nausea
- Orthostatic hypotension
- Paresthesia
- Renal failure
- Tachycardia
- Thrombocytopenia
- Urine retention
- Vomiting

⚠ Except for the ripe fruits, the entire mayapple plant is toxic and should be used only with extreme caution. Severe systemic toxicity can occur following ingestion or topical application. Neuropathy and death have resulted from applying large amounts of the resin to multiple and widespread skin lesions (Rate et al., 1979).

Interactions

None reported.

Contraindications and precautions

Contraindicated in pregnant or breast-feeding patients. Also contraindicated in patients with diabetes, in those using steroids, and in those who have poor circulation. Avoid use of resin to friable, bleeding, unusual warts with hair growing from them, or to recently biopsied warts, moles, or birthmarks.

Use this herb with caution because extremely violent cathartic and CNS effects may occur.

Special considerations
● Monitor for adverse CNS effects.

● Warn the patient to use only FDA-labeled pharmaceutical preparations of mayapple components. Resin and tincture is for external use only and should be guided by a primary healthcare provider. Commercial products are only available by prescription.

● Tell the patient to keep the resin away from the eyes.

● Advise the female patient to avoid use of the herb during pregnancy and when breast-feeding.

● Tell the patient to immediately report signs of unusual bruising, bleeding or infection.

● Tell the patient to keep these products out of the reach of children and pets.

Analysis
Mayapple compounds have many established uses because of documented antimitotic effects. These effects are valuable in treating tumors and venereal warts, but they also contribute to its toxicity. Other claims, including its effectiveness as a liver tonic, lack documentation and require further investigation.

References
Dobb, G.J., et al. "Coma and Neuropathy After Ingestion of Herbal Laxative Containing Podophyllin," *Med J Aust* 140:495, 1984.

Rate, R.G., et al. "Podophyllin Toxicity," *Ann Intern Med* 90:723, 1979.

MEADOWSWEET

BRIDEWORT, DOLLOFF, DROPWORT, *FILIPENDULA*, FLEUR D'ULMAIRE, FLORES ULMARIAE, GRAVEL ROOT, MEADWORT, MEDE-SWEET, QUEEN-OF-THE-MEADOW, SPIERSTAUDE, *SPIRAEAE FLOS* (MEADOWSWEET FLOWER), *SPIRAEAE HERBA* (MEADOWSWEET HERB)

Common trade names
(Available in combination) Arkocaps, Artival, Neutracalm, Rheuma-Tee, Rheumex, Santane, Spireadosa,

Common forms
Available as tablets of dried herb (300 mg), infusion, powder, fluid extract, or tincture.

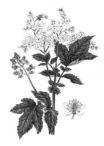

Source

Active components are obtained from the dried flowers and above-ground parts of *Filipendula ulmaria*, a hardy perennial herb native to Europe and Asia and naturalized to the United States as an ornamental plant. A member of the Rose family (Rosaceae), it is also known as *Spiraea ulmaria*.

Chemical components

Meadowsweet contains flavonoids (mainly glycosides of quercetin and kaempherol, spiraeoside in the flowers, and avicularin and hyperoside in the leaves); phenolic glycosides (spiraein in the flowers, monotropin in the flower and leaf, and the primaverosides of salicylaldehyde and methyl salicylate polyphenols), and tannins. The volatile oil contains salicylates (salicylaldehyde, gaultherin, isosalicin, methyl salicylate, monotropitin, salicin, salicylic acid, and spirein), phenylethyl alcohol, benzyl alcohol, anisaldehyde, and methyl salicylate. Other compounds include benzaldehyde, ethyl benzoate, heliotropin, phenylacetate, vanillin, citric acid, mucilage, coumarins (trace), carbohydrates, and ascorbic acid.

Actions

Meadowsweet has traditionally been used for its anti-inflammatory, antiemetic, antiulcer, astringent, antirheumatic, antiflatulent, diuretic, diaphoretic, laxative, sedative, digestive aid, and mild urinary antiseptic properties. In Russian studies with animals, meadowsweet was reported to lower motor activity and rectal temperature, relax the muscles, and potentiate the action of narcotics; prolong life expectancy of mice; lower vascular permeability and prevent stomach ulcers in mice and rats (Barnaulov et al., 1977; Barnaulov and Denisenko, 1980; Yanutsh et al., 1982); increase bronchial tone in cats; potentiate histamine bronchospasm; increase the impact of histamine upon ulcers; increase intestinal tone in guinea pigs; and increase uterine tone in rabbits (Barnaulov et al., 1978). Tannins in meadowsweet have an astringent action that may ease stomach complaints.

Reported uses

Meadowsweet has been used in folk medicine for gastritis, peptic ulcer, arthritis, indigestion, heartburn, cystitis, cancer, irritable bowel syndrome (with other herbs), colds and chills, diarrhea, rheumatic joints and muscles, sprains, and tendonitis. The French use the herb as a diuretic and diaphoretic, and to treat headache and toothache pain. In Belgium, the herb is used for painful articular conditions. Although salicylates are present, they appear to cause less GI irritation than acetylsalicylic acid. In Europe, meadowsweet is used as a natural food flavoring. The FDA lists it as an herb of undefined safety.

Dosage

For treatment of diarrhea, 1 cup decoction b.i.d. or t.i.d. P.O.
Dried flowers: 2.5 to 3.5 g P.O. up to t.i.d.
Dried herb: 2 to 6 g P.O. up to t.i.d.
Liquid extract (1:1 in 25% alcohol): 1.5 to 6 ml P.O. up to t.i.d.
Oral infusion: 100 ml every 2 hours.
Powder: ½ teaspoon with a small amount of water t.i.d.
Tincture (1:5 in 25% alcohol): 2 to 4 ml P.O. up to t.i.d.

Adverse reactions

• Bronchospasm
⚠ Avoid this herb in cases of salicylate sensitivity. Although not substantiated, a link between salicin and birth defects has been reported.

Interactions

None reported.

Contraindications and precautions

Avoid use of the herb in pregnant or breast-feeding patients; effects are unknown. Do not use in patients with asthma or salicylate sensitivity and in children.

Special considerations

• Advise the patient to avoid taking this herb because there are no clinical data to support its use.
• Remind the patient that some contemporary pharmaceuticals have proven antiulcer effects, although efficacy and safety data for meadowsweet are lacking.
• Advise the female patient to avoid use of the herb during pregnancy or when breast-feeding.

Points of interest

• Although meadowsweet was one of the most sacred herbs of the Druids, it is unknown whether it was used medicinally. It was used to flavor mead in the Middle Ages, thus the synonyms meadwort and mede-sweet.
• Meadowsweet was used as source of salicylates for aspirin in the late 1800s. Some sources report that aspirin derived its name from this herb (*Spiraea ulmaria*).

Analysis

The German Commission E reports no known adverse effects or contraindications, except that of salicylate sensitivity, and indicates the use of this herb as supportive therapy for colds. Although its use cannot be recommended currently because of the lack of data, information from the German Commission E suggests that further studies are needed because the herb appears to have potential therapeutic value.

References

Barnaulov, O.D., et al. "Chemical Composition and Primary Evaluation of the Properties of Preparations from *Filipendula ulmaria* (L) Flowers," *Rastit Resur* 13:661-69, 1977.

Barnaulov, O.D., et al. "Preliminary Evaluation of the Spasmolytic Properties of Some Natural Compounds and Galenic Preparations," *Rastit Resur* 14:573-79, 1978.

Barnaulov, O.D., and Denisenko, P.P. "Antiulcerogenic Action of the Decoction from Flowers of *Filipendula ulmaria*," *Pharmakol Toxicol* 43:700-05, 1980.

Yanutsh, A.Y., et al. "A Study of the Antiulcerative Action of the Extracts from the Supernatant Part and Roots of *Filipendula ulmaria*," *Farm Zh* 37:53-56, 1982.

MELATONIN

MEL, N-ACETYL-5-METHOXYTRYPTAMINE

Common trade names
(Various manufacturers; available in combination) Bevitamel, Melatonin, Rapi-Snooze, Tranzone

Common forms
Capsules (extended-release): 3 mg
Liquid: 500 mcg/ml
Tablets: 500 mcg, 1 mg, 1.5 mg, 3 mg

Source
Melatonin is a hormone produced by the pineal gland. It can also be synthesized chemically.

Chemical components
Melatonin has the chemical name of N-2-(5-methoxyindol-3-ethyl) acetamide. Physiologically, melatonin is available when tryptophan is converted to serotonin, which is then enzymatically converted to melatonin in the pineal gland. Commercial products may also contain the inactive ingredients cellulose, lactose, cornstarch, magnesium stearate, and isopropyl alcohol.

Actions
Melatonin release corresponds to sleeping periods. Serum concentrations of melatonin are very low during the day. This would partly explain the role of melatonin in sleep and circadian rhythms. Prolonged intake can reset the sleep-wake cycle. Serum prolactin levels,

growth hormone release, and response to growth-hormone-releasing hormone stimulation increases after acute doses of melatonin. Long-term use may also cause decreases in luteinizing hormone in women. Melatonin has been found to be a free-radical scavenger and may be more effective than mannitol, vitamin E, or glutathione (Brzezinski, 1997).

Reported uses

Melatonin has been studied for many conditions. It has been promoted widely for the prevention and treatment of jet lag and as a hypnotic. (See *Treating jet lag with melatonin,* page 428.) It is thought to induce sleep similarly to benzodiazepines rather than altering sleep cycles. A preliminary study suggests that melatonin supplementation can initiate and maintain sleep in elderly melatonin-deficient patients with insomnia (Haimov et al., 1995).

As an anticancer agent, melatonin may produce partial response in the treatment of solid tumors and stabilization of disease (Lissoni et al., 1991). Larger clinical trials are needed to confirm these results, however. Use of melatonin has also led to significantly less weight loss in patients with cancer (Lissoni et al., 1996). It may also be a future contraceptive option because decreased luteinizing hormone, progesterone, and estradiol levels have been noted.

Dosage

For cancer (solid tumors) as single agent, 20 mg I.M. for 2 months, then 10 mg P.O. daily.
For cancer (with IL-2), 40 to 50 mg P.O. at bedtime, starting 7 days before IL-2.
For chronic insomnia, 75 mg P.O. at bedtime.
For delayed sleep phase syndrome, 5 mg P.O. at bedtime.
For jet lag, 5 mg P.O. daily, starting 3 days before departure and ending 3 days post-departure.
For normalization of nocturnal levels, 4 mcg/hour continuous I.V. for 5 hours.
In blind patients with sleep problems, 5 mg P.O. at bedtime.
In elderly patients with insomnia, 1 to 2 mg P.O. sustained-release, 2 hours before bedtime

Adverse effects

- Altered sleep patterns
- Confusion
- Headache
- Hypothermia
- Pruritus
- Sedation
- Tachycardia

RESEARCH FINDINGS
Treating jet lag with melatonin

Prevention and treatment of jet lag appears to be the most popular indication for using melatonin. Several studies have evaluated melatonin's effect on sleep disturbance, recovery of energy, fatigue, mental alertness, and mood. In most studies, melatonin showed a modest improvement in these outcomes compared with placebo.

In one study, 20 subjects took either placebo or melatonin to prepare for a flight between England and New Zealand. The dosage regimen was 5 mg once daily for 3 days before the flight, during the flight, and 3 days after arrival. The melatonin group required significantly less time to return to normal sleep patterns and energy levels than the placebo group. The study also found that jet lag symptoms were much worse on the return flight, suggesting that melatonin may play an important role during the return portion of a journey (Petrie et al., 1989).

In a subsequent study, the authors compared two dosage regimens and found that 5 mg daily for 5 days after arrival was superior to 5 mg 2 days before departure through 5 days after arrival. The former group experienced significantly less jet lag and sleep disturbance; however, there was no difference in recovery of energy and alertness. An interesting finding was that the melatonin group experienced worse jet lag than the placebo group (Petrie et al., 1993).

In contrast, another study found that melatonin was not statistically superior to placebo in improving sleep quality, morning sleepiness, or mood (Claustraut, 1992).

Interactions
Benzodiazepines: enhanced anxiolytic action. Use cautiously.
DHEA: altered cytokine production in murine studies. Monitor patient.
Magnesium, zinc: additive inhibitory effects on the NMDA receptor (animal studies). Avoid concomitant use.
Methamphetamine: enhanced monoaminergic effects of methamphetamine; may exacerbate insomnia. Avoid concomitant use.
Succinylcholine: potentiates blocking properties of succinylcholine. Avoid concomitant use.

Contraindications and precautions
Contraindicated in patients with hepatic insufficiency, especially cirrhosis because of reduced clearance of the drug. Also contraindi-

cated in patients with a history of cerebrovascular disease, depression, or neurologic disorders. Use cautiously in patients with renal impairment.

Special considerations

● Be aware that the content of commercial melatonin products may not be uniform.

● Comprehensive therapy for sleep disorders may include behavior modification, light-therapy, pharmacology, and counseling.

● Monitor for adverse CNS effects.

Analysis

Melatonin is a popular alternative medication. However, the efficacy rates from clinical trials may lead to conservative recommendation for certain indications.

For jet lag, melatonin appears promising in mitigating symptoms. More controlled trials are needed to determine whether the dosing regimen should be changed to taking the first dose on the departure day rather than for days after. Melatonin is an orphan drug as an aid to blind patients with abnormal circadian rhythms. Larger studies and long-term effects need to be studied.

Theoretically, melatonin may possess contraceptive characteristics. However, trials evaluating whether melatonin can inhibit pregnancy are ongoing. Despite promise as a chemotherapeutic agent, larger studies are needed to define rigid controls in the use of melatonin as an adjunct or single agent for solid tumor treatment. Thus, this drug may be useful in sleep disorders, certain cancers, and as a contraceptive. However, conclusions or recommendations on its use cannot be reached until long-term studies are completed.

References

Brzezinski, A. "Melatonin in Humans," *N Engl J Med* 336:186-95, 1997.

Claustraut, B. "Melatonin and Jet Lag: Confirmatory Result Using a Simplified Protocol," *Biol Psychol* 32:705-11, 1992.

Haimov, I., et al. "Melatonin Replacement Therapy of Elderly Insomniacs," *Sleep* 18:598-603, 1995.

Lissoni, P., et al. "Clinical Results with the Pineal Hormone Melatonin in Advanced Cancer Resistant to Standard Antitumor Therapies," *Oncology* 48:448-50, 1991.

Lissoni, P., et al. "Is There a Role for Melatonin in the Treatment of Neoplastic Cachexia?" *Eur J Cancer* 32A:1340-43, 1996.

Petrie, K., et al. "Effect of Melatonin on Jet Lag after Long Haul Flights," *BMJ* 298:705-07, 1989.

Petrie, K., et al. "A Double-Blind Trial of Melatonin as a Treatment for Jet Lag in International Cabin Crew," *Biol Psych* 33:526-30, 1993.

MILK THISTLE
CARDUUS MARIANUS L., CNICUS MARIANUS, HOLY
THISTLE, LADY'S THISTLE, MARY THISTLE, MARIAN
THISTLE, ST. MARY THISTLE

Common trade names
Beyond Milk Thistle, Milk Thistle Extract, Milk Thistle Phytosol,
Milk Thistle Power, NU VEG Milk Thistle Power, Silymarin

Common forms
Capsules: 50 mg, 100 mg, 175 mg, 200 mg, 505 mg
Tablets: 85 mg (standardized to contain 80% silymarin with the
flavonoid silibinin)
Also available as an extract.

Source
The seeds from *Silybum marianum,* a member of the Asteraceae or
Compositae family (daisies and thistles), are used to formulate milk
thistle preparations. The plant is indigenous to the Mediterranean
area but is also found in Europe, North America, South America,
and Australia.

Chemical components
Milk thistle contains silymarin, which consists of three flavanolig-
nan compounds (silibinin, silidyanin, and silychristin). Other
flavonolignans include dehydrosilybin, siliandrin, silybinome, and
silyhermin. Apigenin, silybonol, linoleic and oleic acids, myristic,
stearic and palmitic acids, betaine, histamine, triamine also are
found.

Actions
Silymarin exerts hepatoprotective and antihepatotoxic actions
over liver toxins, such as *Amanita phalloides* or other cyclopeptide-
containing mushrooms (*Galerina* and *Lepiota* species). Silymarin alters the outer liver membrane cell structure so that toxins cannot
enter the cell; it also stimulates RNA polymerase A, which enhances
ribosome protein synthesis and leads to activation of the regenera-
tive capacity of the liver through cell development. Another suggested protective mechanism is the inhibition of lipid peroxidation
through silymarin's free-radical-scavenging properties.

Reported uses
Milk thistle seeds or seed extracts are believed to be useful as a liver
"cleansing" agent. The extracts have been used as an antidote after
the accidental ingestion of *A. phalloides* and other poisonous mush-

rooms. Successful outcomes were noted in two human trials using silymarin after hepatotoxic mushroom ingestion (Flora, 1998).

In patients with psychotropic-drug-induced hepatic damage, silymarin improved liver function test results and blunted halothane hepatotoxicity. Data exist regarding the use of extracts in both acute and chronic liver disease. (See *Milk thistle and liver disease,* page 432.) There is anecdotal evidence about its use in hepatitis C and by liver transplant patients.

Dosage
The doses evaluated ranged from 420 to 800 mg P.O. daily as a single dose, or divided into two to three doses. The German Federal Institute for Drugs and Medical Devices recommends 200 to 400 mg of silymarin P.O. daily, calculated as the silibinin component.

Adverse reactions
- Mild laxative effect (with standardized extracts)
- Uterine and menstrual stimulation

Interactions
None reported.

Contraindications and precautions
Contraindicated in pregnant or breast-feeding patients. Use cautiously in patients with hypersensitivity to plants belonging to the Asteraceae family.

Special considerations
- Monitor liver function test results during therapy with milk thistle.
- Advise the patient to consult with a medical professional specialized in liver disease before pursuing this therapy.
- Advise the female patient to report planned or suspected pregnancy.
- Instruct the patient to report unusual symptoms immediately.

Points of interest
- The German Federal Institute for Drugs and Medical Devices approves the use of milk thistle for toxic liver and as supportive treatment in chronic inflammatory liver disease and hepatic cirrhosis.

Analysis
Recent studies and the traditional use of milk thistle for liver disorders in Europe suggest that this agent may play a role in preventing acute toxin-induced hepatic damage. Because there are no allopath-

RESEARCH FINDINGS
Milk thistle and liver disease

Milk thistle extract has been studied in the treatment of acute and chronic liver disease. In patients with acute alcoholic hepatitis, the extract caused more patients to normalize (as measured by hepatic transaminase concentrations) than controls and significantly reduced the time to normalization (Fintelmann and Albert, 1980). In a double-blind study, varying doses of silymarin improved liver function test results, reduced complications, hastened recovery, and shortened hospital stays in patients with acute viral hepatitis compared with placebo (Flora et al., 1998).

During a 6-month treatment period in patients with chronic alcoholic hepatitis, liver function test results normalized and liver histology improved compared with placebo (Feher et al., 1989; Salmi and Sarna, 1982). In a third trial of biopsy-confirmed cirrhotics, laboratory findings were not statistically different; however, mortality was significantly reduced in the treated group, and more so in certain patient groups. The largest trial involved over 2,500 patients with chronic liver disease and showed improvement in both objective and subjective parameters of liver function (Albrecht et al., 1992).

Most data supporting the use of silymarin in liver dysfunction are from foreign studies. These trials were flawed in design; they were inconsistent in measuring parameters of hepatic dysfunction and including a control group, sometimes failed to control alcohol intake, included patients with varied etiology and severity of disease, had small study populations in some trials, and used inconsistent definitions of endpoints and variable dosing regimens. Moreover, adverse effects of milk thistle extract are largely undefined.

Despite these limitations, the future of silymarin appears promising in the treatment of liver disease.

ic alternatives available that are hepatoprotective or antihepatoxic, a trial use of milk thistle may be warranted in life-threatening situations.

References

Albrecht, M., et al. "Therapy of Toxic Liver Pathologies with Legalon," *Z Klin Med* 47:87-92, 1992.

Feher, J., et al. "Hepatotprotective Activity of Silmarin (Legalon) Therapy in Patients with Chronic Liver Disease," *Orv Hetil* 130:2723-27, 1989.

Fintelmann, V., and Albert, A. "Nachweis der therapeutischen Wirksamkeit von Legalon bei Toxischen Lebererkrankungen im Doppelblindversuch," *Therapiewoche* 30:5589-94, 1980.

Flora, K., et al. "Milk Thistle *(Silybum marianum)* for the Therapy of Liver Disease," *Am J Gastroenterol* 93:139-43, 1998

Salmi, A., and Sarna, S. "Effect of Silymarin on Chemical, Functional, and Morphological Alterations of the Liver," *Scard J Gastroenterol* 174:517-21, 1982.

MINT

BALM MINT, BRANDY MINT, GREEN MINT, LAMB MINT, OUR LADY'S MINT, PEPPERMINT, SPEARMINT

Common trade names
(Various manufacturers) Ben-Gay, Rhuli Gel, Robitussin Cough Drops, Vicks VapoRub

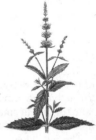

Common forms
Peppermint and spearmint are both available as liquid extracts, tea, oil, and inhalant preparations. Peppermint oil is also available as enteric-coated capsules. Menthol is an active component of several topical analgesics, anesthetics, and antipruritics; it is also available as an antitussive ointment, lozenge, and throat spray.

Source
The two best known and most cultivated members of the fragrant mint family are peppermint and spearmint. Peppermint *(Mentha x piperita)* is a hybrid between *Mentha spicata* (spearmint) and *M. aquatica* (watermint). The essential oils of peppermint and spearmint are extracted from the leaves and flowering tops of these plants. Both are members of the mint family (Labiatae), native to Europe and widely cultivated in the United States and Canada.

Chemical components
Peppermint oil is a volatile oil composed primarily of menthol. Menthol stereoisomers include neomenthol, menthone, menthofuran, eucalyptol, and limonene. Other components are methyl acetate, piperitone, tannins, flavonoids, and tocopherols. More than 100 other chemical components are found, but vary with growth stage, cultivation method, and geographic location. Spearmint oil contains carvone, limonene, phellandrene, and pinene; menthol is absent. Fresh leaves are reported to contain as much vitamin C as oranges and more provitamin A than carrots.

Actions

Peppermint essential oil is reported to have in vitro antibacterial and antiviral activity. It also relaxes the sphincter of Oddi and stimulates bile flow in animals; this choleretic effect is attributed to flavonoid components.

Most of peppermint's pharmacologic activity is due to menthol which, in concentrations of 0.1% to 1%, depresses sensory cutaneous receptors and alleviates itching and irritation. In higher concentrations, it acts as a counterirritant by stimulating the nerves that perceive cold while depressing the nerves that perceive pain and itching. When applied to the skin, menthol causes an initial feeling of coolness, followed by a sensation of warmth. The cooling effect may result from direct desensitization of warmth receptors, and warming follows vasodilation of small blood vessels under the skin (Jacknowitz, 1996).

Menthol also has a direct spasmolytic effect on smooth muscles of the digestive tract. Its spasmolytic activity is reportedly mediated through a calcium antagonist effect. Azulene (cyclopentacycloheptane) occurs in small amounts in peppermint oil and exerts antiinflammatory and antiulcerogenic effects in animals.

The medicinal action of spearmint is not documented in the literature. Although it is reported to have antispasmodic and antiflatulent properties similar to peppermint, its effects are weaker.

Reported uses

Peppermint is a popular medicinal and commercial mint with several uses. It is considered an antiflatulent, diaphoretic, stimulant, digestive aid, antiseptic, anesthetic, antiemetic, aromatic, and flavoring agent. The leaf is also a classic folk remedy for stomach cancer. Peppermint's antiflatulent and antispasmodic activities have been used for dyspepsia, flatulence, colic, diarrhea, indigestion, and abdominal pain. The enteric-coated capsules are reported to be effective for irritable bowel syndrome; however, efficacy data from European studies are inconclusive.

Menthol has been used traditionally to relieve the pain of rheumatism, neuralgia, headache, throat infections, and toothache by acting as a local anesthetic, vascular stimulant, disinfectant, antipruritic, antiseptic, and counterirritant. It is used externally in ointments, rubs, and liniments to treat itching, minor pain of sunburn, and musculoskeletal pain of neuralgia, rheumatism, and arthritis.

Menthol is also used in inhalant preparations to alleviate chest complaints, cold, cough, laryngitis, bronchitis, and nasal congestion. As a local anesthetic, menthol is used in sprays and lozenges for sore throat, and it is occasionally used to anesthetize gastric nerve endings in motion sickness and nausea.

Peppermint oil is widely used in flavoring, pharmaceuticals, cosmetics, toothpastes, and mouthwashes, as well as in local antiseptic, anesthetic, and antipruritic preparations. It is also gaining popularity in aromatherapy and is used to increase concentration and stimulating the mind and body.

Spearmint is mainly used as a flavoring agent, but it is also considered a milder antispasmodic and antiflatulent for colic and other digestive problems, and is claimed to be useful in tumors and stomach cancer. Spearmint is thought to whiten teeth, cure mouth sores, alleviate nausea and vomiting, heal the bites of a rabid dog, relieve pain of wasp stings, and repel rodents. Because its effects are less powerful than those of peppermint, it is considered to cause fewer problems in children.

Dosage

No consensus exists for spearmint preparations. Dosages below are for peppermint:

Capsules (enteric-coated): 1 to 2 capsules (0.2 ml/capsule) P.O. t.i.d. for irritable bowel syndrome.

Spirits (10% oil and 1% leaf extract): 1 ml (20 drops) with water.

Tea: 1 to 1.5 g (1 tablespoon) leaves in 160 ml boiling water, P.O. b.i.d. or t.i.d.

Topicals: apply t.i.d. or q.i.d.; for external use only.

The fatal dose of menthol in humans is estimated to be 1,000 mg/kg body weight (Murray, 1995).

Adverse reactions

- Allergic reactions (flushing, headache, heartburn, irritation of mucous membranes, muscle tremor, rash; with internal use)
- Contact dermatitis (with external use)
- Laryngeal or bronchial spasms (in infants, small children; with menthol in teas)
- Relaxation of lower esophageal sphincter and GI smooth muscle, worsened symptoms of gastroesophageal reflux disease and hiatal hernia

Interactions

None reported.

Contraindications and precautions

Use with caution; menthol can also cause sensitization and allergic reactions in adults and children. Symptoms include urticaria, erythema and other cutaneous lesions.

Special considerations

⚠ Peppermint oil has been shown to cause dose-related neurotoxicity and brain lesions in rats fed up to 100 mg/kg/day for 28 days (Olsen and Thorup, 1984).

⚠ Applying a mentholated ointment to an infant's nostrils for cold relief may cause a syncopal event.

• Warn the patient not to give peppermint or spearmint products to infants or small children.

• Caution the patient against applying topical mentholated products to broken skin.

• Instruct the patient not to use topical menthol preparations with a heating pad because skin damage may occur.

• Warn the patient to avoid prolonged use of peppermint oil as an inhalant.

• Advise the patient with gastroesophageal reflux disease to avoid taking mint products internally.

• Advise the female patient to avoid use of the herb during pregnancy or when breast-feeding.

Points of interest

• Peppermint-flavored toothpaste has been reported to exacerbate asthma symptoms in a young adult (Jacknowitz, 1996).

• Peppermint oil was dropped from nonprescription drug status in 1990 by the FDA Advisory Review Panel on OTC Miscellaneous Internal Drug Products because it lacked safety and efficacy information for use internally as a digestive aid.

Analysis

Peppermint and spearmint are used extensively as flavoring agents in foods, and in pharmaceuticals and cosmetics. Menthol is generally recognized as safe and effective when used externally as a local analgesic or anesthetic and as an antipruritic. Menthol is also approved as a topical antitussive agent and as an inhalant. The internal use of peppermint and spearmint for purposes other than flavoring is not recommended. Although these extracts have been reported to be beneficial for the treatment of some GI disorders, safety and efficacy data are still lacking. Similarly, there are no safety and efficacy data for the use of these agents in children.

References

Jacknowitz, A.I. "External Analgesic Products," in *Handbook of Nonprescription Drugs,* edited by Covington, T.R., et al. Washington, D.C.: American Pharmaceutical Association, 1996.

Murray, M. *The Healing Power of Herbs.* Rocklin, Calif.: Prima Publishing, 1995.

Olsen, P., and Thorup, I. "Neurotoxicity in Rats with Peppermint Oil and Pulegone," *Arch Toxicol Suppl* 7:408-09, 1984.

MISTLETOE

Common trade names
Iscador

Common forms
Available as dried leaves, capsules, infusion, liquid extract, tablets, and tincture.

Source
Active components are derived from the leaves, branches, and berries of European mistletoe, *Viscum album,* and related species *V. abietis* and *V. austriacum.* These plants live as parasites on tree branches and are native to England, Europe, and Asia. North American mistletoes, including *Phoradendron flavescens, P. serotinum,* and *P. tomentosum*, are primarily used as Christmas greens. They are also parasitic and commonly occur on fruit trees, poplars, and oaks.

Chemical components
Mistletoe plants contain amines, acetylcholine, choline, beta-phenylethylamine, histamine, tyramine, phoratoxins, viscotoxins, flavonoids, flavonol derivatives (quercetin), lectins, terpenoids, alkaloids, and acids. Other compounds include mucilage, polyols, sugars, starch, tannins, and syringin.

Actions
Mistletoe is claimed to have hypotensive, cardiac depressant, and sedative effects. Recent in vitro studies with *V. album* showed antineoplastic activity. The phoratoxins, viscotoxins, and various lectins display cytotoxic activity. Lectins are reported to increase the secretion of some interleukins and tumor necrosis factor (Hajto et al., 1990).

Iscador, prepared from the crude juice, caused a slight improvement in patients with colon malignancies and appeared to prolong survival in a patient with small-cell carcinoma of the lung (Bradley et al., 1989). Because the extract has relatively weak antineoplastic activity, it may be useful as an adjuvant therapy with surgery or radiotherapy. Other effects demonstrated by mistletoe include dose-dependent hypotension and hypertension, bradycardia, increased uterine activity, and increased GI motility.

Reported uses

Mistletoe has been claimed to be beneficial in treating malignancies, hypertension, arteriosclerosis, nervousness, tachycardia, hypertensive headache, epilepsy, tension, insomnia, depression, urinary disorders, sterility, and ulcers.

Dosage

Dried leaves: 2 to 6 g P.O. t.i.d.
Liquid extract (1:1 solution in 25% alcohol): 1 to 3 ml P.O. t.i.d.
Tincture (1:5 solution in 45% alcohol): 0.5 ml P.O. t.i.d.

Adverse effects

- Bradycardia
- Dehydration
- Delirium
- Diarrhea
- Gastroenteritis
- Hallucinations
- Hepatitis
- Hypotension, hypertension
- Mild pyrexia, mild leukocytosis
- Mydriasis
- Myosis
- Nausea
- Seizures
- Vomiting

⚠ Coma or cardiac arrest

Interactions

Antihypertensives: possible enhanced hypotensive effects of antihypertensive drugs. Avoid use together.
Cardiac drugs: possible increased cardiac depression. Avoid concomitant use.
CNS depressants: enhanced sedative effects. Avoid concomitant use.
Immunosuppressants: cytotoxic and immunostimulant effects. Do not use together.

Contraindications and precautions

Avoid use of the herb in pregnant or breast-feeding patients; two types of mistletoe have shown uterine stimulant activity in animals.

Special considerations

⚠ Know that all plant parts of mistletoe are toxic. Institute supportive emergency treatment for symptomatic patients.

• Monitor the patient taking mistletoe for dehydration or electrolyte imbalances.

• Warn the patient about the potential GI, cardiac, and CNS toxicity of this herb.

• Advise the patient taking mistletoe for malignancies that conventional treatments should be considered first.

⚠ Advise parents to keep mistletoe out of reach of children.

Analysis

Despite its known toxic effects, mistletoe continues to be used as a natural remedy. Some components have shown antineoplastic activity. However, additional clinical investigation is required to assess the plant's efficacy and long-term safety profile. Because I.V. mistletoe preparations are not standardized in the United States, it is unlikely that mistletoe will be considered for use as an antineoplastic agent in the near future.

References

Bradley, G.W., et al. "Apparent Response of Small Cell Lung Cancer to an Extract of Mistletoe and Homeopathic Treatment," *Thorax* 44:1047-48, 1989.

Hajto, T., et al. "Increased Secretion of Tumor Necrosis Factors Alpha, Interleukin 1, and Interleukin 6 by Human Mononuclear Cells Exposed to Beta-Galactoside-Specific Lectin from Clinically Applied Mistletoe Extract," *Cancer Res* 50:3322-26, 1990.

MOTHERWORT

I-MU-TS'AO, LION'S-EAR, LION'S-TAIL, LION'S-TART, THROWWORT

Common trade names
None known.

Common forms
Available as dried leaves and extracts.

Source
Extracts are obtained primarily from the seeds or nutlets contained in the dry and spinose flowering heads of *Leonurus cardiaca*. Active components of *L. artemisia* are extracted from the dried leaves. These members of the mint family (Labiatae) have been naturalized to the United States and Canada from Europe. Other species that may be referred to as motherwort include *L. glaucescens, L. hetero-phyllus, L. quinquelobatus,* and *L. sibiricus.*

Chemical components

Extracts of various *Leonurus* species have yielded active substances, such as alkaloids, cardanolides, flavones, saponins, and phenyl-propanoid glycosides (from *L. artemisia*). Furanoids derivatives have been purified from *L. cardiaca,* nitrate compounds have been isolated from *L. quinquelobatus,* and guanidine derivatives have been isolated from *L. sibiricus.*

Actions

Few data exist on the therapeutic action of *L. cardiaca.* The herb possesses CV effects, including inhibition of pulsating myocardial cells in vitro, improving coronary and microcirculation in rats, and having platelet-aggregation inhibitory effects in rats (Xia, 1983). *L. quinquelobatus* may exert CNS effects in animals, including slowing the heart rate and increasing the force of cardiac contractility. *L. artemisia* has shown uterotonic effects in the rat uterus in vitro.

Human studies performed with *L. heterophyllus* noted decreased blood viscosity and fibrinogen volume, increased RBC flexibility, and decreased platelet aggregation (Zou, 1989). It is possible that the anticoagulant effect may be attributed to prehispanolone, a motherwort component.

Anti-inflammatory and antineoplastic activity has also been noted in animal models. A Russian study reported possible antioxidant properties in humans (Bol'shakova, 1997).

Reported uses

This herb has long been used as a remedy for cardiac conditions such as palpitations; hence the name *cardiaca.* It has also been used as a uterotonic to assist in childbirth and as a pain reliever for menstrual cramping. These claims have not been confirmed by human therapeutic trials.

Dosage

No consensus exists.

Adverse reactions

- Increased bleeding time
- Photosensitivity (at high doses)

Interactions

Beta blockers, digoxin, other cardiac medications: decreased heart rate and increased contractility (in animals). Avoid concomitant use.
Heparin, warfarin: risk for increased bleeding effects. Avoid concomitant use.

Contraindications and precautions
Contraindicated during pregnancy because of its potential utero-tonic and prostaglandin synthesis effects. Also contraindicated in patients with thrombocytopenia.

Special considerations
• Advise the patient using this herb to avoid direct sunlight.
• Tell the patient to report signs of unusual bruising or bleeding.

Analysis
Although some studies suggest that motherwort may have promising antineoplastic and antioxidant properties, further investigation and clinical trials are needed to support any therapeutic claims.

References
Bol'shakova, I.V. "Antioxidant Properties of a Series of Extracts from Medicinal Plants," *Biofizika* 42:480-83, 1997.
Xia, Y.X. "The Inhibitory Effect of Motherwort Extract on Pulsating Myocardial Cells In Vitro," *J Tradit Chin Med* 3:185-88, 1983.
Zou, Q.Z. "Effect of Motherwort on Blood Viscosity," *Am J Chin Med.* 17:65-70, 1989.

MUGWORT

AI YE, FELON HERB, ST. JOHN'S PLANT, *SUMMITATES ARTEMISIAE*, WILD WORMWOOD

Common trade names
None known.

Common forms
Available as dried leaves and roots, fluid extract, infusion, and tincture.

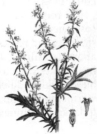

Source
The dried herb is obtained from the leaves and roots of *Artemisia vulgaris,* a shrubby perennial and member of the daisy family (Compositae) native to North America. The herb should not be confused with wormwood (*Artemisia absinthium*).

Chemical components
The volatile oil contains camphor, thujone, linalool, 1,8-cineole, 4-terpineol, borneol, spathulenol, alpha-cadinol, and monoterpene. Other components include sesquiterpenes, sesquiterpene lactones

(including the eudesmane derivative vulgarin, also known as tau-remisin), psilostachyin, psilostachyin C, flavonol glycosides (including quercetin and rutin), coumarins (including aesuletin, aesculin, umbelliferone, scopoletin, coumarin, and 6-methoxy-7,8-methyl-ene-dioxycoumarin), polyacetylenes, pentacyclic triterpenes, sitosterol, stigmasterol, and carotenoids.

Actions

Mugwort is reported to have analgesic, anthelmintic, antibacterial, antiflatulent, antifungal, antirheumatic, antiseptic, aphrodisiac, appetite stimulant, bile stimulant, CNS depressant, counterirritant, diaphoretic, digestive, diuretic, emetic, expectorant, hemostatic, laxative, sedative, uterine stimulant, and uterine vasodilator activities.

Reported uses

Mugwort was used similarly to wormwood (*A. absinthium*), namely as an anthelmintic and for amenorrhea and dysmenorrhea. It is used in Chinese traditional medicine for *moxa* treatments (moxibustion), in which small cones of dried mugwort leaves are burned in cups on certain points of the body, many of which coincide with acupuncture points. Moxibustion is growing in popularity in the United States.

Mugwort is also used to treat GI conditions such as colic, diarrhea, constipation, cramps, and weak digestion. It has also been used to treat hysteria, epilepsy, persistent vomiting, seizures in children, circulatory problems, menopausal and menstrual complaints, chills, fever, rheumatism, mild depression, and stress.

The roots are claimed to be useful as a tonic and for psychoneuroses, neurasthenia, depression, hypochondria, neuroses, general irritability and restlessness, insomnia, and anxiety. Other uses include anorexia, asthma, dermatitis, dysentery, flatulence, gout, headache, hematemesis, hemoptysis, infertility, muscle spasm, neuralgia, nosebleed, opium addiction, pinworms, roundworm, snakebite, threadworms, and whitlow. The essential oil is purported to have antibacterial and antifungal properties.

Dosage

For stress, 5 ml P.O. root tincture taken 30 minutes before bedtime.
For heavy menstruation, infusion of 15 g of dried herb added to 500 ml water P.O., or as tincture, up to 2.5 ml P.O. t.i.d.
As an appetite stimulant, 150 ml boiling water poured over 1 to 2 teaspoons of the dried herb, allowed to steep for 5 to 10 minutes, and then strained. Two to three cups of the tea is taken before meals.
For other complaints, 1 to 4 ml tincture P.O. t.i.d.

Adverse reactions
• Anaphylaxis
• Contact dermatitis
⚠ Mugwort may have significant uterine stimulant effects.

Interactions
Anticoagulants: may potentiate effects of the anticoagulant. Avoid concomitant use.

Contraindications and precautions
Contraindicated in pregnant or breast-feeding patients and in those with bleeding abnormalities. Avoid use in patients with previous sensitization or hazelnut allergy. Use cautiously in patients with reflux disease.

Special considerations
• Be aware that mugwort pollen is a known allergen contributing to hay fever in some patients. It has caused IgE cross-reactivity with hazelnut (Caballero et al., 1997).
• Know that patients with a sensitivity to mugwort pollen may be allergic to other foods in the Compositae family (Garcia Ortiz et al., 1996).
• Caution the patient taking anticoagulants against use of this herb.
• Warn the pregnant or breast-feeding patient to avoid use of mugwort.
• Inform the patient about the lack of clinical safety and efficacy data of mugwort.

Analysis
Because there are no clinical data to support mugwort's several therapeutic claims, it cannot be recommended for any use.

References
Caballero, T., et al. "IgE Crossreactivity Between Mugwort Pollen (*Artemisia vulgaris*) and Hazelnut (*Abellana nux*) in Sera from Patients with Sensitivity to Both Extracts," *Clin Exp Allergy* 27:1203-11, 1997. Abstract.
Garcia Ortiz, J.C., et al. "Allergy to Foods in Patients Monosensitized to *Artemisia* Pollen," *Allergy* 51:927-31, 1996.

MULLEIN
AARON'S ROD, BUNNY'S EARS, CANDLEWICK, FLANNEL-LEAF, GREAT MULLEIN, JACOB'S-STAFF

Common trade names
Mullein Flower Oil, Mullein Leaves, Verbascum Complex

Common forms

Capsules: 290 mg, 330 mg (leaf)
Flower oil: 1 oz, 2 oz
Liquid extract: 250 mg (2 oz)

Source

The crude drug is obtained from the dried leaves and flowers of *Verbascum thapsus,* a tall, biennial herb of the Snapdragon family (Scrophulariaceae). The plant is native to Europe and Asia and naturalized to the United States; it is easily noted by its characteristic fuzzy leaves and yellow flower spikes.

Chemical components

Mullein contains saponins, an iridioid glycoside (verbascoside), and several carbohydrates. Bitter amorphous substances and mucilage are found in the leaves; the seeds contain hemolytic saponins but no alkaloids. Flavonoids have also been noted.

Actions

The pharmacology of verbascoside, an iridoid glycoside isolated from *V. thapsus,* is being studied. Preliminary studies suggest that it may have significant antioxidant, anti-inflammatory, and antitumor effects. The presence of four phenolic hydroxyl groups in the structure of verbascoside may contribute to its antioxidant activity (Zheng et al, 1993).

Because verbascoside also inhibits 5-lipooxygenase, the enzyme that catalyzes formation of inflammatory leukotrienes, it may play a role in inflammatory and allergic diseases. Some glycosides of *V. thapsus* also have documented antitumor effects. One in vitro study found that verbascoside has cytotoxic effects on rat hepatoma and sarcoma cells and cytostatic activity on human epithelial carcinoma cells (Saracoglu et al., 1995).

Reported uses

Therapeutic claims for mullein include use as a demulcent, expectorant, and antitussive. It is believed to tone the mucous membranes of the respiratory system, increasing fluid production and thus promoting a productive cough. It has been combined with white horehound, coltsfoot, and lobelia for bronchitis; elder and red clover for coughs; and with gumweed for asthma. An extract of mullein prepared with olive oil and applied externally is used for healing and soothing inflamed surfaces. This oil has also been used in the ear to stimulate secretion of cerumen and systemically to control painful urination in lithemia, chronic cystitis, and urinary calculi.

Dosage

Capsules: two 290-mg capsules with two meals daily, or as needed.
Flower oil: 5 to 10 drops.
Leaves: mix 1 cup of boiling water with 1 to 2 teaspoons of the dried leaves and let steep for 10 to 15 minutes. Decant and drink tea t.i.d.

Adverse reactions

• Contact dermatitis
• Sedation

Interactions

None reported.

Contraindications and precautions

Avoid use of the herb in children and in pregnant or breast-feeding patients; effects are unknown. Also contraindicated in patients who have developed hypersensitivity reactions to the herb.

Special considerations

• Advise the female patient to avoid use of the herb during pregnancy or when breast-feeding.
• Remind the patient that clinical data about mullein products are lacking.

Points of interest

• During the 19th century, dried flowers or roots of mullein were smoked for treatment of respiratory diseases and asthma symptoms, a practice copied from the Mohegan and Penobscot Indians.

Analysis

Clinical data do not support use of mullein for the treatment of chronic respiratory conditions or for the other therapeutic claims made. Although preliminary data suggest that glycosides might have therapeutic value, human studies have not confirmed initial results. Because of the lack of information regarding treatment, this herb cannot be recommended for routine use.

References

Saracoglu, I., et al. "Studies on Components with Cytotoxic and Cytostatic Activity of Two Turkish Medicinal Plants," *Biol Pharm Bull* 18:1396-400, 1995.

Zheng, R.L., et al. "Inhibition of the Autooxidation of Linoleic Acid by Phenyl-propanoid Glycosides from *Pedicularis* in Micelles," *Chem Phys Lipids* 65:151-54, 1993.

MUSTARD

BLACK MUSTARD, BROWN MUSTARD, CALIFORNIA RAPE,
CHARLOCK, CHINESE MUSTARD, INDIAN MUSTARD,
WHITE MUSTARD, WILD MUSTARD

Common trade names
(Available in combination) Act-On Rub, Musterole

Common forms
Available as a tea, ground mustard seeds (mustard flour), and mustard oil.

Source
The active component is the volatile oil, derived from the seeds by steam distillation or expression. Black and white mustard plants (*Brassica nigra* and *B. alba*) are native to the southern Mediterranean area. Other *Brassica* species occur in eastern Europe, India, and the Middle East. White mustard is also referred to as *Sinapis alba*.

Chemical components
Components include sinigrin (potassium myronate), myrosin, sinapic acid, sinapine, fixed oils (erucic, eicosenoic, arachic, oleic, and palmitic acid glucosides), globulins, and mucilage. Most mustards contain allyl isothiocyanate and p-hydroxybenzyl isothiocyanate precursors in their volatile oils. Sinigrin releases allyl isothiocyanate when in contact with myrosin.

Actions
Potent local irritant effects allow mustard to serve as a rubefacient when applied topically. Irritation and copious tearing in the eyes can be attributed to allyl isothiocyanate. Isothiocyanate compounds have produced goiter in animals. The volatile mustard oil has strong antimicrobial properties. Sinigrin has been reported to have antilarvicidal properties against some insects.

Mustard oil has been reported to exhibit anticarcinogenic effects in animals with arsenic-induced chromosomal aberrations. This effect was greater than that seen with garlic extract (Choudhury et al., 1997).

Reported uses
Anecdotally, mustard has been used in footbaths for rheumatism and arthritis of the feet, and topically to alleviate muscle aches and pains. The herb has also been used as a stimulant, diuretic, emetic, and antiflatulent, and both orally and topically to the chest to relieve pulmonary congestion.

Dosage

As a footbath, mix 1 tablespoon of mustard seeds with 1 L of hot water as a soak.

As a topical rubefacient, prepare a paste with 120 g (4 oz) of ground black mustard seeds in warm water. Irritant effect can be eased by applying olive oil after the paste is removed.

Adverse reactions

• Severe contact irritation of skin and mucous membranes

Contraindications and precautions

Contraindicated in pregnant or breast-feeding patients; effects are unknown. Use cautiously in patients with pulmonary disease because inhalation may aggravate airways.

Special considerations

⚠ Because of its toxic nature, volatile mustard oil should never be tasted or inhaled in undiluted form.

• Caution the patient to use care when preparing mustard herbal products and to wash hands after using products to avoid contact with eyes.

• Warn the patient not to apply mustard preparations to mucous membranes.

• Advise parents to keep mustard products out of the reach of children and pets.

Points of interest

• Mustard flour typically lacks the characteristic pungent aroma when dry, but the aroma is released upon contact with water, which frees allyl isothiocyanate by hydrolysis.

• White mustard does not contain the toxic allyl isothiocyanate.

• The highest average maximum level of mustard oil in foods is about 0.02%.

• Topical application of white mustard seed as a poultice is approved in Germany for pulmonary congestion and joint and soft-tissue inflammation.

Analysis

The unique pungent properties of mustard entice people to use it as an herbal remedy. However, if not handled properly, mustard can damage the tissues. Although white mustard has been used in Germany, data regarding its use are not available.

References

Choudhury, A.R., et al. "Mustard Oil and Garlic Extract as Inhibitors of Sodium Arsenite-Induced Chromosomal Breaks in Vivo," *Cancer Lett* 121:45-52, 1997.

MYRRH

African myrrh, Arabian myrrh, bal, bol, bola, gum myrrh, heerabol, Somali myrrh, Yemen myrrh

Common trade names
Astring-O-Sol, Myrrh Gum, Odara
Also available in combination with Goldenseal.

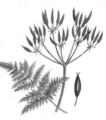

Common forms
Available in capsules (525 mg, 650 mg), salves, mouthwashes, tinctures, and fluid extracts.

Source
Myrrh is a mixture of volatile oil, gum, and resin (oleo-gum-resin) obtained from *Commiphora molmol* and other *Commiphora* species. These shrubs belong to the Bursera family (Burseraceae) and are native to Ethiopia, Somalia, and the Arabian Peninsula.

Chemical components
Myrrh is composed of volatile oils (dipentene, cadinene, heerabolene, limonene, pinene, eugenol, m-creosol, cinnamaldehyde, cuminaldehyde, cumic alcohol), resin (commiphoric acid), steroids (campesterol, cholesterol, beta-sitosterol), terpenoids (particularly alpha-amyrin), and gum.

Actions
Myrrh is reported to have antimicrobial, astringent, antiseptic, antiflatulent, and expectorant properties. Anti-inflammatory and antipyretic activity has been noted in rodents. Myrrh extracts, alone and with other plants, have shown hypoglycemic activity, perhaps by involving increased target cell glucose use and decreased gluconeogenesis (Al-Awadi and Gumaa, 1987).

A lipid (guggulipid) from a related plant, *Commiphora mukul,* appeared to reduce serum cholesterol and associated lipid parameters in some patients (Malhotra and Ahuja, 1971) and to affect thyroid metabolism in baby chicks (Tripathi et al., 1975).

Reported uses

Myrrh has been used for aphthous ulcers, gingivitis, pharyngitis, pulmonary congestion, wounds, and abrasions. It has also been incorporated into salves used externally for hemorrhoids, bed sores, and wounds. Myrrh is primarily used today as a fragrance and flavoring agent.

Anecdotally, myrrh has been used with *Echinacea* for infections, and in mouthwash to treat ulcers. It has also been combined with witch hazel for external use. External preparations with myrrh, golden seal root powder, and marigold flowers have been claimed to be useful for their antimicrobial activity in patients with HIV infection or AIDS.

Dosage

Tea: add 1 to 2 teaspoons resin to 1 cup boiling water, allow to steep for 10 to 15 minutes and take P.O. t.i.d.
Tincture: dissolve resin in alcohol; 1 to 4 ml of the tincture can be applied externally t.i.d.

Adverse reactions

- Dermatitis (conflicting reports)
- Hiccups, diarrhea, restlessness (reported with *C. mukul*)

Interactions

Insulin, sulfonylureas: may enhance hypoglycemic effects when used together. Monitor serum glucose.

Contraindications and precautions

Avoid use of the herb in pregnant or breast-feeding patients, effects are unknown.

Special considerations

- Monitor the patient prone to hypoglycemia closely if this herb is being used.
- Explain that few clinical data exist on human use of myrrh.
- Tell the patient to immediately report signs and symptoms of hypoglycemia.
- Advise the female patient to avoid use of the herb during pregnancy or when breast-feeding.

Points of interest

- The Federal Register recommended that myrrh tincture not be recognized as safe and effective. It should be considered misbranded if labeled as an item for oral health care.

Analysis

Insufficient human data exist to support any therapeutic application of myrrh. Potential applications in HIV infection require thorough clinical investigation. A related plant, *C. mukul,* appears to reduce serum lipids, but this also requires further study.

References

Al-Awadi, F.M., and Gumaa, K.A. "Studies on the Activity of Individual Plants of an Antidiabetic Plant Mixture," *Acta Diabetol Lat* 24:37-41, 1987.

Malhotra, S.C., and Ahuja, M.M. "Comparative Hypolipidemic Effectiveness of Gum Guggulu (*Commiphora mukul)* Fraction, Alpha-ethyl-p-chlorophenoxyisobutyrate, and Cica-13437-Su," *Indian J Med Res* 59:1621-32, 1971.

Tripathi, S.N., et al. "Effect of a Keto-Steroid of *Commiphora mukul* on Hypercholesterolemia and Hyperlipidemia Induced by Neomercazole and Cholesterol Mixture in Chicks," *Indian J Exp Biol* 13:15-18, 1975.

MYRTLE

BRIDAL MYRTLE, COMMON MYRTLE, DUTCH MYRTLE, JEW'S MYRTLE, MIRTIL, ROMAN MYRTLE

Common trade names

None known.

Common forms

Available as extracts.

Source

Active components are derived from the seeds and leaves of *Myrtus communis*, a plant native to the Mediterranean and the Middle East. This plant should not be confused with Madagascar myrtle (*Eugenia jambolana)* or common periwinkle (*Vinca minor).*

Chemical components

The volatile oil contains myrtol or gelomyrtol as well as eucalyptol, dextro-pinene, and camphor. Tannins and polyphenolic compounds have also been found in the leaves.

Actions

An alcoholic extract of myrtle demonstrated weak anti-inflammatory activity in animal models (Al-Hindawi et al., 1989). Myrtle extract showed unique hypoglycemic properties in mice (Elfellah et al., 1984). A leaf tincture may minimize antibiotic resistance to some pathogenic staphylococci (Pochinok et al., 1968).

Reported uses

Myrtle has been used as an astringent antiseptic for wounds, a pulmonary decongestant, and a tonic for digestive and urinary disorders. Although myrtle has been investigated as an antidiabetic agent, this effect has not been adequately documented in humans. Phytohemagglutinins from myrtle seeds have been used to reduce turbidity of lipemic sera, enabling spectrophotometric determination of serum glucose, bilirubin, uric acid, hepatic transaminases, and other components of the sera (Ortega and Rodenas, 1979).

Dosage

Suggested dosage is 1 to 2 ml essential oil P.O. daily.

Adverse reactions

- Allergic reactions
- Hypoglycemia

Interactions

Drugs undergoing significant detoxification through the cytochrome P-450 system of the liver: may enhance hepatic microsomal enzyme function (in animals). Monitor response to drug therapy.
Insulin, oral sulfonylureas: may potentiate hypoglycemic effects. Use cautiously.

Contraindications and precautions

Avoid use of the herb in pregnant or breast-feeding patients; effects are unknown. Use cautiously in diabetic patients.

Special considerations

- Tell the patient not to take the essential oil internally except under the supervision of the health care provider.
- Advise the female patient to avoid use of the herb during pregnancy or when breast-feeding.
- Monitor blood glucose levels and liver function tests.
- Warn the diabetic patient that myrtle may enhance hypoglycemic therapy and affect the metabolism of other drugs.

Points of interest

- Myrtle is used as a dye in some regions of Greece.

Analysis

Although myrtle shows some promise as an antidiabetic agent in animals, human clinical data are lacking. Therefore, this herb cannot be recommended for any therapeutic use.

References

Al-Hindawi, M.K., et al. "Anti-inflammatory Activity of Some Iraqi Plants Using Intact Rats," *J Ethnopharmacol* 26:163-68, 1989.

Elfellah, M.S., et al. "Anti-hyperglycemic Effect of an Extract of *Myrtus communis* in Streptozotocin-Induced Diabetes in Mice," *J Ethnopharmacol* 11:275-81, 1984.

Ortega, M., and Rodenas, S. "*Myrtus communis* L. Phytohemagglutinins as a Clarifying Agent for Lipemic Sera," *Clin Chim Acta* 92:135-39, 1979.

Pochinok, V., et al. "Possibility of Control of Resistance to Antibiotics of Pathogenic Staphylococci by the Tincture of *Myrtus communis* Leaves," *Farm Zh* 23:72-74, 1968. Abstract.

NETTLE

COMMON NETTLE, GREATER NETTLE, STINGING NETTLE

Common trade names
Nettles Capsules, Nettles Liquid Extract

Common forms
Available as capsules (150 mg, 300 mg) and dried leaf and root extract or tincture.

Source
The active chemical components are found in the leaves, stems, and roots of *Urtica dioica,* a perennial herb of the nettle family (Urticaceae). It is one of three species native to Europe, and is naturalized throughout the United States and parts of Canada.

Chemical components
Nettle roots and flowers contain scopoletin, steryl derivatives, lignan glucosides, and flavonol glycosides. In addition, the roots contain phenylpropanes and lignans, and the plant has B-group vitamins as well as C and K, and steroid-related compounds such as sitosterol. The stinging, hairlike projections on the stems contain amines, such as histamine, serotonin, and choline, and formic acid. The lectin found in the roots is specific to this plant and may help to standardize preparations.

Actions
Nettle acts primarily as a diuretic by increasing urine volume and decreasing systolic blood pressure. It has been observed to stimulate uterine contractions in rabbits, although the mechanism is unknown.

Other compounds identified have known pharmacologic activity. The *Urtica dioica* agglutinin (UDA), a lectin protein, has immunostimulating activity. Scopoletin has anti-inflammatory activity. A 20% methanolic extract of stinging nettle roots inhibited benign prostatic hyperplasia (BPH) in mice (Lichius and Muth, 1997). The plant extract was effective in reducing urine flow, nocturia, and residual urine in human patients.

Reported uses

Nettle has been used to treat rheumatism and is claimed to be help-ful as an antispasmodic and expectorant. The leaves have been smoked to treat asthma. Nettle tea has been used to treat cough and tuberculosis. The juice has been applied to the scalp to stimulate hair growth. The plant's styptic or astringent action has been useful for treating nosebleeds and uterine bleeding. Other claims include treatment of diabetes, gout, cancer, and eczema and for wound heal-ing.

Nettle's diuretic properties have prompted its use in hyperten-sion, heart failure, and urinary, bladder, and kidney disorders. It was studied with other herbs as a bladder irrigant for the treatment of prostatic adenoma in humans and was found to reduce postopera-tive blood loss, bacteriuria, and inflammation. The German Com-mission E recognizes this irrigant for the treatment of urinary tract inflammation and prevention and treatment of kidney gravel. Nettle is widely used in Germany for the early treatment of BPH and has been shown to be effective for treating allergic rhinitis (Mittman, 1990).

Dosage

For allergic rhinitis, 150 to 300 mg capsules P.O.
Tea: mix 1 to 2 teaspoons dried herb in 1 cup boiling water; take up to 2 cups daily.
Tincture: ¼ to 1 teaspoon up to b.i.d.

Adverse reactions

• Contact urticaria (leaves)
With internal use:
• Decreased urine volume
• Diarrhea
• Edema
• Gastric irritation
• Oliguria
• Stomach irritation

Interactions

Diuretics: may potentiate effects. Avoid concomitant use.

Contraindications and precautions

Contraindicated in pregnant or breast-feeding women because of its diuretic and uterine stimulation properties. Also contraindicated in children under age 2. Use cautiously, and in reduced doses, in older children and adults over age 65.

Special considerations
- Advise the patient to eat foods high in potassium, such as bananas and fresh vegetables, to replenish electrolytes lost through diuresis.
- Caution the patient against self-medicating with nettle for BPH or to relieve fluid accumulation associated with heart failure without approval and supervision of a health care professional.

⚠ If rubbed against the skin, nettles can cause intense burning for up to 12 hours or more. Tell the patient to wash thoroughly with soap and water, use antihistamines and steroid creams, and wear heavy gloves if the plant is to be handled.

Points of interest
- The FDA considers this herb to be of "undefined safety."
- Nettle plants were used in weaving in the Bronze Age; archeologists have found burial shrouds made of nettle fabric.
- Nettle juice was an ingredient in hair-growth preparations in the 19th century.
- Native American women believed nettle tea eased delivery and stopped uterine bleeding after childbirth

Analysis
Despite its traditional use for several conditions, the only proven pharmacologic action of nettle is as a diuretic. It is considered relatively safe in the amounts recommended and adverse effects from the oral form are rare. The herb has been studied in the treatment of BPH and allergic rhinitis and as a component in postoperative bladder irrigation. More studies are needed to determine its role in BPH and allergic rhinitis.

References
Lichius, J.J., and Muth, C. "The Inhibiting Effects of *Urtica dioica* Root Extracts on Experimentally Induced Prostatic Hyperplasia in the Mouse," *Planta Med* 63:307-10, 1997.

Mittman, P., "Randomized, Double-Blind Study of Freeze-Dried *Urtica dioica* in the Treatment of Allergic Rhinitis," *Planta Med* 56:44-47, 1990.

NIGHT-BLOOMING CEREUS
CACTUS GRANDIFLORUS, *CEREUS GRANDIFLORUS*, LARGE-FLOWERED CACTUS, QUEEN OF THE NIGHT, SWEET-SCENTED CACTUS, VANILLA CACTUS

Common trade names
(Various manufacturers; available in combination) Cactus Grandiflorus, Cactus-Hawthorn Compound, Cereus Grandiflorus, Night-Blooming Cereus

Common forms
Available as liquid extract and tincture.

Source
Active components are derived from stems and flowers of *Seleni-cereus grandiflorus,* which is native to tropical and subtropical America, including the West Indies.

Chemical components
The plant contains a digitalis-like glycoside, either cactine or horde-nine (N,N-dimethyl-4-hydroxy-beta-phenethylamine). Other re-ported components include betacyanin, isorhamnetin-3-glucoside, narcissin, rutin, cacticine, kaempferitrin, grandiflorine, hyperoside, isorhamnetin-3-beta-galactosyl-rutinoside, and isorhamnetin-3-beta-xylosyl-rutinoside.

Actions
Night-blooming cereus is thought to elevate arteriolar tension by increasing the muscular energy of the heart and causing arteriolar contraction. However, this theory has not been confirmed by hu-man data. Early research with commercial preparations of the active compound proved it to be physiologically inert. More recently, in studies with rats and dogs, hordenine showed a positive inotropic effect on the heart, with increased systolic and diastolic blood pres-sures and peripheral blood flow volume (Hapke, 1995). Flavonoids and their derivatives (rutin, rutinoside, and kaempferitrin) are thought to improve capillary function by decreasing abnormal leak-age (Wadworth and Faulds, 1992).

Reported uses
In Europe, the liquid plant extract has been used to treat angina pectoris, irritable bladder, heart palpitations, kidney congestion, nervous headache, and prostatic diseases. The herb has been used as an antirheumatic and cardiotonic in Cuba. Other indications for its use include cystitis, edema, dyspnea, endocarditis, and myocardi-tis. Anecdotal reports claim the herb to be valuable as a cardiac stimulant and partial substitute for digitalis in heart disorders relat-ed to dyspepsia, neurasthenia, anemia, Graves' disease, and tobacco toxicity.

Dosage
Liquid extract: 0.7 ml (12 minims) P.O. every 4 hours.
Tincture: 1 to 1.8 ml (15 to 30 minims) P.O. every 4 hours.

Adverse reactions
• Burning sensation in the mouth

- Diarrhea
- Nausea
- Vomiting

Interactions
Cardiac glycosides: may potentiate the actions of digoxin or digitoxin within the heart. Avoid concomitant use.
Other cardiac drugs (ACE inhibitors, antiarrhythmics, beta blockers, calcium channel blockers): may enhance effect. Avoid concomitant use.

Contraindications and precautions
Contraindicated during the first three months of pregnancy.

Special considerations
- Monitor the patient's heart rate and blood pressure if other prescription cardiac drugs are being taken.
- Emphasize that patients with CV disorders should be evaluated by a health care professional and, if necessary, receive prescribed medications. Because the use of night-blooming cereus as a substitute for digitalis has not been confirmed by human clinical trials, it should not be used by itself for heart-related disorders.
- Warn the patient to immediately report heart-related adverse effects (palpitations, increased heart rate, or blood pressure changes) to his health care professional.
- Instruct the female patient to report planned or suspected pregnancy.
- Advise the female patient to avoid use of the herb during pregnancy or when breast-feeding.

Analysis
Although night-blooming cereus contains a digitalis-like glycoside, its use as a substitute for digitalis preparations (digoxin or digitoxin) or treatment of heart-related disorders has not been evaluated in humans. Patients with such conditions should strongly be encouraged to seek professional medical advice. Additionally, patients currently taking prescription digitalis or other cardiac medications should avoid concurrent use of this herb.

References
Hapke, H.J. "Pharmacological Effects of Hordenine," *DTW - Deutsche Tierarztliche Wochenschrift* 102:228-32, 1995. Abstract in English.
Wadworth, A.N., and Faulds, D. "Hydroxyethylrutosides: A Review of Pharmacology and Therapeutic Efficacy in Venous Insufficiency and Related Disorders," *Drugs* 44:1013-32, 1992.

NUTMEG
MACE, MACIS, MUSCADIER, MUSKATBAUM, MYRISTICA,
NOZ MOSCADA, NUEZ MOSCADA, NUX MOSCHATA

Common trade names
(Various manufacturers; available in combination) Agua del Carmen, Aluminum Free Indigestion, Incontinurina, Klosterfrau Magentonikum, Melisana, Nervospur, Vicks Vaporub

Common forms
Available as capsules (200 mg), powders, and essential oil.

Source
Nutmeg is the dried kernel of seeds of the nutmeg tree, *Myristica fragrans*. Inside the fruit lies a netlike substance, the aril, from which another spice (mace) is produced. The aril is wrapped around the brittle shells containing the nutmeg kernel. Nutmeg trees grow in Sri Lanka, the West Indies, and the Molucca Islands.

Chemical components
Nutmeg seeds contain a fixed oil (nutmeg butter), consisting of myristic acid and glycerides of lauric, tridecanoic, stearic, and palmitic acids. Also present is an essential oil composed of d-camphene, dipentene, myristicin, elemicin, and small amounts of iso-elemicin, gerianiol, eugenol, isoeugenol, d-pinene, l-pinene, borneol, safrole, limonene, sabinene, cymene alpha-thujene, gamma-terpinene, lysergide, and monoterpene alcohols.

Actions
Nutmeg's components eugenol and isoeugenol may cause inhibition of renal prostaglandin synthesis in rats (Misra et al., 1978). Much preliminary data surround nutmeg's claim as an antidiarrheal agent (Barrowman et al., 1975; Shafran and McCrone, 1975). Components of nutmeg have been shown to impair release of toxins from *Escherichia coli* bacteria. The herb may have value in veterinary medicine as an antidiarrheal agent in cattle.

Total cholesterol levels were found to be significantly reduced, and platelet aggregation inhibited in albino rabbits after receiving an ethanolic extract of nutmeg for 60 days (Ram et al., 1996). Nutmeg's potent hallucinogenic effect is thought to be attributed to lysergide, borneol, eugenol, geraniol, and safrol (Giannini et al., 1986); it is often sought by recreational drug users when stronger chemicals, such as LSD, cannot be obtained.

Reported uses

Commonly used as a cooking spice, nutmeg has also been used as an antiemetic or aphrodisiac, and for indigestion and other gastric disorders, chronic nervous disorders, and kidney disorders. The essential oil is claimed to be useful for rheumatic pain, toothaches, and bad breath. Although nutmeg is used for GI disorders in Germany, its use is controversial. Homeopathy supports the use of nutmeg for anxiety or depression.

Dosage

Some suggested doses are within the hazardous range.
For nausea, gastric upset, and chronic diarrhea, 1 to 2 capsules of nutmeg "kernel" P.O. as a single dose, or 3 to 5 drops of essential oil on a sugar lump or a teaspoon of honey P.O., or 4 to 6 tablespoons powder P.O. daily (for diarrhea).
For toothache, 1 to 2 drops of essential oil applied to gum around aching tooth until dental visit.

Adverse effects

• Euphoria, hallucinations, delusions (with excessive doses)
With ingestion of nutmeg oil or doses over 5 g:
• Confusion
• Constipation
• Dry mouth
• Flushing
• Nausea
• Stupor
• Tachycardia
• Vomiting
⚠ Miscarriage
⚠ Seizures
⚠ Death has occurred. Symptoms of overdose include hypothermia, faint pulse, confusion, nausea, vomiting, chest or abdominal pressure, and extended periods of alternating bouts of delusions and somnolence. Anticholinergic hyperstimulation, palpitations, and psychosis may also occur. Treatment consists of gastric lavage and supportive therapy (Abernethy and Beckel, 1992).

Interactions

Antidiarrheals: may cause additive effects. Monitor bowel function.
Neuroleptic agents (haldol, thiothixene, olanzapine, clozapine): possible loss of symptom control in patients taking these drugs or interference with existing therapy for psychiatric illnesses. Avoid concomitant use.

Contraindications and precautions

Contraindicated in pregnant or breast-feeding patients; nutmeg may cause a miscarriage. Use cautiously in patients with psychiatric illnesses.

Special considerations

- Monitor patient for CNS effects.
- Monitor patient's bowel habits if used as an antidiarrheal.
- Know that nutmeg has been abused and misused.
- Instruct the female patient to report planned or suspected pregnancy.
- Advise the patient to avoid hazardous activities until the herb's CNS effects are known.
- Caution the patient against consuming large amounts of nutmeg because of its toxic potential.
- Warn the patient to keep nutmeg products out of reach of children and pets.
- Explain that nutmeg may precipitate symptoms associated with disease in a patient with psychiatric illness.
- Counsel the patient taking nutmeg for antidiarrheal effects to consider less toxic agents, such as bulk laxatives, milk of magnesia, or casanthrol with docusate sodium.

Points of interest

- Nutmeg is most popular for its uses as a spice in foods and drinks and as a fragrance in cosmetics and soaps.
- Nutmeg is one of the active ingredients in Aromatic Ammonia Spirits NF, which causes reflex stimulation when inhaled.

Analysis

Despite nutmeg's interesting pharmacologic profile, its therapeutic use is limited because of the risk of toxicity and abuse or misuse. Death has resulted from ingestion of excessive quantities. There are less toxic agents available for treating diarrhea. Nutmeg cannot be recommended for any indication because of its risks.

References

Abernethy, M.K., and Beckel, L.B. "Acute Nutmeg Intoxication," *Am J Emerg Med* 10:429-30, 1992.

Barrowman, J.A., et al. "Diarrhea in Thyroid Medullary Carcinoma: Role of Prostaglandins and Therapeutic Effect of Nutmeg," *BMJ* 3:11-12, 1975.

Giannini, A.J., et al. "Contemporary Drugs of Abuse," *AFP* 33:208, 1986.

Misra, V., et al. "Role of Nutmeg in Inhibiting Prostaglandin Biosynthesis," *Indian J Med Res* 67:482, 1978.

Ram, A., et al. "Hypolipidaemic Effect of *Myristica fragrans* Fruit Extract in Rabbits," *J Ethnopharmacol* 55:49-53, 1996.

Shafran, I., and McCrone, D. "Nutmeg and Medullary Carcinoma of Thyroid," *N Engl J Med* 293:1266, 1975. Letter.

OAKS

BRITISH OAK, BROWN OAK, COMMON OAK, CORTEX
QUERCUS, ECORCE DE CHENE, EICHERINDE,
EICHENLOHE, ENCINA, ENGLISH OAK, GRAVELIER,
NUTGALL, OAK APPLES, OAK BARK, OAK GALLS, STONE
OAK, TANNER'S BARK

Common trade names

(Various manufacturers; available in combination) Conchae Compound, Eichenrinden-Extrakt, Entero-Sanol, Hamon No. 14, Kernosan Elixir, Menodoron, Peerless Composition Essence, Pektan N, Silvapin, Tisanes de l'Abbe, Tonsilgon-N, Traxaton

Common forms

Available as capsules, decoctions, extracts, ointments, ooze (a tea of oak bark), tincture, unground or powdered oak bark, or oak galls. Oak bark is also sometimes included in prepared herbal mixtures and several commercially prepared GI remedies, such as Enterosanol.

Source

Oak bark is obtained from the English oak, *Quercus robur*, and the durmast oak, *Q. petraea,* members of the Beech family (Fagaceae). Oaks are slow-growing deciduous trees occurring in Eurasia, North America, and Australia. The bark is taken from young branches and twigs and is up to 4 mm thick, grayish brown on the outside and brownish red on the inner surface.

Oak galls are abnormal growths produced on oak stems and leaves, primarily by insects and nematodes. Many galls are rich in tannins. The leading gallmakers are tiny gall-wasps belonging to the genus *Cynips* (Cynipidae family). The insect pierces the shoots and young boughs of the oak and deposits its egg in the wound. After hatching from the egg, the larva secretes an enzyme-containing fluid that changes starch in adjacent oak cells into sugar, which the larva consumes as a food source. This sugar is also used by growing plant cells, which form large, protective growths around the developing insects. The insects reach the adult stage and eat their way out of the galls.

Chemical components

Oak bark contains tannins, including quercitannic acid and varying amounts of catechin, ellagitannin, and proanthocyanidin. The galls contain tannic acid, gallic acid, resin, calcium oxalate, and starch. Acorns contain primarily tannic acid, gallic acid, and pyrogallol. The content of the tree components varies and depends on the time of harvesting and age of the branches, galls, or acorns. Other compounds found in the bark and galls include beta-sitosterol, friedelin, leucocyanidin, leucodelphinidin, levulin, pectin, quercetin, quercin, quercitol, and the glycoside quercitrin.

Actions

The active ingredients associated with oak bark and galls are the tannins. These are highly astringent compounds that act locally by precipitating proteins and decreasing cell membrane permeability. Tannic acid also exerts astringent action on the mucous membranes of the GI tract; it can also be absorbed from damaged skin and mucous membranes. Although several properties have been reported for other components of oak, these chemicals exist in trace amounts and are unlikely to have clinical effects.

Quercitrin and quercetin have been reported to exert a vasodilating effect. However, recent studies have found that quercetin is extensively bound to cellular proteins, and that it has no effect on CV or thrombogenic risk factors (Boulton et al., 1998; Conquer et al., 1998).

Reported uses

Traditionally, oak bark has been used as an astringent, antiseptic, and anti-inflammatory agent. Although oak galls may be used in small quantities instead of the bark, their use internally is not recommended. Astringent compresses were often applied to treat eczema and contact dermatitis in their early, "weeping" stages. Decoctions, such as vaginal douches, were used to treat leucorrhea; they were also used externally to treat varicose veins, hemorrhoids, foot odor, inflamed eye conditions, anal fissures, small burns, and other dermatologic conditions. The decoction was also reportedly used as a gargle to treat sore throats, tonsillitis, laryngitis, and bleeding gums.

Powdered oak bark was used as a snuff to treat nasal polyps and sprinkled on weeping eczema to dry the affected area. The German Commission E recommends external use of oak bark for inflammatory skin diseases, and internal use for the local treatment of acute diarrhea and mild inflammatory conditions of the oral cavity and pharyngeal region, as well as the urogenital areas.

Tannic acid has been used in suppositories for hemorrhoids, and locally for sore throat, stomatitis, and to harden nipples during nursing. It has recently been shown to inhibit gastric enzyme activity in pigs, an effect attributed to its antisecretory and antiulcerogenic properties (Murakami et al., 1992).

Other claims advanced for tannic acid include use as an antimutagenic, antinephritic, antioxidant, antiviral, bactericidal, cancer-preventive, hepatoprotective, immunosuppressant, psychotropic, and viricide.

Dosage

As an antidiarrheal, German Commission E recommends 3 g of the powdered oak bark or equivalent preparations P.O. daily. If diarrhea persists for over 3 to 4 days, consult a health care professional. Alternatively, 1 cup of tea P.O. t.i.d., made by adding 1 g finely cut or coarsely powdered drug or 1 to 2 teaspoons of chopped bark to 500 ml water, or 1 teaspoon bark per 250 ml water, boiling for 15 minutes, strained, cooled, and used undiluted.

Baths: 5 g of drug per 1 L water. Several ready-to-use oak bark extracts are available; typically, 1 to 3 teaspoons is added to a partial bath.

Capsules: 2 capsules P.O. with meals t.i.d.

Compress, rinse, gargle: prepare fresh decoction daily by boiling 20 g of drug per 1 L water for 10 to 15 minutes. Use strained liquid undiluted; apply compresses loosely to affected area to enable free evaporation. External application should typically be needed for only a few days and should not exceed 3 weeks.

Tincture: 1 to 2 ml P.O. t.i.d.

Adverse reactions

● Nausea, vomiting, gastric irritation, gastroenteritis, abdominal pain, constipation (with possible fecal impaction), hepatic necrosis (with more than 1 g tannins).

● Nephritis, respiratory failure (with tannic or gallic acid in animals)

⚠ Hepatotoxicity, possible death (with tannic acid enemas, prolonged skin application)

Interactions

Alkaloids, glycosides, heavy metal salts: precipitation and reduced absorption of drugs. Avoid concomitant use internally.

Contraindications and precautions

Avoid use of the herb in pregnant or breast-feeding patients; effects are unknown. External use is contraindicated if extensive skin surface damage is present. Full baths are contraindicated, according to the German Commission E, in patients with discharging, extensively large eczema and skin injuries; febrile and infectious diseases; New York Heart Association (NYHA) classes III and IV; and hypertonia state IV (World Health Organization).

Special considerations
• Instruct the patient to avoid contact with areas of extensive skin damage, large areas of the body, or the eyes. Tell the patient to flush with tepid water for at least 15 minutes if contact with the eyes occurs.
• Instruct the patient to wash the exposed areas with soap and water if contact with areas of extensive skin damage or contact with large areas of healthy skin occurs.
• Advise the female patient to avoid use of the herb during pregnancy or when breast-feeding.
• Inform the patient to avoid full-body baths with the herb.
• Advise the patient not to take the herb internally for more than a few weeks.

Points of interest
• Oaks have a long history of medical use. (See *Use of oak in history*.)
• Tannic acid was included in barium enemas at one time. However, due to reports of some deaths from hepatic necrosis, such use is no longer recommended.
• White oak bark (*Q. alba*) makes a yellowish tea with a slightly bitter, astringent taste.

Analysis
Limited external use of oak decoctions may provide some relief for certain forms of dermatitis such as eczema, contact dermatitis, and minor burns. Although there are anecdotal reports of the herb's use internally for diarrhea, clinical studies are lacking. This treatment is not recommended until safety and efficacy data are available.

References
Boulton, D.W., et al. "Extensive Binding of the Bioflavonoid Quercetin to Human Plasma Proteins," *J Pharm Pharmacol* 50:243-49, 1998.

Conquer, J.A., et al. "Supplementation With Quercetin Markedly Increases Plasma Quercetin Concentration Without Effect on Selected Risk Factors for Heart Disease in Healthy Subjects," *J Nutr* 128:593-97, 1998.

Dobelis, I.N., ed. *Magic and Medicine of Plants.* Pleasantville, N.Y.: Reader's Digest Association Inc., 1986.

Murakami, S., et al. "Inhibitory Effect of Tannic Acid on Gastric H^+, K^+, -ATPase," *J Natl Prod* 55:513-16, 1992.

OATS

GROATS, HAVER, HAVER-CORN, HAWS, OATMEAL

Common trade names
Aveeno Cleansing Bar, Aveeno Colloidal, Aveeno Dry, Aveeno Lotion, Aveeno Oilated Bath, Aveeno Regular Bath, Oats and Honey, Oat Bran, Oat Straw Tea, Quaker Oat Bran

Common forms
Tablets: 850 mg, 1,000 mg
Whole grains, cereals, wafers: 750 mg
Also available as soaps, gels, teas, powders, lotions, and bath preparations.

Source
Oat extracts are derived from the grains of *Avena sativa*. Oats are cultivated mainly in the United States, Russia, Canada, and Germany.

Chemical components
Oats contain saponins, carotenoids, gluten, polyphenols, monosaccharides, oligosaccharides, various minerals (such as iron, manganese, and zinc), fiber, and cellulose.

Actions
Oat products have emollient properties when applied topically to dry and pruritic skin. Oat bran cereals and oatmeal contain significant quantities of soluble and insoluble fiber. Dietary fiber is be-

lieved to lower plasma cholesterol by binding bile acids and cholesterol in the intestines, thus preventing their absorption. Although insoluble fiber is less effective, both forms of dietary fiber appear to reduce serum cholesterol.

Reported uses

Oat extracts have long been used as topical treatments for minor skin irritations and pruritus associated with common skin disorders. Oat-herb teas are claimed to be valuable as sedatives and antigout agents.

Regular intake of dietary fiber from oats can lower serum cholesterol in patients with elevated and normal serum cholesterol levels. When combined with other fiber-rich foods, these reductions are further increased (Van Horn et al., 1986). Epidemiologic evidence supports a relationship between oat bran intake and CV risk as measured by body mass index, blood pressure, and high density lipoproteins (He et al., 1995). Oat extracts and oat bran bread products also appear to lower serum glucose, insulin, and cholesterol levels (Pick, 1996; Hallfrisch et al., 1995).

Oat derivatives, such as green oat decoction (tea), may be useful in the treatment of chemical addictions (Anand, 1971a), and the extract is being evaluated in smoking cessation programs (Anand, 1971b; Bye et al., 1974).

Dosages

For lowering cholesterol, studies used 50 to 100 g daily of dietary fiber from oat bran.
For topical use, apply once or twice daily.

Interactions

None reported.

Adverse reactions

- Bloating, fullness, increased defecation
- Contact dermatitis (oat flour)
- Flatulence
- Perineal irritation

Contraindications and precautions

Contraindicated in patients with celiac disease because oats contain gluten. Use with caution in patients with bowel obstruction or other bowel dysmotility syndromes.

Special considerations

- Advise the patient taking oat bran to regulate bowel habits and to drink plenty of fluids.

• Advise the patient using colloidal oat products for baths to avoid contact with eyes and acutely inflamed areas. The products should be washed off with water.
• Inform the patient that increased bowel movements and flatulence may occur with oat products.

Points of interest
• Like other grains, oats have sometimes been contaminated with aflatoxin, a fungal toxin linked with some cancers.

Analysis
Oats provide an important source of dietary fiber. Evidence supports the use of oat extracts as a dietary adjunct for reducing CV risk factors (cholesterol, glucose) and postoperative constipation. Oatmeal baths are known for use in minor skin conditions; however, clinical data supporting this therapeutic application are sparse.

References
Anand, C.L. "Treatment of Opium Addiction," *BMJ* 3:640, 1971a.

Anand, C.L. "Effect of *Avena sativa* on Cigarette Smoking," *Nature* 233:496, 1971b.

Bye, C., et al. "Lack of Effect of *Avena sativa* on Cigarette Smoking," *Nature* 252:580, 1974.

Hallfrisch, J., et al. "Diets Containing Soluble Oat Extracts Improve Glucose and Insulin Responses of Moderately Hypercholesterolemic Men and Women," *Am J Clin Nutr* 61:379-84, 1995.

He, J., et al. "Oats and Buckwheat Intakes and Cardiovascular Disease Risk Factors in an Ethnic Minority of China," *Am J Clin Nutr* 61:366-72, 1995.

Pick, M.E. "Oat Bran Concentrate Bread Products Improve Long-Term Control of Diabetes: A Pilot Study," *J Am Diet Assoc* 96:1254-61, 1996.

van Horn, L.V., et al. "Serum Lipid Response to Oat Product Intake with a Fat-Modified Diet," *J Am Diet Assoc* 86:759-64, 1986.

OCTACOSANOL

OCTOCOSONOL, 1-OCTACOSANOL, 14C-OCTACOSANOL, N-OCTACOSANOL, OCTACOSYL ALCOHOL, POLICOSANOL

Common trade names
Octacosanol Concentrate, Super Octacosanol

Common forms
Capsules: 3,000 mcg, 8,000 mcg
Capsules (softgel): 3,000 mcg
Tablets: 1,000 mcg, 6,000 mcg

Source
Policosanol, and subsequently octacosanol, can be isolated from sugar cane wax, other vegetable waxes, and wheat germ oil. Octacosanol has also been isolated from *Eupolyphaga sinensis*, some *Euphorbia* species, *Acacia modesta*, *Serenoa repens*, and other plants.

Chemical components
Octacosanol is primarily a 28-carbon long-chain alcohol. The term has also been used to describe other long-chain 8- to 36-polycarbon alcohols.

Actions
Octacosanol is taken up by muscle tissue, liver, and digestive tract. One study suggested that octacosanol increased muscle endurance in exercising rats because of higher stores of the agent in exercised rather than resting muscle. These researchers also suggested enhanced lipolysis in muscle and suppressed lipid accumulation in adipose tissue by octacosanol (Kabir and Kimura, 1995). In another study, some lipoprotein lipase activity was enhanced in rats fed octacosanol and a high-fat diet (Kato et al., 1995). Significant lipid-lowering effects, mostly of low-density lipoprotein cholesterol, were found in rabbits fed policosanol (Arruzazabala et al., 1994). Earlier studies in animals suggest the agent has androgenic effects and improved exercise tolerance.

There may also be a role for octacosanol in CV disorders. Varying doses of policosanol inhibited some mechanisms of platelet activation and aggregation in rats (Arruzazabala et al., 1993). In a drug-induced model of a myocardial infarction, pretreatment with policosanol promoted significant reductions in infarct size and decreased the numbers of polymorphonuclear cells and mast cells compared with control rats.

Reported uses
Although regular use of octacosonal is claimed to enhance athletic performance, there are no supporting data. Anecdotal reports of success in treating amyotrophic lateral sclerosis (ALS) with octacosanol have not been achieved in research studies. Octacosanol has also been evaluated in Parkinson's disease (Snider, 1984). (See *Octacosanol in parkinsonism*.)

Dosage
Most sources suggest 40 to 80 mg P.O. daily.

RESEARCH FINDINGS
Octacosanol in parkinsonism

Octacosanol was evaluated in patients with mild to moderate idiopathic parkinsonism because of its apparent ability to improve muscle endurance. Ten patients received 5 mg octacosanol in a wheat germ oil base P.O. t.i.d. or placebo for 6 weeks.

The patients rated themselves weekly on activities of daily living (ADLs), mood, physical endurance, and parkinsonian symptoms.

Only three patients improved significantly at the study's end. Some responded slightly or did not have disease progression during treatment. Although ADLs and mood improved significantly, changes in other measurements were not significant. One patient experienced mild positional nonrotational dizziness, and two others experienced exacerbation of dyskinesias. The investigators believed that the octacosanol dosage might have been excessive for these patients. They concluded that octacosanol may be beneficial for patients with mild Parkinson's disease. However the benefit is likely to be small, and less than that exerted by existing antiparkinsonian agents (Snider, 1984)

Adverse effects
- Exacerbation of dyskinetic movements
- Nervousness
- Orthostatic hypotension

Interactions
Carbidopa/levodopa: may promote worsening of dyskinesias. Avoid concomitant use.

Contraindications and precautions
Avoid use in pregnant or breast-feeding patients; effects are unknown.

Special considerations
- Monitor severity and frequency of dyskinetic events in patients taking both octacosanol and carbidopa/levodopa.
- Inform the patient that long-term clinical data for octacosanol use are lacking.
- Explain that existing clinical evidence does not support a role for octacosanol as an ergogenic aid for athletes.
- Advise the female patient to avoid use of this agent during pregnancy or when breast-feeding.

Analysis

Current data for octacosanol do not support its use for any condition. Although it may be useful in CV or Parkinson's disease, more research is needed. Long-term risks have not been adequately assessed.

References

Arruzazabala, M.L., et al. "Cholesterol-Lowering Effects of Policosanol in Rabbits," *Biol Res* 27:205-8, 1994.

Arruzazabala, M.L., et al. "Effects of Policosanol on Platelet Aggregation in Rats," *Thromb Res* 69:321-27, 1993.

Kabir, Y., and Kimura, S. "Tissue Distribution of 8-14C-octacosanol in Liver and Muscle of Rats After Serial Administration," *Ann Nutr Metab* 39:279-84, 1995.

Kato, S., et al. "Octacosanol Affects Lipid Metabolism in Rats Fed on a High-Fat Diet," *Br J Nutr* 73:433-41, 1995.

Snider, S. "Octacosanol in Parkinsonism," *Ann Neurol* 16:723, 1984. Letter.

OLEANDER

ADELFA, LAURIER ROSE, ROSA FRANCESA, ROSA LAUREL, ROSE BAY

Common trade names

None known.

Common forms

Available as a tincture and leaf extract.

Source

Although active components are found in all parts of *Nerium oleander,* they are primarily extracted from the leaves. Oleander is a popular ornamental shrub native to the Mediterranean and widely grown in the South and in California.

Chemical components

Oleander contains several cardiac glycosides including oleandrin, neriin, oleandroside, nerioside, digitoxigenin, gentiobiosyloleandrin, and odoroside A. Other pharmacologically active compounds include folinerin, rutin, rosagenin, cornerine, and oleandomycin. The plant also contains hydrocyanic and ursolic acids, and traces of vitamins A, K, and C.

Actions

The cardioactive glycosides in oleander act similarly to the cardiac glycosides used in the treatment of heart failure. Their pharmacologic similarities suggest that these compounds enhance the force and velocity of myocardial contractions through inhibition of the sodium, potassium-ATPase pump in the sarcolemmal membrane (Clark et al., 1991). The flavonal glycosides influence vascular permeability and have diuretic actions. Cornerine improves myocardial function in clinical trials and is effective in cardiac conditions. Oleandrin, the principal cardiac glycoside, acts as a diuretic and stimulates the heart. In vivo analysis suggests that it lacks anticancer activity, but retains weak macrophage-mediated cell toxicity and weak mitogenic activity.

Reported uses

Despite its well-recognized toxicity, oleander claims of use center around cardiac illnesses, asthma, corns, dysmenorrhea, epilepsy, cancer, and skin eruptions. Folk remedies claim actions as an emetic, insecticide, parasiticide, cathartic, diuretic, menstrual stimulant, abortifacient, and cardiotonic. In Curaçao, the sap is applied to warts, added to beverages, and used as an anthelmintic. In Venezuela, the leaves are boiled and the steam inhaled to alleviate sinus problems. The leaves are also used as poultices for skin diseases and to kill skin parasites or maggots in wounds.

Dosage

No consensus exists. The ingestion of oleander is not recommended. A single ingested leaf may produce fatal poisoning in an adult (Howard and DeWolf, 1974).

Adverse reactions

- Abdominal pain
- Anorexia
- Contact dermatitis
- Cramps
- Depression
- Hyperkalemia
- Nausea
- Severe irritation (smoke inhalation)
- Tachypnea
- Vertigo
- Vomiting

⚠ All parts of the oleander plant are toxic. Death has occurred in adults and children following ingestion of the flowers, leaves, and nectar, and from using oleander twigs as skewers to roast foods. Fatalities have also occurred after oral and rectal administration of the extract (Clark et al., 1991). Smoke from the burning wood and water in which the plant has been immersed can also be toxic.

⚠ Symptoms of oleander toxicity may mimic digitalis toxicity, and include nausea, vomiting, colic, appetite loss, dizziness, drowsiness, hyperkalemia, ventricular tachycardia or fibrillation, heart block, mydriasis (dilated pupils), bloody diarrhea, seizures, syncope, and slow, irregular pulse. Death usually results from heart failure or respiratory paralysis. A canine model suggests that digoxin antibody fragments (such as Digibind) may be valuable in treating oleander toxicity (Clark et al., 1991)

Interactions
Digoxin, digitoxin: may increase risk of toxicity and fatal outcomes. Avoid concomitant use.

Contraindications and precautions
Because of its extremely poisonous nature, avoid use of oleander in any form.

Special considerations
• Know that the cross-reactivity between digoxin and oleander glycosides enables radioimmunoassays to measure serum digoxin levels in oleander poisoning. Assays for serum digoxin levels may not reflect the severity of the toxicity.

⚠ Manage oleander toxicity aggressively and treat as for digitalis poisoning. Treatment includes gastric lavage, emetics, and activated charcoal. Monitor serum potassium levels and ECG. Systemic hyperkalemia induced by the plant may worsen cardiac function and may be treated with potassium exchange resins. Treat conduction deficits with atropine, phenytoin, pacemakers, or antiarrhythmics. Do not use digitalis preparations for oleander poisoning (Clark et al., 1991).

• Monitor heart rate and rhythm.
• Monitor serum potassium levels.
• Caution the patient to keep the plant and products out of the reach of children and pets.
• Advise the patient to take precautions to prevent accidental ingestion.
• Advise the patient to avoid burning oleander branches or other plant parts in poorly ventilated areas to avoid toxic smoke.

Points of interest
• Birds may die from consuming less than 1,000 mg of the plant. A fatal dose in a large animal such as a cow or horse may be 10 to 20 g.
• Oleander is cultivated mainly as an ornamental shrub. The bush grows to about 20 feet in height, has long, narrow, pointed leaves and produces small clusters of red, pink, or white blossoms.

Analysis

Oleander's extreme toxicity precludes any therapeutic use. Although it has been used in traditional medicine, there are no clinical trials to support the efficacy and safety of this herb.

References

Clark, R.F., et al. "Digoxin-Specific Fab Fragments in the Treatment of Oleander Toxicity in a Canine Model," *Ann Emerg Med* 20:1073-77, 1991.

Howard, R.A., and DeWolf, G. P., Jr. *Poisonous Plants Arnoldia* 34:73, 1974. Reprint

OREGANO

MOUNTAIN MINT, ORIGANUM, WILD MARJORAM

Common trade names
(Also available in combination) Oil of Oregano, Oregamax, Oregano

Common forms
Capsules: 450 mg
Oil: 0.45 fl oz
Also available as a spice.

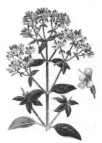

Source
Oregano is derived from dried aboveground parts of *Origanum vulgare,* a member of the mint family (Labiatae). It should not be confused with its close relative, marjoram (*O. majorana*).

Chemical components
The plant contains hydrolyzable tannins, including gallic acid, an iron-binding phenolic substance, and tocopherols.

Actions
Oregano may have significant antioxidant properties that may be attributed to the high levels of tocopherol. An oregano extract showed antimutagenic activity against a dietary carcinogen (Kanazawa et al., 1995). Gamma-tocopherol also occurs in high concentrations. This tocopherol homologue is reported to be most active next to alpha-tocopherol regarding antioxidant activity (Lagouri and Boskou, 1996).

Phenolic compounds (such as gallic acid in oregano) may bind with iron and decrease its absorption in the gut (Brune et al., 1989). Oregano inhibited mycelial growth of *Aspergillus parasiticus,* a common food mold (Tantaoui-Elaraki and Beraoud, 1994).

Reported uses

Herbalists have used oregano as a mild tonic, diaphoretic, and menstrual stimulant. It is used as a flavoring agent and preservative in the kitchen. The antibacterial and antioxidant properties of oregano have led modern herbalists to recommend its use for superficial and systemic infections.

Dosage

As a dietary supplement, 2 capsules P.O. once or twice daily, preferably with meals, or add a few drops of oil of oregano to milk or juice.

For topical use, apply oil of oregano directly to affected region once or twice daily. As a shampoo, add a small amount of oil of oregano to commercial shampoo. After shampooing, allow it to remain for a few minutes, then rinse hair. Add to pump soaps and use during showering and hand washing as an antiseptic cleanser.

Adverse reactions

⚠ A hypersensitivity reaction manifested by pruritus, facial edema, dysphagia, dysphonia, and upper respiratory distress was described. Cross-sensitivity to plants in the Labiatae (thyme, hyssop, basil, marjoram, mint, or sage) family may occur (Benito et al., 1996).

Interactions

Iron supplements: may reduce iron absorption. Separate administration of oregano by at least 2 hours when taken with iron supplements or iron-containing foods.

Contraindications and precautions

Contraindicated in patients with previous hypersensitivity reactions to oregano or other herbs of the Labiatae family. Use cautiously in patients with anemia secondary to iron deficiency.

Special considerations

• Tell the patient that previous hypersensitivity to herbs in the Labiatae family may indicate a reaction with oregano.
• Instruct the patient to discontinue use of oil of oregano if rash or irritation occurs.
• Tell the patient to avoid taking oregano within 2 hours of iron-containing foods or supplements.

Points of interest

• Oregano is a wild, coarse plant with sprawling stems, pink or white flowers, and a balsamic aroma.

• The Greeks crowned newlyweds with the herb and planted it on graves. In ancient times, the herb was used as a remedy for narcotic poisonings and seizures.

Analysis

Oregano shows some promise as an antiseptic, antifungal, and antioxidant. Because clinical human data are lacking, its use for these indications is not recommended.

References

Benito, M., et al. "Labiatae Allergy: Systemic Reactions Due to Ingestion of Oregano and Thyme," *Ann Allergy Asthma Immunol* 76:416-18, 1996.

Brune, M., et al. "Iron Absorption and Phenolic Compounds: Importance of Different Phenolic Structures," *Eur J Clin Nutr* 43:547-58, 1989.

Kanazawa, K., et al. "Specific Desmutagens in Oregano Against a Dietary Carcinogen, Trp-P-2, are Galengin and Quercetin," *J Agric Food Chem* 43:404-09, 1995.

Lagouri, V., and Boskou, D., "Nutrient Antioxidants in Oregano," *Int J Food Sci Nutr* 47:493-97, 1996.

Tantaoui-Elaraki, A., and Beraoud, L., "Inhibition of Growth and Aflatoxin Production in *Aspergillus parasiticus* by Essential Oils of Selected Plant Materials," *J Environ Pathol Toxicol Oncol* 13:67-72, 1994.

OREGON GRAPE

HOLLY-LEAVED BARBERRY, MOUNTAIN GRAPE

Common trade names
Mountain Grape, Oregon Grape Root

Common forms
Capsules: 400 mg
Fluid extract (tincture): 1 oz, 2 oz
Also available as powder and tincture.

Source
Active components are obtained from the bark of the roots and stems of *Mahonia aquifolium,* a bushy shrub native to the western United States. Do not confuse with the common barberry, *Berberis vulgaris.*

Chemical components
Mountain grape contains several alkaloids. The three major alkaloids contributing to the herb's pharmacologic activity are berberine, berbamine, and oxyacanthine. The plant also contains other alkaloids (canadine, corypalmine, hydrastine, isocorydine, oxyberberine, corytuberine, columbamine, and mahonine), resin, and tannin.

Actions

Although most *Mahonia* alkaloids have antibacterial properties, berbine also possesses amebicidal and trypanocidal properties. This alkaloid has anticonvulsant and uteronic actions, and has shown sedative and hypotensive effects in animals. Alkaloids isolated from *M. aquifolium* have demonstrated strong lipoxygenase-inhibitory and antioxidant properties (Bezakova et al., 1996; Misik et al., 1995).

These compounds also exert antiproliferative properties, suggesting a possible therapeutic role in treating diseases such as psoriasis in which lipoxygenase is involved (Müller et al., 1995). Root extracts have exhibited antifungal properties (McCutcheon et al., 1994).

Reported uses

The fruits, called "Oregon grapes," are edible, dark-purple berries that have been used in wines and brandies. Oregon grape is claimed to have aphrodisiac, antiseptic, astringent, bile-stimulating, cleansing, diuretic, expectorant, fever-reducing, cathartic, and tonic properties. The root has been used for gall bladder diseases, diarrhea, dyspepsia, dysuria, fever, urinary stones, and leucorrhea. The tincture has been claimed to be useful in treating acne, arthritis, bronchitis, congestion, eczema, hepatitis, herpes, psoriasis, rheumatism, syphilis, and vaginitis.

Dosage

Tincture: 2 to 4 ml P.O. t.i.d.
Powder: 0.5 to 1 g P.O. t.i.d.

Adverse reactions

⚠ Possible poisoning and death have been associated with excessive doses of berberine.

Interactions

None reported.

Contraindications and precautions

Avoid use of the herb in pregnant or breast-feeding patients; effects are unknown. Also contraindicated in persons with allergies to this or related plant species.

Special considerations

• Instruct the patient to avoid getting the preparation in the eyes. If contact occurs, tell the patient to flush the eyes well with water.
• Warn the patient that intense pain may occur with skin contact.
• Advise the patient that clinical evidence for therapeutic claims is lacking.

Points of interest

• Oregon grape is similar to, but should not be confused with, the common barberry (*Berberis vulgaris*). Several components found in Oregon grape also occur in goldenseal (*Hydrastis canadensis*).

Analysis

Although recent studies suggest that the active components of mountain grape or *Mahonia aquifolia* may be useful for psoriasis or other diseases involving the products of lipoxygenase metabolism (antioxidation), human studies are needed. There is limited information regarding the safety and efficacy of this herb.

References

Bezakova, L., et al. "Lipoxygenase Inhibition and Antioxidant Properties of Bisbenzylisoquinoline Alkaloids Isolated from *Mahonia aquifolium*," *Pharmazie* 51:758-61, 1996.

McCutcheon, A.R., et al. "Antifungal Screening of Medicinal Plants of British Columbian Native Peoples," *J Ethnopharmacol* 44:157-69, 1994.

Misik, V., et al. "Lipoxygenase Inhibition and Antioxidant Properties of Protoberberine and Aporphine Alkaloids Isolated from *Mahonia aquifolium*," *Planta Med* 61:372-73, 1995.

Müller, K., et al. "The Antipsoriatic *Mahonia aquifolium* and Its Active Components II. Antiproliferative Activity Against Cell Growth of Human Keratinocytes," *Planta Med* 61:74-75, 1995.

PANSY

FIELD PANSY, HEARTSEASE, JOHNNY-JUMP-UP, JUPITER FLOWER, LADIES'-DELIGHT, WILD PANSY

Common trade names
None known.

Common forms
Available as an extract.

Source
Active components are obtained from the flowers of *Viola tricolor*.

Chemical components
The stems and leaves contain flavonoids, salicylate derivatives, terpenes and triterpenes, carbohydrate derivatives, sterines, a polysaccharide, and magnesium tartrate. Vitamin F and other fatty acids have also been detected (Pápay et al., 1987). Other compounds include violanthin, rutin, violaquercitrin, resin, saponin, gums, and mucilage.

Actions
Physiologic mechanisms of action are poorly described. Salicylates may be responsible for anti-inflammatory properties due to prostaglandin inhibition. Although not a major component of pansy, rutin has been shown to exert many pharmacologic effects; the most well-known of which is its ability to affect capillary permeability. Herbals with high levels of rutin were thought to be useful for bleeding events. Other effects of rutin include inhibition of angiotensin II and prostaglandin E_2.

Reported uses
This agent is claimed to be useful in treating skin cancer, bronchitis, rheumatism, and whooping cough. One Hungarian study indicates possible use in preventing heart spasms and as an anti-inflammatory agent (Pápay et al., 1987).

Dosage
Dosage is 2 to 4 ml of tincture or tea P.O. t.i.d.

Adverse reactions
• Cathartic effects (seeds)
• Diarrhea

Interactions
Salicylates: possible additive effects. Use cautiously.

Contraindications and precautions
Avoid use of the herb in pregnant or breast-feeding patients; effects are unknown.

Special considerations
• Monitor the patient for diarrhea.
• Advise the female patient to avoid use of the herb during pregnancy or when breast-feeding.
• Advise the patient that there are no clinical data to support use of this herb for any medical condition.

Analysis
Without clinical data supporting the use of pansy for medical purposes, use of the herb cannot be recommended.

References
Pápay, V., et al. "Study of Chemical Substances of *Viola tricolor* L.," *Acta Pharm Hung* 157:153-58, 1987.

PAPAYA

MELON TREE, PAPAIN, PAWPAW

Common trade names
Papaya Enzyme, Papaya Enzyme with Chlorophyll, Papaya Leaf

Common forms
Tablets (chewable): 25 mg
Tablets: 5 mg
Also available as a tea.

Source
Components are usually extracted from the leaves, seeds, pulp, and latex of *Carica papaya*, which is native to Mexico and Central America but also grows in other tropical areas.

Chemical components

Papaya is composed primarily of proteolytic enzymes, including papain and chymopapain. Papain (also know as vegetable pepsin) occurs in the leaves and fruit latex. The alkaloid carpaine has also been isolated from the leaves. The seeds contain the glycosides caricin and myrosin.

Actions

Meat, seeds, and plant pulp of unripe papaya have demonstrated antioxidant properties and exerted weak bacteriostatic activity in vitro. Latex from papaya sap has inhibited the growth of *Candida albicans* in culture (Giordani et al., 1996).

Reported uses

Papain is classified as a debriding agent for necrotic tissue. Chymopapain is approved for intradiscal injection in patients with herniated lumbar intervertebral discs who don't respond to conventional therapy.

Papaya was used for athletic injuries and showed improved anti-inflammatory response and speedy recovery (Holt, 1969). It was also helpful in reducing postoperative edema and ecchymosis following nasal plastic surgery (Vallis and Lund, 1969). In patients requiring head and neck surgery, papaya reduced postoperative edema slightly (Lund and Royer, 1969).

Papain is claimed to be useful as an anthelmintic and in treating digestive disorders. The latex has been effective against intestinal nematodes in mice.

Dosage

For inflammation, clinical trials suggest 10 mg P.O. q.i.d. for 7 days.

Adverse reactions

• Carotenemia
• Dermatitis
• Hypersensitivity reactions (plant parts, extracts)
• Paralysis, decreased heart rate and CNS activity (carpaine)
⚠ Perforation of the esophagus and severe gastritis (with ingestion of excessive papaya or papain)
⚠ Anaphylactic shock has been reported after injection of chymopapain.

Interactions

None reported.

Contraindications and precautions

Avoid use of the herb in pregnant or breast-feeding patients; effects are unknown. Use cautiously in patients with a history of atopy or those prone to contact dermatitis reactions from the herb.

Special considerations

● Monitor the patient with hypersensitivity for reactions to papaya.
● Warn the patient against prolonged use because of the risk for severe gastritis and allergic hypersensitivity reactions. Explain that the latex in the plant may induce dermatitis.
● Advise the female patient to avoid use of the herb during pregnancy or when breast-feeding.

Points of interest

● Papaya is a source of flavoring used in candies and ice cream.
● Papain is used in some facial creams to soften skin and is also used as a meat tenderizer.

Analysis

Human clinical trials suggest that papaya may be useful in the treatment of inflammation due to trauma or surgical procedures. In vitro studies have documented bacteriostatic effects against enteropathogens, but human clinical trials need to be conducted to verify these claims. Because allergic reactions have been caused by plant parts and extracts, papaya should be used cautiously in patients with a history of hypersensitivity reactions.

References

Giordani, R., et al. "Fungicidal Activity of Latex Sap from *Carica papaya* and Antifungal Effect of D(+)-Glucosamine on *Candida Albicans* Growth," *Mycoses* 39:103-10, 1996.

Holt, H. "*Carica papaya* as Ancillary Therapy for Athletic Injuries," *Curr Ther Res Clin Exper* 11:621-24, 1969.

Lund, M., and Royer, R. "*Carica papaya* in Head and Neck Surgery," *Arch Surg* 98:180-82, 1969.

Vallis, C., and Lund, M. "Effect of Treatment with *Carica papaya* on Resolution of Edema and Ecchymosis Following Rhinoplasty," *Curr Ther Res Clin Exper* 11:356-59, 1969.

PAREIRA

PAREIRA BRAVA, PAREIRA RADIX

Common trade names

(Available in combination) Pareira Complex

Common forms

Available as dried roots and stems, and as powders or granules. Pareira is often combined with other plant species in homeopathic preparations (such as Pareira Complex).

Tubocurarine chloride, an alkaloid present in pareira, is available as a prescription injectable in the United States and contains 3 mg/ml active drug. Each 3 mg is equivalent to approximately 20 units of crude curare extract. This injectable drug should not be confused with dietary supplements containing pareira.

Source

Pareira is obtained from roots and stems of *Chondrodendron tomentosum*, a tropical, woody vine native to rain forests of the upper Amazon, Ecuador, and Panama. Root and stem sections are cleaned, cut into transverse segments, and dried. Commercial supplies of pareira come mainly from Rio de Janeiro and Bahia, Brazil.

Chemical components

Pareira contains various alkaloids, including delta-tubocurarine (also referred to as d-tubocurine), d-chondrocurine, d-isochondrodendrine, d-isochondrodendrine dimethyl ether, l-curarine (also referred to as l-curine or l-bebeerine), chondrofoline, and cycleanine. Only tubocurarine has the physiological activity characteristic of curare, a potent muscle relaxant.

Actions

Several actions have been reported for pareira, including analgesic, anticonvulsant, antimalarial, antiaggregant, antiarthritic, anti-inflammatory, antipyretic, antitumor, cytotoxic, dopamine-receptor inhibitor, ganglionic blocker, hepatoprotective, histaminic, hypotensive, and vagolytic. None of these actions are supported by clinical data regarding oral administration of pareira.

Reported uses

Traditional use of pareira by oral and topical routes appears less hazardous as long as it is not introduced into the bloodstream. The herb is bitter and slightly sweet, and it is claimed to be a mild laxative, tonic, diuretic, and antiseptic, and reportedly also acts to induce menstruation. It has been used to relieve chronic inflammation of the urinary tubules, and has been recommended for calculi, leucorrhea, rheumatism, jaundice, generalized edema, and gonorrhea. It is also used in Brazil for snakebites.

Pareira extracts have long been used as arrow poisons. Tubocurarine's ability to cause muscle paralysis has been extensively researched, and this agent is now commonly used in Western medicine. Tubocurarine chloride is used mainly to produce skeletal muscle relaxation during surgery, after induction of general anesthesia. It may also be used to facilitate endotracheal intubation, increase pulmonary compliance during assisted or controlled respiration, and as an adjunct during pharmacologically or electrically induced convulsive therapy (Osol and Farrar, 1955).

Dosage

For snake bites, infusion (tea) of the root taken P.O.; bruised leaves applied externally.

For other disorders, 2 to 4 ml fluid extract P.O.; 10 to 20 grains solid extract P.O.; or 1 to 4 fluid oz infusion P.O.

Adverse reactions

None reported for oral preparation; with tubocurarine injection:
• Apnea (prolonged), residual muscle weakness
• Ganglionic blockade leading to decreased GI motility and tone
• Hypotension, pulmonary effects (wheezing, bronchospasm), cutaneous effects (flushing, erythema, pruritus, urticaria, wheal formation; associated with histamine release)
• Malignant hyperthermia (with parenteral administration of tubocurarine chloride; rare).

Interactions

None reported for oral preparation.

Drugs known to cause or enhance neuromuscular blockade (aminoglycosides, lidocaine, neuromuscular blockers, polymyxin antibiotics): may increase risk of paralysis. Avoid concomitant use.

Contraindications and precautions

Tubocurarine is contraindicated in patients for whom histamine release may be hazardous and in patients who are hypersensitive to the drug. The same cautions and precautions should be taken with oral administration of pareira. Also contraindicated in patients with oral, gastric, and duodenal ulcers.

Use with caution in patients with respiratory depression and in those with impaired hepatic, renal, endocrine, CV, or pulmonary function.

Special considerations

⚠ Examine mucous membranes to ensure they are intact before the patient takes this agent. If there are cuts or sores in the mouth, the potential exists for the tubocurarine components of the plant to enter the bloodstream, resulting in the physiologic activity characteristic of curare.

⚠️Warn the patient about the symptoms of curare exposure, and advise him to seek emergency medical help immediately if needed. The first symptoms of muscle relaxation following parenteral administration of tubocurarine typically include blurred vision, bilateral drooping of the lids, heaviness of the face, and relaxation of the jaws; next, generalized weakness and heaviness of the neck muscles, inability to raise the head, and weakness or complete paresis of the spinal muscles, legs, and arms; and finally, shallow respiration.

• Tell the patient to use pareira only under supervision of a health care professional.

• Advise the patient to keep the herb away from injured skin or mucous membranes.

Points of interest
• Pareira is famous for being the source of the arrow poison curare. The term "curare" comes from an Amazon Indian word for poison. Amazonian and other South American Indians tipped a dart or spear with curare to paralyze game animals.

Analysis
As a prescription medication, tubocurarine has a definite role as a nondepolarizing neuromuscular blocking agent. However, pareira lacks clinical data to substantiate its claims for topical and oral use or of its safety and efficacy. The potential risks associated with oral ingestion of the plant parts outweigh any potential and, as yet unproven, therapeutic benefits.

References
Osol, A., and Farrar, G.E. *Dispensatory of the United States of America.* 25th ed. Philadelphia: Lippincott-Raven Pubs., 1955.

PARSLEY

COMMON PARSLEY, GARDEN PARSLEY

Common trade names
(Also available in combination) Insure Herbal, Parsley Herb, Parsley Leaves

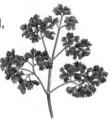

Common forms
Capsules: 430 mg, 450 mg, 455 mg
Liquid: 1 oz
Also available as teas.

Source

Leaves from *Petroselinum crispum* are most commonly used for parsley, although the roots, seeds, and oil are also used. The plant grows wild in parts of the Mediterranean but is cultivated in herb gardens worldwide. Germany, France, Belgium, Hungary, and California are the largest producers of parsley oils. The plant is sometimes labeled as *Apium petroselinum, Carum petroselinum,* or *Petroselinum sativum.*

Chemical components

Parsley contains several vitamins and minerals, such as calcium, iron, vitamin A, a significant amount of B vitamins, and vitamin C. It also contains glycosides (apigenin and luteolin), furanocoumarins (bergapten, methoxypsoralen, psoralen, oxypeucedanin), proteins, carbohydrates, and an oleo-resin. The volatile oil contains apiol, myristicin, tetramethoxyallylbenzene, terpene aldehydes, ketones, and alcohols.

Actions

In animals, parsley has demonstrated a significant hypotensive effect (Petkov, 1979; Opdyke, 1975); an increase in smooth muscle tone in the bladder, uterus, and intestines (Opdyke, 1975); and stimulation of hepatic regeneration (Gershbein, 1977). Myristicin, a component of the chemical that shares structural similarity with sympathetic amines, is thought to exhibit MAO inhibitor-like properties. When given to pregnant women, parsley oil has been reported to increase the levels of circulating plasma proteins, serum calcium, and diuresis (Buchanan, 1978). Aprolol and myristicin are uterine stimulants.

Reported uses

During the Middle Ages, parsley was claimed to be useful in treating the plague, asthma, kidney and liver dysfunctions, GI complaints, and edematous conditions. In folk medicine it has been used as an antiflatulent, menstrual stimulant, expectorant, antirheumatic, diuretic, antispasmodic, antimicrobial, and a digestive aid.

Parsley is a popular phytotherapy agent for hypertension in regions of Morocco (Ziyyat et al., 1997). More recently, it has been reportedly prescribed for female patients with bladder problems.

Dosage

Tea: 2 to 6 g P.O. of the leaf or root.
Liquid extract (1:1 in 25% alcohol): 2 to 4 ml P.O. t.i.d.

Adverse reactions
• Arrhythmias
• Contact dermatitis and photosensitivity (psoralen components)
With parsley seed oil:
• Fatty liver, hepatotoxicity (apiole and myristicin components)
• GI bleeding
• Hypotension
• Pulmonary vascular congestion
• Renal epithelial cell damage (apiole component)
• Smooth muscle contraction (bladder, uterus, intestine)

Interactions
Antihypertensive agents: may enhance hypotensive effects of these agents. Monitor patient.
MAO inhibitors in combination with certain antidepressants (selective serotonin reuptake inhibitors, some tricyclics), dextromethorphan, lithium, narcotic analgesics (meperidine): may promote or produce serotonin syndrome. Avoid concomitant use.

Contraindications and precautions
Avoid use of the herb in pregnant or breast-feeding patients; effects are unknown. Use parsley oil with extreme caution, if at all, in pregnant patients because of risk of increased uterine contractions. Use cautiously in patients prone to arrhythmias, hypotension, coronary insufficiency, heart failure, renal failure, peptic ulcer disease, or liver disease.

   Also use cautiously in patients receiving other agents known to precipitate serotonin syndrome.

Special considerations
• Inform the patient with multiple health problems to avoid using this herb.
• Counsel the patient receiving medications that may interact with parsley to avoid use of this herb.
• Explain that there is little clinical evidence for any medicinal use of parsley.
• Advise the female patient to avoid use of parsley during pregnancy or when breast-feeding.

Points of interest
• Parsley is well known as a garnish for various culinary dishes. Parsley and parsley oils are used in small quantities in various baked goods, sauces, stews, packaged meats, soups, and other processed foods. The highest quantity (1.5%) is found in processed vegetables.
• In ancient Greece, parsley was often used at funerals. Wreaths for

graves were made from parsley, and it is said that before the advent of embalming, the corpses were sprinkled with parsley to mask the smell.

Analysis
Although parsley has shown some useful actions in animals, until human clinical trials are available to support these claims, consumption of parsley beyond that normally found in food is not recommended.

References

Buchanan, R.L. "Toxicity of Spices Containing Methylenedioxybenzene Derivatives: A Review," *J Food Safety* 1:275-95, 1978.

Gershbein, L.L. "Regeneration of Rat Liver in the Presence of Essential Oils and Their Components," *Food Cosmet Toxicol* 15:171-81, 1977.

Opdyke, D.L.J. "Parsley Seed Oil," *Food Cosmet Toxicol* 13(Suppl):897-98, 1975.

Petkov, V. "Plants with Hypotensive, Antiatheromatous and Coronarodilating Action," *Am J Chin Med* 7:197-236, 1979.

Ziyyat, A., et al. "Phytotherapy of Hypertension and Diabetes in Oriental Morocco," *J Ethnopharmacol* 58:45-54, 1997.

PARSLEY PIERT

FIELD LADY'S MANTLE, PARSLEY BREAKSTONE, PARSLEY PIERCESTONE

Common trade names
(Also available in combination) Parsley Piert

Common forms
Liquid extract: 1:1 in 25% alcohol
Tincture: 1:5 in 45% alcohol
Also available as dried herb.

Source
Aphanes arvensis (also known as *Alchemilla arvensis* or *A. microcarpa)* is a low-growing hairy annual growing to 4 inches (10 cm) and is native to Europe, North Africa, and North America. The aerial parts of the herb are harvested when the flower is in bloom in the summer, and they are used either fresh or dried.

Chemical components
A related species *Alchemilla vulgaris* (lady's mantle) is reported to contain 6% to 8% tannins. Although the exact composition is unknown, it is claimed to contain an astringent compound (Newall et al., 1996).

Actions

Parsley piert is claimed to have diuretic and astringent properties. Tannins are highly astringent compounds that act locally by precipitating proteins. Tannic acid coagulates protein and exerts an astringent action on the mucous membranes of the GI tract.

Reported uses

The herb has been used to treat kidney and bladder disorders, especially calculi, dysuria, and edema of renal and hepatic origin. It is also claimed to be a useful remedy for cystitis and recurrent urinary tract infections. No clinical studies with parsley piert have been reported.

Dosage

Dried herb: 2 to 4 g P.O. or by infusion P.O. t.i.d.
Liquid extract: 2 to 4 ml P.O. t.i.d.
Tincture: 2 to 10 ml P.O. t.i.d.
Tea: mix a handful of the herb in 1 pint of boiling water; 3 or 4 cups P.O. daily.

Adverse reactions

None reported.

Interactions

None reported.

Contraindications and precautions

No known contraindications. Avoid use of the herb in pregnant or breast-feeding patients; effects are unknown.

Special considerations

• Advise the patient that there are no clinical data to support use of this herb for any medical condition.
• Advise the female patient to avoid use of the herb during pregnancy or when breast-feeding.

Analysis

There is little, if any, chemical or clinical information on parsley piert. The herb cannot be recommended for use until safety and efficacy data are available.

References

Newall, C.A., et al. *Herbal Medicines: A Guide for Healthcare Professionals.* London: Pharmaceutical Press, 1996.

PASSION FLOWER

APRICOT VINE, GRANADILLA, JAMAICAN HONEYSUCKLE, MAYPOP, PASSION FRUIT, WATER LEMON

Common trade names
None known.

Common forms
Liquid extract: 1:1 in 25% alcohol
Tincture: 1:8 in 45% alcohol, or containing 0.7% flavonoids
Also available as crude extract, dried herb, and in several homeopathic remedies.

Source
Active components are extracted from dried flowering and fruiting tops of *Passiflora incarnata,* a perennial climbing vine found in tropical and subtropical areas of the Americas. This plant should not to be confused with its close relative, the cultivated blue passion flower (*P. caerulea*), which does not contain cyanogenic glycosides (Hegnauer, 1993).

Chemical components
Passion flower contains 2.5% flavonoids such as vitexin, coumarin, and umbelliferone. It also includes harmala alkaloids such as harman, harmaline, harmine, and harmalol. A pyrone derivative, maltol, has also been found in the plant.

Actions
The agent exerts both stimulatory and depressant CNS effects. The harman alkaloids are known to stimulate CNS activity through MAO inhibition. The sedative effects of maltol mask the stimulatory effects of the alkaloids. A depressant effect and other sedative actions were seen when injected in mice (Aoyagi et al., 1974). For maltol and its derivatives, anticonvulsant effects and reductions in spontaneous motor activity have been documented in mice (Aoyagi et al., 1974; Kimura et al., 1980).

Reported uses
Passion flower is claimed to be effective as a sedative and is approved in Germany to treat nervousness.

Dosage
For Parkinson's disease, 10 to 30 drops P.O. (0.7% flavonoids) t.i.d.
Dried herb: 0.25 to 1 g P.O. t.i.d.
Liquid extract: 0.5 to 1 ml P.O. t.i.d

Tea: 4 to 8 g (3 to 6 teaspoons) daily P.O. in divided doses.
Tincture: 0.5 to 2 ml P.O. t.i.d.

Adverse reactions
● CNS depression (with large doses)
No adverse effects were noted when given I.V. to mice. No human toxicity has been reported.

Interactions
MAO inhibitors: may potentiate action. Monitor patient.
Other CNS depressants: possible additive effects. Use cautiously.

Contraindications and precautions
Contraindicated in pregnant or breast-feeding patients; harman alkaloids have shown uterine stimulant activity in animal models.

Special considerations
● Monitor the patient for possible adverse CNS effects.
● Counsel the female patient to report planned or suspected pregnancy.
● Advise the female patient to avoid use of the herb during pregnancy or when breast-feeding.
● Warn the patient of potential sedation if considering consumption of this herb.

Points of interest
● Passion flower is collected almost entirely for export (Ramstad, 1959).
● The herb was patented in a chewing gum form in Romania in 1978.
● Passion flower is found in sedative-hypnotic drug mixtures in Europe.
● The herb is listed by the Council of Europe as a natural food flavoring.

Analysis
There are no clinical data to support use of this herb for any medical condition. Despite the lack of toxicity data, use of this herb without efficacy data is not recommended.

References
Aoyagi, N., et al. "Studies on *Passiflora incarnata* Dry Extract. I. Isolation of Maltol and Pharmacological Action of Maltol and Ethylmaltol," *Chem Pharm Bull* 22:1008-13, 1974.

Hegnauer, R. *Chemotaxonomie der Planzen*, Vol 5: 295. Cited in Tyler, V., *The Honest Herbal,* 3d ed. Binghamton, N.Y.: Pharmaceutical Products Press, 1993, p. 238.

Kimura, R., et al. "Central Depressant Effects of Maltol Analogs in Mice," *Chem Pharm Bull* 28:2570-79, 1980.

Ramstad, E. *Modern Pharmacognosy.* London: McGraw Hill, 1959.

PAU D'ARCO

IPE ROXO, IPE, IPES, LA PACHO, LAPACHO COLORADO, LAPACHO, LAPACHOL, LAPACHO MORADO, PURPLE LAPACHO, RED LAPACHO, ROXO, TAHEEBO, TAJIBO, TRUMPET BUSH, TRUMPET TREE

Common trade names
(Various manufacturers; available in combination) Advance Defense System Tablets, Brazilian Herbal Tea, Candistroy, Cat's Claw Defense Complex, Cellguard Coq 10 Nac, Healthgard With Echinacea, Immuno-Nourish, Pau D'arco, Pau D'arco Inner Bark, Ultra Multiple Vitamin, Wellness Formula Vitamin, Wellness Multiple Max Daily, Women's Ut Formula

Common forms
Available as capsules (460 mg), tablets, skin salve, extracts, and teas.

Source
Pau d'arco products are made from the bark of *Tabebuia impetiginosa* (also known as *T. avellanedae* or *Tecoma curialis*). These evergreen flowering trees belong to the Bignonia family (Bignoniaceae) and are native to Florida, the West Indies, Mexico, Central America, and South America.

Chemical components
Approximately 15 quinone compounds have been found in the heartwood of *Tabebuia impetiginosa*, including lapachol, B-lapachone (both naphthoquinones), and tabebuin (an anthroquinone). *Tabebuia* naphthoquinones are extracted from plant material with organic solvents. Lapachol or xyloidone (dehydro-B-lapachone) were not found in the bark of *T. impetiginosa*, the part of the tree usually sold as pau d'arco; however, both were present in the heartwood of related species. An analysis of 12 taheebo products available in Canada revealed that only one contained lapachol (Awang, 1988).

Actions
Lapachol and xyloidone have been extensively investigated for antimicrobial activity. Xyloidone was found to be active against only

Brucella and *Candida* (Awang, 1988). Gram-positive bacteria were sensitive to lapachol and its isomer lapachone, but only *Pseudomonas aeruginosa* and *Brucella melitensis* were sensitive among the gram-negative organisms (Guiraud et al., 1994).

Although lapachol and B-lapachone are both fungistatic, the presumed mechanisms of action suggest that these compounds may be too toxic for medical use (Guiraud et al., 1994). Aqueous pau d'arco extracts have shown no activity against *Candida* cultures. Lapachol also has some effect as an antimalarial (Awang, 1988) and antischistosomal agent.

Human clinical trials have been inconclusive regarding the use of lapachol as an anticancer agent (Block et al., 1974; Awang, 1988). Recent in vitro studies showed antineoplastic activity, but this action was inhibited by vitamin K_1 (Dinnen and Ebisuzaki, 1997). The anti-inflammatory properties have also been demonstrated for a rat paw edema model.

Reported uses

Tabebuia species have been used in Latin American and Caribbean folk medicine as aphrodisiacs and for the treatment of anemia, backache, bedwetting, boils, colds, dysentery, dysuria, fever, gonorrhea, headache, incontinence, snakebite, sore throat, syphilis, toothache, and external wounds. The tea or topical extracts are claimed to be useful for *Candida albicans* infections, despite evidence that they are ineffective (Awang, 1988).

Other therapeutic claims include treatment of lupus, hernia, cancer, diabetes, inflammation, smoker's cough, warts, infection, ulcers, rheumatism, allergies, AIDS, and liver disease. The agent has also been touted as a "blood purifier," with the ability to cleanse the blood of pathogens and chemical contaminants; however, clinical evidence in support of these claims is lacking.

Dosage

Some packages do not specify the quantity of pau d'arco contained in the product.

Capsules: 1 to 2 capsules b.i.d. (with water or as a tea) at meals, or 3 to 4 capsules t.i.d. for no more than 7 days.

Lapachol (unspecified product): 1 to 2 g daily.

Lapachol tea: boil 15 to 20 g of bark in 16 oz of water for 10 minutes to make a tea with a lapachol content of about 3%.

Adverse reactions

- Nausea
- Pink-colored urine
- Reversible anticoagulant effects
- Vomiting

Interactions
Anticoagulants: may potentiate effects. Avoid concomitant use.

Contraindications and precautions
Contraindicated in patients receiving medications that interfere with blood clotting and in those with coagulation disorders (such as hemophilia, severe liver disease) or other hemorrhagic diseases (such as von Willebrand's disease, or thrombocytopenia). Also contraindicated in pregnant or breast-feeding patients and in children under age 18; effects are unknown.

Special considerations
• Caution the patient against using this herb instead of conventional medical treatment.
• Advise the female patient to avoid use of the herb during pregnancy or when breast-feeding.

Points of interest
• "Taheebo" is a South American Indian word for the hard, durable wood of these trees from which the Indians made bows for hunting. The Portuguese, who first colonized Brazil, named the tree pau d'arco, meaning "bow stick." The Spanish name for these trees is *lapacho* (Awang, 1988).

Analysis
There are no clinical data to support the use of this herb for any medical condition. Besides lapachol and xyloidone, other chemical components of pau d'arco have not been studied. Because hydroquinone compounds are known to possess toxic effects, pau d'arco should be considered potentially toxic. Therefore, its use cannot be recommended.

References
Awang, D.V.C. "Commercial Taheebo Lacks Active Ingredient," *Can Pharm J* 5:323-26, 1988.

Block, J.B., et al. "Early Clinical Studies with Lapachol (NSC-11905)," *Cancer Chemotherapy Reports* Part 2. 4:27-28, 1974.

Dinnen, R.D., and Ebisuzaki, K. "Search for Novel Anticancer Agents: A Differentiation-Based Assay and Analysis of a Folklore Product," *Anticancer Res* 17:1027-34, 1997.

Guiraud, P., et al. "Comparison of Antibacterial and Antifungal Activities of Lapachol and B-Lapachone," *Planta Med* 60:373-74, 1994.

PEACH

AMYGDALIN, *AMYGDALIS PERSICA*, LAETRILE, *PERSICA VULGARIS*, VITAMIN B-17

Common trade names
Laetrile, Vitamin B-17

Common forms
Available as persic oil, peach kernel oil, peach bark, leaves, and seeds. Crushed seeds are marketed as health foods, cancer remedies, and vitamin supplements. None of these preparations are standardized as to the amount of active ingredient.

Source
Active components are obtained from the leaves, bark, and seeds or kernels of the fruit of *Prunus persica*, a fruit tree belong to the rose family (Rosaceae). The fruit (peach) is fleshy and succulent and surrounds a hard, deeply pitted stone or pit, which in turn envelops a seed or kernel. The leaves are typically gathered in the summer and dried. The bark is harvested from young trees in the spring and dried. Peach kernel oil is expressed from the kernels of seeds of the pit. The oil is also referred to as persic oil; however, persic oil may be obtained from either the peach kernel or the apricot kernel (*Prunus armeniaca*).

Chemical components
The leaves, seeds, flowers, and bark contain amygdalin, which on hydrolysis yields hydrocyanic acid. Phloretin is found in the bark and leaves. Numerous other minerals and compounds have been isolated from the bark, flower, fruit, leaf, seed, and root of the plant.

Actions
Peach kernel oil is used as a pharmaceutical oil; it has also demonstrated in vitro fungicidal properties (Mishra and Dubey, 1990). Various parts of the peach tree are claimed to irritate and stimulate the GI tract. Phloretin from the bark and leaves is an antibiotic effective against gram-positive and gram-negative bacteria. Leaves and bark also have soothing, sedative, diuretic, laxative, and expectorant actions. Amygdalin is known to be a highly toxic cyanogenic glycoside.

Reported uses
Traditionally, peach leaves and bark have been used as an analgesic, antitussive, astringent, cathartic, demulcent, diuretic, expectorant, sedative, and anthelmintic. They have been used topically for blis-

ters, boils, bruises, burns, eczema, warts, and minor wounds. They have also been used to treat bronchitis, constipation, generalized edema, dysentery, dysmenorrhea, dyspepsia, earache, halitosis, headache, hemorrhage, hypertension, lockjaw, pneumonia, scurvy, shingles, and sore throat.

Laetrile, also called amygdalin or vitamin B_{17}, has often been promoted as a cancer preventative and cure. It is obtained from the kernels of apricots, peaches, plums, cherries, nectarines, apples, and almonds. However, extensive testing by the National Cancer Institute has failed to confirm the drug's anticancer effect (Moertel et al., 1982). Moreover, laetrile has been banned by the FDA because of the risk of poisoning from its cyanide content.

Dosage
Tea: ½ oz of dried bark or 1 oz of dried leaves and 1 pint of boiling water; steep for 15 minutes; take P.O. t.i.d.

Adverse reactions
• Allergic reactions to outer skin of the fruit.
⚠ Risk of cyanide poisoning. Cyanogenic glycosides are poisonous and are found in the seeds, leaves, flowers, and bark of the peach tree. The peach pit contains approximately 2.6 mg hydrocyanic acid per gram of seed. A lethal dose of hydrocyanic acid is 50 to 60 mg in adults (equivalent to about 20 g of peach seeds) (Holzbecher et al., 1984). Several fatalities have been reported from peach pit consumption.

Symptoms following cyanide poisoning include sudden, severe vomiting and epigastric pain followed by syncope, lethargy, coma, and seizures. Chronic consumption of plants high in cyanogenic glycosides has resulted in optic atrophy, nerve deafness, spastic paraparesis, ataxia, clonus, and peripheral neuropathy.

Interactions
None reported.

Contraindications and precautions
Contraindicated in pregnant or breast-feeding patients because risk profiles are still uncertain.

Special considerations
• Warn the patient to keep the dangerous parts of the peach (pits, kernels) away from children and pets.
• Warn the patient to avoid consuming pits or kernels because of their potential cyanide toxicity.
• Advise the patient to wear gloves if hypersensitive to the fruit and when handling is necessary.

Analysis

Although there are several anecdotal reports of the use of peach leaves or bark tea, clinical safety and efficacy data are lacking. Therefore, this treatment cannot be recommended. Consumption of peach kernels is potentially fatal, and there are no valid clinical studies documenting the effectiveness of hydrocyanic acid in the prevention or treatment of cancer. The potential risks associated with the consumption of peach kernels outweigh any potential benefits, and their use should be discouraged.

References

Holzbecher, M.D., et al. "The Cyanide Content of Laetrile Preparations, Apricot, Peach , and Apple Seeds," *Clin Toxicol* 22:341-47, 1984.

Mishra, A.K., and Dubey, N.K., "Fungitoxic Properties of *Prunus persica* Oil," *Hindustan Antibiot Bull* 32:91-93, 1990. Abstract.

Moertel, C.G., et al. "A Clinical Trial of Amygdalin (Laetrile) in the Treatment of Human Cancer," *N Engl J Med* 306:201-06, 1982.

PENNYROYAL

AMERICAN PENNYROYAL, EUROPEAN PENNYROYAL, MOSQUITO PLANT, SQUAWMINT

Common trade names

(Available in combination) Aloe Herbal Horse Spray, Miracle Coat Spray-On Dog Shampoo, Pennyroyal, Pennyroyal Essential Oil

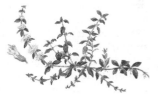

Common forms

Available as an oil, dried leaves, and flowers.

Source

Active components are obtained from the dried leaves and flowering tops of the American pennyroyal (*Hedeoma pulegioides)* and the European pennyroyal (*Mentha pulegium)*. Both belong to the mint family (Labiatae).

Chemical components

The leaves and flowering tops of *H. pulegioides* are the main source of pennyroyal oil. The oil consists chiefly of a monoterpene (pulegone), which ranges from 9% in Brazilian varieties, 16% to 30% in American varieties, and 80% to 94% in European varieties of the plant. Other components of pennyroyal oil are hedeomal, tannins, alpha-pinene, beta-pinene, limonene, 3-octanone, *p*-cymene, 3-octylacetate, 3-octanol, 1-octen-3-ol, 3-methylcyclohexanone, menthone, piperitenone, and paraffins. Dried seeds of *H. pulegioides* contain protein, fat, ash, and small amounts of calcium, sodium, and potassium.

Actions
Pulegone is thought to be responsible for the toxic organ effects of pennyroyal oil in animals and humans. It is metabolized by the cytochrome P-450 enzyme system to form a toxic metabolite, methofuran. The monoterpene is also oxidized to several other metabolites that may be involved in toxicity. Once formed, methofuran, other pulegone metabolites, and uncharged pulegone can deplete hepatic glutathione, leading to liver failure. Pulegone is a potent liver toxin. It also acts as an insect repellent.

Pennyroyal oil is most commonly known for its abortifacient properties. It is believed that the oil causes irritation of the uterus with resultant uterine contractions (Sullivan et al., 1979). These effects are not consistent, however, and use of pennyroyal oil as an abortifacient has sometimes resulted in hemorrhaging and even death.

Reported uses
Pennyroyal has been used for several ailments, most notably as an abortifacient. The whole plant was once used for fibroids and indurations of the uterus. The root, ground with vinegar, has also been used to treat tumors.

The plant has a strong, pungent odor similar to spearmint. The oil has a scent of citronella and has been used for scenting soaps and detergents and as an insect repellent. Some herbalists use pennyroyal oil to induce menstruation and to treat symptoms of premenstrual syndrome. As a hot infusion (tea), this herb has also been used for the treatment of colds, fevers, and the flu because it promotes sweating. Other uses of pennyroyal include management of colic, toothache, and chest congestion.

Dosage
Oil: 1 to 8 drops (for topical use only, as an insect repellent or in aromatherapy).
Tea: steep 1 to 2 teaspoons of dried pennyroyal leaves in 1 cup boiling water for 10 to 15 minutes, or mix 1 tablespoon dried herb with 1 cup warm water. Drink up to 2 cups daily.

Adverse reactions
- Abdominal cramping
- Confusion
- Dizziness
- Hallucinations
- Hematemesis

- Lethargy
- Liver failure
- Malaise
- Nausea
- Renal failure
- Respiratory depression
- Rigors
- Seizures
- Vomiting

⚠Coma and death have been reported.

⚠Pennyroyal oils and teas continue to be promoted for several ailments. However, these products are potentially toxic and should not be ingested except under medical supervision of a health care professional. (See *Pennyroyal poisoning.*)

Interactions

Inhibitors of the cytochrome P-450 system (amiodarone, azole antifungals, cimetidine, macrolide antibiotics, omeprazole): may change the rate of formation of toxic metabolites of pennyroyal. Monitor patient.

Contraindications and precautions

Contraindicated in pregnant or breast-feeding patients; abortive effects have been documented. Also contraindicated in children, patients with known seizure disorders, and in those with renal or hepatic insufficiency. Use with extreme caution because of the lack of data and risk of toxicity.

Special considerations

- Be aware that hepatic toxicity may be prevented by early administration of acetylcysteine (Anderson et al., 1996).
- Know that pennyroyal induces abortion in lethal or near-fatal doses. Therefore, it should never be used as an abortifacient.
- Warn the patient not to take the oil internally.
- Advise the patient still wishing to take pennyroyal not to exceed recommended doses and to avoid taking it for longer than 1 week.
- Warn the patient not to use the herb if unusual symptoms occur.
- Advise the female patient to avoid use of the herb during pregnancy or when breast-feeding.
- Advise the patient to keep pennyroyal preparations out of reach of children and pets.

Points of interest

- In ancient times, pennyroyal was hung in the rooms of convalescents and was believed to hasten recovery. Worn around the head, garlands of pennyroyal were also claimed to alleviate dizziness

RESEARCH FINDINGS
Pennyroyal poisoning

Pennyroyal poisoning continues to occur regularly and with relatively small doses; as little as 1 tablespoon of the oil has been reported to cause death. Other toxic effects, including seizures, have been reported after ingestion of less than 1 teaspoonful of the oil. Because 50 to 100 g of leaves are needed to produce 1 ml of oil, 1 teaspoon may be equivalent to 0.5 kg of leaves (Mack, 1997).

One case report described a 24-year-old woman who repeatedly ingested extracts of pennyroyal and black cohosh root for 2 weeks to induce abortion. The patient experienced abdominal cramps, chills, vomiting, syncope, rigors and difficulty walking. About 7.5 hours after ingestion, the patient was in cardiopulmonary arrest. On arrival in the emergency room, physical examination showed coma and a rigid abdomen. A computed tomographic scan of the abdomen suggested a possible ruptured ectopic pregnancy. Throughout the initial 12 hours of hospitalization, the patient's course was marked by hemodynamic shock, decreased hematocrit, hepatic failure, and a clinical picture consistent with disseminated intravascular coagulation. The patient died 46 hours after her last pennyroyal ingestion (Anderson et al., 1996).

In another case, a 12-week-old infant died after being given acetaminophen, a brompheniramine/phenylpropanolamine cold remedy, and 4 oz of pennyroyal tea. In some of the other toxicity cases reported, individuals did not exceed the "recommended" doses.

and headache. Use of pennyroyal as an abortifacient dates back to ancient Rome at the time of Pliny the Elder (23-79 A.D.).

● Pennyroyal's scientific name stems from the Latin term for flea, "pulex," which refers to the plant's use as an insect repellent. People have reportedly rubbed the leaves on their clothes or skin for this effect.

Analysis

Although pennyroyal has many therapeutic claims, there are no clinical data to support use of this herb. Together with the herb's toxicity, the medicinal use of pennyroyal cannot be recommended.

References

Anderson, I.B., et al. "Pennyroyal Toxicity: Measurement of Toxic Metabolite Levels in Two Cases and Review of the Literature," *Ann Intern Med* 124:726-34, 1996.

Mack, R.B. "'Boldly They Rode...Into the Mouth of Hell': Pennyroyal Oil Toxicity," *NCMJ* 58:456-57, 1997.
Sullivan, J.B., et al. "Pennyroyal Oil Poisoning and Hepatotoxicity," *JAMA* 242:2873-74, 1979.

PEPPER, BLACK

BIBER, FILFIL, HU-CHIAO, LADA, KOSHO, KRISHNADI, PEPE, PEPER, PFEFFER, PHI NOI, PIMENTA, PJERETS, POIVRE, THE MASTER SPICE, THE KING OF SPICES

Common trade names
(Various manufacturers; available in combination) Curry Powder, Galat Dagga, Garam Masala, Lowrey, McCormick, Panch Phoron, Quatre Epices, Ras El Hanout, Sambaar Podi, Trikatu

Common forms
Available as powder (ground into different grades of coarseness).

Source
Piper nigrum, the pepper plant, is a woody vine that grows up to 20 feet and is indigenous to Southeast Asia. First cultivated by Indian colonists in Indonesia, it has been transplanted to many equatorial climates, notably Brazil, Malaysia, Sumatra, and China.

Slow drying of the unripe fruit creates black pepper, whereas quick drying creates green pepper. White pepper is obtained by washing the ripe fruit down to the seed core and then drying.

Chemical components
The main active ingredients in pepper are the alkaloids, particularly piperine. Other alkaloids include piperlongumine, piperyline, piperanine, piperidine, and piperettine. These alkaloids, along with chavicin, give pepper its pungent qualities.

Essential oils give pepper its aromatic qualities. Most of these oils consist of monoterpenes, terpenes (sabinen, carvone, alpha-and beta-pinene, myrcene, limonen, borneol, carvacrol, and linalool), and sesquiterpenes (beta-caryophyllene, humelene, and beta-bis-abolone). Other substances include safrol, myristicine, eugenol, beta-sitosterol, and five phenolic amides.

Actions
Pepper increases gastric secretions and bile flow and stimulates diuresis. Five phenolic amides have been identified, and all have greater antioxidant activity than alpha-tocopherol in vitro.

Minor anti-infective activity has been shown against several infectious agents by *Piper* species.

Black pepper's carcinogenic properties have also been studied. Safrole and tannic acids, both found in black pepper, caused tumors in several organs in mice. However, when another component of black pepper was added, the carcinogenicity of the other two substances was reduced. Therefore, it appears that black pepper might have its own built-in protectant.

The anti-inflammatory activity of piperine has been shown, although the mechanism of action was not clear (Mujumdar et al., 1990). Black pepper might have the ability to block pain impulses and cause pain relief. Antifertility and abortive qualities were also shown in pregnant mice given piperine. It inhibited delayed labor, exhibited abortive action (depending on the period of gestation), reduced uterine contractions, and caused bloody discharge. Fetal mortality was significantly increased.

Piperine's ability to affect hepatic enzyme systems and increase drug bioavailability has been reported (Bano et al., 1991). Other studies have confirmed it to be a noncompetitive inhibitor of the P-450 mixed oxidase systems.

Reported uses

Claims include use as an antiflatulent and digestive aid, to increase gastric juices, stimulate appetite and diuresis, and to treat constipation, diarrhea, colic, indigestion, heartburn, ulcers, dysentery, and abdominal pain. A product called Trikatu, which contains black pepper, is popular in India for treating digestive ailments and for cold and flu symptoms, rhinorrhea, congestion, diabetes, obesity, and tumor control.

The oil vapors have helped stop the craving for cigarettes in heavy smokers compared with placebo or a menthol dispensing product. Somatic symptoms of anxiety have also been significantly reduced (Rose and Behm, 1994).

Black pepper is thought to clear phlegm and mucous in respiratory conditions, but no studies are available to support these claims. The herb is used also in muscular conditions, for arthritis, rheumatism, sprains, stiffness, and pain. Pain relief with black pepper is being studied in animals and humans.

It is used as an aromatic stimulant in weakness due to cholera, coma, or vertigo; to clear the mind; help memory; alleviate mental exhaustion; and lift spirits. No studies were found analyzing the aromatic oil's effect on mental status.

Dosage

No consensus exists.

Adverse reactions

● Some carcinogenic activity (safrole and tannins are known carcinogens). More information is needed due to conflicting studies and the possibility that protectant components may negate the carcinogenic potential.

⚠ A few fatal cases of apnea in children have been reported when a handful of black pepper has been ingested.

Interactions

Drugs metabolized by the cytochrome P-450 system: piperine is a nonspecific inhibitor of the cytochrome P-450 system and proven to affect the metabolism of a few drugs. Use caution regarding the amount ingested in patients taking medications that have a narrow therapeutic index (such as theophylline, warfarin).

Smoking cessation aids: additive effects. Monitor patient response.

Contraindications and precautions

Use cautiously in pregnant or breast-feeding patients; effects are unknown.

Special considerations

● Monitor the patient for changes in effects of drugs he may be taking that are metabolized by the cytochrome P-450 system.

● Be aware that generally, moderate doses do not show many adverse reactions. The FDA has given this herb a "Generally Recognized as Safe" status.

● Explain to the patient that evidence for smoking cessation is inadequate to support therapeutic application in this regard. Refer the patient to appropriate smoking cessation treatment.

Points of interest

● The common form is a result of drying the unripe fruit (berries) slowly, and grinding into different grades of coarseness. Also utilized are essential oils, ground root, and ethanol extracts, which are then ground into a powder and mixed with other types of peppers.

● Peppers used to be named according to the port they were shipped from, giving some hint as to the grade and potency of the product. Malabar used to indicate the best peppercorns in India; also from India, Tellicherry was a particularly bold version of Malabar pepper. However, all Indian pepper is now called "Malabar."

● Black pepper has been used for medicinal purposes world wide since Hippocrates, but nowhere is it used more than in India, where it occurs in almost every medicinal preparation.

• Black pepper is used as an insecticide, as a flavoring in brandy, in perfumes, and has tremendous value as a spice in food, drinks, and desserts.

Analysis
Black pepper is the most widely used spice in the world and does have some pharmacologic properties. Although most claimed uses lack supporting evidence, studies in animals may indicate some validity to these claims. It shows promise as an aid for smoking cessation and as a vehicle for enhancing drug bioavailability. However, studies in humans are needed before any anecdotal claim can be seriously supported.

References
Bano, G., et al. "Effect of piperine on Bioavailability and Pharmacokinetics of Propranolol and Theophylline in Healthy Volunteers." *Eur J Clin Pharmacol* 41:615-17, 1991.

Mujumdar, A.M., et al. "Anti-inflammatory Activity of Piperine." *Jpn J Med Sci Biol* 43:95-100, 1990.

Rose., J.E., and Behm., F.M. "Inhalation of Vapor from Black Pepper Extract Reduces Smoking Withdrawal Symptoms," *Drug Alcohol Depend* 34:225-92, 1994.

PEYOTE

ANHALONIUM, BIG CHIEF, BUTTONS, CACTUS, MESC, MESCAL, MESCAL BUTTONS, MESCALINE, MEXC, MOON, PAN PEYOTE, PEYOTE BUTTON

Common trade names
None known.

Common forms
Basic pan peyote: chloroform extract of ground peyote
Button: 45 mg of mescaline
Mescaline hydrochloride or sulfate: 375 mg of hydrochloride salt equals 500 mg of the sulfate salt
Soluble peyote: hydrochloride extract of basic pan peyote used for injection
Tincture: 70% alcohol extract of peyote

Source
The crude drug is obtained from the dried tops or whole plants of *Lophophora williamsii*, a small cactus native to Mexico and south Texas. Mescaline, the chief active ingredient of the cactus, has been synthesized.

Chemical components

Several chemical compounds have been isolated and may play a role in the hallucinogenic actions of this plant. The main active constituent is the alkaloid mescaline, or 3,4,5-trimethoxyphenylethylamine. Other components include N-methylmescaline, N-formylmescaline, N-acetylmescaline, 3-demethylmescaline, N-formyl-3-demethylmescaline, N-acetyl-3-demethylmescaline, 3,4-dimethoxyphenthylamine, tyramine, N-methyltyramine, hordenine, candicine, anhalamine, N-formylanhalamine, N-acetylanhalamine, anhaladine, and anhalanine.

Actions

Mescaline achieves its affects by stimulating adenylate cyclase activity at central dopaminergic receptors in the anterior limbic structures. It specifically acts on the pons and pontine raphe nuclei, decreasing neuronal firing and serotonin turnover. It also acts on the catecholamine and indolamine systems. It has been suggested that it may inhibit cholinergic neuromuscular transmission by blocking release of acetylcholine and affecting potassium conductance. Mescaline is also thought to have affinity for the $5-HT_{1A}$, $5-HT_{2A}$, and $5-HT_{2C}$ receptors (Ghansah et al., 1993; Monte et al., 1997).

Reported uses

Peyote has long been used in Native American religious ceremonies. It has also reportedly been used as an antibiotic, cardiotonic, hallucinogenic, intoxicant, narcotic, poison, psychedelic, sedative, and tonic. Folk remedies involve use of the herb for alcoholism, paralysis, and angina; as a painkiller for arthritis, backache, burns, and corns; and for fever, headache, rheumatism, snakebite, sunstroke, and throat irritation.

Dosage

Mescaline doses of 5 mg/kg produce physical effects and hallucinations.

Adverse reactions

⚠ Hypotension, bradycardia, vasodilatation, and respiratory depression (mescaline doses over 20 mg/kg)

⚠ Nausea and vomiting are noted within 30 to 60 minutes after ingestion. Diaphoresis, mild tachycardia, hypertension, mydriasis, and hyperreflexia are common. Other symptoms may include photophobia, ataxia, nystagmus, tremors, and muscle fasciculations. The user may experience anxiety, paranoia, and emotional lability. Auditory hallucinations are infrequent. Visual hallucinations and intensified color and texture perception follow, peaking at approximately 4 to 6 hours and lasting up to 14 hours. They usually include complex geometric patterns that seem to follow the user (Giannini et al., 1986).

Interactions
Other drugs that act on CNS (alcohol, marijuana, narcotic analgesics, psychedelics): may potentiate or aggravate effects. Avoid concomitant use.

Contraindications and precautions
Avoid use of the herb in pregnant or breast-feeding patients; effects are unknown. Use cautiously in CNS disorders.

⚠ Be aware that the peyote has been mixed with phencyclidine (PCP or "angel dust") or other illicit drugs that may worsen the patient's condition.

Special considerations
● Be aware that both mescaline and peyote are considered schedule I controlled substances. Because peyote is CSA schedule I, it is considered to have no accepted medicinal use and a high abuse potential. Know that peyote is used as a sacramental rite in the Native American Church, and its members are, therefore, exempt from prosecution under the Controlled Substances Act.
● Be aware that peyote is not thought to cause physical dependence, and it is not known if it can cause psychological dependence. Tolerance does occur and can cross over to LSD (lysergic acid diethylamide) and DMT (dimethyltryptamine).
● Know that death from high doses is less common than traumatic fatalities resulting from altered perception. Treatment is supportive until the effects have worn off. Place the patient in a semidarkened room and "talk down," if necessary. Diphenhydramine or a mild tranquilizer, such as diazepam, can be given if needed. Avoid use of antipsychotics because the psychosis will resolve spontaneously.

Analysis
Besides the fact that it is illegal, peyote has no valid medicinal use at this time.

References
Ghansah, E., et al. "Effects of Mescaline and Some of Its Analogs on Cholinergic Neuromuscular Transmission," *Neuropharmacol* 32:169-74, 1993.

Giannini, A.J., et al. "Contemporary Drugs of Abuse," *Am Fam Phys* 33:207-16, 1986.

Monte, A.P., et al. "Dihydrobenzofuran Analogues of Hallucinogens. 4. Mescaline Derivatives," *J Med Chem* 40:2997-3008, 1997.

PILL-BEARING SPURGE

ASTHMA WEED, CATSHAIR, EUPHORBIA, GARDEN
SPURGE, MILKWEED, QUEENSLAND ASTHMAWEED,
SNAKE WEED

Common trade names
(Various manufacturers; available in combination) As-Comp,
Ephedra Plus, Euphorbia, *Euphorbia hirta,* Sinus and Catarrh
Complex

Common forms
Available as capsules, dried plant (powder), liquid extract, tablets,
and tincture.

Source
The crude drug is obtained from the dried plant of *Euphorbia pilu-
lifera* (also called *E. hirta* or *E. capitata*). It is an annual herb native
to India and Australia. In the United States, it occurs from Texas to
Arizona.

Chemical components
The plant contains choline, shikimic acid, flavonoids (quercitrin,
quercetin, leuococyanidin), triterpenes (taraxerol, taraxerone esters,
alpha- and beta-amyrin), sterols (campesterol, euphosterol, sitosterol), alkanes (hentriacontane), phenolic acids, *l*-inositol, sugars,
and resins. Tannins have also been reported.

Actions
Rodents given an extract of *E. hirta* intraperitoneally exhibit dose-
dependent analgesic, antipyretic, and anti-inflammatory properties.
Higher doses produce sedative effects, whereas lower doses exert
anxiolytic effects (Lanhers et al., 1991). These plant extracts may
have antibacterial activity, and in vitro amebicidal activity against
Entamoeba histolytica has also been reported. Shikimic acid has
shown mutagenic activity in mice.

Choline is a cholinergic agonist similar to acetylcholine but with
less activity. Shikimic acid is the precursor of phenylalanine, tyrosine, tryptophan, and several plant alkaloids. In guinea pigs, choline
administration results in contraction of the ileum, whereas shikimic
acid causes relaxation of the ileum. Quercetin, the aglycone of quercitrin, showed antidiarrheal properties in mice (Galvez et al., 1993).
In addition, quercetin decreases platelet aggregation in humans.

Reported uses
Therapeutic claims for pill-bearing spurge include treatment of
asthma, hay fever, coughs, bronchitis, diarrhea, dysentery, intestinal

amebiasis, gonorrhea, thrush, snakebites, and ophthalmic disorders (Watt and Breyer-Brandwijk, 1962).

Dosage
Dried plant: 120 to 300 mg P.O. or by infusion P.O. t.i.d.
Liquid extract (1:1 in 45% alcohol): 0.12 to 0.3 ml P.O. t.i.d.
Tincture (1:5 in 60% alcohol): 0.6 to 2 ml P.O t.i.d.

Adverse reactions
- Cholinergic symptoms (with overdose)
- Contact dermatitis
- Emesis
- Gastric irritation

Interactions
ACE inhibitors: may potentiate antihypertensive effects. Use together cautiously.
Anticholinergics (atropine, ipratropium, scopolamine, other belladonna-type alkaloids): choline may decrease their effect. Use together cautiously.
Anticoagulants: may potentiate effects. Use together cautiously.
Barbiturates: may potentiate central hypnotic effects. Use together cautiously.
Disulfiram: disulfiram reaction may occur if herbal form contains alcohol. Avoid concomitant use.
Muscarinic agonists (arecoline, methacholine, muscarine), cholinesterase inhibitors (donepezil, edrophonium, physostigmine): additive effect when combined, and increased risk of toxicity. Use together cautiously.
Other medications metabolized by CYP3A enzymes (cyclosporine, erythromycin): may inhibit cytochrome P-450-3A enzymes. Use together cautiously.

Contraindications and precautions
Contraindicated in pregnant or breast-feeding patients because it causes both contraction and relaxation of smooth muscle. Use cautiously with patients receiving anticoagulants and in those with bleeding disorders because platelet aggregation may be reduced.

Special considerations
- Warn the patient to recognize toxic symptoms associated with excessive cholinergic stimulation (sweating, lacrimation, salivation, vomiting, hypotension, bradycardia) and to stop using the herb if these occur.

• Advise the patient with allergies that dermatologic reactions may result from handling products containing *E. hirta*.
• Warn the patient taking disulfiram not to take herbal form containing alcohol.

Points of interest
• The herb is not recognized by the FDA as being safe and effective for certain OTC use, such as asthma.

Analysis
This herb has shown possible analgesic, antipyretic, anti-inflammatory, sedative, and anxiolytic activity in animals, as well as antibacterial action against certain strains of *Shigella* species. However, human clinical data are lacking. The FDA has ruled that products containing *E. hirta* are neither safe nor effective for treating asthma; therefore, the herb should not be used to treat respiratory conditions. Because of the risk of drug interactions, use cautiously if taking concurrently with prescription medications.

References
Galvez, J., et al. "Antidiarrheic Activity of *Euphorbia hirta* Extract and Isolation of an Active Flavonoid Constituent," *Planta Med* 59:333-36, 1993.
Lanhers, M.C., et al. "Analgesic, Antipyretic, and Anti-inflammatory Properties of *Euphorbia hirta*," *Planta Med* 57:225-31, 1991.
Watt, J.M., and Breyer-Brandwijk, M.G. *The Medicinal and Poisonous Plants of Southern and Eastern Africa,* 2nd ed. Edinburgh and London: E and S Livingston LTD., 1962.

PINEAPPLE

ANANAS, GOLDEN ROCKET, SMOOTH CAYENNE PINEAPPLE

Common trade names
Ananase

Common forms
Available as juices, syrups, candy, whole fruit, and extracts.

Source
Active components are derived from the juice and fruiting portion of *Ananas comosus,* a member of the bromeliad family (Bromeliaceae) native to South America. Pineapple is now cultivated widely in tropical regions, especially Hawaii and Thailand.

Chemical components
The fruit contains citric acid, malic acid, vitamin A, and ascorbic acid. The leaves contain a steroidal compound, and a volatile oil contains aromatic compounds. All plant parts contain bromelain and several other proteolytic enzymes.

Actions
Juice from unripe pineapples reportedly produces violent cathartic action. The root and ripe fruit are claimed to have diuretic activity. Bromelain is moderately well absorbed from the intestine after oral administration. Bromelain's actions are reported to enhance serum fibrinolytic activity, inhibit fibrinogen synthesis, degrade fibrin and fibrinogen, and influence prostaglandin synthesis. It also is reported to lower serum tissue levels of kininogen and bradykinin (Lotz-Winter, 1990). Consumption of pineapple juice reduces endogenous production of nitrogenous compounds in humans, implying a reduction in the risk of cancer (Helser et al., 1992).

Reported uses
Claims for pineapple include treatment of constipation, jaundice, obesity, and prevention of ulcers. Bromelain has been claimed to be useful in reducing local inflammation and edema after topical application. Bromelain may also act to hasten wound healing (Rowan et al., 1990).

Dosage
No consensus exists.

Adverse reactions
With excessive amounts of juice:
● Angular stomatitis
● Diarrhea
● Nausea
● Rash (dermal sensitization)
● Uterine contractions
● Vomiting

Interactions
ACE inhibitors: may antagonize effects on bradykinin. Don't use together.
Anticoagulants: may prolong bleeding time. Avoid concomitant use.

Contraindications and precautions
Contraindicated in pregnant or breast-feeding patients.

Special considerations
• Advise the patient to avoid consumption of excessive amounts of juice because significant GI distress may occur.
• Advise the pregnant patient to avoid consumption of large quantities of juice during pregnancy (sometimes used in fad diets) because it may promote uterine contractions.

Points of interest
• Bromelain is used as a meat tenderizer in the food industry.
• Use of bromelain for burns and stings has declined because of the lack of documented support for its use.

Analysis
Pineapple is a reasonable source for obtaining bromelain, a useful proteolytic enzyme. However, there are insufficient data to support therapeutic uses for the plant. Ingestion of quantities above that normally obtained in foods is not recommended.

References
Helser, M.A., et al. "Influence of Fruit and Vegetable Juices on the Endogenous Formation of N-Nitrosproline and N-Nitrosthiozolidine-4-Carboxylic Acid In Humans on Controlled Diets," *Carcinogenesis* 13:2277, 1992.

Lotz-Winter, H. "On the Pharmacology of Bromelain: An Update with Special Regard to Animal Studies on Dose-Dependent Effects," *Planta Med* 56:249, 1990.

Rowan, A.D., et al. "Debridement of Experimental Full-Thickness Skin Burns of Rats with Enzyme Fractions Derived from Pineapple Stem," *Burns* 16:243, 1990.

PIPSISSEWA

GROUND HOLLY, PRINCE'S-PINE, SPOTTED
WINTERGREEN, WINTERGREEN

Common trade names
None known.

Common forms
Available as crude extracts.

Source
Active components are obtained from the dried leaves of *Chimaphila umbellata*, a creeping perennial herb belonging to the heath family (Ericaceae) that is native to Eurasia and northern North America.

Chemical components

Pipsissewa contains arbutin, chimaphilin, chlorophyll, ericolin, minerals, pectic acid, tannins, and urson. Isohomarbutin, reinfolin, homogentisic acid, toluquinol, hyperoside, taraxasterol, nonacosane, methyl salicylate, resins, gums, starches, and sugars have also been identified.

Actions

Pipsissewa is reported to have hypoglycemic action in animals (Segelman and Farnsworth, 1969). Arbutin and chimaphilin reportedly act as urinary antiseptics.

Reported uses

Therapeutic claims for pipsissewa include use as a diuretic, astringent, diaphoretic, antispasmodic, and antiepileptic; for nervous disorders; and externally for sores and ulcers. Tea made from pipsissewa has also shown antidiuretic properties. Tannins make the herb potentially useful for treating diarrhea.

Dosage

No consensus exists.

Adverse reactions

- Diarrhea
- GI irritation
- Nausea
- Skin eruptions
- Vomiting

Interactions

Minerals, including iron rich foods and supplements: reduced mineral absorption. Take 2 hours apart from meals or mineral supplements because tannins may form complexes with these agents.

Contraindications and precautions

Avoid use of the herb in pregnant or breast-feeding patients; effects are unknown. Use cautiously or avoid use in GI disorders (ulcerative colitis, gastroesophageal reflux disease, stomach or duodenal ulcers), iron deficiency, and malabsorptive disorders.

Special considerations

- Advise the patient that there is insufficient evidence to recommend use of this herb.
- Warn the patient taking this herb to immediately report unusual signs or symptoms and to stop use of the herb.

Analysis

Because this herb lacks clinical data on safe doses and therapeutic claims, it should not be consumed.

References

Segelman, A.B., and Farnsworth, N.R. "Biological and Phytochemical Evaluation of Plants IV. A New Rapid Procedure For the Simultaneous Determination of Saponins and Tannins," *Lloydia* 32:5695, 1969.

PLANTAINS

BLOND PLANTAGO, BROADLEAF PLANTAIN, BUCKHORN, CART TRACT PLANT, COMMON PLANTAIN, ENGLISH PLANTAIN, FLEA SEED, FRENCH PSYLLIUM, GREATER PLANTAIN, INDIAN PLANTAGO, LANTEN, NARROWLEAF PLANTAGO SEED, PLANTAIN, PLANTAIN SEED, PSYLLIUM, RIBWORT, RIPPLE GRASS, SNAKEWEED, SPANISH PSYLLIUM, TRACT PLANT, WAY-BREAD, WHITE MAN'S FOOT, WILD PLANTAIN, WILD SASO

Common trade names

(Various manufacturers) Effer-Syllium, Hydrocil, Konsyl, Metamucil, Perdeim

Common forms

Available as psyllium supplied as seeds or powder or tablet. Also available as liquid extracts (1:1 in 25% alcohol) and tincture (1:5 in 45% alcohol) of the leaves of other plantain species.

Source

Active components are derived from leaves of *Plantago lanceolata* and *P. major*, and from seeds and husks of *P. psyllium* and *P. ovata*. These plants are members of the buckwheat family (Polygonaceae) and are distributed worldwide.

Chemical components

Various plantain species contain plant acids, alkaloids, amino acids, and flavonoids. Sugars and polysaccharides have been found in the mucilaginous layer of the seed coat, including galactose, glucose, xylose, arabinose, and rhamnose. Protein, fiber, oil (oleic, linoleic, and linolenic acids), tannins, and iridoids can also be found in the seeds. Polysaccharides have been found in leaf mucilage. Psyllium, commonly used as a bulk laxative, is produced from the outer coat or husk of the plantain seed. This outer coat contains 10% to 30% of mucilage or hydrocolloid.

Actions

The pharmacologic effects of plantain extracts have been studied. Topical application of two phenylethanoids from *P. lanceolata* (acteoside and plantamajoside) has been found to have significant anti-inflammatory activity on mouse ear edema (Murai et al., 1995). Antinephritic and immunosuppressive effects have also been reported with acteoside.

Diuretic effects of several Vietnamese herbal remedies, including *P. major,* given alone and in combination, were found not to have significant activity (Du Dat et al., 1992). Clinical trials have shown psyllium to have a modest effect on lowering total cholesterol and low-density lipoprotein cholesterol (Chan and Schroeder, 1995).

At least 16 antigens have been found in *P. lanceolata,* and six are potentially allergenic (Baldo et al., 1982). Minor antibacterial activity in vitro and weak bronchodilatory effects in animals have been documented. Hypotensive activity has been shown in dogs.

Reported uses

Leaf extracts of *P. major* and *P. lanceolata* have been used topically as an astringent for burns and wounds, for treatment of poison ivy, and for inflammation of mucous membranes and skin. Decoctions of the leaves and seeds have been used orally for the treatment of dysentery or chronic diarrhea, for cough, as a gargle for throat irritation, as a diuretic, and for urinary tract disorders. In addition, there have been some reports of extracts of *P. major* and *P. lanceolata* having anticancer or immunotropic activity.

Psyllium, derived from the seeds of *P. psyllium* and *P. ovata,* is used primarily as a bulk laxative and also to lower serum cholesterol levels. One foreign trial lends support to the application of plantago for chronic bronchitis (Koichev, 1983).

Dosage

Leaf extracts or decoctions have been used orally and topically.
As a laxative, 7.5 g plantain seeds P.O. with large amounts of water.

Adverse reactions

- Abdominal distention
- Dermatitis
- Diarrhea
- Flatulence
- GI obstruction
- Hypersensitivity reactions
- Hypotension

⚠ Anaphylaxis to psyllium seed has been reported in individuals with no previous allergy and in those with a history of occupational exposure to plantain (Lantner et al., 1990; Ford et al., 1992).

Interactions

Carbamazepine, lithium: psyllium seed has been reported to inhibit GI absorption of lithium and carbamazepine. Avoid concomitant use.

Cardioactive drugs, (beta blockers, calcium channel blockers, digitalis): enhanced digitalis effects. Avoid concomitant use.

Contraindications and precautions

Contraindicated in pregnant or breast-feeding patients because of reported urotonic activity in vitro. Also contraindicated in patients with a history of intestinal obstruction. Use plantain-derived products cautiously in patients with a history of allergy to other weed pollens or a history of occupational exposure to plantain.

Special considerations

• Know that studies have shown that many patients with a positive skin prick test reaction to weed pollens also react positively to plantain pollen extracts.

• Monitor the patient for signs of allergic reactions (dermatitis, skin eruptions).

• Know that a patient with anorexia or bulimia may abuse laxatives including this agent.

• Advise the patient to separate consumption of this herb from other medications to avoid changes in absorption.

• Suggest more standard forms of bulk laxatives than plantain.

Points of interest

• Recently, the FDA has reported that some plantains are contaminated with cardiac glycosides.

Analysis

Plantain species have been claimed to be useful for many disorders, including inflammation of the skin and mucous membranes, and for GI and urinary tract disorders. Psyllium has long been used as a cathartic and may achieve modest reductions in serum cholesterol. Research indicates various pharmacologic effects from plantain derivatives. The plants are also allergenic in some persons. Plantain and derived products should be used cautiously in patients with a history of allergy to other weed pollens. Although plantains may be intriguing plants, they currently have no valid role in therapeutic treatment of disease. Additional clinical research is needed.

References

Baldo, B.A., et al. "Allergens from Plantain (*Plantago lanceolata*)," *Int Arch Allergy Appl Immunol* 68:295-304, 1982.

Chan, E.K., and Schroeder, D.J., "*Psyllium* in Hypercholesterolemia," *Ann Pharmacother* 29:625-27, 1995.

Du Dat, D., et al. "Studies on the Individual and Combined Diuretic Effects of Four Vietnamese Traditional Herbal Remedies (*Zea mays, Imperata cylindrica, Plantago major,* and *Orthosiphon stamineus*)," *J Ethnopharmacol* 36:225-31, 1992.

Ford M.A, et al. "Delayed Psyllium Allergy in Three Nurses," *Hosp Pharm* 27:1061-62, 1992.

Koichev, A. "Complex Evaluation of the Therapeutic Effect of a Preparation From *Plantago major* in Chronic Bronchitis," *Probl Vatr Med* 11:61-69, 1983.

Lantner R.R., et al. "Anaphylaxis Following Ingestion of a Psyllium-Containing Cereal", *JAMA* 264:2534-36, 1990.

Murai, M., et al. "Phenylethanoids in the Herb of *Plantago lanceolata* and Inhibitory Effect on Arachidonic Acid-Induced Mouse Ear Edema," *Planta Med* 61:479-80, 1995.

POKEWEED

CANCER JALAP, CANCER ROOT, CHANGRAS, COAKUM, CROWBERRY, GARGET, PIGEONBERRY, POCON, POKEBERRY, POKE SALAD, POKEWEED ROOT, REDINK PLANT, REDWOOD, SCOKE, TXIU KUB NYUG, VIRGINIA POKE

Common trade names
None known.

Common forms
Available as an extract (1:1 in 45% alcohol) and tincture.

Source
The active components occur in the roots, stems, leaves, and berries of *Phytolacca americana*. This weedy perennial subshrub grows throughout eastern North America.

Chemical components
The toxic agents of pokeweed are glycoside saponins (such as phytolaccigenin), a glycoprotein mitogen consisting of five glycoproteins, phytolaccatoxin, triterpenes, asparagine, and oxalic acid. The root contains three mitogenic lectins. A tannin and a resin are contained in the plant. Pokeweed shoots contain protein, fat, carbohydrate, ascorbic acid, niacin, beta-carotene equivalent, calcium, phosphorus, and iron.

Actions
In humans, pokeweed appears to induce central and peripheral cholinergic stimulation. Other pharmacologic actions reported in-

clude anti-inflammatory, cardioinductive, diuretic, abortifacient, and antineoplastic. The PL-B lectin has the highest amount of mitogenic and hemagluttinating activity, whereas the PL-C has the least hemagluttinating activity. Phytolaccigenin, one of the primary saponins, acts as a powerful parasiticide.

Reported uses
Pokeweed is said to possess emetic and laxative effects and to be useful for itching and rheumatism (Roberge et al., 1986). Other therapeutic claims include cough, tonsillitis, laryngitis, swollen glands, mumps, mastitis, mammary abscesses, and as a "lymphatic system cleanser." Mitogens and a recently discovered protein (pokeweed antiviral protein) are being studied as antineoplastic agents against certain leukemias and osteosarcomas (Jansen et al., 1992; Anderson et al., 1995; Myers et al., 1997).

Pokeweed has long been known and used as an edible green vegetable, but only the young shoots are safe to eat and only after boiling (Fernald and Kinsey, 1958).

Dosage
Dried root: 60 to 300 mg as an emetic.
Extract: 0.1 to 0.5 ml P.O.

Adverse reactions
- Blurred vision
- Confusion
- Contact dermatitis
- Diarrhea
- Dizziness
- Eye irritation
- Excessive salivation
- Headache
- Hematologic aberrations (eosinophilia, B and T cell disruption)
- Incontinence
- Nausea
- Sneezing
- Sore throat
- Sweating
- Syncope
- Tremor
- Vomiting
- Weakness

⚠ Deaths in children and heart block have been reported (Roberge et al., 1986; Hamilton and Shih, 1995). Seizures, coma, tachycardia, hypotension, and respiratory depression occur rarely.

Interactions
CNS depressants: additive effects. Avoid concomitant use.
Disulfiram: disulfiram reaction if patient takes herbal form containing alcohol. Avoid concomitant use.
Oral contraceptives, fertility medications: may cause menstrual cycle abnormalities and uterine stimulation. Avoid concomitant use.

Contraindications and precautions
Contraindicated in pregnant or breast-feeding women because of possible teratogenicity. Use cautiously in patients with a history of atopy and in those prone to contact dermatitis.

Special considerations
• Instruct the female patient to report planned or suspected pregnancy.
• Advise the female patient to avoid use of the herb during pregnancy or when breast-feeding.
• Caution the patient to avoid hazardous activities until effects on CNS are known.
• Warn the patient taking disulfiram not to take an herbal form containing alcohol.
• Advise the patient to keep pokeweed and its preparations out of reach of children and pets.
• Warn the patient about the potential toxicity of this herb.
• Instruct the patient to wear gloves if the plant is to be handled because of its potential for systemic toxicity if it contacts abraded skin.
• Advise the patient that there are no clinical data to support use of this herb.

Points of interest
• The FDA has classified pokeweed as an herb of undefined safety because of its narcotic-like effects.

Analysis
All plant parts of pokeweed appear to be toxic. Although the plant shows some promise as an anticancer agent, there are insufficient clinical data to support use of this herb for any condition.

References
Anderson, P.M., et al. "In Vitro and In Vivo Cytotoxicity of an Anti-osteosarcoma Immunotoxin Containing Pokeweed Antiviral Protein," *Cancer Res* 55:1321-27, 1995.

Fernald, M.L., and Kinsey, A.C., *Edible Wild Plants of Eastern North America.* New York: Harper & Brothers, 1958.

Hamilton, R.J., and Shih, R.D. "Mobitz Type I Heart Block After Pokeweed Ingestion," *Vet Human Toxicol* 37: 66-67, 1995.

Jansen, B., et al. "Establishment of a Human T(4;11) Leukemia in Severe Combined Immunodeficient Mice and Successful Treatment Using Anti-CD19 (B43)-Pokeweed Antiviral Protein Immunotoxin," *Cancer Res* 52:406-12, 1992.

Myers, D.E., et al. "Large Scale Manufacturing of TXU (Anti-CD7)-Pokeweed Antiviral Protein (PAP) Immunoconjugate for Clinical Trials," *Leuk Lymphoma* 27:275-302, 1997.

Roberge, R., et al. "The Root of Evil: Pokeweed Intoxication," *Ann Emerg Med* 15:470-73, 1986.

POMEGRANATE

GRANATUM

Common trade names
None known.

Common forms
Available as the crude herb or extract.

Source
Active components are derived from the bark, root, stem, peel, and fruit of *Punica granatum,* a shrub native to northwestern India and cultivated in many tropical areas.

Chemical components
The plant contains alkaloids (pelletierine, methylpelletierine, pseudopelletierine, and isopelletierine), mannite, various phenols, ellagic acid, and gallic acid. The bark and rinds contain approximately 20% tannins, including punicalin, punicalagin, granatins A and B, gallagyldilactone, casuarinin, pedunculagin, tellimagrandin I, and corilagin.

Actions
In vitro studies have shown *P. granatum* to have notable antimicrobial activity against *Staphylococcus aureus, Pseudomonas aeruginosa,* and *Candida albicans* (Navarro et al.,1996). Other studies have shown similar activity against various GI pathogens, supporting the folkloric use of pomegranate to treat diarrhea. Tannins from pomegranate have shown antiviral activity against the herpes simplex-2 virus. Pomegranate components also showed anthelmintic activity against *Entamoeba* species (Segura et al., 1990), and a uterine stimulant effect has been observed in animals (Farnsworth et al., 1975).

Reported uses
Pomegranate is claimed to be useful as an anthelmintic, and it is used as an antidiarrheal in Asia and South America. Although in

vitro studies appear to support these uses, human clinical trials are lacking.

Dosage
No consensus exists. Infusions (tea) or extracts of plant parts are often the source of pomegranate studied during in vitro evaluations.

Adverse reactions
- Hepatotoxicity (related to high tannin component)
- Hypersensitivity reactions
- Nausea
- Vomiting

⚠ Possible carcinogenicity. Pomegranate seeds and peels may increase the risk of some cancers. Women in northern Iran have the highest rate of esophageal cancer, attributed to a local food called "majum" or "majoweh" used during pregnancy. Majum is a crushed mixture of sour pomegranate seeds, black pepper, dried raisins, and sometimes garlic. This mix of harsh ingredients appears to cause esophageal trauma. Other local practices, such as consuming foods at higher than usual temperatures, preserving food by sun-drying, and the relative lack of fruits and vegetables in the diet, may also be factors (Ghadirian, 1987). Dried pomegranate peel has been shown to contain excessive amounts of aflatoxin B-1, a compound known to increase the risk of certain cancers (Selim et al., 1996).

Interactions
None reported.

Contraindications and precautions
Contraindicated in pregnant or breast-feeding patients and in those with asthma or atopy. Use cautiously, if at all, in patients with liver disease.

Special considerations
- Monitor liver function in patients taking this herb.
- Explain that continued use of this herb may increase the risk of certain cancers.
- Advise the female patient to avoid use of the herb during pregnancy or when breast-feeding.
- Warn the patient with a history of atopy (allergic reactions) or asthma not to use pomegranate preparations.

Analysis
The use of the herb for diarrhea is supported by studies showing in vitro activity against common causative organisms only; clinical confirmation is lacking. Other studies suggest activity against fungi,

viruses, and helminths. However, few human clinical studies are known. Because of a possible link with some cancers, the herb cannot be recommended for internal use until more data are available.

References

Farnsworth, N.R., et al. "Potential Value of Plants as Sources of New Antifertility Agents I.," *J Pharm Sci* 64:535-98, 1975.

Ghadirian, P. "Food habits of the people of the Caspian Littoral of Iran in Relation to Esophageal Cancer," *Nutr Cancer* 9:147-57, 1987.

Navarro, V., et al. "Antimicrobial Evaluation of Some Plants Used in Mexican Traditional Medicine for the Treatment of Infectious Diseases," *J Ethnopharmacol* 53:143-47, 1996.

Segura, J.J., et al. "Growth Inhibition of *Entamoeba histolytica* and *E. invadens* Produced by Pomegranate Root," *Arch Invest Med* 21:235-39, 1990.

Selim, M.I., et al. "Aflatoxin B-1 in Common Egyptian Foods," *J AOAC Int* 79:1124-29, 1996.

POPLAR

American aspen, black poplar, quaking aspen, white poplar

Common trade names
None known.

Common forms
Available as dried powdered bark or liquid extract.

Source
Active components are obtained from the bark of white poplar (*Populus alba*), quaking aspen (*P. tremuloides*), and black poplar (*P. nigra*). Exudates from poplar leaf buds have also been evaluated.

Chemical components
The phenolic glycosides salicin and the salicin benzoate salts (populin, tremuloidin, and tremulacin) are isolated from poplar species. Other components include tannins, triterpenes including fats, waxes, alpha- and beta-amyrin, glucose, fructose, and various trisaccharides. *P. nigra* also contains the lignan (+)-isolariciresinol mono-beta-D-glucopyranoside, and 3-methyl-but-2-enyl caffeate. *P. tremuloides* also contains flavonoids and ubiquiteric phenolic carboxylic acids, including p-coumaric acid.

Actions
Because salicin is a salicylate precursor, its actions are likely to be similar to other salicylates. These effects may be clinically relevant.

A compound found in exudates of poplar leaf buds is thought to have antiviral properties (Amoros et al., 1994).

Reported uses
Traditionally, poplar has been used as an antirheumatic or anti-inflammatory agent. The herb is also claimed to be useful for treating diarrhea, cystitis, stomach and liver disorders, and the common cold.

Dosage
Liquid extract (1:1 in 25% alcohol): 1 to 3 ml P.O. t.i.d.
Powdered bark: 1 to 5 g P.O. or by decoction t.i.d.

Adverse reactions
- Asthma
- Contact dermatitis (propolis product)
- GI bleeding, irritation (similar to salicylates)
- Hepatotoxic potential (related to tannin component)
- Pruritus
- Renal dysfunction
- Tinnitus

Interactions
Anticoagulants, other antiplatelet agents: may enhance risk of bleeding. Avoid concomitant use.
Salicylates: may cause GI symptoms. Avoid concomitant use.

Contraindications and precautions
Avoid use of the herb in pregnant or breast-feeding patients; effects are unknown. Use cautiously in patients with a history of plant allergies, salicylate hypersensitivity, GI bleeding, nasal polyps, bronchial asthma, renal disease, or peptic ulcer disease.

Special considerations
- Explain that consumption of poplar may increase bleeding risk in peptic ulcer disease or if anticoagulants or antiplatelets are also being taken.
- Advise the patient not to use poplar for a viral illness because of the risk of developing Reye's syndrome.
- Tell the patient to avoid OTC medications containing aspirin while taking the herb.
- Advise the patient taking prescription drugs containing aspirin to avoid use of poplar.
- Advise the female patient to avoid use of the herb during pregnancy or when breast-feeding.

Points of interest
● Propolis, a resinous plant product collected by honeybees, is largely composed of 3-methyl-but-2-enyl caffeate. Bees collect this material from the bud exudates of various trees, especially the poplar species. It has been well established that topically applied propolis and poplar bud exudate can cause severe contact dermatitis (Hausen et al., 1987a, 1987b).

Analysis
Because of the lack of animal and human clinical data, medicinal use of poplar cannot be recommended.

References
Amoros, M., et al. "Comparison of the Anti-Herpes Simplex Virus Activities of Propolis and 3-methyl-but-2-enyl Caffeate," *J Natl Prod* 57:644-47, 1994.

Hausen, B.M., et al. "Propolis Allergy. (I) Origin, Properties, Usage, and Literature Review," *Contact Dermatitis* 17:163-70, 1987a.

Hausen, B.M., et al. "Propolis Allergy. (II) The Sensitizing Properties of 1,1,-dimethylallyl Caffeic Acid Ester," *Contact Dermatitis* 17:171-77, 1987b.

PRICKLY ASH

ANGELICA TREE, HERCULES' CLUB, NORTHERN PRICKLY ASH, SOUTHERN PRICKLY ASH, SUTERBERRY, TOOTHACHE TREE

Common trade names
None known. Available in combination.

Common forms
Available as tincture (1:5 in 45% alcohol), berry liquid extract (1:1 in 25% alcohol) and the bark.

Sources
Active components are obtained from the bark of the northern prickly ash (*Zanthoxylum americanum*), and the southern prickly ash (*Z. clava-herculis*). Both trees belong to the rue (Citrus) family (Rutaceae) and are native to the United States.

Chemical components
Coumarin derivatives (xanthyletin, xanthoxyletin, allo-xanthoxyletin) have been isolated from the bark of *Z. americanum*, but have not been found in *Z. clava-herculis*. Other components found in the bark include tannins, resins, an acrid volatile oil, and the alkaloids nitidine and laurifoline.

Actions
The pharmacologic activity of prickly ash is relatively unknown. Natural coumarins possess anticoagulant vasodilatory, hepatotoxic, and diuretic properties.

Neuromuscular blocking effects have been observed in animals due to toxins isolated from *Z. clava-herculis*. Laurifoline has been reported to lower blood pressure and magnoflorine has been associated with neuromuscular blocking activity (Newall et al., 1996).

Reported uses
Prickly ash has been used as an antiflatulent, as well as a diaphoretic agent, antipyretic, and circulatory stimulant. The bark of prickly ash has also been used as a commercial product in the past for treating rheumatism and as a GI tract stimulant.

Dosage
A decoction of 15 g of bark in 600 ml of water, or up to 5 ml of the tincture P.O. t.i.d. has been suggested.

Adverse reactions
- Photosensitivity
- Risk of increased bleeding (coumarins)
- Toxicity (in sheep and cattle)

Interactions
Anticoagulants: may potentiate effects. Avoid concomitant use.
Aspirin, NSAIDs: enhanced anticoagulant effect. Avoid concomitant use.
Disulfiram: disulfiram reaction if herbal form contains alcohol. Avoid concomitant use.

Contraindications and precautions
Avoid use of the herb in pregnant or breast-feeding patients; effects are unknown. Also contraindicated in patients with allergies to this herb or related plant species.

Special considerations
- Advise the female patient to report planned or suspected pregnancy.
- Warn the patient taking disulfiram not to take an herbal form containing alcohol.
- Advise the patient to watch for signs of unusual bruising or bleeding.
- Warn the patient that few safety and efficacy data exist on this herb.

• Instruct the patient to discontinue use of this herb and to notify a primary health care professional if unusual symptoms occur.
• Advise the female patient to avoid use of the herb during pregnancy or when breast-feeding.

Points of interest
• Prickly ash is called the "toothache tree" in folk medicine because the bark is chewed to relieve toothache pain.
• Ingestion of parts of the northern prickly ash tree has been suspected to cause death in sheep and cattle in Indiana. Ingestion of the bark of the southern prickly ash tree has also caused death and symptoms of toxicosis (blindness, dysphagia, high-stepping gait, inability to drink water) in beef cattle in Georgia.

Analysis
Despite its many uses in folklore medicine, there is very little clinical information to support the use of prickly ash in humans. At this time, its use cannot be recommended for any condition.

References
Newall, C.A., et al., eds. *Herbal Medicines. A Guide for Health Care Professionals.* London: Pharmaceutical Press, 1996.

PRIMROSE, EVENING

KING'S-CURE-ALL

Common trade names
(Various manufacturers; available in combination)
Efamol, Epogram, Evening Primrose Oil, Mega Primrose Oil, My Favorite Evening Primrose Oil, Primrose Power

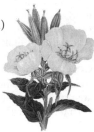

Common forms
Capsules: 50 mg, 500 mg, 1,300 mg
Gelcaps: 500 mg, 1,300 mg

Source
The oil is extracted from the seeds of *Oenothera biennis,* a biennial herb that is cultivated or grows wild in parts of North America and Europe.

Chemical components
Evening primrose oil is comprised primarily of essential fatty acids, including linoleic acid, gamma linolenic acid, oleic acid, palmitic acid, and stearic acid.

Actions

The therapeutic action of evening primrose oil stems from essential fatty acids that are important as cellular structural elements and as precursors of prostaglandin synthesis. Linoleic acid cannot be manufactured by the body and therefore must be provided through dietary intake. The body relies on the metabolic conversion of linoleic acid (LA) to gamma linoleic acid (GLA). Deficient conversion, which has been observed in such disorders as diabetes, CV disease, hypercholesterolemia, viral infections, cancer, and skin conditions, affects prostaglandin-E_1 and E_2 synthesis. It is claimed that LA and GLA supplementation from dietary sources maintains a balance between the inflammatory and noninflammatory prostaglandins that may, in turn, be useful in treating these disorders.

Reported uses

Evening primrose oil has been used as a vegetable with a peppery flavor. An infusion using the whole plant is reported to have sedative and astringent properties. Traditionally, it has been used for asthmatic cough, GI disorders, whooping cough, eczema, breast pain, premenstrual syndrome (PMS), psoriasis, multiple sclerosis, rheumatoid arthritis, hypercholesterolemia, asthma, Raynaud's disease, Sjögren's syndrome, diabetic neuropathy, and as a sedative and analgesic (Barber, 1988; Briggs, 1986). Poultices made with evening primrose oil have been used to speed wound healing.

Patients with atopic dermatitis and eczema have an enzymatic defect for the conversion of LA to GLA. A meta-analysis of nine clinical trials showed an improvement in pruritic symptoms with GLA administration. Two large clinical trials have shown no evidence of benefit (Kleijnen, 1994).

Placebo-controlled studies have suggested that GLA is superior in the treatment of breast pain and tenderness associated with PMS and benign breast disease (Briggs, 1986). Animal studies have shown that diabetic neuropathy can be prevented or reversed through GLA supplementation with evening primrose oil.

Evening primrose oil has been studied alone and with fish oils versus placebo in rheumatoid arthritis. These trials showed an improvement in the patient's symptoms, based on the reduced need for pain medication. There was no evidence, however, of evening primrose oil having a disease-modifying action (Briggs, 1986).

Although LA can reduce elevated serum cholesterol, GLA's cholesterol-lowering activity is about 100 times that of LA. GLA has been reported to reduce hypertension and decrease platelet aggregation in both animals and humans.

Hyperactive children are thought to have abnormal levels of essential fatty acids. Supplementation of evening primrose oil has produced controversial results. One trial saw no improvement in the behavioral patterns of children and blood fatty acid levels. However, another study showed a calming effect in two-thirds of children treated with evening primrose oil (Briggs, 1986).

Animal studies have indicated that evening primrose oil produced significant reductions in mammary tumors from baseline size. In vitro experiments found a dose-related inhibition of the growth rate in malignant tumors. High levels of essential fatty acids are toxic to several cancers but not lethal to normal cells. Human studies are currently underway to assess supplementation of essential fatty acids on the growth of cancer cells.

Dosage

The following dosages are based on a standardized GLA content of 8%.

For eczema, 320 mg to 8 g P.O. daily in adults. In children ages 1 to 12, 160 mg to 4 g P.O. daily; continue for 3 months.

For mastalgia, 3 to 4 g P.O. daily.

No consensus exists for all other disorders.

Adverse reactions

- Headache
- Inflammation, thrombosis, and immunosuppression may occur due to slow accumulation of tissue arachidonate after use of GLA for over 1 year (Kleijnen, 1994).
- Nausea
- Rash

⚠ Temporal lobe epilepsy may occur, especially in schizophrenic patients or those taking epileptogenic drugs such as phenothiazines.

Interactions

Phenothiazines: may increase the risk of seizures. Avoid concomitant use.

Contraindications and precautions

Avoid use of the herb in pregnant patients; effects are unknown. Also use cautiously, if at all, in schizophrenic patients and in those taking epileptogenic drugs.

Special considerations

- Instruct the patient with a seizure disorder to reconsider use this herb.
- Caution parents to use this herb for a hyperactive child only under supervision of a primary health care provider.

Analysis

Evening primrose oil is not approved for the treatment of any specific condition. Although the underlying mechanisms of essential fatty acid metabolism in health and disease may justify its alleged therapeutic uses, more clinical studies are needed to confirm the value of this oil for treating these conditions.

References

Barber, H.J. "Evening Primrose Oil: A Panacea?" *Pharm J* 240:723-25, 1988.
Briggs, C.J. "Evening Primrose, La Belle de Nuit, The King's Cure-all," *Can Pharm J* 249-54, 1986.
Kleijnen, J. "Evening Primrose Oil," *BMJ* 309:824-25, 1994.

PULSATILLA

CROWFOOT, EASTER FLOWER, KUBJELLE, MEADOW ANEMONE, PASQUE FLOWER, PRAIRIE ANEMONE, *PULSATILLAE HERBA*, SMELL FOX, STOR, WINDFLOWER

Common trade names

(Available in combination) Ana-Sed, Biocarde, Calmo, Cicaderma, Cirflo, Eviprostat, Eviprostat N, Hemolual, Histo-Fluine P, Mensuosedyl, Nytol Herbal, Premantaid, Pulsatilla Med Complex, Viburnum Complex, Yeast-X

Common forms

Available as a dried herb, liquid extract, tincture, and in homeopathic remedies.

Source

Active components are derived from dried leaves, stems, and flowers of *Anemone pulsatilla* (also known as *Pulsatilla vulgaris*), a perennial plant native to southern Europe.

Chemical components

Ranunculin is a lactonic glucoside present in the undamaged, fresh plants. When the plants are crushed, the aglycone protoanemonin is enzymatically liberated. Protoanemonin dimerizes to form anemonin, anemoninic acid, and anemonic acid. Anemonin is highly volatile, and much of it is lost during drying. Other plant components include saponins, tannins, volatile oil, chelidonic and succinic acids (as calcium salts), flavonoids, and glucose. Delphinidin and pelargonidin glycosides also occur in the flowers.

Actions

Protoanemonin causes stimulation followed by paralysis of the CNS in animals. In the fresh plant, it has antibacterial and local irritant properties; however, the dimer anemonin lacks these actions. Pulsatilla can be a powerful CNS and cardiac depressant. Protoanemonin-containing plants have caused abortions and teratogenic effects in grazing animals.

Reported uses

Pulsatilla has traditionally been claimed to be useful for earaches; spasmodic disorders of the genitourinary tract; nervous, circulatory, and gynecologic disorders; and as a diuretic, menstrual stimulant, expectorant, sedative, and analgesic. It has also been used internally to treat inner eye conditions such as iritis, scleritis, diseases of the retina, cataract, and glaucoma. Its use in homeopathic medicine ranges from coughs and colds to digestive and gynecologic disorders.

Although pulsatilla and other homeopathic remedies have been claimed to be superior to conventional treatments for otitis media in children (Friese et al., 1997), several design flaws make the data suspect.

In France, pulsatilla is used in the symptomatic treatment of nervous disorders, especially minor sleep disorders, and coughs. The German Commission E monographs list the potential uses of pulsatilla as disorders of genital organs, the GI tract, and the urinary tract; inflammatory and infectious diseases of the skin and mucosa; neuralgia; migraine; and general restlessness.

Dosage

Dried herb: 0.1 to 0.3 g in infusion P.O. t.i.d. Alternatively, ½ teaspoon dried herb added to 1 cup boiling water; steeped for 10 to 15 minutes and taken P.O. t.i.d.
Liquid extract (1:1 in 25% ethanol): 0.1 to 0.3 ml P.O. t.i.d.
Tincture (1:10 in 25% ethanol): 0.5 to 3 ml P.O. t.i.d.

Adverse reactions

• Burning of the throat and tongue (if chewed)
• Irritation of the kidneys and urinary tract, gastroenteritis, vomiting (large doses); albuminuria and hematuria (from kidney irritation)
⚠ Direct contact of the fresh plant parts with the skin or mucous membranes may result in severe irritation.

Interactions

None reported.

Contraindications and precautions

Contraindicated in pregnant or breast-feeding patients because of abortive and teratogenic effects in animals.

History of *Anemone pulsatilla*

The scientific name for pulsatilla comes from Greek legends. Windflower, the English term for anemone, refers to the flowers of the plant that appear to be blown open by the wind. Greek legends held that Anemos, god of winds, sent anemones to herald his coming in early spring. The name "pasque flower," a synonym of pulsatilla, is derived from the Old French pasque, or Easter, and refers to various floral emblems of Easter as *A. patens*, *A. pratensis*, and *A. pulsatilla*.

The anemone was once regarded by various cultures as an ill omen; the Chinese called it the "Flower of Death." Other cultures regarded it as a charm against disease (Dobelis, 1986).

Pulsatilla has been used for centuries in traditional medicine. Dioscorides (A.D. 40 to 90), a well-known Roman physician, used pasque flower to treat ocular conditions. Native Americans have used pulsatilla for several conditions: they prepared a poultice of crushed, fresh leaves for rheumatism and neuralgia; inhaled the dried, pulverized leaves for headaches; and took a decoction of the root for pulmonary problems.

The sepals of the flower open wide in sunshine, but close and fold over the stamens when evening approaches or when rain threatens. This folding of the sepals has been likened to a tent; various legends have held that fairies used these "tents" for shelter from the elements.

Special considerations
• Advise the female patient to avoid use of the herb during pregnancy or when breast-feeding.
• Warn the patient not to use or handle fresh plant parts.
• Advise the patient to immediately report unusual symptoms, such as painful urination or blood in the urine.
⚠ Pulsatilla is a potential poison. Symptoms in animals include visual impairment and loss of vision, irritation of the nose and throat, sneezing, paralysis, seizures, dizziness, ulceration of the mouth and throat, vomiting, abdominal pain, diarrhea, excessive salivation, renal damage, blisters, hyperpigmentation, polyuria, and painful urination.

Points of interest
• Pulsatilla has a long history of use among many cultures. (See *History of* Anemone pulsatilla.)

Analysis

Until clinical studies are performed documenting the safety and efficacy of pulsatilla in humans, this plant cannot be recommended for use. The potential for adverse effects outweighs any therapeutic benefit at this time.

References

Dobelis, I.N., ed. *Magic and Medicine of Plants.* Pleasantville, N.Y.: Reader's Digest Association, Inc., 1986.

Friese, K.H., et al. "The Homeopathic Treatment of Otitis Media in Children–Comparisons with Conventional Therapy," *Int J Clin Pharmacol Ther* 35:296-301, 1997.

PUMPKIN

CUCURBITA, PUMPKINSEED OIL, VEGETABLE MARROW

Common trade names
(Various manufacturers; available in combination) Action Super Saw Palmetto Plus, Hain Pumpkin Seed Oil Caps, Max Nutrition System, Mega Men Men's Vitapak, Men's Multiple Formula, Proleve 40, Prost-Answer Alcohol-Free, Pumpkin Seed Shield, Saw Palmetto Formula, Saw Palmetto Pygeum Plus, Ultimate Oil

Common forms
Available as seeds (whole or crushed), seed extract or oil, tablets, and tea.

Source
The seeds of various species of the *Cucurbita* genus (Family Cucurbitaceae), commonly known as pumpkin, squash, or gourd, are used. *Cucurbita pepo* (pumpkin, pepo, or vegetable marrow), *C. maxima* (autumn squash or red gourd), and *C. moschata* (crookneck squash, Canadian pumpkin, or Indian gourd), have been cultivated for medicinal use, as well as nutritional and other practical uses. *C. pepo*, the pumpkin, seems to be used most often for the preparation of medicinal products available in the United States.

Chemical components
Cucurbitin, or (-) 3-amino-3-carboxypyrrolidine, a water-soluble amino acid, has been isolated as the pharmacologically active component of pumpkin seeds (Mihranian and Abou-Chaar, 1968). *Cucurbita* seed oil has been found to contain unsaturated fatty acids, including approximately 25% oleic acid and 55% linoleic acid. The presence of these fatty acids and phytosterols may account for effects on prostatic hypertrophy, though scientific evidence is lacking.

Actions

Cucurbitin inhibits the growth of immature *Schistosoma japonicum* in vivo (Mihranian and Abou-Chaar, 1968). Extracts of seeds and fruit of several pumpkin relatives show anthelmintic activity against pinworms and tapeworms in mice (Elisha et al., 1987).

The beneficial effects of pumpkin seeds on the prostate gland are often attributed to the unsaturated fatty acid content, claimed to have a diuretic effect that increases urine flow and lessens the appearance of urinary retention without reducing prostatic enlargement. Curbicin, a preparation of pumpkin seeds and dwarf palm plants, was evaluated in patients with symptoms of benign prostatic hyperplasia (BPH) and was found to significantly improve urinary flow, micturition time and frequency, and residual urine compared with controls (Carbin et al., 1990). However, another study found no evidence of inhibitory effect on further prostate growth (Bracher, 1997).

Reported uses

Pumpkin has been used in the symptomatic treatment of BPH. For centuries, the seeds have been used to expel tapeworms and other intestinal worms and parasites. However, large doses are required for anthelmintic activity to occur. Because cucurbitin content varies among species, and even within species, pumpkin seeds are ineffective for the treatment of *Taenia* infections. The availability of more reliable and effective medical treatments has resulted in a decreased use of pumpkin for this purpose.

Dosage

For anthelmintic activity, some sources report 60 to 500 g of pumpkin seed in three divided doses, as tea or emulsion of the crushed seeds, in powdered sugar and milk or water (Elisha et al., 1987). In many cultures, daily consumption of small amounts of seed is recommended to prevent worm infestations. In Bulgaria, Turkey, and Ukraine, the daily consumption of a handful of pumpkin seeds is popular for treating prostatic hypertrophy.

Adverse reactions

• Potential electrolyte loss from diuretic effects

Interactions

Diuretics: increased effects. Use together cautiously.

Contraindications and precautions

Contraindicated in patients when the cause of prostatic hypertrophy is unknown. Also contraindicated in pregnant or breast-feeding patients; effects are unknown.

Special considerations
• Monitor the patient for adverse diuretic effects such as electrolyte loss.
• Monitor response to pumpkin if used as an anthelmintic.
• Advise the patient to seek medical attention for proper diagnosis and treatment of BPH. Symptoms may herald more serious disease, including other GI disorders, infection with intestinal parasites, or prostate cancer. Urinary tract outflow obstruction may also result in serious complications including acute renal failure.

Points of interest
• *Cucurbita* seeds, and the oils and extracts made from them, are sold throughout the world for medicinal purposes; the roasted seeds are often sold as snacks.
• The sale of all OTC drugs for the treatment of prostate enlargement was banned by the FDA in 1990 because of the risk of serious adverse effects and complications.

Analysis
Although several small studies indicate a potential benefit of pumpkin seeds, seed extracts, and oils, these products vary widely in their active ingredients. Treatment failure can occur because a large dose is needed for anthelmintic activity, and even supplements contain only trace amounts of active component.

These agents have not been proven to have significant effect on prostatic hypertrophy. It is advisable to check the ingredients for other toxic compounds before use.

References
Bracher, F. "Phytotherapy of Benign Prostatic Hyperplasia," *Urologe A* 36:10-17, 1997. In German; abstract used.

Carbin, B.E., et al. "Treatment of Benign Prostatic Hyperplasia with Phytosterols," *Br J Urol* 6:639-41, 1990.

Elisha, E.E., et al. "The Anthelmintic Activity of Some Iraqi Plants of the Cucurbitaceae," *J Crude Drug Res* 25:153-57, 1987.

Mihranian, V.H., and Abou-Chaar, C.I. "Extraction, Detection and Estimation of Cucurbitin in Cucurbita Seeds," *Lloydia* 31:23-29, 1968.

QUEEN ANNE'S LACE

BEE'S NEST, BIRD'S NEST, DEVIL'S PLAGUE, MOTHER'S
DIE, OIL OF CARROT, WILD CARROT, WILD CARROT SEED

Common trade names
None known.

Common forms
Available as a crude extract and in teas.

Sources
The active ingredients are obtained from the leaves, roots, and seeds
of the *Daucus carota* subspecies *sativas*, which typically grows wild
in various parts of North America.

Chemical components
The fruits and leaves of *D. carota* contain aglycones and glycosides,
which are flavonoids (apigenin, chrysin, luteolin) and porphyrins.
Furanocoumarins (methoxypsoralens) are also found in the plant.
The volatile oil contains many components (pinenes, geraniol, limonene, terpinens, carophyllene, carotol, daucol, and asarone). *D. carota* seeds consist predominantly of unsaturated fatty acids (oleic acid,
linolenic acid, and palmitic acid) and myristicin. *D. carota* contains
choline, ethanol, xylitol, coumarin, formic acid, and oxalic acid.

Actions
The tertiary base of the seeds has papaverine-like, nonspecific antispasmodic activity. However, only about one-tenth the antispasmodic activity of papaverine was found in animals (Gambhir et al.,
1979). In vitro, spasmodic actions have been observed in both
smooth muscle and skeletal muscle, and have been attributed to the
choline component of Queen Anne's lace.

The petroleum ether extract and fatty acids of *D. carota* seeds were
found to halt the normal estrogen cycle and decrease ovary weight
in adult mice (Majumder et al., 1997). Seed extracts produced weak
estrogenic activity and inhibited implantation of embryo (Prakash,
1984).

Pretreatment of *D. carota* extract on carbon tetrachloride-induced
acute liver damage in mice showed decreased serum enzyme levels

of glutamate oxaloacetate transaminase, glutamate pyruvate transaminase, glutamate dehydrogenase, lactate dehydrogenase, alkaline phosphatase, and sorbitol, and also reduced elevated serum bilirubin and urea (Bishayee et al., 1995).

Minimal antifungal activity has also been suggested. Terpinen-4-ol is a documented component of other plants and is known to produce diuresis by renal irritation. Various CV effects of wild carrot have been noted in animal models (Gilani et al., 1994); other studies in animals have reported hypotensive and cardiac depressant effects, and CNS and respiratory depression at high doses.

Reported uses

D. carota is claimed to be useful as an aphrodisiac, abortifacient, diuretic, and hypoglycemic agent. It has been reported anecdotally to treat cancer, dysentery, dyspepsia, gout, heart and kidney disease, menstrual abnormalities, night blindness, ulcers, uterine pain, and worms. There are no controlled clinical trials supporting any of these claims.

Dosage

No consensus exists.

Adverse reactions

- Cardiac depression
- CNS depression
- Contact dermatitis, photosensitization (especially with wet leaves because of methoxypsoralen content)
- Diuresis
- Hypotension

Interactions

Analgesics, anxiolytics, sedative-hypnotic agents: potential enhanced CNS depression. Monitor patient.
Antihypertensives: potential enhanced hypotensive effect. Use cautiously.
Digitalis, other rate-controlling agents: potential heightened depressant effects on myocardium. Monitor vital signs.
Muscle relaxants, other agents that affect muscle function: potential for altered musculoskeletal contraction. Monitor patient.

Contraindications and precautions

Avoid use in pregnant or breast-feeding patients; effects are unknown. The seeds have been reported by some to have abortifacient action (Farnsworth et al., 1975).

Special considerations

• Tell the patient there are insufficient data to support use of this herb.

⚠ Inform the patient that some poisonous plants appear similar to, and may be confused with, *D. carota,* including water hemlock (*Cicuta maculata*), poison hemlock (*Conium maculatum*), and fool's parsley (*Aethusa cynapium*).

• Advise the female patient to report planned or suspected pregnancy.

• Advise the patient to avoid hazardous activities until CNS effects are known.

• Encourage the photosensitive patient to avoid exposure to sunlight by wearing sunblock, a hat, sunglasses, and appropriate clothing.

Points of interest

• *D. carota* is known as Queen Anne's lace because of its intricately patterned, flat flower cluster.

• The herb is also known as mother's die because of the superstition, "If you bring it into your home, your mother will die."

• The orange root of *D. carota* subspecies *carota* (the cultivated carrot), is consumed either cooked or raw, and is different from *D. carota* subspecies *sativas.*

• *D. carota* is used as a dye, fragrance, and flavoring agent.

Analysis

Data from studies in animals suggest that *D. carota* has antispasmodic, antisteroidogenic, antifungal, and hepatoprotective properties. However, there are no data supporting the therapeutic use of *D. carota* for any of these claims. Contact with the leaves has been associated with dermatitis, and neurologic effects occur when the seeds are taken in high doses. Additional data are needed to determine the therapeutic potential for components of *D. carota.*

References

Bishayee, A., et al. "Hepatoprotective Activity of Carrot (*Daucus carota* L.) Against Carbon tetrachloride Intoxication in Mouse Liver," *J Ethnopharmacol* 47:69-74, 1995.

Farnsworth, N.R., et al. "Potential Value of Plants as Sources of New Antifertility Agents I," *J Pharm Sci* 64:535-98, 1975.

Gambhir, S.S., et al. "Antispasmodic Activity of the Tertiary Base of *Daucus carota,* Linn. Seeds," *Indian J Physiol Pharmacol* 23:225-28, 1979.

Gilani, A.H., et al. "Cardiovascular Actions of *Daucus carota,*" *Arch Pharmacol Res* 17:150-53, 1994.

Majumder, P.K., et al. "Anti-steroidogenic Activity of the Petroleum Ether Extract and Fraction 5 (Fatty Acids) of Carrot (*Daucus carota* L.) Seeds in Mouse Ovary," *J Ethnopharmacol* 57:209-12, 1997.

Prakash, A.O. "Biological Evaluation of Some Medicinal Plant Extracts for Contraceptive Efficacy," *Contracep Deliv Syst* 5-9, 1984.

QUINCE

COMMON QUINCE, *CYDONIA VULGARIS*, GOLDEN APPLE, *PYRUS CYDONIA*

Common trade names
None known.

Common forms
Available as fruit syrup, decoctum cydoniae, B.P. (decoction from seeds), mucilage of quince seeds.

Source
The fruit and seeds of *Cydonia oblonga* are used in preparing the medicinal products of quince.

Chemical components
The seeds contain fixed oil, protein, and a small amount of amygdalin, and its coat contains mucilage. The fruit pulp contains malic acid. Beta-D-glucopyranosyl-(1,6)-beta-D-glucopyranoside of 3-hydroxy-beta-ionol has also been isolated in the fruit.

Actions
Tertiary literature suggests astringent, demulcent, emollient, restorative, diuretic, and cardiac effects. A decoction of *C. oblonga* has been shown in vitro to have a bactericidal effect against *Vibrio cholerae* (Guevara et al., 1994).

Reported uses
Traditionally, quince fruit syrup has been commonly added to beverages to treat sore throat, diarrhea, and dysentery. The decoction from the seeds is taken internally in the treatment of dysentery, gonorrhea, and thrush; it is also used as an adjunct in boric-acid eye lotions, and in skin lotions and creams. Anecdotal data exist for these uses; there are no clinical human data available. The mucilage of quince seeds has been used as a suspending agent in pharmaceutical and toilet preparations such as mouthwashes for canker sores, gum problems, and sore throats. Although the quince seeds are thought to be useful in the treatment of cancer (Moertel et al., 1982)—probably due to the cyanogenetic action of amygdalin—no studies have confirmed this effect.

Dosage
For diarrhea, dysentery, gonorrhea, and thrush, sources suggest "large quantities" of decoctum cydoniae (2 drams of quince seed boiled in 1 pint of water for 10 minutes) P.O.

No dosages have been reported for the external use of mucilage preparations.

Adverse reactions
• None reported for the fruit syrup, decoction, or mucilage.
⚠ Quince seeds are potentially toxic because of their amygdalin (laetrile) content.

Interactions
None reported.

Contraindications and precautions
Avoid use in pregnant or breast-feeding patients; effects are unknown.

Special considerations
• Advise the patient taking quince for GI symptoms that other agents with known safety and efficacy data are available.
• Caution the patient to keep quince out of reach of children and pets.

Points of interest
• Other varieties of quinces, especially the Japanese quince, *Cydonia japonica*, are not used medicinally.
• Japanese quince is a popular ornamental plant grown all over the world.

Analysis
Preparations made from the fruit or the mucilage derived from the seed coat may provide minor relief from diarrhea and sore throat because of their astringent and demulcent properties. Although a quince decoction has been shown to have an in vitro bactericidal effect against *V. cholerae*, there are no clinical reports suggesting its value in the treatment of cholera. The amygdalin (laetrile) component of quince is toxic and not effective as a cancer treatment and should not be consumed.

References
Guevara, J.M., et al. "The *In Vitro* Action of Plants on *Vibrio cholerae*," *Rev Gastroenterol Peru* 14:27-31, 1994.
Moertel, C.G., et al. "A Clinical Trial of Amygdalin (Laetrile) in the Treatment of Human Cancer," *N Engl J Med* 306:201-06, 1982.

RAGWORT

CANKERWORT, COCASHWEED, COUGHWEED, DOG STANDARD, FALSE VALERIAN, GOLDEN RAGWORT, GOLDEN SENECIO, LIFEROOT, RAGWEED, St. JAMES WORT, STAGGERWORT, STAMMERWORT, STINKING NANNY, SQUAW WEED, SQUAWROOT

Common trade names
None known.

Common forms
Available as fresh and dried herb.

Source
The leaves, seeds, and flowers of *Senecio jacobae* are commonly used. Ragwort is a member of the daisy family (Compositae) and is native to North America.

Chemical components
Limited information exists on the chemical composition of *Senecio* species. The volatile oil has been described for some species (Dooren et al., 1981). Pyrrolizidine alkaloids (floridanine, florosenine, otosenine, and senecionine) are the chief components isolated from the leaves, seeds, and flowers.

Actions
Several texts report that ragwort has an astringent, cooling, and analgesic effect when applied topically or gargled. It is also claimed to have diuretic, weak expectorant, and uterine stimulant properties.

Reported uses
Emollient poultices have been made from leaves. Plant "juice" has been used as a wash for burns, bee stings, rheumatism, cancerous ulcers, and as a gargle for ulcerations in the throat and mouth. Additionally, claims for use of the plant have been made for the treatment of functional amenorrhea and menopausal neurosis. These claims lack sufficient clinical trial data to validate their application.

Dosage

Only external use of the herb is recommended. Poultices are made by applying the bruised, fresh plant directly on the affected area. Dried herb can be used by soaking it in warm water before applying. Gargle is made by soaking the plant in warm water and then straining.

Adverse reactions

- Nausea
- Pulmonary edema or effusion
- Vomiting

⚠ Hepatotoxicity; pyrrolizidine alkaloids are metabolized to hepatotoxic pyrrolic compounds. Death resulting from liver failure has been reported in animals and humans.

Interactions

Hepatotoxins: increased risk of hepatotoxicity if used in combination. Avoid concomitant use.

Contraindications and precautions

Contraindicated in patients susceptible to liver dysfunction. Avoid use of the herb in pregnant or breast-feeding patients; effects are unknown.

Special considerations

- Monitor liver function tests.
- Advise the patient to report signs and symptoms of liver dysfunction (jaundice, fatigue, fever, abdominal pain).
- Advise the female patient to avoid use of the herb during pregnancy or when breast-feeding.

Points of interest

- In South Africa, some *Senecio* species are used as food.

Analysis

Because there are well-documented cases of human and animal poisonings, ragwort presents an unacceptable risk and should not be used for any medicinal purpose.

References

Dooren, B., et al. "Composition of Essential Oils of Some *Senecio* Species," *Planta Med* 42:385-89, 1981.

RASPBERRY

BLACK RASPBERRY (*RUBUS OCCIDENTALIS*),
BLACKBERRY (*R. FRUTICOSUS, R. FRONDOSUS, R. HISPIDUS, R. MACROPETALUS*), BRAMBLE, BRAMBLE OF MOUNT IDA, HINDBERRY, RASPBIS, RED RASPBERRY (*R. IDAEUS*), *RUBUS*

Common trade names
Red Raspberry Leaves

Common forms
Capsules: 384 mg, 400 mg
Liquid: 1 oz, 2 oz

Source
The red raspberry comes from the *Rubus idaeus* plant; other raspberries species exist, mostly referred to as blackberries. The berries are commonly red, but they may also be yellow. The leaves and berries, and sometimes the root, are used for medicinal purposes.

Chemical components
The *R. idaeus* leaves contain tannin, gallic and ellagic acids, flavonoids, fragarin, organic acids, and vitamin C. The fruit of the raspberry plant contains pectin, fructose, aromatic compounds, and vitamin C (less than that found in the leaves).

Actions
The tannins contained in the leaves of the raspberry plant have an astringent action, whereas the leaves have been used in teas to treat diarrhea and dysentery.

The most common medical claim of the raspberry is its use in pregnancy and childbirth. A tea prepared from the leaves has been used to prevent miscarriage, ameliorate morning sickness, aid in childbirth, and relieve menstrual cramps because it has a slight oxytocic property (reportedly from the fragarin component), which is said to both relax *and* stimulate the uterus. Some sources recommend that pregnant women in their last trimester partake in the fruit to "ease and speed" delivery.

Raspberry may also be useful in treating diabetes; it has lowered blood glucose levels in animals (Briggs and Briggs, 1997).

Reported uses
The leaves of the raspberry plant are reported to have diuretic, expectorant, and anti-inflammatory properties. A tea made from the leaves has been used as a mouthwash and to clean wounds. Because

of the acidity of the juice, the fruits are considered useful for urinary conditions and also to break up and aid in the expulsion of kidney stones and gallstones. When mixed with sugar and boiled into a syrup, the juice has also been used as a gargle for inflamed tonsils.

Because of the presence of tannic and gallic acids, the roots are claimed to have antibiotic action. A tea prepared from the roots may be used for sore throats and cankers and in wound cleansing. All these claims are based on traditional or anecdotal data; human clinical trial data are lacking. The fruit is most commonly used for culinary purposes.

Dosage
Dried red raspberry leaf powder or tablets: 4 to 8 g P.O. t.i.d.
Liquid extract (1 g leaf per ml of 25% ethanol): 4 to 8 ml P.O. t.i.d.

Adverse reactions
None reported.

Interactions
Antidiabetic agents: increased effectiveness of hypoglycemic action. Use cautiously.
Disulfiram: disulfiram reaction may occur if herbal product contains alcohol. Do not use together.

Contraindications and precautions
Use the raspberry leaf or preparations made from it with caution during pregnancy because they may initiate labor.

Special considerations
• Monitor the glucose level in a patient with diabetes.
• Warn the patient taking disulfiram not to take any preparation that contains alcohol.
• Tell the female patient to report planned or suspected pregnancy. Advise the patient who wishes to become pregnant not to exceed moderate consumption of the fruit.

Points of interest
• Raspberry syrup is often used to mask the taste of bitter-tasting drugs.

Analysis
Because the raspberry fruit is a common food item, it appears to be harmless when consumed in moderation. Plant extracts or products containing the leaves should be used with caution and under med-

ical supervision in pregnant women because of their oxytocic effects. Despite its common use as a food, there is currently no acceptable medicinal use of raspberry.

References
Briggs, C.J., and Briggs, K. "Raspberry," *Can Pharmaceutical J* 130:41-43, 1997.

RAUWOLFIA
INDIAN SNAKEROOT, *RAUVOLFIA*, SNAKEROOT

Common trade names
Harmonyl (deserpidine, U.K.), Raudixin, Rauwiloid (alseroxylon fraction), Serpasil (reserpine)

Common forms
Tablets: 50 mg (Raudixin)
Injection (reserpine): 250 mg/ml
Also available as crude root, tea, and liquid and powdered extract.

Source
Of more than 100 species of rauwolfia growing in India, Thailand, South America, Asia, and Africa, the root of *Rauvolfia serpentina* is notable for its medicinal effects.

Chemical components
There are more than 50 alkaloids found in *R. serpentina;* reserpine has been extensively studied in clinical evaluations. Other alkaloids include rescinnamine, deserpidine, syrosingopine, ajmaline (rauwolfine), ajmalinine, ajmalicine, isoajmaline, serpentine, rauwolfinine, and sarpagine.

Actions
Reserpine is known to have hypotensive, depressant, and sedative properties. It produces a catecholamine-depleting effect in the brain and peripheral sympathetic neurons.

Reported uses
Rauwolfia alkaloids have been used to lower fevers, calm noisy babies, cure diarrhea and dysentery, and treat some psychiatric illnesses.

   Much evidence exists that proves the rauwolfia alkaloids' success in the treatment of hypertension and psychiatric conditions. Although the use of rauwolfia alkaloids in hypertensive patients has decreased significantly in the United States because of the adverse effects of the drugs, reserpine is still used in countries such as Spain—usually with a thiazide diuretic (Capella et al., 1983).

Dosage

For hypertension, daily doses of Raudixin 200 mg, Rauwiloid 4 mg, or reserpine 0.25 mg P.O. (100 mg of crude root corresponds to 2 mg alseroxylon fraction, which corresponds to 0.1 mg reserpine). Average daily dose is 600 mg, which corresponds to 6 mg total alkaloids.

Adverse reactions

The following adverse reactions of reserpine may occur with higher doses of rauwolfia:

- Bradycardia
- Decreased libido
- Depression and suicidal ideations
- Edema, weight gain
- GI complaints, diarrhea
- Hypotension (more common with parenteral than oral)
- Increased appetite
- Nasal congestion
- Nightmares, hallucinations
- Peptic ulcer
- Premature ventricular beats
- Unsteady gait and Parkinsonian-like syndrome (rare)

⚠ Breast cancer. Several reports have attempted to link the development of breast cancer with consumption of rauwolfia derivatives (O'Fallon et al., 1975; Armstrong et al., 1976; Schyve et al., 1978). Many reports have failed to verify this association, but the issue remains controversial.

Interactions

Antihypertensives, nitrates: additive hypotensive effects. Use cautiously.

Barbiturates, CNS depressants: pronounced CNS effects and toxicity when rauwolfia alkaloids are used with barbiturates (Pfeifer et al., 1976). Avoid concomitant use.

Cardiac glycosides: lowered heart rate. Monitor patient.

Levodopa: reduced effectiveness of levodopa. Avoid concomitant use.

NSAIDs, tricyclic antidepressants: possible reduced hypotensive effectiveness of rauwolfia derivatives. Monitor patient.

Sympathomimetics: initial increase in blood pressure. Monitor patient.

Contraindications and precautions

Rauwolfia is contraindicated in active peptic ulcer disease and ulcerative colitis because it increases gastric acid secretion. Use cautiously in patients with current diagnosis or past history of breast cancer and during pregnancy.

Special considerations

- Know that the patient should discontinue rauwolfia ingestion at least 2 weeks before undergoing electroconvulsive therapy.
- Monitor the patient's blood pressure.
- Counsel the patient with a history of depression or at risk for depression to avoid use of rauwolfia derivatives.
- Advise the patient with a history of cancer (especially breast cancer) or peptic ulcer to avoid use of rauwolfia derivatives.
- Caution the patient to avoid hazardous activities until CNS and hypotensive effects of rauwolfia derivatives are known.
- Explain that the adverse effects of rauwolfia alkaloids limit their use. Other proven agents exist for the treatment of hypertension or psychiatric illnesses.

Analysis

Rauwolfia alkaloids have proven to be valuable in the treatment of hypertension and some psychoses; the most popular and most studied is reserpine. Extensive application of rauwolfia derivatives is limited by the adverse reactions of the drugs. Other safe, and equally effective, agents are available.

References

Armstrong, B., et al. "Rauwolfia Derivatives and Breast Cancer in Hypertensive Women," *Lancet* 2:8-12, 1976.

Capella D., et al. "Utilization of Antihypertensive Drugs in Certain European Countries," *Eur J Clin Pharmacol* 25:431-35, 1983.

O'Fallon, W.M., et al. "Rauwolfia Derivatives and Breast Cancer. A Case/Control Study in Olmsted County, Minnesota," *Lancet* 2:292-96, 1975.

Pfeifer H.J., et al. "Clinical Toxicity of Reserpine in Hospitalized Patients: A Report from the Boston Collaborative Drug Surveillance Program," *Am J Med* 271:269-76, 1976.

Schyve, P.M., et al. "Neuroleptic-Induced Prolactin Level Elevation and Breast Cancer; An Emerging Clinical Issue," *Arch Gen Psychiatry* 35:1291-1301, 1978.

RED CLOVER

BEEBREAD, COW CLOVER, MEADOW CLOVER, MISSOURI MILK VETCH, PURPLE CLOVER, TREFOIL, WILD CLOVER

Common trade names

(Available in combination) Red Clover Blossoms, Red Clover Cleanser, Red Clover Combo, Red Clover Plus, Red Clover Tops

Common forms

Tablets: 100 mg
Capsules: 200 mg, 354 mg, 375 mg, 430 mg

Liquid: 1 oz, 2 oz
Also available as a tea and in raw sprouts

Source
The aerial parts of the plant, specifically the rose-colored flower head, are used. *Trifolium pratense,* or red clover, was naturalized to the United States from its native Europe.

Chemical components
More than 125 chemicals have been identified in the red clover plant. The notable components include the elemental constituents (aluminum, calcium, copper, iron, magnesium, manganese, potassium), several carbohydrates (arabinose, glucose, xylose, rhamnose), two coumarins (coumarin, medicagol), various flavonoids and iso-flavonoids, saponins, coumaric acid, salicylic acid, clovamide compounds, and fats.

Actions
In animals, isoflavonoid components are thought to be responsible for estrogen-like actions (Kelly et al., 1979). Components of red clover have altered vaginal cytology, increased follicle-stimulating hormone, and altered luteinizing hormone serum levels in animal models (Wilcox et al., 1990; Zava et al., 1998).

Preliminary information reported that red clover possessed a carcinogen-protective effect in vitro (Cassady et al., 1988).

Reported uses
There are several claims for red clover—the more popular include uses as an estrogen replacement for postmenopausal women, treatment for chronic skin diseases, and to suppress whooping cough.

Dosage
For skin diseases, apply compress b.i.d.
Tincture: 2 to 6 ml P.O. t.i.d.
Infusion made by pouring hot water over 1 to 3 teaspoons of dried herb. Let stand for 10 to 15 minutes, and take P.O. t.i.d.

Adverse reactions
• Estrogen-like effects; breast tenderness and enlargement, change in menses, weight gain and redistribution
• Infertility and growth disorders (with large doses; reported in animals)
• Potentiated growth of estrogen receptor-positive neoplasia

Interactions

Anticoagulants (heparin, warfarin), antiplatelet agents (aspirin, clopidogrel, ticlopidine): possible enhanced risk of bleeding. Red clover contains some coumarin and coumarin-like compounds. Monitor patient closely.

Oral contraceptives: possible enhanced effects by increasing estrogen components. Use cautiously.

Contraindications and precautions

Avoid use in pregnant or breast-feeding patients; effects are unknown. Also avoid use in patients with estrogen receptor-positive neoplasia. Use cautiously in patients susceptible to bleeding problems or in those taking anticoagulants.

Special considerations

• Monitor the patient for signs and symptoms of bleeding.
• Alert the pathology laboratory reviewing Papanicolaou smear that patient is taking red clover.
• Explain that few data exist about the use of red clover in humans. Other proven estrogen products exist and should be pursued first.
• Counsel the female patient to avoid use of red clover if pregnancy is desired.
• Advise the patient with a history of estrogen receptor-positive malignancy to avoid use of red clover.

Points of interest

• Red clover has long been implicated as a cause of infertility in livestock (Hoffman et al., 1997).

Analysis

Although many uses for red clover have been reported, only animal and in vitro data exist. Because efficacy evidence in humans is lacking and the toxicity of the herb is essentially undescribed, consumption of red clover cannot be recommended. There are numerous estrogen products currently available; the need for the herb's estrogen-like effects is questionable.

References

Cassady, J.M., et al. "Use of a Mammalian Cell Culture Benzo(a)pyrene Metabolism Assay for the Detection of Potential Anticarcinogens from Natural Products: Inhibition of Metabolism by Biochanin A, an Isoflavone from *Trifolium pratense* L," *Cancer Res* 48:6257-61, 1988.
Hoffman, P.C., et al. "Performance of Lactating Dairy Cows Fed Red Clover or Alfalfa Silage," *J Dairy Sci* 80: 3308-15, 1997.
Kelly, R.W., et al. "Formononentin Content of Grasslands Pawera Red Clover and Its Estrogenic Activity in Sheep," *N Z J Exp Agricult* 7:131-34, 1979.

Wilcox, G., et al. "Estrogenic Effects of Plant Foods in Postmenopausal Women," *BMJ* 301:905-06, 1990.

Zava, D.T., et al. "Estrogen and Progestin Bioactivity of Foods, Herbs, and Spices," *Proc Soc Exper Biol Med* 217:369-78, 1998.

RED POPPY

CORN POPPY, CORN ROSE, FIELD POPPY, FLANDERS POPPY, *PAPAVER RHOEAS*

Common trade names
None known.

Common forms
Available as capsules.

Source
Red poppy, *Papaver rhoeas*, is an annual plant of the Papaveraceae family. It is native to Europe, North Africa, and temperate areas of Asia; it has been naturalized in North America and South America. The bright red-colored flowers are used.

Chemical components
Red poppy contains many alkaloids, including papaverine, rhoea-dine, and isorhoeadine. It has been reported that the alkaloid content is similar to that of the opium poppy, *Papaver somniferum*, which contains morphine, noscapine, and codeine. Controversy exists regarding the presence of significant pharmacologically active narcotic constituents. Other constituents of red poppy include meconic acid, mekocyanin, mucilage, and tannin.

Actions
The actions of the various components of red poppy have not been studied in animals or humans.

Reported uses
Similar to opium poppy, red poppy is claimed to be mildly analgesic and sedative. It has been primarily used as a cough suppressant and expectorant; however, its effectiveness for any use has not been evaluated in controlled clinical human trials.

Dosage
No consensus exists.

Adverse reactions
• Potential CNS depressant effects
• A case of allergic contact dermatitis has been reported (Gamboa et al., 1997).

Interactions
Analgesics, CNS depressants: potential additive effects of these agents. Avoid concomitant use.

Contraindications and precautions
Avoid use in pregnant or breast-feeding patients; effects are unknown. Also, avoid use in patients with allergy to morphine or codeine. Use cautiously in patients with a history of allergic contact dermatitis.

Special considerations
• Monitor CNS effects.
• Advise the patient that few data exist with regard to red poppy.

Points of interest
• Members of the Papaveraceae family may contain potentially toxic alkaloids, such as morphine, codeine, papaverine, noscapine, and thebaine. Because red poppy contains unknown quantities of these substances, toxic doses of red poppy cannot be estimated.

Analysis
Unlike opium poppy, there is little information about the red poppy. Its components are not well characterized, and the actual quantities contained are unknown. Red poppy has not been demonstrated to be therapeutically useful, and its toxic potential is unclear. Therefore, its use cannot be recommended at this time.

References
Gamboa, P.M., et al. "Allergic Contact Urticaria from Poppy Flowers (*Papaver rhoeas*)," *Contact Dermatitis* 37:140-41, 1997.

RHATANY

KRAMERIA ROOT, MAPATO, PERUVIAN RHATANY, PUMACUCHU, RAIZ PARA LOS DIENTES, RATANHIAWURZEL, RED RHATANY, RHATANHIA

Common trade names
(Various European manufacturers) Echtrosept-GT, Encialina, Gengivario, Parodontax, Repha-OS

Common forms

Available as a tincture, mouthwash, lozenge, powder, syrup, and solution.

Source

The active ingredients are extracted from the dried root of *Krameria triandra,* also known as pumacuchu or mapato.

Chemical components

The agent is composed primarily of 10% to 20% tannins. Rhataniatannic acid, also known as krameria tannic acid, is the principal tannin extracted from the plant.

Actions

Rhatany is a tannin-containing herb that functions as an astringent. The primary mechanism of action for astringents is through the coagulation of surface proteins of cells (Swinyard and Pathak, 1985), which decreases cell permeability and reduces secretions of inflamed tissues. The coagulated surface proteins function as a protective barrier on skin surfaces and helps promote growth of new tissue underneath. In areas of inflammation, astringents cause vasoconstriction and reduce blood flow. Astringents cool and dry skin surfaces when applied as wet dressings; they also clean the skin of surface exudates and debris.

Reported uses

Therapeutic claims for rhatany are derived from the plant's astringent properties. They are claimed to be useful in treating conditions involving irritations of the skin, mucous membranes, and gingiva. Both internal and external preparations of rhatany are thought to have medicinal uses. Specific applications have included treatment of inflammatory disorders of the oropharynx, bleeding gums, pyorrhoea, canker sores, diarrhea, dysentery, urinary incontinence, and bowel and bladder bleeding. However, clinical trials supporting the safety and efficacy of rhatany in treating these conditions are lacking.

Dosage

Numerous doses involving several forms have been prepared. However, clinical trials establishing standard doses of rhatany are lacking. The German Commission E recommends the decoction to be taken P.O. (1 g in 1 cup of water) or 5 to 10 drops of tincture in 1 glass of water.
For topical use, apply b.i.d. to t.i.d.

Adverse reactions
⚠ Acute hepatotoxicity (with tannic acid)

Interactions
Disulfiram: disulfiram reaction if the tincture product contains alcohol. Avoid concomitant use.

Contraindications and precautions
Contraindicated in patients with a history of hypersensitivity to products containing the plant or its components. Avoid use of rhatany-containing products that are highly astringent. Tannic acid-containing products are generally considered unsafe and ineffective; frequent application of such products could result in absorption of tannic acid from the GI tract, denuded mucosal surfaces, and mucous membranes sufficient enough to produce toxicity.

Special considerations
• Monitor liver function tests.
• Advise the patient taking disulfiram not to take the tincture.
• Advise the patient to report signs and symptoms of liver dysfunction (jaundice, fatigue, fever).

Points of interest
• Only two astringent solutions, aluminum acetate and witch hazel, are considered safe and effective by the FDA for treating minor skin irritations (West and Nowakowski, 1996). The FDA has ruled that no ingredient in rhatany is generally recognized as safe and effective for use as an OTC oral wound healing agent (Flynn, 1996).

Analysis
Rhatany is a tannin-containing plant claimed to have several medicinal applications as an astringent. However, well-controlled clinical trials supporting its safety and efficacy are lacking. Internal and external use of rhatany are best avoided.

References
Flynn, A.A. "Oral Health Products," in *Handbook of Nonprescription Drugs*, 9th ed. Edited by Covington, T.R., et al. Washington, D.C.: United Book Press, Inc., 1996.

Swinyard, E.A., and Pathak, M.A. "Locally Acting Drugs," in *Goodman and Gilman's: The Pharmacological Basis of Therapeutics*, 7th ed. Edited by Goodman, L.S., et al. New York: Macmillan Publishing Company, 1985.

West, D.P., and Nowakowski, P.A. "Dermatitis," in *Handbook of Nonprescription Drugs*, 9th ed. Edited by Covington, T.R., et al. Washington, D.C.: United Book Press, Inc., 1996.

ROSE HIPS
DOG ROSE FRUIT, DOG BRIER FRUIT, HIPBERRIES, WILD
BRIER BERRIES

Common trade names
(Various manufacturers; available in combination) Rose Hips,
Vitamin C with Rose Hips

Common forms
Available as capsules, tablets, syrup, tincture, teas, cream, and extracts in combination with vitamin preparations.

Source
The "rose hip," or fruit of *Rosa canina*, is usually dried and processed before use. The plant grows widely in North America after having been naturalized from Europe and Asia. Although *R. canina* is the major source of rose hips, other Rosaceae plants have also been used.

Chemical components
Rose hips contain vitamin C, tannins, pectins, and carotene (carotenoids).

Actions
The *R. canina* flower petal extract containing anthocyans was shown to have a protective effect on radiation-induced cell damage in Chinese hamster cells (Akhmadieva et al., 1993). The roots of *R. canina* showed anti-inflammatory effects in vitro. This anti-inflammatory activity was also exhibited by several plant extracts used in Turkish traditional medicine, when they exerted effects on either tumor necrosis factor or interleukin-1 (Yesilada et al., 1997).

Although rose hips is claimed to have a diuretic effect, this effect was not seen in rats (Grases et al., 1992). An infusion of *R. canina* may have some benefit on calcium oxalate urolithiasis.

Reported uses
A "natural" source of vitamin C (Brand et al., 1982), rose hips has been claimed to be useful as a laxative, capillary strengthener, and boost to the immune system to prevent illness. Although vitamin C has been studied for these effects, studies on rose hips are lacking. Some herbal references claim that the leaves have been used as a poultice to heal wounds.

Dosage
No consensus exists.

Adverse reactions
● Allergic reactions (Kwaselow et al., 1990)
● Diarrhea
● Renal dysfunction (poorly documented)

Interactions
None reported.

Contraindications and precautions
Avoid use of the herb in pregnant or breast-feeding patients; effects are unknown. Use cautiously in patients with atopy or plant allergies.

Special considerations
● Know that in diabetic patients, high-dose vitamin C may interact with the home glucose monitoring tests.
● Advise the patient to take sources of vitamin C from reliable manufacturers; rose hips (after processing) may represent only a minor and variable source of vitamin C.
● Advise the patient with plant allergies to pursue other sources of vitamin C.

Points of interest
● Rose hips contains more vitamin C per milligram than many citrus fruits and raw broccoli. However, much of the vitamin C contained in rose hips (over 50%) may be destroyed during processing. More than 100 g of actual rose hips may be needed to obtain 1,200 mg of vitamin C. Thus, many products containing rose hips are supplemented with synthetically prepared vitamin C.
● Although a German monograph supported the use of rose hips for preventing colds and flu, the data appear questionable.

Analysis
Despite the herb's vitamin C content, large quantities of rose hips must be ingested to obtain commonly available amounts of vitamin C in tablet form.

References
Akhmadieva, A.Kh., et al. "The Protective Action of a Natural Preparation of Anthocyan (Pelargonidin-3,5-diglucoside)," *Radiobiologia* 33:433-35, 1993.
Brand, J.C., et al. "An Outstanding Food Source of Vitamin C," *Lancet* 16:873, 1982. Letter.
Grases, F., et al. "Effect of *'Rosa canina'* Infusion and Magnesium on the Urinary Risk Factors of Calcium Oxalate Urolithiasis," *Planta Med* 58:509-12, 1992.
Kwaselow, A., et al. "Rose Hips: A New Occupational Allergen," *J Allergy Clin Immunol* 85:704-08, 1990.

Yesilada, E., et al. "Inhibitory Effects of Turkish Folk Remedies on Inflammatory Cytokines: Interleukin-1alpha, Interleukin-1beta, and Tumor Necrosis Factor," *J Ethnopharmacol* 58:59-73, 1997.

ROSEMARY

COMPASS PLANT, INCENSOR, OLD MAN

Common trade names
Rosemary Oil

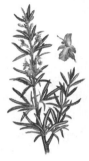

Common forms
Available as volatile oil, infusion, or tea, and in bath and toiletry products.

Source
The leaves, twigs, or flowering tops are typically pursued for active medicinal components of *Rosemarinus officinalis*. Rosemary is native to the Mediterranean region, but is commonly cultivated indoors and in mild climates of North America.

Chemical components
The leaves contain a volatile oil, from which several compounds have been isolated (monoterpene hydrocarbons, camphor, borneol, and cineole). The leaves also contain the flavonoid pigments diosmin, diosmetin, and genkwanin. Numerous volatile and aromatic compounds are also present.

Actions
Several pharmacologic effects have been described for rosemary or its components. Antibacterial and antifungal properties have been demonstrated for the volatile oil. Various gram-positive and gram-negative organisms commonly responsible for food spoilage are inhibited by the presence of rosemary oil. The antioxidant properties are thought to be related to the carnosol and ursol components of rosemary oil.

Several sources report that diosmin reduces capillary permeability and fragility, whereas a derivative of rosemaricine is capable of inducing smooth muscle and analgesic effects in vitro.

I.V. administration of rosemary oil has demonstrated spasmolytic action on the Oddi muscle sphincter of guinea pigs. Rabbit models of septic shock have shown that I.V. rosemarinic acid suppresses endotoxin-mediated activation of the sequence of steps leading to septic shock. It also suppresses release of thromboxane A_2, formation of prostacyclin, thrombocytopenia, and hypotension (Bult et al., 1985).

Although these effects are believed to be the result of the inhibitory effect of rosmarinic acid on complement (a component of blood), other studies have suggested other mechanisms of anti-inflammatory activity (Parnham and Kesselring, 1985).

Rosmarinic acid has also been touted as the component responsible for successful prevention of adult respiratory distress syndrome in rabbit models (Parnham and Kesselring, 1985). Additional rodent studies of rosemary oil and rosmarinic acid have demonstrated increased locomotor effects and antigonadotropic effects, respectively.

In recent years, a number of studies have been published that suggest potential anticancer properties of the plant. These preliminary studies suggest that rosemary components have the potential to decrease activation and increase detoxification of important human carcinogens. Rosemary components might have potential as chemoprotectants, but studies in humans are necessary (Huang et al., 1994; Oxford et al., 1997).

Reported uses
The clinical effects of rosemary are not well known; few studies have been conducted in humans. Rosemary is widely used as a spice in cooking. It has been claimed to be of use in traditional medicine for its astringent, tonic, antiflatulent, antispasmodic, and diaphoretic properties.

Rosemary extract and the volatile oil have been used through the centuries to promote menstrual flow and as an abortifacient. Rosemary oil has been used topically and taken internally to improve chronic circulatory weakness and hypotension, although a few tertiary references warn against internal consumption of the undiluted volatile oil. Rosemary has also been used for ingestion and rheumatic disorders; efficacy is yet to be demonstrated.

A lotion consisting of rosemary has been suggested to stimulate hair growth and prevent baldness, although this has not yet been proven.

Dosage
Therapeutic doses of rosemary have not been defined, although the following have been promoted:
Liquid extract (1:1 in 45% alcohol): 1 to 4 ml P.O. t.i.d.
Tea: 1 to 4 g of the leaf as a tea P.O. t.i.d.
Essential oil in an ointment preparation may also be used externally.

Adverse reactions
• Antifertility effects (Rosemary oil may prevent implantation but does not appear to interfere with the normal development of the fertilized ova after implantation [Lemonica et al., 1996].)
• Dermatitis and photosensitivity in hypersensitive individuals

• Erythema (possible with preparations meant for bathing)
• Stomach and intestinal irritation, renal damage (with large quantities of volatile oil)

Interactions
Disulfiram: disulfiram reaction if herbal product contains alcohol. Do not use together.

Contraindications and precautions
Avoid use of the herb in pregnant or breast-feeding patients; effects are unknown. Use with caution in persons who have experienced a prior plant sensitivity reaction.

Special considerations
• Inform the patient that therapeutic efficacy has not been demonstrated for rosemary or its components for any disease.
• Warn the patient that the undiluted oil should not be taken internally until its safety can be established.
• Warn the female patient wishing to become pregnant to avoid consumption of this herb.
• Advise the patient taking disulfiram not to take a form of this drug that contains alcohol.

Points of interest
• German health authorities have approved rosemary for internal use for indigestion and as a supportive treatment for rheumatic disorders. It is also approved for external use for circulatory disorders.

Analysis
Rosemary is widely used in both cooking and cosmetics. Several components of rosemary oil have been shown to possess pharmacologic activity; however, enthusiasm for some interesting pharmacologic effects seen in animals must be interpreted in light of the fact that studies in humans are unavailable. Until studies are conducted in humans, this herb cannot be recommended for any therapeutic application. Future areas of research will likely focus on the potential of rosemary in the treatment of acute inflammatory conditions, such as adult respiratory distress syndrome and septic shock, or as a chemotherapeutic agent.

References
Bult, H., et al. "Modification of Endotoxin-Induced Hemodynamic and Hematologic Changes in the Rabbit by Methylprednisolone, F(ab')2 Fragments and Rosmarinic Acid," *Biochem Pharmacol* 35:1397-1400, 1985.
Huang, M.T., et al. "Inhibition of Skin Tumorigenesis by Rosemary and Its Constituents Carnosol and Ursolic Acid," *Cancer Res* 54:701-08, 1994.

Lemonica, I.P., et al. "Study of the Embryotoxic Effects of an Extract of Rosemary (*Rosemarinus officinalis* L.)," *Br J Med Biol Res* 29:223-27, 1996. Abstract.

Oxford, E.A., et al. "Mechanisms Involved in the Chemoprotective Effects of Rosemary Extract Studied in Human Liver and Bronchial Cells," *Cancer Lett* 114:275-81, 1997.

Parnham, M.J., and Kesselring, K. "Rosmarinic Acid," *Drugs Future* 10:756-57, 1985.

ROYAL JELLY

QUEEN BEE JELLY

Common trade names
Royal Jelly

Common forms
Available in 100-mg ampules and capsules, topical cream, ointment, lotion, and soap.

Source
Royal jelly is a milky-white secretion formulated by worker bees of *Apis mellifers* and fed to the queen bee to induce her growth and development.

Chemical components
Royal jelly consists of a mixture of complex proteins, sugars, fats, water, fatty acids, carbohydrates, and variable amounts of vitamins (A, B, C, and E) and minerals (potassium, calcium, zinc, iron, manganese, and acetylcholine). The B vitamins are especially prominent, with pantothenic acid expression predominating (Vittek, 1995). Royal jelly also provides approximately 20 amino acids and contains gamma globulin. A substance known as 10-hydroxy-trans-(2)-decanoic acid (HDA) has been identified and is thought to play an important role in bee growth and regulation.

Actions
Clinical trials have noted some antimicrobial activity in royal jelly, attributed to HDA and gamma globulin. The activity is found to be 25% less effective than penicillin and 20% less active than chlortetracycline.

Preliminary studies found antitumor activity in experimental mouse leukemias using royal jelly. Published reports suggest royal jelly may be effective in preventing atherosclerosis. It significantly influences lipid metabolism in rats and prevents atherosclerosis in rabbits fed cholesterol-rich diets.

Serum cholesterol was reduced up to 25% in humans. Because of an abundance of phytosterols (mainly beta-sitosterol), royal jelly is thought to decrease the resorption of cholesterol in the GI tract. (Both beta-sitosterol and cholesterol compete for binding sites.) Researchers have reported a significant reduction in total blood serum lipids, cholesterol levels, and normalization of high-density lipoproteins and low-density lipoprotein levels (Vittek, 1995).

Reported uses

Queen bees are twice the size of worker bees, are fertile (worker bees are sterile), and live 5 to 8 years longer than worker bees, all of which may contribute to the purported claims of royal jelly. However, royal jelly does not provide any estrogenic effects that promote fertility, growth, or longevity. The agent's effectiveness in rejuvenating the skin and slowing the aging process (erasing wrinkles and facial blemishes) has not been completely substantiated.

Although there is no evidence for it, royal jelly has also been claimed to be useful for treating male pattern baldness and menopause and for improving sexual performance. A cholesterol-lowering action has been reported in humans. Although royal jelly has demonstrated in vitro antimicrobial activity, no clinical trials have been reported for this indication.

Dosage

For lowering cholesterol, 50 to 100 mg P.O. daily.
For cosmetic use, apply royal jelly topically b.i.d. or t.i.d.

Adverse reactions

- Allergic reactions (can be severe)
- Exacerbation of asthma
- Hyperglycemia

⚠ Life-threatening bronchospasm has occurred in asthmatic patients after ingestion of royal jelly. Royal jelly has been responsible for IgE-mediated anaphylaxis, leading to death in a least one individual (Bullock et al., 1994; Harwood et al., 1996).

Interactions

Antidiabetic agents: may lead to loss of glycemic control in diabetic patients. Avoid concomitant use.

Contraindications and precautions

Avoid use of royal jelly in pregnant or breast-feeding patients; effects are unknown. Use cautiously in patients susceptible to allergic reactions or asthma and in those taking antidiabetic agents.

Special considerations
● Monitor blood glucose levels closely because royal jelly may contribute to loss of glycemic control in diabetic patients.
● Counsel the patient with atopy against use of this agent.
● Inform the asthmatic patient that life-threatening bronchospasm has occurred after ingestion of this agent.
● Advise the female patient to report planned or suspected pregnancy.

Analysis
Death has occurred by bronchospasm with the use of royal jelly in asthmatic patients. The agent may reduce cholesterol in humans; however, long-term evidence is lacking and the availability of clinically proven agents limits royal jelly's usefulness for this condition. Insufficient data and poorly documented risk profiles for royal jelly make it unsuitable for use at this time.

References
Bullock, R.J., et al. "Fatal Royal Jelly Induced Asthma," *Med J Aust* 160:44, 1994.
Harwood, M., et al. "Asthma Following Royal Jelly," *N Z Med J* 23:325, 1996.
Vittek, J. "Effect of Royal Jelly on Serum Lipids in Experimental Animals and Humans with Atherosclerosis," *Experientia* 51:927-35, 1995.

RUE
HERB-OF-GRACE, HERBYGRASS, *RUTA*, RUTAE HERBA, VINRUTA

Common trade names
(Various manufacturers; available in combination) Joint and Muscle Relief Cream, Rue

Common forms
Available as crude herb, capsules, extracts, and creams.

Source
Rue, or *Ruta graveolens,* is a member of the Rutaceae family. Although cultivated in Europe, America, Asia, and Africa, rue is native to the Mediterranean region. It is generally considered to have a disagreeable odor. Both the leaves and root have been used.

Chemical components
Numerous specific chemical entities have been isolated from *R. graveolens*, including quinoline alkaloids, furocoumarins, gamma-eagarine, lignanes, volatile oils, and psoralens.

Actions

Rue extracts have shown antimicrobial effects and mutagenic and cytotoxic actions in several cellular models. Studies in mammals have demonstrated an antifertility action, mediated by decreased implantation (Ghandi et al., 1991). An abortifacient action has also been noted. Components of rue nonselectively block potassium and sodium channels in myelinated nerves (Bethge et al., 1991).

Rue has also demonstrated CV effects in rats. It exhibits positive chronotropic and inotropic effects in isolated rat atria (Chui and Fung, 1997). It acts as a hypotensive agent in normotensive animals, presumably through a direct vasodilatory mechanism. The alkaloids have demonstrated antispasmodic effects. Rue also exhibits analgesic properties in mice (Atta and Alkofahi, 1998).

Reported uses

Rue has traditionally been promoted as a spasmolytic and abortifacient. It has also been used for its sedative effects and to promote lactation. Based on anecdotal data and studies in animals, the herb is currently being promoted for the treatment of sports injuries, arthritis, bruising, sprains and strains, and other joint and muscle disorders. However, there are no human clinical trial data available for these uses.

Other claims for which there are no supporting data include use in neuralgia, eye strain, earache, edema, dysmenorrhea, amenorrhea, and digestive disorders, and as an anthelmintic. Rue has also been used by Chinese herbalists for snake and insect bites.

Dosage

For earache, a few drops of infused oil on a cotton plug placed over the ear.
Extract: ¼ to 1 teaspoonful P.O. t.i.d. with water and food.
Capsule: 1 capsule P.O. t.i.d. with water and food.
Cream: applied as needed.

Adverse reactions

• Allergic skin reactions (erythema, hyperpigmentation, and severe blistering) with topical use
• Hypotension
• Increased risk of spontaneous abortion
• Photosensitivity

Interactions

Antihypertensives: possible increased vasodilatory effects. Use with caution.
Digoxin, dobutamine: enhanced inotropic effects. Use with caution.

Fertility agents: possible counteraction of therapy. Avoid concomitant use.

Contraindications and precautions
Avoid use in pregnant patients because of the risk of abortion. Use cautiously in patients with a history of heart failure or arrhythmias and in those receiving antihypertensive medications.

Special considerations
• Monitor for cumulative effects in patients taking antihypertensives.
• Rue is thought to be a powerful antidote at low doses; larger doses are toxic.
• Caution the patient that there is insufficient information regarding the effects of rue in humans. The risks of use outweigh the benefits.
• Advise the female patient to report planned or suspected pregnancy.
• Instruct the patient to discontinue use of the herb and to notify the health care professional of allergic skin reactions.

Analysis
Preliminary studies in animals show that rue has many interesting pharmacologic effects. Insufficient testing in humans makes any therapeutic application premature. The strong potential for contact dermatitis severely restricts topical use of this agent. In Germany, rue is considered ineffective and unsafe. At present, rue cannot be recommended for any use.

References
Atta, A.H., and Alkofahi, A. "Anti-nociceptive and Anti-inflammatory Effects of Some Jordanian Medicinal Plant Extracts," *J Ethnopharmacol* 60:117-24, 1998.

Bethge, E.W., et al."Effects of Some Potassium Channel Blockers on the Ionic Currents in Myelinated Nerve," *Gen Physiol Biophys* 10:225-44, 1991.

Chui, K.W., and Fung, A.Y. "The Cardiovascular Effects of Green Beans (*Phaseolus aureus*), Common Rue (*Ruta graveolens*), and Kelp (*Laminaria japonica*) in Rats," *Gen Pharmacol* 29:859-62, 1997.

Ghandi, M., et al. "Post-coital Antifertility Action of *Ruta graveolens* in Female Rats and Hamsters," *J Ethnopharmacol* 34:49-59, 1991.

SAFFLOWER

Common trade names
(Various manufacturers; available in combination) Safflower Oil, Saffron

Common forms
Available as tea, extracts, 390-mg capsules, and 8.5-oz liquid.

Source
Carthamus tinctorius is indigenous to the Middle East. However, it is cultivated throughout Europe and the United States for its edible oil, which is obtained from the seeds.

Chemical components
The oil consists of unsaturated fatty acids, including linoleic acid (75%), oleic acid (13%), palmitic acid (6%), steric acid (3%), and a mixture of saturated fatty acids. The flowers of the plant contain a dye, carthamin. Seven antioxidant compounds have been isolated from *C. tinctorius.*

Actions
Safflower oil is considered a long-chain triglyceride (LCT), which may exert an effect on the reticuloendothelial system. The linoleic acid portions of the oil (polyunsaturated fatty acids) are converted into immunosuppressants, prostaglandin E_2, and prostaglandin I_2 within the prostaglandin pathway (Sax, 1990).

Reported uses
Safflower is thought to treat fevers and constipation. The oil has been compounded with glycerin, rose oil, polysorbate 80, benzyl alcohol, and water to produce an external massage lotion. The topical administration of safflower oil in patients with essential fatty acid deficiency failed to show improvement in critically ill patients; however, previous studies have supported this use in stable outpatients and chronically ill patients (Sacks et al., 1994). A diet high in safflower oil has been shown to reduce some lipid levels (Wardlaw et

al., 1991). In Chinese herbal medicine, safflower has been used to treat menstrual disorders.

Dosage
Fresh flower: 1 to 2 tablespoon P.O. t.i.d.
Dried flower: 2 to 3 g P.O. t.i.d.
Extract: 3 g dried flower in 15 ml alcohol and 15 ml water P.O. t.i.d.

Adverse reactions
None reported.

Interactions
None reported; however, in theory, use of safflower oil may enhance immunosuppressive effects of other immunosuppressive agents (azathioprine, cyclosporine, tacrolimus). Also avoid concurrent use of herb and administration of vaccines.

Contraindications and precautions
Use with caution in immunosuppressed patients, especially burn or septic patients and transplant recipients. Avoid excessive consumption of safflower in pregnant or breast-feeding patients; effects are unknown. Murine models have shown it to be a uterine stimulant (Shi et al., 1995).

Special considerations
• Do not administer vaccines to patients using safflower because of its potential immunosuppressive effects.
• Explain that studies have failed to support therapeutic applications for safflower oil.
• Counsel the patient using safflower oil for its lipid-lowering effects to change to other proven cholesterol-lowering therapies.

Points of interest
• Safflower oil or linoleic acid may be a component of commercially available lipid emulsions.
• Safflower (*C. tinctorius*) should not be confused with the true saffron (*Crocus sativus*).

Analysis
Safflower is used primarily as a source of edible polyunsaturated oil. It has been used in teas to reduce fevers by inducing sweating, and as a laxative; however, there is no supporting evidence for these uses. Although a diet rich in safflower oil has been shown to lower cholesterol, it has not been proven to reduce the incidence of CV mortality; therefore, safflower oil remains an adjunct to other proven therapies.

References

Sacks, G.S., et al. "Failure of Topical Vegetable Oils to Prevent Essential Fatty Acid Deficiency in a Critically Ill Patient Receiving Long-Term Parenteral Nutrition," *JPEN* 18: 274-77, 1994.

Sax, H.C. "Practicalities of Lipids: ICU Patient, Autoimmune Disease, and Vascular Disease," *JPEN* 14:223S-25S, 1990.

Shi, M., et al. "Stimulating Action of *Carthamus tinctorius* L., *Angelica sinensis*, (Oliv) Diels and *Leonurus sibiricus* L. on the Uterus," *Chung Kuo Chung Yao Tsa Chih* 20:173-75,192, 1995.

Wardlaw, G.M., et al. "Serum Lipid and Apolipoprotein Concentrations in Healthy Men on Diets Enriched in Either Canola Oil or Safflower Oil," *Am J Clin Nutr* 54:104, 1991.

SAFFRON

INDIAN SAFFRON, TRUE SAFFRON

Common trade names
None known.

Common forms
Available as crude powder.

Source
This agent is derived from the dried stigmas and tops of styles of *Crocus sativus,* which is indigenous to southern Europe and Asia Minor.

Chemical components
Saffron contains several compounds, including carotenoids such as crocines, crocetins, picrocrocin, and dimethyl-crocetin. Hydrolysis of the agent results in the production of safranal and glucose. An essential oil may also be produced.

Actions
The components of saffron have been shown to be cytotoxic in vitro to human carcinoma, sarcoma, and leukemia cells (Escribano et al., 1996; Nair et al., 1995). This effect is believed to be dose-dependent and is attributed to the carotenoid components, specifically dimethyl-crocetin.

The crocetin component of saffron appears to increase the diffusion of oxygen in plasma, possibly by as much as 80% (Grisolia,1974). This action may prevent atherosclerosis secondary to vascular wall hypoxia, and a subsequent decrease in RBC diffusion of oxygen. This agent is reported also to have immunomodulating effects, but supporting data are lacking.

Reported uses

Saffron has been used as an expectorant, a diaphoretic, and a sedative. In some parts of Asia, this agent has been made into a paste and used to treat dry skin. It is also thought to have some aphrodisiac effects. Clinical trials supporting these claims do not exist. Its use is primarily as a coloring and flavoring agent.

Dosage

No consensus exists in humans. Saffron may be ingested by mixing the powder with food or brewing it as a tea.

Adverse reactions

None reported with culinary doses (under 1.5 g); the following have been documented with doses above 5 g:
- Bradycardia
- Epistaxis
- Flushing of face
- Menorrhagia (less frequent)
- Spontaneous abortion (rare)
- Vertigo
- Vomiting

Interactions

None reported.

Contraindications and precautions

Contraindicated in pregnant women because of the risk of spontaneous abortion. Avoid use of this compound in breast-feeding patients; effects are unknown.

Special considerations

- Recommend that the patient maintain doses of less than 5 g daily to minimize risk of adverse effects.
- Ask the patient to immediately report unusual signs or symptoms to the primary health care provider.
- Explain that evidence to support therapeutic applications for saffron is insufficient, and that its risks are not well described.

Points of interest

- A combination of saffron with quinine and opium has received a patent in Germany for inhibiting premature ejaculation.

Analysis

Although saffron has been used safely as a food additive for many years, its use as a medicinal agent remains to be determined. Until adequate human trials can be conducted, the use of saffron to prevent or treat cancer or CV conditions cannot be recommended.

References

Escribano, J., et al. "Crocin, Safranal, and Picrocrocin from Saffron (*Crocus sativus* L.) Inhibit the Growth of Human Cancer Cells In Vitro," *Cancer Lett* 100:23-30, 1996.

Grisolia, S. "Hypoxia, Saffron and Cardiovascular Disease," *Lancet* 7871:41, 1974.

Nair, S.C., et al. "Saffron Chemoprevention in Biology and Medicine: A Review," *Cancer Biother* 10:257-64, 1995.

SAGE

DALMATIAN, GARDEN SAGE, MEADOW SAGE, SCARLET SAGE, TREE SAGE

Common trade names
None known.

Source
Active components are extracted from the *Salvia officinalis* plant. It is a perennial plant with violet-blue flowers that was originally native to Southern Europe but has come to be cultivated in North America.

Chemical components
Components include caffeic, carnosol, chlorogenic, ellagic, ferulic, garlic, rosemarinic, tannins, picrosalvin, and salvin. A total of 1% to 2.8% of the plant is composed of volatile oil, and 30% to 50% of that oil is either alpha- or beta-thujones.

Actions
Sage extract and oil have been shown to have antispasmodic activity in the guinea pig ileum, hypotensive activity in cats, and CNS depressant effects in mice (Todorov et al., 1984). The herb's antimicrobial activity in vitro is attributed to the alpha- and beta-thujone component. The antimicrobial action was evident for the following organisms: *Escherichia coli*, *Shigella sonnei*, *Salmonella* species, *Klebsiella ozanea*, *Bacillus subtilis*, and various fungi species (Meier et al., 1994).

One study conducted in rabbits showed a hypoglycemic effect from sage ingestion (Cabo et al., 1985).

Reported uses
Sage has been used as an astringent, antioxidant, and antispasmodic. It is also claimed to be therapeutic for dysmenorrhea, diarrhea,

gastritis, sore throats, gingivitis, and galactorrhea. However, clinical trial data are lacking to support these claims.

Sage has been used for many years as a food flavoring and fragrance for soaps and perfumes. Sage is listed by the Council of Europe as a natural source of food flavoring.

Dosage
For sore throat, 1 to 4 g leaf as a gargle P.O. t.i.d.
For menstrual disorders, 1 to 4 ml leaf extract (1:1 in 45% alcohol) P.O. t.i.d.

Adverse reactions
• Chelilitis, stomatitis (with high doses or chronic use)
• Local irritant
• Tonic-clonic seizures

Interactions
Anticonvulsants: lowered seizure threshold. Avoid concomitant use.
Disulfiram: disulfiram reaction if herbal product contains alcohol. Do not use together.
Insulin, other antidiabetic agents: antagonized glycemic control, necessitating adjustment of therapy. Monitor blood glucose closely.

Contraindications and precautions
Avoid use in pregnant patients because the herb may cause spontaneous abortion. Use cautiously in patients prone to hypoglycemia (such as diabetics). Also use cautiously in patients receiving anticonvulsants because loss of seizure control may occur.

Special considerations
• Caution the diabetic patient against use of this herb because it may worsen condition and promote loss of control of disease.
• Advise the epileptic patient to avoid use of this herb because it may worsen condition and promote loss of control of disease.
• Warn the patient taking disulfiram not to take an herbal product containing alcohol.

Analysis
There is little clinical information available to recommend the medicinal use of sage at this time. Animal and toxicity data suggest that consumption of sage may lessen control of seizures in epileptic patients as well as reduce glycemic control of diabetic patients.

References
Cabo, J., et al. "Accion hipoglucemiante de prepardos fitoterapicos que contienen especies del genero salvia," *Ars Pharmaceutica* 26:239-49, 1985.

Meier, S., et al. "The Antimicrobial Activity of Essential Oils and Essential Components Towards Oral Bacteria," *Oral Microbiol Immunol* 9:202-08, 1994.

Todorov, S., et al. "Experimental Pharmacological Study of Three Species from Genus *Salvia*," *Acta Physiol Pharmacol Bulg* 10:13-20, 1984.

ST. JOHN'S WORT

AMBER, AMBER TOUCH-AND-HEAL, CHASSEDIABLE, DEVIL'S SCOURGE, GOATWEED, GOD'S WONDER PLANT, GRACE OF GOD, *HYPERICUM*, KLAMATH WEED, MELLEPERTUIS, ROSIN ROSE, SAINT JOHN'S WORT, WITCHES' HERB

Common trade names
(Various manufacturers; available in combination) Hypercalm, Hypericum, Kira, Mood Support, St. John's Wort, Nutri Zac, Tension Tamer

Common forms
Available as capsules, sublingual capsules, and liquid tinctures. Solid dosage forms are available as 100 mg, 300 mg, 500 mg (standardized to 0.3% hypericin) and 250 mg (standardized to 0.14% hypericin).

Source
St. John's wort is obtained from the flowering tops of the perennial plant *Hypericum perforatum* L. The plant is endemic to Europe and Asia, and was brought to the United States by European colonists.

Chemical components
The chemical composition of St. John's wort is related to the harvesting, drying process, and storage of plant material. The biologic activity is probably attributable to several components rather than a single component. Active components include the naphthodianthrones (hypericin, pseudohypericin), flavonoids (hyperin, hyperoside, isoquercetrin, kaempferol, luteolin, quercetin, quercitrin, rutin), biflavonoids (amenotoflavone, I3,II8-biapigenin), and phloroglucinols (adhyperforin, hyperforin). The aboveground plant parts contain tannin, which may account for wound-healing effects.

Actions
The exact mechanism of antidepressant effects has not been determined. Early in vitro studies demonstrated that hypericin inhibited type-A, and to a lesser extent type-B, MAO (Suzuki et al., 1984). However, a purer form of hypericin did not inhibit MAO (Cott,

1995). High concentration of St. John's wort affects serotonin reuptake in vitro (Perovic et al., 1995), although the level required was much higher than achieved with usual therapeutic doses. Other studies have demonstrated that St. John's wort is a weak inhibitor of norepinephrine uptake and minimally inhibits catechol-O-methyltransferase (COMT). St. John's wort affects receptor affinity of adenosine, benzodiazepine, gamma aminobutyric acid (GABA)-A, GABA-B, and inositol triphosphate in vitro (Chavez, 1997). A recent study found that hypericin has modest binding affinity for muscarinic cholinergic and for nonselective sigma receptors (Raffs, 1998).

Other demonstrated biologic activities include inhibition of stress-induced increase in corticotropin-releasing hormone, adrenocorticotropic hormone, and cortisol; increase in nocturnal melatonin plasma levels; and modulation of cytosine expression, particularly interleukin-6. St. John's wort and hypericin also have antiviral activity, including action against retroviruses (Chavez, 1997).

Reported uses

St. John's wort has long been used to treat depression, bronchial inflammation, burns, cancer, enuresis, gastritis, hemorrhoids, hypothyroidism, insect bites and stings, insomnia, kidney disorders, and scabies, and has been used as a wound healing agent (Bombardelli et al., 1995; Chavez, 1997). Hypericin is being studied for treatment of HIV infection as well as topically for phototherapy of skin diseases, including psoriasis, cutaneous T-cell lymphoma, warts, and Kaposi's sarcoma (Chavez, 1997). St. John's wort is currently used for treatment of mild to moderate depression. (See *Studies of St. John's Wort*.)

Dosage

For depression, 300 mg standardized extract preparations (standardized to 0.3% hypericin) P.O. t.i.d. for 4 to 6 weeks. Or, 2 to 4 g tea that has been steeped in 1 to 2 cups of water for about 10 minutes and taken P.O. daily for 4 to 6 weeks.
For burns and skin lesions, cream applied topically; strength is not standardized.

Adverse reactions

Adverse reactions are uncommon.
• Allergic hypersensitivity
• Constipation
• Dizziness
• Dry mouth
• GI distress
• Restlessness
• Sleep disturbances

RESEARCH FINDINGS
Studies of St. John's wort

A meta-analysis of 23 randomized, clinical trials involving 1,757 outpatients with depressive disorders was published in the *British Medical Journal* (Linde et al., 1996). Sample size ranged from 30 to 162 patients, and the duration of treatment ranged from 4 to 12 weeks. A total of 15 trials were placebo controlled, and eight trials compared St. John's wort with other drugs (amitriptylline, bromazepam, desipramine, diazepam, imipramine, and maprotiline).

St. John's wort was found to be more effective than placebo and as effective as standard antidepressants. The incidence of adverse effects was greater in patients receiving standard antidepressants (52.8%) than St. John's wort (19.8%). However, there were many flaws associated with these trials, including inadequate diagnostic criteria, inclusion of patients with only mild to moderate disease (patients with severe depression were not included), lack of information about the randomization process, lack of compliance control, variable dosage of St. John's wort (more than sixfold), low dosage of antidepressants, short duration of treatment, lowered placebo response rate than other clinical trials, lack of statistical analysis information, and failure to perform an intent-to-treat analysis.

Another study of controlled trials of St. John's wort extract for the treatment of mild to moderate depression was recently published (Volz, 1997). This review evaluated the methodologic considerations of 12 published placebo-controlled trials, three of which compared St. John's wort with synthetic antidepressants. The authors reported mostly positive benefit with St. John's wort, although antidepressant dosage was not adequate. Similar to the meta-analysis, most of the studies evaluated had methodologic flaws and the author concluded that further studies are needed.

⚠ Phototoxicity has occurred in grazing animals that consumed large amounts of St. John's wort. Until recently there was no report of phototoxicity in humans. Systemic photosensitivity of recurring elevated erythematous lesions occurred in light-exposed areas in a woman who took an unknown dose of St. John's wort for 3 years (Golsch et al., 1997). Pure hypericin has resulted in phototoxicity when given I.V. and P.O. in clinical trials patients with AIDS (Chavez, 1997).

Interactions
Alcohol, MAO inhibitors, narcotics, OTC cold and flu medications, sympathomimetics, tyramine-containing foods: may enhance MAO inhibition activity. Avoid concurrent use.

Paroxetine: may result in sedative-hypnotic intoxication with concurrent ingestion of the herb (Gordon, 1998).
Serotonergic drugs (amphetamines, serotonin reuptake inhibitors, trazodone, tricyclic antidepressants): serotonin syndrome may occur when used in combination with these agents. Use cautiously together.

Contraindications and precautions

Contraindicated in patients with a history of allergy to St. John's wort or its components. Avoid use in children and in pregnant or breast-feeding patients; effects are unknown.

Special considerations

• The patient's depression should be evaluated by a health care professional. Conventional therapy may be prudent for a more moderate to severe disorder.
• Educate the patient to purchase herbs only from a reputable source and that products and their contents may vary among different manufacturers.
• Caution the patient against using the herb with alcohol and OTC cold and flu medications.
• Advise the patient to take precautions against sun exposure.

Points of interest

• In spring 1998, the National Institutes of Health began a 3-year, multicenter clinical study to investigate the efficacy of St. John's wort for the treatment of major depressive disorders. The study includes 336 subjects and compares a standardized extract of St. John's wort with a selective serotonin reuptake inhibitor (SSRI) and placebo. After evaluating efficacy at 8 weeks, patients who respond to treatment will continue for an additional 18 weeks. The study includes a 4-month follow-up period to assess long-term effects.
• St. John's wort oil is prepared by extracting the flowers with olive oil.

Analysis

There are numerous case reports and clinical trials evaluating the efficacy and safety of St. John's wort. The herb is mostly better than placebo for treatment of mild to moderate depression and as effective as standard antidepressants, but causes fewer adverse effects. Recently, a study evaluated the efficacy of St. John's wort for severe depression and reported that St. John's wort is equally effective as imipramine, with significantly fewer adverse effects (Vorbach, 1997). Although most clinical trials contained design flaws, overall they indicate that St. John's wort may be valuable for the treatment of depressive disorders. However, additional well-designed studies are needed. The United States Pharmacopoeia expert advisory panel has determined that there is insufficient evidence in the scientific literature to support the use of St. John's wort for the treatment of mild to moderate depression.

References

Bombardelli, E., et al. "*Hypericum perforatum,*" Fitoterapia 66:43-68, 1995.

Chavez, M.L. "Saint John's Wort," *Hosp Pharm* 32:1621-32, 1997.

Cott, J. "Medicinal Plants and Dietary Supplements: Sources for Innovative Treatments or Adjuncts?" *Psychopharmacol Bull* 31:131-37, 1995.

Golsch, S., et al. "Reversible Increase in Photosensitivity to UV-B caused by St. John's Wort Extract," *Hautarzt* 48:249-52, 1997.

Gordon, J.B. "SSRIs and St. John's Wort: Possible Toxicity?" *Am Fam Physician* 57:950-53, 1998.

Linde, K., et al. "St. John's Wort for Depression:An Overview and Meta-analysis of Randomized Clinical Trials," *BMJ* 313:253-58, 1996.

Perovic, S., et al. "Effect on Serotonin Uptake by Postsynaptic Receptors," *Arzneimittelforschung* 45:1145-48, 1995.

Raffs, R.B. "Screen of Receptor and Uptake-Size Activity of Hypericin Component of St. John's Wort Reveals Sigma Receptor Binding," *Life Sci* 62:265-70, 1998.

Suzuki, O., et al. "Inhibition of Monoamine Oxidase by Hypericin," *Planta Med* 50:272-74, 1984.

Volz, H.P. "Controlled Clinical Trials of Hypericum Extracts in Depressed Patients — An Overview," *Pharmacopsychiatry* 30(Suppl):72-76, 1997.

Vorbach, E.U. "Efficacy and Tolerability of St. John's Wort Extract LI 160 Versus Imipramine in Patients with Severe Depressive Episodes According to ICD-10," *Pharmacopsychiatry* 30(Suppl):81-85, 1997.

SANTONICA

LEVANT WORMSEED, SEA WORMWOOD, SEMEN CINAE, SEMEN SANCTUM, WORMSEED

Common trade names
(Available in combination only)

Common forms
Available as dried powdered santonin and oral tablets.

Source
The flowers and seeds of *Artemesia cina* (a distinct variety of *Artemesia maritima*), a member of the Compositae family, is found in most parts of Asia.

Chemical components
Santonin, the active ingredient, is a lactone glycoside extracted from unopened flowers. It is bitter tasting and odorless, and occurs as a colorless to white crystalline powder. Other ingredients include artemisin and a volatile oil.

Actions
Some references claim that this agent has anthelmintic properties and is effective against roundworms and threadworms, but not tapeworms.

Reported uses
Santonica has been used anecdotally throughout history as an anthelmintic for adults and especially children. Russia exported the crude powder to the United States during World War II, until the United States was able to produce a domestic supply itself (Pratt and Youngken, 1951). Santonica was used for pertussis in the 1700s (Hocking, 1997).

Dosage
Powder, tablets, oral lozenges: 2 to 5 grains in varying dosages.

Adverse reactions
• Epileptiform seizures
• Headache
• Nausea
• Visual disturbances (including aberrations of color vision)
• Vomiting
⚠ Death has occurred from poisonings.

Interactions
Anticonvulsants: may lower seizure threshold. Avoid concomitant use.

Contraindications and precautions
Avoid use of herb in pregnant or breast-feeding patients; effects are unknown. Use with caution in patients prone to seizures.

Special considerations
• Caution the patient to use care when driving and performing other hazardous activities until CNS effects of the herb are known.
• Tell the female patient to report planned or suspected pregnancy.
• Instruct the patient to keep the herb out of reach of children and pets.
• Advise the patient not to take this herb without medical supervision.

Analysis

Historically, santonica has seen wide traditional use as an anthelmintic. It was an official product in the National Formulary and British Pharmacopeia into the 1950s. Its value cannot be discounted, but more contemporary anthelmintics are likely to be less toxic and more effective against a wider range of worm infestations.

References

Hocking, G.M. *A Dictionary of Natural Products.* Medford, N.J.: Plexus Publishing, Inc., 1997.

Pratt, R., and Youngken, H.W. *Pharmacognosy The Study of Natural Drug Substances and Certain Allied Products,* 3rd ed. Philadelphia: Lippincott-Raven Pubs., 1951.

SARSAPARILLA

ECUADORIAN SARSAPARILLA, HONDURAN SARSAPARILLA, JAMAICAN SARSAPARILLA, MEXICAN SARSAPARILLA, SALSAPARILHA, SALSEPAREILLE, SARSA, SARSAPARILLA ROOT, *SMILAX*

Common trade names
(Various manufacturers; available in combination) Sarsaparilla, Sarsaparilla Root Extract

Common forms
Available as capsules (455 mg), tablets, teas, dried root powder, liquid, and solid root extract.

Source
The dried roots and rhizomes of various *Smilax* species (*S. aristochiifolia, S. regelii, S. febrifuga, S. ornata*) are used in commercial products. *Smilax* species are cultivated in Mexico, Jamaica, and South America.

Chemical components
Saponins constitute 1% to 3% of the chemical components of sarsaparilla, with the three main saponins being sarsaponin (parillin), smilasaponin (smilacin), and sarsaparilloside. Other saponins include sarsapogenin (parigenin), smilagenin, diosgenin, tigogenin, aspergenin, and laxogenin. Phytosterols, resins, starch, trace volatile oils, and cetyl alcohol constitute the remainder of the compound.

Actions
The herb's pharmacologic effects have been attributed to the saponins, which are claimed to be "blood purifiers" or tonics that supposedly remove unwanted toxins from the body. This idea might have

arisen from the supposed diuretic and diaphoretic effects of sarsaparilla. Other claims for saponins include an ability to bind serum cholesterol in the GI tract and a hemolytic effect if administered I.V. These pharmacologic effects of sarsaparilla are not well documented.

Sarsaparilla has shown in vitro activity against common dermatophytes (*Epidermophyton floccosum, Trichophyton rubrum, Trichophyton mentagrophytes*) (Caceres et al., 1991). Significant anti-inflammatory activity and prevention of chemically induced hepatocellular damage has been noted in rodents (after pretreatment with sarsaparilla) (Ageel et al., 1989; Rafatullah et al., 1991). Sarsaparilla was found not to have any beneficial effects for improving healing of bone fractures in rats.

Reported uses

Sarsaparilla root is claimed to be useful for skin diseases such as psoriasis, rheumatism, and renal disease. Older research attempts to substantiate sarsaparilla for use in psoriatic disease.

The most notable trial involved patients with psoriasis vulgaris who received sarsaponin (a major component of sarsaparilla) or placebo (Thermon, 1942). Although the study showed favorable results in terms of improved symptoms, duration of benefit, and reduced disease exacerbations, problems with study design led to questions regarding the final conclusions reached.

Because of its steroidal components, sarsaparilla has also been touted as an athletic performance-enhancing agent. However, these steroids have not been proven to be anabolic and, therefore, this claim remains unsubstantiated. Sarsaparilla has been promoted as a diuretic agent and as an agent to aid appetite and digestion. Its extract has been evaluated as adjunctive therapy in leprosy (Rollier, 1959). Currently, sarsaparilla is accepted by the FDA as a flavoring agent.

The 1992 German Commission E monograph advocates the use of sarsaparilla in the treatment of psoriasis, rheumatic complaints, and kidney ailments, and for diuresis and diaphoresis.

Dosage

For psoriasis, 1 to 4 g of dried root, 8 to 30 ml of concentrated sarsaparilla compound decoction, and 8 to 15 ml of liquid extract, P.O. t.i.d. has been suggested.

Adverse reactions

- Asthma (inhalation of root dust)
- Diarrhea
- GI irritation
- Hemolysis (I.V. use)
- Renal damage

Interactions

Certain hypnotic agents: enhanced elimination. Monitor for lack of effectiveness.

Digitalis: enhanced absorption. Do not use together.

Oral medications: altered absorption; saponins may affect absorption of other medications. Take other medications 2 hours before or after taking sarsaparilla.

Contraindications and precautions

Avoid use in pregnant or breast-feeding patients; effects are unknown.

Special considerations

● Tell the patient that claims for sarsaparilla for any condition are only weakly substantiated.

● Advise the patient with asthma to avoid inhalation of sarsaparilla root dust or root particles.

● Caution the patient already taking a diuretic about excessive diuretic effects, fluid and electrolyte imbalances, and hypotension.

Points of interest

● Since the 16th century, sarsaparilla was thought to be an effective treatment for syphilis. It gained popularity in the Old West of the United States and was the drink of choice for cowboys. It was even listed for such uses in the U.S. Pharmacopoeia from 1820 to 1910. Activity against syphilis, however, is not pharmacologically substantiated.

Analysis

The use of sarsaparilla for any condition needs further research. Mechanisms and properties are not clearly documented or adequately researched. The most notable clinical trial evaluated the herb's use in psoriasis, but poor study design and the presence of confounding variables placed the conclusions in question.

References

Ageel, A..M., et al. "Experimental Studies on Antirheumatic Crude Drugs Used in Saudi Traditional Medicine," *Drugs Exp Clin Res* 15:369-72, 1989.

Caceres, A., et al. "Plants Used in Guatemala for the Treatment of Dermatophytic Infections," *J Ethnopharmacol* 31:263-76, 1991.

Rafatullah, S., et al. "Hepatoprotective and Safety Evaluation Studies on Sarsaparilla," *Int J Pharmacognosy* 29:296-301, 1991.

Rollier, R. "Treatment of Lepromatous Leprosy by a Combination of DDS and Sarsaparilla (*Smilax ornata*)," *Int J Leprosy* 27:328-40, 1959.

Thermon, F.M. "The Treatment of Psoriasis with a Sarsaparilla Compound," *N Engl J Med* 227:128-33, 1942.

SASSAFRAS

AGUE TREE, BOIS DE SASSAFRAS, CINNAMON WOOD,
FENCHELHOLZ, LIGNUM FLORIDUM, LIGNUM SASSAFRAS,
ROOT BARK, SALOOP, SASSAFRASHOLZ, SAXIFRAS

Common trade names
None known.

Common forms
Available as crude bark, liquid extract, oil, tea, and powder.

Source
The sassafras tree, *Sassafras albidum,* is native to the eastern region of North America. The oil and teas are extracted from the roots and bark of the sassafras tree.

Chemical components
Sassafras alkaloids include isoquinoline-type 0.02%, aporphine, benzylsoquinoline derivatives, boldine, isoboldine, norboldine, cinnabolaurine, norcinnamolaurine, and reticuline. Other components include volatile oils, safrole (a highly aromatic oil), anethole, apiole, asarone, camphor, elemicin, eugenol, menthone, myrisicin, pinene apiole, thujone, magnolol, isomagnolol, tannins, resins, mucilage, and wax. The pleasant-tasting oil is a 2% portion of the roots and 6% to 9% component of the root bark.

Actions
Most studies have focused on the investigation of sassafras toxicity. Sassafras root bark is 5% to 9% safrole. Safrole has been demonstrated to be hepatocarcinogenic in rodents (Borchert et al., 1973). Sassafras has also been shown to induce hepatic enzymes P-450 and P-488. The oil has been used topically as an antiseptic and pediculicide, and to relieve flatulence.

Reported uses
Sassafras has been used primarily as a tonic or performance-enhancing agent. Tea prepared from the bark has also been used as a diuretic and diaphoretic agent to treat visceral obstruction, dermatologic conditions, cachexia, rheumatism, and venereal disease. Although the herb was originally recommended as a cure for syphilis, its effectiveness has never been demonstrated. Traditionally, the herb has been favored as a remedy for cutaneous eruptions, gout, and rheumatic pain.

Dosage
For dermal conditions and venereal diseases, dosages vary with formulation.
Bark: 2 g to 4 g P.O. by infusion t.i.d.
Powder: tea is prepared by adding ¼ teaspoon of the powder to 1 cup (8 oz) boiling water, and infusing for 15 minutes.
Oil: applied topically.
Extract (1:1 in 25% alcohol): 2 to 4 ml P.O. t.i.d.

Adverse reactions
Adverse reactions are often attributed to safrole component.
- Ataxia
- CNS depression
- CV collapse
- Dermatitis
- Diaphoresis, hot flashes
- Hallucinogenic effects
- Hepatic carcinogen
- Hypersensitivity to touch
- Hypothermia
- Paralysis
- Ptosis
- Spasm
- Spontaneous abortion
- Stupor
- Vomiting

⚠ Death has resulted with a few drops of oil (in children) and 1 teaspoon (in adults) (Craig, 1953).

Interactions
None reported; however, safrole is a potent inhibitor (and inducer) of certain hepatic microsomal enzymes systems (P-450, P-488) and may, theoretically, potentiate toxicity of drugs metabolized by these enzyme systems, including some cardiac, immunosuppressant, and antidepressant medications (Opdyke, 1974).

Contraindications and precautions
Avoid use in pregnant or breast-feeding patients; effects are unknown.

⚠ Avoid prolonged internal or external use (over 2 weeks) of sassafras. Safrole, the major constituent of the oil of sassafras, is a liver carcinogen; even some safrole-free extracts have been reported to produce tumors in animal models.

Special considerations
• Monitor for hepatic dysfunction in patients using sassafras.
• Caution the patient regarding known adverse reactions, particularly CNS effects when driving or performing activities that require alertness.
• Warn the patient about the carcinogenic effects of the herb.
• Advise patients, especially pregnant or breast-feeding women, to avoid internal and external use of sassafras.
• Explain that consumption of sassafras may interfere with the elimination of other drugs being taken.

Points of interest
• The volatile oil and safrole were banned by the FDA for use as food additives or flavor-enhancing agents. A safrole-free sassafras extract is approved for food use in the United States.

Analysis
Sassafras has traditionally been used for several conditions, including dermatologic and rheumatic illnesses, as well as a flavoring agent in select beverages. Despite extensive evidence of toxicity and carcinogenesis and legal restrictions, sassafras continues to be readily available in natural product stores and other facilities in the United States. The herb may interfere with the metabolism of many prescription drugs. Therefore, use sassafras or its components cannot be recommended.

References
Borchert, P., et al. "The Metabolism of the Naturally Occurring Hepato-carcinogen Safrole to 1'-hydroxysafrole and the Electrophilic Reactivity of 1'-acetoxysafrole." *Cancer Res* 33:575-89, 1973.
Craig, J.O. "Poisoning by the Volatile Oils in Childhood," *Arch Dis Child* 28:475-83, 1953.
Opdyke, D.L.J. "Safrole," *Food Cosmet Toxicol* 12:983-86, 1974.

SAW PALMETTO
AMERICAN DWARF PALM TREE, CABBAGE PALM, IDS 89, LSESR, SABAL

Common trade names
Permixon, Propalmex, Strogen

Common forms
Available as tablets, capsules, teas, berries (fresh or dried), and liquid extract.

Source

The brownish-black berry of the American dwarf palm, also known as *Serenoa repens* or *Sabal serrulata*, is used to extract active compounds. The berries contain about 1.5% of an oil. Until a fat-soluble purified extract was produced, it was believed that the extracts of the plant had little effect because they were poorly absorbed.

Chemical components

The active ingredient in commercial preparations is the n-hexane lipidosterolic extract of *S. repens* (LSESR). This extract contains a complex mixture of various compounds, including fatty acids (primarily lauric acid), phytosterols, and polysaccharides. Recently, two biologically active monacylglycerides were also isolated.

Actions

The precise mechanism of action of saw palmetto is not defined. Most research involves animal and human models using prostate tissue or cell lines. Several pharmacodynamic effects have been described in in vitro studies. The LSESR has been shown to inhibit 5-alpha-reductase, the enzyme responsible for conversion of testosterone to dihydrotestosterone (Weisser et al., 1996).

Although controversial, LSESR is believed to have greater potency and to inhibit both subtypes of 5-alpha-reductase, whereas finasteride selectively inhibits type 2. LSESR also appears to have an inhibitory effect on the binding of dihydrotestosterone (DHT) to androgen receptors in the prostate. Other data suggest that LSESR also has an anti-inflammatory effect and inhibits prolactin and growth-factor-induced prostatic cell proliferation (Paubert-Braquet et al., 1996, 1998).

In a recent study, LSESR inhibited hormonally induced prostate enlargement in rats (Paubert-Braquet et al., 1996); this effect was greatest after 60 days of treatment. Decreased levels of DHT and antiestrogenic activity after 3 months of LSESR treatment occurred in men with benign prostatic hypertrophy (BPH) (DiSilverio et al., 1992).

Reported uses

The tea is claimed to be effective in the management of genitourinary problems such as BPH; to increase sperm production, breast size, and sexual vigor; and to act as a mild diuretic. (See *LSESR in the treatment of benign prostatic hypertrophy,* page 580.)

Dosage

For BPH, clinical studies in humans have used 320 mg P.O. daily in two divided doses. Duration of treatment has usually been 3 months,

RESEARCH FINDINGS
LSESR in the treatment of benign prostatic hypertrophy

The effectiveness of the lipidosterolic extract of *Serenoa repens* (LSESR) in the treatment of benign prostatic hypertrophy (BPH) has been studied in several human noncomparative, placebo-controlled trials, and comparative trials with other drugs (Plosker and Brogden, 1996). Most trials involved men between the ages of 60 and 70 and used dosages of 320 mg daily for 1 to 3 months. Of seven placebo-controlled clinical trials, four included at least 50 patients. Three of these larger trials showed that *S. repens* was superior to placebo in reducing night-time and daytime urinary frequency, and in increasing peak flow rate. Significant symptomatic improvement compared to placebo was reported in one study (Champault et al., 1984).

In another well-conducted, large, double-blind, randomized, comparative trial involving 1,098 men, *S. repens* and finasteride demonstrated similar efficacy (Carraro et al., 1996).

No significant difference was found in patient-reported quality of life or objective measures as defined by the International Prostate Symptom Score. *S. repens* had little or no effect on prostate size and PSA levels, suggesting a mechanism other than its proposed antiandrogenic effect. Patients receiving *S. repens* had significantly better sexual function scores compared with those receiving placebo.

S. repens has also been compared to alfuzosin and prazosin in two smaller, double-blind, randomized trials. Objective results such as urinary frequency, post-void residuals, and mean urinary flow favored the alpha$_1$-receptor antagonist in both studies, but the results were not statistically significant.

although both shorter and longer (up to 6 months) trials have been conducted.

Other recommendations include 1 to 2 g fresh saw palmetto berries or 0.5 to 1 g dried berry in decoction P.O. t.i.d.

Adverse reactions
- Abdominal pain
- Back pain
- Constipation
- Decreased libido
- Diarrhea
- Dysuria
- Headache
- Hypertension

- Impotence
- Nausea
- Urine retention

Interactions
None reported.

Contraindications and precautions
Contraindicated during pregnancy and in women of childbearing age because of the herb's potential hormonal effects. Use cautiously in conditions other than BPH because there is a lack of data regarding its effects.

Special considerations
- Be aware that saw palmetto apparently does not alter the size of the prostate. Because of the concern that the herb causes a false-negative prostate-specific antigen (PSA) result, obtain a baseline PSA before starting treatment.
- Know that the herb should be taken with the morning and evening meal to minimize GI effects.
- Inform the patient wishing to use the herb for BPH to do so only after a diagnosis has been made and only on the advice of the primary health care provider.
- Advise the female patient to avoid use of the herb during pregnancy or when breast-feeding.

Points of interest
- Saw palmetto tea was included in the United States Pharmacopoeia and National Formulary from 1906 to 1950 for urogenital ailments.

Analysis
Saw palmetto, specifically LSESR, appears to be well tolerated, and has shown greater efficacy than placebo and equal efficacy to finasteride in improving subjective and objective symptoms of BPH. Its use is supported by many in vitro, in vivo, and clinical studies involving humans. Although LSESR appears to be a safe and effective alternative agent, more comparative studies involving alpha$_1$-receptor antagonists are needed to further delineate the herb's role in the management of BPH.

References
Carraro, J.C., et al. "Comparison of Phytotherapy (Permixon) with Finasteride in the Treatment of Benign Prostate Hyperplasia: A Randomized International Study of 1,098 Patients," *Prostate* 29:231-40, 1996.

Champault, G., et al. "A Double-Blind Trial of an Extract of the Plant *Serenoa repens* in Benign Prostatic Hyperplasia," *Br J Clin Pharmacol* 18:461-62, 1984.

DiSilverio, F., et al. "Evidence that *Serenoa repens* Extract Displays an Anti-estrogenic Activity in Prostatic Tissue of Benign Prostatic Hypertrophy Patients," *Eur Urol* 21:309-14, 1992.

Paubert-Braquet, M., et al. "Effect of *Serenoa repens* Extract (Permixon) on Estradiol/Testosterone-Induced Experimental Prostate Enlargement in the Rat," *Pharmacol Res* 34:171-79, 1996.

Paubert-Braquet, M., et al. "Effect of the Lipodosterolic Extract of *Sernoa repens* (Permixon) and Its Major Components on Basic Fibroblast Growth Factor-Induced Proliferation of Cultures of Human Prostate Biopsies," *Eur Urol* 33:340-47, 1998.

Plosker, G.L., and Brogden, R.N. "*Serenoa repens* (Permixon). A Review of Its Pharmacology and Therapeutic Efficacy in Benign Prostatic Hyperplasia," *Drugs Aging* 9:379-95, 1996.

Weisser, H., et al. "Effects of the *Sabal serrulata* Extract IDS 89 and Its Subfractions on 5 Alpha-Reductase Activity in Human Benign Prostatic Hyperplasia," *Prostate* 28:300-06, 1996.

SCENTED GERANIUM

Common trade names
None known.

Common forms
Available as potpourri, essential oil, and tea flavoring. Scented geranium is commonly used as a house plant.

Source
There are six subfamilies in the Geraniaceae family: Erodium, Hypseocharis, Geranium, Monsonia, Pelargonium, and Sarcocaulon. The scented geraniums are derived from Pelargonium, the largest of the subfamilies. True geranium are found in all continents, but the Pelargonium occur predominantly in South Africa.

Chemical components
Flavonoids and tannins (gernaniin) are the active ingredients in many of the geranium species.

Actions
Although the efficacy of scented geranium has limited documented use in medical literature, several geranium species appear to have antiviral, antifungal, antioxidative, antibacterial, and effective pesticide qualities.

Geranium viscossissimum var. *viscossissimum*, has been found to release ellagic and gallic acids on hydrolysis; these acids exhibit significant growth-inhibitory activity against the larvae of the polyphagous pest insect *Heliothis virescens* (Gegova et al., 1993). Geraniin (tannin from *G. thunbergii*) was found to be protective against oxidative damage in the mouse ocular lens. One study found that the phagocystosis of yeasts was induced by geraniin isolated from peritoneal macrophages with geraniin, isolated from *G. funbergii* (Ivanchera et al., 1992).

The polyphenolic complex of *G. sanguineum* L. showed efficacy against influenza, herpes simplex, vaccinia, and HIV-1 in cell cultures, with its anti-influenza effect being most pronounced (Serkedjieva, 1997).

Reported uses
Scented geranium is reportedly useful as a pesticide. It is also reported to be an antiviral agent, but there are no clinical data to support this claim.

Dosage
No consensus exists. The leaves are commonly used in tea or potpourri preparations, and the essential oils may be used to make tablets and creams.

Adverse reactions
• Allergic reaction
• Contact dermatitis

Interactions
None reported; may potentially interact with flu vaccines.

Contraindications and precautions
Avoid use in pregnant or breast-feeding patients; effects are unknown. Use cautiously in atopic patients

Special considerations
• Scented geraniums are used as ornamental plants in the United States and as natural pesticides in gardens.

Analysis
Most of the information available for the medicinal use of scented geranium comes from foreign language journals and is based on in vitro data and trials in animals. Insufficient data exist to support any therapeutic application of scented geranium in humans. More data are needed to determine the safety of this plant.

References

Gegova, G., et al. "Combined Effect of Selected Antiviral Substances of Natural and Synthetic Origin. II. Anti-influenza Activity of a Combination of a Polyphenolic Complex Isolated from *Geranium sanguineum* L. and rimantadine in vivo," *Acta Microbiol Bulg* 30:37-40, 1993.

Ivancheva, S., et al. "Polyphenols from Bulgarian Medicinal Plants with Anti-infectious Activity," *Basic Life Sci* 59:717-28, 1992.

Serkedjieva, J. "Antiinfective Activity of a Plant Preparation from *Geranium sanguineum* L.," *Pharmazie* 52:799-802, 1997.

SCHISANDRA

GOMISHI, OMICHA, SCHIZANDRA, TJN-101, WU-WEI-ZU

Common trade names
(Various manufacturers) Schisandra Extract, Sheng-mai-san

Common forms
Available as 100-mg capsules, dried fruit, and liquid.

Source
The active components of *Schisandra chinesis* may be extracted using ethanol. Active components are isolated through petroleum ether extraction of the fruit, stems, or kernel. Schisandra are native to China, Russia, and Korea.

Chemical components
The extracts of seeds and fruit are composed of numerous lignans (schizandrins, schizandrols, and schisantherins); malic, tartaric, nigranoic, and citric acids; resins; pectin; vitamins A, C, and E; sterols; and tannins. The fruit contains a volatile oil.

Actions
Schisandra has exhibited antioxidant activity in animals. Studies on the myocardium of rats suggests some protective benefit against hypoxia and reperfusion injuries (Li et al., 1996). Schisandrin A (TJN-101) showed some inhibition of leukotrienes and also decreased artificially induced hepatic damage in rats. Oral dosages of TJN-101 decreased liver injury and mortality in a dose-dependent manner. The proposed mechanism of benefit may result from nonspecific hepatoprotection rather than toxin inhibition. Specifically, schisandra may promote protective effects by stimulating hepatic metabolism and inhibiting leukotriene formation through augmentation of the hepatic glutathione antioxidant and detoxification system (Ko et al., 1995).

A component of schisandra has been found to inhibit reverse transcriptase in vitro (Sun et al., 1996).

Reported uses

This agent is claimed to be of benefit in preventing hepatic injury, although studies only in animals have been conducted. Antioxidant properties may also contribute to this action.

This herb has long been used in Chinese medicine for the treatment of lung, liver, and kidney disorders It is also claimed to be useful for treating ocular disorders, although clinical trials are lacking. Advocacy literature also suggests that schisandra has "adaptogenic" properties (helps the body deal with stress), but this also remains unproven.

Dosage

Dosage of 100 mg extract P.O. b.i.d. has been suggested.

Adverse reactions

• Profound CNS depression (rare)

Interactions

None reported. Because of the effect on the liver, schisandra extracts may interfere with other drugs eliminated through the liver.

Contraindications and precautions

Avoid use of the herb in pregnant or breast-feeding patients; effects are unknown. Use cautiously in patients taking medications extensively metabolized by the liver.

Special considerations

• Inform the patient that little information exists regarding the herb's safety and effectiveness.
• Advise the female patient to avoid use of the herb during pregnancy or when breast-feeding.
• Advise the patient that drugs eliminated by the liver may interact with schisandra. Tell the patient to inform the primary health care provider about any medications (prescription and OTC) that are being taken.

Points of interest

• The Chinese name "wu-wei-zu" means five-flavored herb (or seeds), which refers to the sweet, sour, pungent, bitter, and salty taste of schisandra.

Analysis

Although schisandra has shown a protective effect on the liver in some animals, human data regarding safety and effectiveness are lacking. Claims for treating lung and kidney conditions have also not been studied adequately. Additionally, little is known about the adverse effects and dosage range of schisandra extracts; therefore, this herb cannot be recommended for medicinal use at this time.

References

Ko, K.M., et al. "Effect of a Lignan-Enriched Fructus Schisandrae Extract on Hepatic Glutathione Status in Rats: Protection Against Carbon Tetrachloride Toxicity," *Planta Med* 61:134-37, 1995.

Li, P.C., et al. "*Schisandra chinensis*-Dependent Myocardial Protective Action of Sheng-Mai-San in Rats," *Am J Chin Med* 24:255-62, 1996.

Sun, H.D., et al. "Nigranoic Acid, A Triterpenoid from *Schisandra sphaerandra* that Inhibits HIV-1 Reverse Transcriptase," *J Nat Prod* 59:525-27, 1996.

SEA HOLLY

ERYNGO, SEA HOLME, SEA HULVER

Common trade names

None known.

Common forms

Available as dried roots, extract, and tincture.

Source

The active components are derived from the dried roots of *Eryngium maritimum*. Sea holly is typically found along seashores in temperate regions.

Chemical components

Active components include saponins, coumarins, plant acids, and flavonoids.

Actions

Extracts of sea holly indicated possible anti-inflammatory action in rats, as demonstrated by decreased paw edema (Lisciani et al., 1984).

Reported uses

The herb is used primarily for urologic conditions; it is claimed to act as a diuretic when normal urine flow is inhibited by conditions known to obstruct urinary flow, such as kidney stones, urethritis, cystitis, and enlarged or inflamed prostate. These reported uses are anecdotal and lack supporting evidence (Hiller et al., 1976).

Dosage

For diuretic action, herb may be taken as a decoction (tea) or tincture t.i.d.

Adverse reactions
None reported.

Interactions
Diuretics: potential for increased electrolyte loss. Monitor electrolyte levels closely.

Contraindications and precautions
Avoid use in pregnant or breast-feeding patients; effects are unknown.

Special considerations
- Explain that little information exists for sea holly.
- Warn the patient receiving diuretics against use of this herb.
- Warn the patient that long-term use of the herb may lead to electrolyte imbalance.
- Advise the female patient to avoid use of this herb during pregnancy or when breast-feeding.

Analysis
Despite its long-time use as a urologic remedy, there is insufficient evidence to support the medicinal application of this herb for any disease.

References
Hiller, K., et al. "Saponins of *Eryngium maritimum* L. 25. Contents of Various Saniculoideae," *Pharmazie* 31:53, 1976.
Lisciani, R., et al. "Anti-inflammatory Activity of *Eryngium maritimum* L. Rhizome Extracts in Intact Rats," *J Ethnopharmacol* 12:263-70, 1984.

SELF-HEAL

ALL HEAL, BRUNELLA, CONSUELDA MENOR,
HSIA KU TS'AO, *PRUNELLA INCISA*, *PRUNELLA QUERETTE*,
SICKLEWORT, XIA KU CAO

Common trade names
None known.

Common forms
Available as liquid and fresh plant.

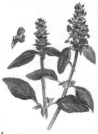

Source
Prunella vulgaris is a perennial weed commonly found in fields, grassy areas, and woods of North America, Asia, and Europe. Various parts of the plant are used.

Chemical components

Components isolated from the whole herb include oleanolic acid, rutin, hyperoside, ursolic acid, caffeic acid, vitamins, tannins, carotenoids, essential oils, and alkaloids. The flowers contain the glycosides of delphinidin, cyanidin, d-camphor, d-fenchone, and ursolic acid. Prunellin, an aqueous extract of the herb, has been identified as an active antiviral compound.

Actions

Antiviral activity of prunellin against the HIV-1 virus has been shown in vitro. Prunellin was more effective than retrovir (AZT) in inhibiting reverse transcriptase activity. Viral replication was completely abolished up to 60 days after exposure in lymphoid and monocytoid cells. When the extract was added after viral adsorption, the aqueous extract achieved partial inhibition of HIV replication. Prunellin was also found to inhibit the binding of glycoprotein 120 to CD4 cells, which was concluded to be its primary mechanism for inhibiting HIV-1 infection (Yao et al., 1992).

Diluted and undiluted aqueous extracts of *P. vulgaris* provided complete coverage against HIV-induced cytotoxicity. Diluted *P. vulgaris* extract with zidovudine or didanosine provided protection of 69% to 74% compared with either agent alone (John et al., 1994).

Patients with herpes simplex type I keratitis given an ophthalmic form of *P. vulgaris* extract experienced clinical cure or improvement (Zheng, 1990). In vitro studies in human lung carcinoma and lymphocytic leukemia showed ursolic acid to have significant cytotoxic activity (Lee et al., 1988). Ursolic acid has shown marginal cytotoxic activity in human colon and mammary tumor cells.

Reported uses

In Chinese folklore medicine, *P. vulgaris* is still used for conditions such as infectious hepatitis, jaundice, tuberculosis, cancer, pleuritis with effusion, and bacillary dysentery (Lee et al., 1988). Prunella has been used for the treatment of sore throat, colic, gas, diarrhea, hemorrhage, and boils. Its main use as recommended by herbalists is for sore throat and GI upset.

Dosage

Because most studies have been in vitro, standard doses are not known. The formulation of the herb appears to be an important aspect with regard to treatment. Aqueous extracts have the most antiviral activity (Yamasaki et al., 1996). An infusion of *P. vulgaris* has been used as a gargle and is prepared by mixing 1 g of the fresh plant in boiling water and then cooled.

Adverse reactions
None reported.

Interactions
None reported.

Contraindications and precautions
No known contraindications.

Special considerations
• Advise the patient that although *P. vulgaris* has been shown to be beneficial in suppression of HIV-1 retroviral activity, it should not be used as a substitute for conventional therapy.
• Tell the patient to use the herb cautiously because its effects on sore throat and GI conditions have not been evaluated.

Points of interest
• *P. vulgaris* was originally called *Brunella vulgaris*, from the German word *bruen*, meaning quinsy. Quinsy is a disorder of the throat for which brunella was considered a cure.

Analysis
P. vulgaris appears to show some benefit against HIV-1 retrovirus and certain cancers. However, it lacks significant in vivo studies in animals or humans. Although *P. vulgaris* appears promising as a medicinal agent, more information is needed to determine its safety and efficacy in humans.

References
John, J.F., et al. "Synergistic Antiretroviral Activities of the Herb, *Prunella vulgaris*, with AZT, ddI and ddC," *Abstr Gen Meet Am Soc Microbiol* 94:481, 1994. Abstract S-27.

Lee, K.H., et al. "The Cytotoxic Principles of *Prunella vulgaris*, *Psychotrial serpens*, and *Hyptis capitata*: Ursolic Acid and Related Derivatives," *Planta Med* 54:308-11, 1988.

Yamasaki, K., et al. "Anti-HIV-1 Activity of Labiatae Plants, Especially Aromatic Plants," *Int Conf AIDS* 11:65, 1996. Abstract Mo.A.1062.

Yao, X.J., et al. "Mechanism of Inhibition of HIV-1 Infection In Vitro by Purified Extract of *Prunella vulgaris*," *Virology* 187 56-62, 1992.

Zheng, M. "Experimental Study of 472 Herbs with Antiviral Action Against the Herpes Simplex Virus," *Chung His I Chieh Ho Tsa Chih* 10:39-41, 1990.

SENEGA

MILKWORT, MOUNTAIN FLAX, NORTHERN SENEGA, POLYGALA ROOT, RATTLESNAKE ROOT, SENECA, SENECA ROOT, SENECA SNAKEROOT, SENEGA ROOT, SENEGA SNAKEROOT

Common trade names
(Available in combination) Enhance, SN-X Vegitabs

Common forms
Available as syrups (various concentrations), lozenges, teas, tinctures, dried powdered root, and extract.

Source
The source of senega preparations is the dried root and rootstock of *Polygala senega*, a perennial herbaceous plant indigenous to southern Canada and the United States. It is made commercially in Canada and Japan.

Chemical components
The active ingredients in the preparations are the root saponins. Senegin is a saponin that hydrolyzes to form the glycosides, presenegin, and then senegenin, a chlorine-containing triterpenoid. Another root saponin is polygalic acid; this may add to the irritant activity of senega. Other compounds include carbohydrates (arabinose, sucrose, and fructose, among others), alpha-spinasterol, polygalitol, resins, valeric acid ester, fatty acids, and salicylic acid and methyl salicylate.

Actions
Senega is claimed to have an expectorant effect through direct irritation of the upper respiratory tract mucosa. This causes secretion of fluid from mucosal cells within the bronchioles as a reflex response to the irritation. A few *Polygala* species have been shown to produce a sedative-like effect in rodents, probably attributed to the saponin components (Carretero et al., 1986). Pharmacokinetic studies in animals show poor oral absorption of senega saponins from the GI tract (Johnson et al., 1986).

Reported uses
Although Native Americans first used senega root for rattlesnake bites, evidence supporting this use is lacking. Herbal practitioners recommend senega root as an expectorant for coughs and in chronic bronchitis, asthma, pneumonia, croup, and pharyngitis (Briggs, 1988). Other claims include its use as a diaphoretic, saliva stimulant, and emetic. Although it was listed as an official drug in the National

Formulary until 1960, no human clinical trials demonstrating its efficacy for these claimed uses is available.

Patent documentation in France suggests senega has activity toward treatment of eczema and psoriasis multiple sclerosis, graft rejection, and inflammation.

Dosage
For respiratory conditions, 2 tablespoons syrup P.O. every 4 hours as needed; 2.5 to 5 ml tincture P.O.; 0.3 to 1 ml extract P.O.; or 0.5 to 1 g dried root P.O. t.i.d.

Adverse reactions
• Abdominal pain
• Anxiety
• GI upset (nausea, irritation, vomiting, diarrhea; with large doses)
• Hemolysis (I.V. administration)
• Mental dullness
• Mouth and throat irritation
• Vertigo
• Vision disturbances

Interactions
Anticoagulants: may prolong bleeding time. Avoid concurrent use.
Antidiabetic agents: may counteract hypoglycemic therapy. Avoid concurrent use.
CNS depressants: may enhance CNS effects. Avoid concurrent use.

Contraindications and precautions
Contraindicated in patients with aspirin or salicylate hypersensitivity. Avoid use of senega in pregnant or breast-feeding patients; effects are unknown.

Special considerations
• Explain that inadequate data exist for any therapeutic use of the herb.
• Tell the diabetic patient to monitor for loss of glycemic control.
• Advise the female patient to avoid use of senega during pregnancy or when breast-feeding.

Analysis
Senega root preparations have been used as expectorants for centuries. Although the herb's efficacy and safety have been reported widely in the lay press, controlled trials are lacking. Compared with other expectorant products currently available, the herb s significant adverse effects and unproven efficacy preclude it from being recommended for any therapeutic use.

References

Briggs, C.J. "Senega Snakeroot — A Traditional Canadian Herbal Medicine," *Can Pharm J* 121:199-201, 1988.

Carretero, M.E., et al. "Etudes Pharmacodymiques Preliminaires de Polygala Microphylla (L.), sur le Systeme Nerveux Central," *Planta Med Phytother* 20:148-54, 1986.

Johnson, I.T., et al. "Influence of Saponins on Gut Permeability and Active Nutrient Transport In Vitro," *J Nutr* 116:2270-77, 1986.

SENNA

ADEN SENNA, *CASSIA ACUTIFOLIA, CASSIA AUGUSTIFOLIA, CASSIA SENNA,* MECCA SENNA, NUBIAN SENNA, TINNEVALLY SENNA

Common trade names

Senekot, Senexon, Senokot-S, Senolax, Senna Leaves

Common forms

Tablets: 187 mg
Capsules: 10 mg, 25 mg, 470 mg
Syrup of senna: 218 minims of fluid extract of senna, 81 minims of coriander, and sufficient syrup (6.5 fluid drams)
Senna tea or infusion of senna: 100 g of senna leaves, 1,000 ml of distilled boiling water, and 5 g of sliced ginger or coriander.
Also available as syrup, granules, suppositories, fluid extract, and teas.

Source

Active compounds are derived from the leaves and pods (fruits) of many *Cassia* species *(C. acutifolia, C. augustifolia,* and *C. senna).* Other species used include *C. obovata, C. lanceolata, C. marilandica, C. chamecrista*, and *C. fistula.*

Chemical components

Many chemical components are isolated from senna. The leaves contain myricyl alcohol, a flavonol containing kaempferol and isormamnetin. Anthroquinone derivatives and their glycosides comprise 3% to 5% of senna.

Sennosides A and B are the major components characterized by a rhein-dianthrone aglycone. Sennosides C and D are characterized by rhein and aloe-emodin aglycone. The leaves also contain chrysophanol and free sugars (fructose, glucose, sucrose, and pinitol). The seeds do not contain anthraquinones. The plant also contains cathartic acid, cathartin, mucilage, phaeoretin, sennacrol, and sennapicrin.

C. augustifolia has a total anthranoid content of 2% to 3% compared with *C. senna,* which has 3.5% to 5%; thus, *C. augustifolia* must be used in higher doses to receive the same action (Dreessen and Lemli, 1982).

Actions
Senna is a prodrug that is cleaved into an active component by intestinal bacteria. *Bacteroides fragilis, Streptococcus faecalis,* and *Streptococcus faecium* have been found to hydrolyze and reduce the glycosides into their active laxative aglycone component (Dreessen and Lemli, 1982). Senna works primarily to increase peristaltic activity in the lower bowel. Its primary site of action is the intestinal wall. It also has antiabsorptive properties and stimulates secretions. Senna passes into the breast milk of breast-feeding women (Morton, 1977).

It is postulated that sennosides may exert part of their laxative action by stimulation of prostaglandin E_2, leading to stimulation of colonic fluid and electrolyte excretion (Beubler and Kollar, 1988).

Reported uses
Senna is valuable as a laxative agent. The herb is used to relieve constipation and cleanse the bowel before diagnostic procedures are performed. The leaves and pods both have this activity.

Other uses are based on the *Cassia* species used. Claims include applying a paste of vinegar and powdered leaves (*C. alata*) for use in skin eruptions, psoriasis, and burns (Morton, 1977). A combination of the leaves, flowers, and pods has been used to allay fever; the leaves have been mixed with rose petals as a purgative; the juice or the powdered leaves have been used for cancerous tumors; the aloe-emodin component is believed to be useful in PS-127 and WA tumors; and the beta-sitosterol component useful in CA,WA, and LL tumors. Senna has also been used to help expel intestinal worms.

Dosage
For constipation, adult dosage is 2 tablets (187 mg) at bedtime (maximum 8 tablets daily); in children weighing over 60 lb (27 kg), 1 tablet at bedtime (maximum 4 tablets daily).
Powdered leaves: 1 dram
Concentrated solution: ½ to 1 dram
Compound or aromatic syrup: 2 fluid drams
Fluid extract: ½ to 2 fluid drams

Adverse reactions
• Cachexia, pigmentation of the colon (with excessive use)
• Colic, cramps, gripping pains
• Dermatitis (due to saponin)

Prolonged use:
- Clubbing of fingers
- Diarrhea
- Hypokalemia
- Melanosis coli
- Tetany

Interactions
Calcium channel blockers, calmodulin antagonists, indomethacin: blocked diarrheal effects. Avoid concomitant use.

Contraindications and precautions
Contraindicated in patients with GI inflammatory conditions, hemorrhoids, and prolapses.

Special considerations
- Explain that senna may cause discoloration of urine.
- Instruct the patient to increase fluid intake and add bulk-containing foods to diet (whole grain breads, grains, fruits, vegetables) to assist in relief of constipation.
- Tell the patient not to use senna if intense abdominal pain or nausea occurs.
- Advise the patient not to take stimulant laxatives for longer than 1 week. When condition resolves, senna should be discontinued.
- Instruct the patient that there are differences in potency between herbal supplements containing sennosides.

Points of interest
- Laxative abuse is a widespread problem for patients with eating disorders and for elderly patients who feel they must have daily bowel movements. Adverse effects that have been associated with excessive ingestion of senna include tetany, hypokalemia, and clubbing of the fingers (Prior and White, 1978).

Analysis
Senna is a widely used laxative agent that may be found in many OTC products. The leaves and pods have been used for the relief of constipation; thus, herbal supplements containing sennosides are believed to be safe and effective when used according to labeling. Many studies comparing senna products with other laxative products find it to be a useful agent for the treatment of constipation. However, overuse of products containing anthranoids has been shown to cause many adverse effects and, therefore, these agents should be used only for temporary relief of constipation.

References

Beubler. E., and Kollar, G. "Prostaglandin-Mediated Action of Sennosides," *Pharmacology* 36(Suppl.1):85-91, 1988.

Dreessen, M., and Lemli, J. "Qualitative and Quantitative Interactions Between the Sennosides and Some Human Intestinal Bacteria," *Pharm Acta Helv* 57:350-52, 1982.

Morton, J.F. *Major Medicinal Plants — Botany, Culture and Uses.* Springfield, Ill.: Charles C. Thomas, Bannerstone House, 1977.

Prior, J., and White, I. "Tetany and Clubbing in Patients Who Ingested Large Quantities of Senna," *Lancet* 2:947, 1978.

SHARK CARTILAGE

Common trade names
Carticin, Cartilade, GNC Liquid Shark Cartilage, Informed Nutrition Shark Cartilage, Natural Brand Shark Cartilage

Common forms
Ampules: 10 ml (containing 80 mg/ml)
Capsules: 750 mg
Tablets: 750 mg
Concentrate: 500 mg/15 ml

Source
Cartilage is obtained from the spiny dogfish shark, *Squalus acanthias,* and the hammerhead shark, *Sphyrna lewini.*

Chemical components
Glycoproteins sphyrnastatin 1 and 2 are obtained from cartilage of the hammerhead shark.

Actions
Cartilage composes 6% of the shark's total body weight, making it an abundant source of cartilage compared with mammalian sources (Hunt and Connelly, 1995).

Shark cartilage extract implanted into rabbit corneas that contained implanted tumors was found to significantly inhibit tumor neovascularization. The inhibitor did not appear to act directly on the tumor itself, because the carcinomas continued to grow slowly (Hunt and Connelly, 1995).

Reported uses
A 16-week Cuban trial attempted to evaluate the efficacy of shark cartilage in 29 patients with cancer; 15 were deemed evaluable and 3 showed response to treatment. However, this trial had design flaws; the types of cancer, definition of response, and reasons for exclusion

of some patients were not documented. The National Cancer Institute (NCI) Division of Cancer Treatment decided not to begin NCI-sponsored clinical trials because of the incomplete and unimpressive data from this study (Hunt and Connelly, 1995).

In another study of cancer patients taking shark cartilage either rectally or orally, 10 of the 20 patients reported an improved quality of life—including decreased pain and increased appetite—after 8 weeks. Additionally, 4 of the 20 patients showed partial or complete response (50% to 100% reduction in tumor mass). However, patient selection criteria, cartilage dose, concomitant antitumor therapy, and the type of cancer studied was not presented (Mathews, 1993).

A 12-week, phase I/II trial on 60 patients with advanced cancer evaluated the safety and efficacy of shark cartilage. The trial concluded that shark cartilage had no anticancer activity and no effect on the quality of life (Miller et al., 1998).

Dosage

For cancer treatment, typical dosages of commercially available shark cartilage dietary supplements range from 500 mg to 4,500 mg daily, depending on the type of preparation and the amount of "pure" shark cartilage contained. However, many of the commercially available shark cartilage food supplements contain only binding agents or fillers. Therefore, without reliable dose-response data and bioavailability studies, it is difficult to determine if these products have true antiangiogenic activity.

The manufacturer of commercially available tablets and capsules recommends the dosing interval to be two to six times daily.
Concentrates: 1 to 2 tablespoons daily.
Ampules: 1 ampule P.O. daily.

Adverse reactions
• Hepatitis (See *Shark cartilage–induced hepatitis.*)

Interactions
None reported.

Contraindications and precautions
Use cautiously in patients with liver disease.

Special considerations
• Advise the patient that there are insufficient data to support the use of shark cartilage for any malignancy.
• Advise the patient to undergo periodic liver function tests if use of shark cartilage is planned.
• Inform the patient that commercially available forms of shark cartilage contain varying amounts of the active ingredient.

A case of shark cartilage-induced hepatitis was reported in a 57-year-old man with a 3-week history of nausea, vomiting, diarrhea, and anorexia. He took no prescription medications but had begun taking shark cartilage dietary supplements 10 weeks before hospitalization. Because of a change in the odor of the supplements, he stopped taking them a few days before his symptoms began. He denied using alcohol or drugs and had no history of blood transfusions.

The patient's evaluation included ultrasonography of the right upper quadrant and computed tomography scan of the abdomen, both of which yielded unremarkable results. Results of hepatitis serologic tests, as well as tests for antinuclear antibody, ferritin, and acetaminophen levels, were also unrevealing. The patient was discharged with a presumed diagnosis of drug-induced hepatitis. A follow-up examination, done 6 weeks after discharge, showed normal liver function (Ashar and Vargo, 1996).

Points of interest
• Following the publication of W. Lane's *Sharks Don't Get Cancer* in 1992, shark cartilage became the newest "cancer cure." Contributing to the media frenzy, *a 60 Minutes* segment in February 1993 spotlighted shark cartilage as a promising treatment, and cancer information offices were swamped with calls about what some believed to be a new weapon against cancer.

Analysis
Because most macromolecules are usually not absorbed by the intestinal tract, it is questionable that oral administration of shark cartilage can release some compounds into the blood. There are no reliable dose-response data or bioavailability studies available.

In addition, no well-controlled clinical studies have been published. The NCI began a trial of shark cartilage in 1994, but it was stopped when each batch of shark cartilage (provided by advocates) was found to be contaminated. Currently, there is no evidence that shark cartilage offers any benefit to patients with cancer.

References
Ashar, B., and Vargo, E. "Shark Cartilage–Induced Hepatitis," *Ann Intern Med* 125:780-81, 1996.

Hunt, T.J., and Connelly J.F. "Shark Cartilage for Cancer Treatment," *Am J Health-Syst Pharm* 52:1756-60, 1995.

Mathews, J. "Media Feeds Frenzy Over Shark Cartilage as Cancer Treatment," *J Natl Cancer Inst* 85:1190-91, 1993.

Miller, D.R., et al. "Phase I/II Trial of the Safety and Efficacy of Shark Cartilage in the Treatment of Advanced Cancer," *J Clin Oncol* 16:3649-55, 1998.

SHEPHERD'S PURSE

CAPSELLA, CASEWEED, MOTHER'S-HEART, SHOVELWEED

Common trade names
None known.

Common forms
Available as dried herb and liquid extract.

Source
The leaves and stems of *Capsella bursa-pastoris* are most commonly sought for their medicinal properties.

Chemical components
Shepherd's purse contains flavonoids (quercetin, diosmetin, luteolin, hesperetin), their glycosides (rutin, diosmin, hesperidin), various amines (acetylcholine, choline, histamine, tyramine), volatile oils (predominantly camphor), carotenoids, fumaric acid, sinigrin (mustard oil glucoside), and vitamins C and K.

Actions
Shepherd's purse is claimed to have antihemorrhagic and urinary antiseptic properties. Some sources suggest the seeds have skin-reddening properties. Ethanolic extracts of shepherd's purse have demonstrated anti-inflammatory and reduced vessel wall permeability effects. Additionally, intraperitoneal injection accelerated recovery of stress-induced gastric lesions in rats. Gastric acid secretion was unaffected (Kuroda and Takagi, 1969).

Hypotensive effects have also been noted in several animal models. Negative inotropic and chronotropic effects have been seen, including effects causing coronary vasodilation (Jurisson, 1971).

Unidentified components have been shown to cause smooth muscle contraction (intestine, uterine, tracheal) and sedative effects in animals (Jurisson, 1971). Weak and limited antibacterial and antineoplastic activities have also been demonstrated with some components of shepherd's purse (Kuroda, 1977; Moskalenko, 1986).

Reported uses
Shepherd's purse has been claimed to be popular therapy for diarrhea, menorrhagia, hematuria, hematemesis, and other bleeding disorders. Scientific evidence of these uses in humans is lacking.

Dosage

Fluid extract: 1 teaspoon fluid extract in 1 glass (8-oz) water P.O. q.i.d.

Dried plant: infusion of 1 oz dried plant in 12 oz boiling water; cool and take P.O. t.i.d.

Adverse reactions

- Ataxia
- Hypotension
- Hypothyroidism with thyroid enlargement (iso-thiocyanate component)
- Mydriasis
- Respiratory paralysis (with toxicity seen in animals)
- Sedation

⚠ Respiratory paralysis leading to death

Interactions

Antihypertensives: possible enhanced hypotensive effects. Don't use together.

Beta blockers, calcium channel blockers, digoxin: added effects on myocardium. Avoid concurrent use.

Sedatives, hypnotic agents: added CNS effects. Avoid concurrent use.

Contraindications and precautions

Avoid use in pregnant or breast-feeding patients; effects are unknown. Use with caution in patients receiving heart rate-modifying drugs or CNS depressants and in those with heart or lung disease.

Special considerations

- Explain that insufficient evidence exists to support a role for any therapeutic application of shepherd's purse.
- Suggest other well-known and well-proven therapies to patients with significant heart or lung disease.

Analysis

Most data regarding shepherd's purse comes from in vitro models or animals. Little or no human clinical trial data exist to support a role for this herb in therapeutic applications. Shepherd's purse may be dangerous for patients with preexisting lung or heart disease.

Despite interesting pharmacologic effects in animals, human clinical data are needed before shepherd's purse can be recommended for use.

References

Jurisson, S. "Determination of Active Substances of *Capsella bursa-pastoris*," *Tartu Riiliku Ulikooli Toim* 270:71-79, 1971.

Kuroda, K. "Neoplasm Inhibitor from *Capsella bursa pastoris*," *Japan Kokai* 41:207, 1977.

Kuroda, K., and Takagi. K. "Studies on *Capsella bursa-pastoris* II. Diuretic, Anti-inflammatory and Anti-ulcer Action of Ethanol Extracts of the Herb. *Arch Int Pharmacodyn Ther* 178:392-99, 1969.

Moskalenko, S.A. "Preliminary Screening of Far-Eastern Ethnomedicinal Plants for Antibacterial Activity," *J Ethnopharmacol* 15:231-59, 1986.

SKULLCAP

HELMET FLOWER, HOODWORT, SCULLCAP

Common trade names
Scullcap Herb, Skullcap

Common forms
Capsules: 425 mg, 429 mg
Liquid extract: 1 oz, 2 oz

Source
The leaves and roots of the plants *Scutellaria laterifolia* and *S. baicalensis* are prepared as hot water or methanolic extracts. Skullcap is native to temperate regions of North America.

Chemical components
Scutellaria species contain flavonoids (apigenin, luteolin, hispidulin, scutellarein, scutellarin, baicalein, baicalin), an iridoid (catalpol), limonene, terpineol, carophyllene, cadinene, and other sesquiterpenes in the volatile oils. Wogonin, lignin, resin, and tannins are also present.

Actions
Skullcap is believed to have anticonvulsant and sedative actions. An aqueous extract was found to have mild anthelmintic properties in vitro. Other studies found bacteriostatic or bacteriocidal effects in vitro.

A root extract of skullcap showed anti-inflammatory action by inhibiting interleukin-1, and inhibited the synthesis of prostaglandin E_2 and leukotriene B_4 (Chung et al., 1995). Another study noted the inhibitory effects of skullcap flavonoids on sialidase—an agent associated with certain cancers—in mice. Skullcap extracts decreased 5-fluorouracil and cyclophosphamide myelotoxicity and decreased tumor cell viability in mice (Razina et al., 1987).

The extracts (flavonoids) of skullcap have demonstrated antiviral effects against the influenza virus and human T-cell leukemia virus type I. The authors thought that the inhibitory effect of the extract was dose dependent (Baylor et al., 1992). Another agent, baicalin, inhibited both HIV-1 infection and replication in human peripheral blood cells (Li et al., 1993). Skullcap may also inhibit Epstein-Barr virus early antigen activation in vitro.

Reported uses

Skullcap has been used traditionally as an anticonvulsant, an agent for movement disorders and spasticity, an anti-inflammatory agent, and a cholesterol-lowering agent. Little, if any, information exists to support the use of this herb in humans.

Skullcap has also been used as an antiviral agent and has demonstrated some effectiveness in animal studies in vitro. One study found that the addition of skullcap to chemotherapy prompted an increase in serum immunoglobulins in patients with lung cancer who were theophylline resistant (Smolianinov et al., 1997). In another study of patients receiving chemotherapy for lung cancer, the addition of a dry skullcap extract promoted hematopoiesis and an increase in the circulating precursors of erythroid and granulocyte colony stimulating units (Goldberg et al., 1997).

Other foreign reports in humans have suggested a role for skullcap in therapy of stroke and cerebral thromboembolism.

Dosage

Dosages have been administered P.O., I.V., and I.M.
Dried herb: 1 to 2 g as a tea P.O. t.i.d.
Liquid extract (1:1 in 25% alcohol): 2 to 4 ml P.O. t.i.d.
Tincture (1:5 in 45% alcohol): 1 to 2 ml P.O. t.i.d.

Adverse reactions

- Hepatotoxicity
Overdoses of tincture:
- Arrhythmias
- Confusion
- Giddiness
- Seizures
- Stupor
- Twitching

Interactions

Disulfiram: disulfiram reaction may occur if herbal form contains alcohol. Avoid concurrent use.
Immunosuppressive agents: possible altered effect on serum immunoglobulins. Do not use together.

Contraindications and precautions

Avoid use in pregnant or breast-feeding patients; effects are unknown.

Special considerations
- Monitor the patient's liver function studies periodically.
- Counsel the patient to avoid "large doses" of skullcap tincture because of possible toxicities.
- Explain that commercial sources of skullcap have been found to be contaminated with other herbs.
- Advise the patient that insufficient evidence exists to recommend skullcap for any condition or disease.
- Advise the female patient to avoid use of skullcap during pregnancy or when breast-feeding.

Points of interest
- Skullcap has been demonstrated to be adulterated with *Teucrium* species. Some species of *Teucrium* (*T. chamaedrys*-Germander) have also been linked with hepatotoxicity.

Analysis
Although several animal and in vitro studies have demonstrated the inhibitory effects of skullcap on pathologic viruses, there is little, if any, clinical trial evidence to support this application in humans. However, human studies have demonstrated some benefit of skullcap consumption in lung cancer, which points out the need for vigorous follow-up clinical investigation.

References

Baylor, N.W., et al. "Inhibition of Human T Cell Leukemia Virus by the Plant Flavonoid Baicalin (7-glucuronic acid, 5,6-dihydroxyflavone)," *J Infect Dis* 165:433-37, 1992.

Chung, C.P., et al. "Pharmacological Effects of Methanolic Extract from the Root of *Scutellaria baicalensis* and Its Flavonoids on Human Fibroblast," *Planta Med* 61:150-53, 1995.

Goldberg, V.E., et al. "Dry Extract of *Scutellaria baicalensis* as a Hemostimulant in Antineoplastic Chemotherapy in Patients with Lung Cancer," *Eksp Klin Farmakol* 60:28-30, 1997.

Li, B.Q., et al. "Inhibition of HIV Infection by Baicalin — A Flavonoid Compound Purified from Chinese Herbal Medicine," *Cell Mol Biol Res* 39:119-24, 1993.

Razina, T.G., et al. "Enhancement of the Selectivity of the Action of the Cytostatics Cyclophosphane and 5-Fluorouracil by Using an Extract of the Baikal Skullcap in an Experiment," *Vopr Onkol* 33:80-84, 1987.

Smolianinov, D.A., et al. "Effect of *Scutellaria baicalensis* Extract on the Immunologic Status of Patients with Lung Cancer Receiving Antineoplastic Chemotherapy," *Eksp Klin Farmakol* 69:49-51, 1997.

SKUNK CABBAGE

DRACONTIUM FOETIDUM, MEADOW CABBAGE, POLE-CAT CABBAGE, SKUNKWEED

Common trade names
None known.

Common forms
Available as powdered root, liquid extract, and tincture.

Source
The rhizome and roots of the *Symplocarpus foetidus* plant are sought for their active ingredients in skunk cabbage.

Chemical components
Skunk cabbage consists of starches, gum-sugar, fixed and volatile oils, resin, tannin, an acrid principal, iron, large amounts of non-specified alkaloids, phenolic compounds, and glycosides. There have been reports of high concentrations of oxalates or salts in the rhizome, consisting of calcium that forms insoluble calcium crystals. Some of these oxalates contain potassium, but these crystals are soluble (Konyukhov et al., 1970).

Actions
Little is known about the components of skunk cabbage and their pharmacologic activity. There have been no documented scientific studies about the pharmacologic and medicinal use of skunk cabbage in vitro, or in animal or human models.

Reported uses
Skunk cabbage has been used for tightness of the chest, irritable tight coughs, and other spasmodic respiratory disorders (asthma, bronchitis, and whooping cough).

It is also claimed to be useful in nervous disorders. Another claim as a diuretic is also unsubstantiated. The Micmac Indians crushed the leaves of skunk cabbage and inhaled the pungent oils of the herb to treat headaches.

Dosage
For coughs, 0.5 to 1 ml extract (1:1 in 25% alcohol) P.O. t.i.d.; 2 to 4 ml tincture (1:10 in 25% alcohol) P.O. t.i.d.; or 0.5 to 1 g rhizome powder mixed with honey t.i.d.

Adverse reactions
• Damaged renal tubules (where the crystals may lodge)
• Dizziness, headache, vertigo, nausea, vomiting (with overdose by inhalation)
• Drowsiness
• Itching, redness, inflammation (skin contact with root)
• Irritation, burning of the mucous membrane (when root is taken orally and calcium oxalate crystals may be embedded in mouth)

Interactions
None reported.

Contraindications and precautions
Avoid use in pregnant or breast-feeding patients; effects are unknown. Avoid use of skunk cabbage in patients with a history of kidney stones because of the presence of high concentrations of oxalates.

Special considerations
• Inform the patient that there is little information regarding this herb.
• Counsel the patient about the available pharmaceutical therapies for the treatment of asthma and bronchitis.
• Advise the female patient to avoid use of skunk cabbage during pregnancy or when breast-feeding.

Points of interest
• Skunk cabbage received its name because of the appearance of its leaf and the distinctive, unpleasant smell it secretes when bruised.
• The root of skunk cabbage is bitter and acrid, with a disagreeable odor.

Analysis
Because of the lack of information regarding the components of skunk cabbage, its pharmacologic activities, and its safety and efficacy, its use as a medicinal therapeutic agent cannot be recommended at this time.

References
Konyukhov, V.P., et al. "Dynamics of the Accumulation of Biologically Active Agents in *Lysichitum camtsochatcense* and *Symplocarpus foetidus*," *Uch Zap Khabarovsk Gos Pedagog Inst* 26:59-62, 1970.

SLIPPERY ELM

AMERICAN ELM, INDIAN ELM, MOOSE ELM, RED ELM, SWEET ELM

Common trade names
None known.

Common forms
Available as powdered bark and liquid extract (1:1 in 60% alcohol).

Source
The inner bark of *Ulmus rubra* Muhl. (*Ulmus fulva* Mich.) is used for medicinal purposes. Slippery elm is a member of the Ulmaceae (Elm) family, which can be found throughout North America. The pieces of bark are flat (about 2 to 4 mm thick) and oblong in shape. The outer surface of the bark is light-yellowish to reddish brown in color, whereas the inner side of the bark is much paler.

Chemical components
The major therapeutic component in slippery elm bark is a mucilaginous material that consists of hexoses, pentoses, methylpentoses, at least two polyuronides, glucose, galacturonic acid, *l*-rhamnose, *d*-galactose, and fructose (trace). Other components include tannins, phytosterols (phytositosterol, citrostadienol, dolichol), sesquiterpenes, calcium oxalate, and cholesterol.

Actions
Slippery elm has largely been used as a soothing agent. It has demulcent and emollient activity (Locock, 1997). The tannin components may impart some astringent activity to slippery elm.

Reported uses
Although this plant was once listed in the *U. S. Pharmacopoeia*, there is no clinical study data available to support its use. Its soothing effects have been long described and have been accepted by many herbalists. Slippery elm has therefore been used as a skin emollient, antitussive agent, and an agent to soothe GI ailments. Some pharmacognosy textbooks have added that a poultice of powdered slippery elm bark has been used for inflammation of the skin or GI tract.

Dosage
For GI discomfort, powdered bark as a 1:8 decoction of 4 to 16 ml P.O. t.i.d., or 4 g in 500 ml boiling water P.O. t.i.d.; or 5 ml liquid extract P.O. t.i.d.
For topical use as a skin emollient, poultice made of coarse powdered bark in boiling water.

Adverse reactions
• Spontaneous abortion (with whole bark preparations)

Interactions
None reported.

Contraindications and precautions
Avoid use in pregnant or breast-feeding patients and in those with a hypersensitivity to slippery elm or its components.

Special considerations
• Explain that insufficient data exist to describe risks and benefits of slippery elm.
• Advise the female patient to avoid use of slippery elm during pregnancy or when breast-feeding.
• Tell the patient to avoid whole bark preparations of slippery elm because there is very little evidence to support the herb's use.

Points of interest
• Small quantities of slippery elm powdered bark have been included in the multiherbal decoction known as Essiac. Anecdotal reports supported the notion that this formulation had anticancer activity, but a clinical trial could not show any benefit.

Analysis
There are not enough published data available to recommend internal use of this agent. Proven contemporary therapies should be used instead of this herb.

References
Locock, R.A. "Essiac," *Can Pharm J* 14:18-19, 51, 1997.

SOAPWORT

BOUNCING BET, BRUISEWORT, CROW-SOAP, FULLER'S HERB, LATHERWORT, SOAP ROOT, SWEET BETTY, WILD SWEET WILLIAM

Common trade names
None known.

Common forms
Available as dried root and leaves, decoction, extract, fluid extract, inspissated juice.

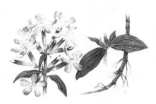

Source

Medicinal formulations are extracted from the root and leaves of *Saponaria officinalis,* which is indigenous to Asia and has become naturalized to eastern North America.

Chemical components

Chemical components of soapwort include saponin, sapotoxin, saponarin, several saporins (ribosome-inactivating proteins), resin, gum, woody fiber, and mucilage.

Actions

Soapwort is claimed to alter metabolism and have diaphoretic, tonic, and astringent effects. Saponins derived from *S. officinalis* have been shown to reduce the rate of bile salt absorption in vivo in rats. Dietary saponins may also be useful for controlling plasma cholesterol and nutrient absorption.

Saporins have been shown to be powerful cytotoxic agents in vitro, especially when conjugated to molecular targeting antibodies or protein ligands (Soria, 1989). Saporins, alone or with targeting molecules, have shown cytotoxic action in vitro to human lymphoma, leukemia, melanoma, and breast cancer cells (Gasperi-Campani et al., 1991; Siena et al., 1989; Tecce et al., 1991).

Reported uses

Soapwort has been used externally for its sudsing action as an ingredient in herbal shampoos. Historically, soapwort preparations were taken internally for itching associated with dandruff and dermatitis, rheumatism, gout, and cutaneous symptoms associated with syphilis. It has also been used for jaundice and intestinal problems. Human clinical trials are lacking for any medicinal uses.

Soapwort has been used as an expectorant and laxative in small doses, and for skin conditions such as psoriasis, acne, boils, and eczema; human studies are lacking for these uses.

Dosage

Decoction: 2 to 4 fl oz P.O. t.i.d. or q.i.d.
Extract (or inspissated juice): 10 to 20 grains P.O.
Fluid extract: ¼ to 1 dram P.O.

Adverse reactions

- GI irritation (severe), nausea, vomiting (oral administration)
- GI ulceration (oral administration)
- Hepatotoxicity (Stripe et al., 1987)
- Nephrotoxicity
- Neurotoxicity (Chan et al., 1995)

⚠ Some components of soapwort, notably saponin, sapotoxin, and the saporins, are potentially gastrotoxic; therefore, high doses of the herb for prolonged periods (over 2 weeks) should be avoided.

Interactions
None reported.

Contraindications and precautions
Avoid use in pregnant or breast-feeding patients; effects are unknown. Because of the numerous toxicities associated with ingestion of soapwort, its use is contraindicated in many patients.

Special considerations
• Periodically monitor hepatic and renal function of patients using this herb.
• Advise the patient to avoid oral consumption of soapwort because of its strong cathartic effects.

Points of interest
• The Egyptian soapwort root, *Gypsophila struthium*, has been rarely used medicinally as a substitute for soapwort (*S. officinalis*). It contains saponin and some of the same components as *S. officinalis*.
• Saponins are known for their ability to produce foam or suds in solution. The term *saponification* refers to the process of making soap. The taste of plant products high in saponin components is said to be much like soap. Soapwort was once popular as a cleaning and sizing agent in the textile industry. This process, known as "fulling," is how soapwort came to be referred to as "fuller's herb."
• Soapwort is commonly included as an ingredient in herbal shampoos.

Analysis
Soapwort has traditionally been used to treat symptoms associated with syphilis, and for the treatment of jaundice and intestinal complaints. The presence of potentially toxic components makes this root or its preparations a poor choice as a general tonic or for supportive therapy. Although purified saponins have been shown to be cytotoxic to cancer cells in vitro, there is no clinical evidence for their use. Because of the availability of safer, more effective medications, soapwort cannot be recommended for any indication.

References
Chan, T.Y., et al. "Neurotoxicity Following the Ingestion of a Chinese Medicinal Plant, *Alocasia macrorrhiza*," *Hum Exp Toxicol* 14:727-28, 1995.
Gasperi-Campani, A., et al. "Inhibition of Growth of Breast Cancer Cells In Vitro by the Ribosome-Inactivating Protein Saporin 6," *Anticancer Res* 11:1007-11, 1991.

Siena, S., et al. "Activity of Monoclonal Antibody-Saporin-6 Conjugate Against B-Lymphoma Cells," *Cancer Res* 49:3328-32, 1989.

Soria, M. "Immunotoxins, Ligand-Toxin Conjugates and Molecular Targeting," *Pharmacol Res* 21(Suppl 2):35-46, 1989.

Stripe, F., et al. "Hepatotoxicity of Immunotoxins Made with Saporin, a Ribosome-Inactivating Protein from *Saponaria officinalis*," *Virchows Arch* 53: 259-71, 1987.

Tecce, R., et al. "Saporin 6 Conjugated to Monoclonal Antibody Selectively Kills Human Melanoma Cells," *Melanoma Res* 1:15-23, 1991.

SORREL

CUCKOO SORROW, CUCKOO'S MEATE, DOCK, GARDEN SORREL, GREENSAUCE, GREEN SORREL, SOUR DOCK, SOURGRASS, SOUR SAUCE, SOURSUDS

Common trade names
None known.

Common forms
Available as teas and juice from fresh plants.

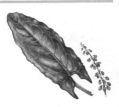

Source
Garden sorrel is known as *Rumex acetosa;* the popular sorrel is the sheep sorrel (*Rumex acetosella*). All sorrel species belong to the Polygonaceae family, which is native to Europe and northern Asia and has been naturalized in North America. Several parts of the sorrel plant have been used for their medicinal value, such as the leaves, flowers, roots, and seeds.

Chemical components
Oxalates, particularly potassium oxalate (a soluble oxalate salt), is a constituent of the sorrel plant. Although it occurs in the soluble oxalate form and especially in the leaves, the content of oxalates in the plant varies with geographic location and season. Other compounds include tartaric acid, anthracene, oxymethylanthraquinone, and tannins. Ascorbic acid has also been identified in high concentrations in the leaf and berry. The active chemical compounds have not been isolated.

Actions
Because of the poisonous nature of the soluble oxalates found in the plant, a wide range of toxicity in humans and animals has been described. Soluble oxalate salts are absorbed without causing irritation to the mucosa. The onset of symptoms occurs from 2 to 48 hours after the ingestion of soluble oxalate salts (Sanz and Reig, 1992). Oxalates are excreted unchanged in the urine within 24 to 36 hours after ingestion.

Reported uses

Various claims for the therapeutic effect of sorrels have contributed to its medical use as an antiseptic and diuretic, and for treating scurvy. It has also been used in the treatment of diarrhea because of its astringent properties.

Dosage

No consensus exists. The leaves and flowers are made into a tea. Juice from the plant may be diluted with water and taken P.O.

Adverse reactions

• Dermatitis (with fresh herbal products)
• Gastroenteritis; renal damage; hypocalcemia with resultant tetany; brain, myocardial, and liver damage (due to soluble oxalate salts)
⚠ After ingesting 500 g of garden sorrel (*R. crispus*) in a soup, a patient experienced vomiting, diarrhea, metabolic acidosis, and hypocalcemia, leading to extensive liver necrosis and death (Farre et al., 1989).

Interactions

Diuretics: additive effects. Avoid concomitant use.
Other renal or hepatotoxic drugs: additive toxic effects. Avoid concomitant use.

Contraindications and precautions

Contraindicated in children and in pregnant or breast-feeding patients. Also contraindicated in patients prone to developing, or with a history of, kidney stones.

Special considerations

• Inform the patient to change the water that the sorrel plant leaves are cooked in at least once to decrease the herb's potency; otherwise, the herb is toxic.
• Tell the patient to use the herb with caution because the oxalates contained in the plant may be toxic.
• Instruct the patient to keep the herb away from children and pets.

Points of interest

• The estimated fatal dose of oxalic acid is 15 to 30 g; as little as 5 g may cause death.
• The concentration of soluble oxalates in the leaves varies depending on the season and geographic location of the sorrel plant.
• The herb was used in the 16th century for the treatment of fevers. The medicinal value of sorrel was recognized through the 19th century, but concern over the plant's poisonous nature limited its use (Crellin and Philpott, 1990).

Analysis
Therapeutic claims for the use of sorrel to treat fevers or diarrhea, and as a diuretic, lack supporting evidence. There appears to be no data regarding efficacy in animals or humans. Toxicity and death in animals and humans have been documented in the literature.

References
Crellin, J.K., and Philpott, J. *A Reference Guide to Medicinal Plants: Herbal Medicine Past and Present.* Durham and London: Duke University Press, 1990.

Farre, M., et al. "Fatal Oxalic Acid Poisoning from Sorrel Soup," *Lancet* 2:1524, 1989.

Sanz, P., and Reig, R. "Clinical and Pathological Findings in Plant Oxalosis: A Review," *Am J Forensic Med Pathol* 13:342-45, 1992.

SOUTHERNWOOD

APPLERINGIE, BOY'S LOVE, GOD'S TREE, LAD'S LOVE, MAIDEN'S RUIN, OLD MAN

Common trade names
None known.

Common forms
Available as teas, oil, and extracts.

Source
Southernwood is a strongly aromatic, shrubby perennial native to southern Europe. The leaves, tops, shoots, and seeds are used.

Chemical components
The volatile oil of southernwood is composed primarily of absinthol. Other components include abrotanin, adenosine, adenine, choline, calycanthosides, guanines, essential oils, malates, nitrates of potassium, isofraxidine, resin, scopolin, scopoletin, tannins, succinic acid, and umbelliferone.

Actions
The extraction process of *A. abrotanum* isolated four flavonols, namely three coumarins (umbelliferone, scopoletine, and isofraxidine) and one sesquiterpene (hydroxyflavanone). These flavonols showed a dose-dependent relaxing effect on the carbacholine-induced contraction of guinea-pig trachea. These components inhibit the cAMP phosphodiesterase and the spasmolytic flavone 7-O-methyleriodictyol. More studies and assays are needed to determine the extent of spasmolytic effects of this herb. Human studies

are necessary to determine this herb's place in medicinal use (Bergendorff and Sterner, 1995).

One German abstract describes the choleretic effects of isofraxidine, scopoletine, and umbelliferone, with isofraxidine being the most potent (Nieschulz and Schmersahl, 1968).

Reported uses

Medicinal use of southernwood is limited and sparsely documented. Anecdotal claims include use as a digestive aid, anthelmintic, and diuretic. Others include use as a cure for fevers and wounds, antiseptic detergent, promotion of menstruation, and uterine stimulant. The ash of southernwood mixed with an ointment is thought to promote hair regrowth in balding men. None of these claims are supported by published trials.

Dosage

Dried herb: 2 to 4 g in hot water; take P.O. t.i.d.
Extract (1:1 in 25% alcohol): 2 to 4 ml P.O. t.i.d.

Adverse reactions

None reported.

Interactions

None reported.

Contraindications and precautions

Avoid use in pregnant or breast-feeding patients; effects are unknown.

Special considerations

● Explain that very little information exists to discuss benefits or dangers of herbal use.
● Advise the female patient to avoid use of southernwood during pregnancy or when breast-feeding.

Points of interest

● *Artemisia* is thought to come from Artemis, the Greek goddess of hunting and of chastity. Artemis was identified with Diana, who is the goddess of nature, the forests, and the moon.
● There are more than 180 species of *Artemisias*, including *A. absinthium (wormwood), A. vulgaris (mugwort)*, and *A. abrotanum (southernwood)*.
● Southernwood's obnoxious odor fends off moths and insects, leading to the name *Garde Robe*. It has been placed in clothes and on the skin for this purpose. The branches and leaves have been used to produce a yellow dye for coloring wool.

Analysis

There is little documentation in clinical trials supporting the use of southernwood for medicinal purposes. The emergence of other *Artemisia* species for use in herbal preparations has made southernwood a less favorable option. The most likely use for this agent appears to be as a stimulant for menstruation and as a possible spasmolytic agent. Use of southernwood should be avoided until clinical studies support these therapeutic claims and the herb's safety and efficacy can be established.

References

Bergendorff, O., and Sterner, O. "Spasmolytic Flavonols from *Artemisia abrotanum*," *Planta Med* 61: 370-71, 1995.

Nieschulz, V.O., and Schmersahl, P. "Uber choleretische Wirkstoffe aus *Artemisia abrotanum L.*," *Arzneimittelforschung* 18:1330-36, 1968.

SPIRULINA

BLUE-GREEN ALGAE, DIHE, TECUITLATL

Common trade names

Spirulina

Common forms

Capsules: 500 mg, 750 mg
Tablets: 250 mg, 380 mg, 500 mg, 750 mg
Powders: 20 mg
Supplemental fruit drinks: 20 mg
Also available as fresh plant for consumption as food.

Source

Spirulina belongs to the Oscillatoriaceae family of algae that occur in high-salt, alkaline waters in subtropical and tropical areas. There are approximately 35 *Spirulina* species. They appear blue-green because of the chlorophyll (green) and phycocyanin (blue) pigments in their cells and take the form of microscopic, corkscrew-shaped filaments.

Chemical components

Spirulina has a high nutritional content. Protein represents 60% to 70% of its sample, even in dry weight. The protein content includes 22 amino acids, 47% of which represent essential amino acids (such as phenylalanine). Although spirulina is one of the richest protein sources of plant origin, 15% of the crude protein is derived from nonprotein nitrogen. Spirulina also contains fats, carbohydrates, B complex vitamins (especially B_{12}), vitamins A and E, trace elements (manganese, selenium, and zinc), minerals (calcium, potassium, and magnesium), and iron. The bioavailability of the iron is 60% more absorbable than commercially available iron supplements. Spirulina also contains gamma-linolenic acid (GLA) and a sulfolipid fraction; GLA is a rich source of omega-6 essential fatty acid.

Actions
Because of its high nutritional content, spirulina has been used as a supplement for malnourished and starving adults and children. A study of malnourished children ages 5 to 12 months who were fed spirulina, milk, or soy milk found that despite a lower protein digestibility (spirulina 60% and soy 70%), nitrogen retention was higher with spirulina (40%) than with soy (30%) (Dillon, 1995).

Because phenylalanine is thought to act on the brain's appetite center to alleviate hunger pangs, spirulina was used to promote weight loss. However, the FDA advisory committee on OTC drugs has ruled that phenylalanine lacks safety and efficacy data supporting its use in weight control (Popovich, 1982).

A sulfated polysaccharide called calcium spirulan has been formulated from the algae's lipid content, and it exhibits antiviral properties. The compound was found to have a high selectivity index for inhibiting the replication of all enveloped viruses, including human cytomegalovirus, measles virus, mumps virus, herpes simplex virus, influenza A virus, and HIV-1. Research is currently directed toward a detailed structure of the complex and also the relationship between molecular conformation and bioavailability (Hayashi et al., 1996).

Reported uses
Spirulina has been used in diet and weight-loss products for its high nutritional value and claimed action on appetite suppression. Although there are reports of its use instead of dietary supplements, its cost does not justify use in this manner. In developing countries, such as Peru, India, Vietnam, and Togo and other African countries, spirulina is used to help fight protein and vitamin A malnutrition. In industrialized countries, the GLA content is thought to contribute to the prevention of CV disease.

Other reported uses for spirulina include diabetes, anemia, liver disease, peptic ulcers, pancreatitis, glaucoma, hair loss, and stress. None of these uses have been supported through clinical trials.

Dosage
The usual dose is 3 to 5 g P.O. daily before meals. In malnourished infants, 3 to 15 g P.O. daily has resulted in rapid weight gain.

Adverse reactions
None reported. Nutritional tests have established spirulina as non-toxic for humans.

Interactions
None reported.

Contraindications and precautions
Contraindicated in patients in whom the risk of heavy metal poisoning is not outweighed by benefit of use. Use cautiously in pregnant or breast-feeding patients.

Special considerations
• Know that spirulina can contain significant amounts of mercury depending on where it is grown. Consumption of 20 g of spirulina daily may produce a mercury consumption above the maximum 180-mcg safety limit. Reported mean heavy metal levels include arsenic, cadmium, lead, and mercury.
• Be aware that spirulina may also contain minute amounts of radioactive di- and trivalent metallic ions, depending on where the product was manufactured.
• Tell the patient that spirulina has a mild marine odor that is stronger than its taste.

Points of interest
• The content of GLA in spirulina is 25% to 30% compared with other sources, such as evening primrose oil or blackcurrant berry (10% to 15%).
• Algae have long been regarded as promising sources of protein if food shortages occur in the future.
• In regions not familiar with its use, the algae's color may present a problem, especially when used in baby foods. Decolorizing the product can be accomplished conveniently.

Analysis
There is no question regarding the nutritional value of spirulina; however, there are more economical means of providing protein and nutrients to the body than through algae. Supplementation with commercially available vitamins does not include the potential risk of heavy metal poisonings or exposure to radioactive ions. Spirulina cannot be recommended for any medical use until clinical research details its benefits.

References
Dillon J.C., et al., "Nutritional Value of the Alga Spirulina," *World Rev Nutr Diet* 77:32-46, 1995.

Hayashi, T., et al. "Calcium Spirulan, an Inhibitor of Enveloped Virus Replication, from a Blue-Green Alga *Spirulina platensis*," *J Nat Prod* 59:83-87, 1996.

Popovich, N.G. "Spirulina," *Am Pharm* 22:8-10, 1982.

SQUAW VINE

CHECKERBERRY, DEERBERRY, *MITCHELLA REPENS*, *MITCHELLA UNDULATA*, ONE-BERRY, PARTRIDGE BERRY, RUNNING BOX, SQUAWBERRY, TWIN BERRY, TWO-EYED BERRY, TWO-EYED CHECKERBERRY, WINTER CLOVER

Common trade names
Mitchella repens, Partridge Berry, Squaw Vine

Common forms
Available as whole leaves, dried plant (powder), liquid extract, and tincture.

Source
Squaw vine is the dried plant of *Mitchella repens* Linne (Rubiaceae family), common to the woodlands of the central and eastern United States. The plant blooms in July and is usually harvested in late summer.

Chemical components
The leaves of the plant contain resin, wax, mucilage, dextrin, and tannin. The leaves are also thought to contain glycosides and saponins (Chevallier, 1996).

Actions
Tannic acid has local astringent properties that act on the mucosa of the GI tract, which is thought to occur through binding and precipitation of proteins. Tannic acid also forms insoluble complexes with select heavy metal ions, alkaloids, and glycosides. It has also been shown to have antiulcerogenic and antisecretory effects within the GI tract due to an inhibitory action on the gastric enzyme system. Saponins are usually nontoxic to humans after oral ingestion; however, when administered I.V., they act as potent hemolytics (Budavari, 1996).

Reported uses
Squaw vine has been used as an astringent, diuretic, and tonic. Because its tonic properties are thought to work primarily on the uterus, squaw vine has been used extensively as an aid in labor and childbirth. Native Americans were the first to use the plant to make

parturition safer and easier. It has also been used in cases of abnormal menstruation, heavy bleeding, and abdominal pain associated with menstruation (Chevallier, 1996). Other claims include its use as a remedy for amenorrhea, diarrhea, edema, dysentery, dysuria, gonorrhea, kidney stones, hysteria, polyuria, and vaginitis (Duke, 1985). Crushed squaw vine berries have been mixed the with myrrh and used for sore nipples (Chevallier, 1996). The use of squaw vine is based on traditional and anecdotal reports, not on controlled human clinical trials.

Dosage
Squaw vine (dried): 30 to 60 grains (2 to 4 g) P.O.
Fluid extract: ¼ to 1 teaspoon P.O. t.i.d.
Tincture: 1 to 2 ml P.O. t.i.d.

Adverse reactions
• Burning of GI tract
• Irritated mucous membranes
⚠ Hepatotoxicity (rare)

Interactions
Cardiac glycosides: potential increased effect. Use cautiously.
Disulfiram: disulfiram reaction may occur if herbal form contains alcohol. Do not use together.
Alkaloid-related substances (atropine, scopolamine), iron-containing products: tannic acid may slow metabolic breakdown. Monitor patient.

Contraindications and precautions
Contraindicated during the first 6 months of pregnancy. Use cautiously in patients with preexisting hepatic diseases or complications.

Special considerations
• Know that it has been suggested that "due to its extensive use, squaw vine should be considered potentially dangerous, and anyone consuming large amounts of the leaves should be watched and treated symptomatically."
• Be aware that saponin glycosides have a bitter taste and are irritating to the mucous membranes.
• Monitor liver function tests. If abnormal increases in liver transaminases occur, discontinue use of the plant immediately.
• Tell the female patient to report planned or suspected pregnancy.
• Advise the patient to report symptoms of hepatic injury immediately (right upper-quadrant pain, jaundice, fever).

● Warn the patient taking disulfiram not to take an herbal form that contains alcohol.

Analysis
Although there appears to be widespread use of squaw vine as a medicinal herb, none of these claims have been studied or proven in animals or humans.

References
Budavari, S. *The Merck Index: An Encyclopedia of Chemicals, Drugs, and Biologicals,* 12th ed. Whitehouse Station, N.J.: Merck & Co., 1996.

Chevallier, A. *The Encyclopedia of Medicinal Plants,* 1st ed. New York: DK Publishing, Inc., 1996.

Duke, J.A. *CRC Handbook of Medicinal Herbs.* Boca Raton, Fla.: CRC Press, 1985.

SQUILL
European squill, Indian squill, Mediterranean squill, red squill, sea onion, sea squill, white squill

Common trade names
Not commercially available.

Common forms
Available as dried roots, extract, and tincture.

Source
The active components are derived from the bulbous portion of the base and the dried inner scales of the bulb of *Urginea maritima.*

Chemical components
The herb contains several steroidal cardioactive glycosides, including scillaren A and B, proscillaridin A, glucoscillaren, scillaridin A, and scilliroside, as well as several different flavonoids (Wartburg et al., 1968).

Actions
Squill has demonstrated peripheral vasodilatory, as well as heart-rate lowering properties in rabbits. In humans, the herb exhibits inotropic and chronotropic effects on the heart similar to digitalis, but less potent (Stauch et al., 1977). In low doses, squill is a mucolytic (improves the flow of secretions), whereas at higher doses it acts as an emetic by both centrally mediated and local gastric irritant mechanisms (Court, 1985).

Reported uses

The herb is well-known for its cardiac effects and, before the discovery of the more effective cardiac glycosides, was used to treat symptoms related to heart failure. It is also used for its expectorant and diuretic effects (Orita, 1996). Red squill rich in scilliroside is commercially known as a highly effective rat poisoning.

Dosage

Dose is 0.06 to 0.25 g of bulb P.O. t.i.d. Decoction is made by mixing hot water over ½ to 1 teaspoon of bulb; allow to steep for 10 to 15 minutes. Refrigerate and take 1 cup P.O. t.i.d. Tincture is taken ½ to 1 ml P.O. t.i.d.

Adverse reactions

- CNS stimulation
- Gastric irritation and emesis

⚠ Seizures; life-threatening cardiac toxicity (heart block, arrhythmia, asystole) if ingested in sufficient doses (Tuncok et al., 1995)

Interactions

Antiarrhythmics, beta blockers, calcium channel blockers, digoxin: may cause enhanced cardiac effects and toxicity. Monitor patient closely.
CNS stimulants: potential for additive effects. Avoid using together.
Disulfiram: disulfiram reaction may occur if herbal product contains alcohol. Avoid use together.
Glucocorticoids, laxatives: may cause increased effects and adverse reactions. Avoid concomitant use.

Contraindications and precautions

Contraindicated in pregnant or breast-feeding patients and in those with potassium deficiency. Use cautiously in patients with cardiac disorders and in those receiving agents that may interact with squill, such as digoxin, beta blockers, calcium channel blockers, and antiarrhythmics.

Special considerations

- Monitor the patient for adverse CNS reactions.
- Monitor vital signs, including cardiac rhythm, of patient also taking cardiac drugs.
- Explain that insufficient data exist to support the herb's use as a therapeutic agent.
- Warn the cardiac patient to avoid use of this herb because it may promote disease exacerbation or contribute to cardiotoxicity.
- Advise the patient to avoid hazardous activities until the herb's CNS effects are known.

• Caution the patient receiving disulfiram against taking an herbal product that contains alcohol.

• Instruct the female patient to report planned or suspected pregnancy.

• Tell the patient to keep the herb out of reach of children and pets.

Analysis

Squill extracts are used today primarily as expectorants. Squill's use as a cardiac stimulant declined after the discovery of cardiac glycosides. Its use for cardiac effects cannot be recommended.

References

Court, W.E. "Squill-Anergetic Diuretic," *Pharm J* 235:194-97, 1985.

Orita, Y. "Diuretics," *Nippon Jinzo Gakkai Shi* 38:1-7, 1996.

Stauch M, et al. "Effect of Proscillaridin-4í-methylether on Pressure Rise Velocity in the Left Ventricle of Patients with Coronary Heart Disease." *Klin Wochenschr* 55:705-06, 1977.

Tuncok, Y., et al. "*Urginea maritima* (Squill) Toxicity." *J Toxicol Clin Toxicol* 33:83-86, 1995.

Wartburg, A. von , et al. "Cardiac Glycosides from White Sea Onion or Squill. The Constitution of the Scilliphaeosides and Glucoscilliphaeosides," *Helv Chim Acta* 51:1317-28, 1968.

STONEROOT

HEAL-ALL, HORSE BALM, HORSEWEED, KNOB ROOT, KNOB WEED, KNOT ROOT, OX BALM, RICH LEAF, RICH WEED

Common trade names
Tincture Collinson

Common forms
Available as tincture of the root.

Source
Stoneroot is derived from the rhizome and root of *Collinsonia canadensis,* which belongs to the Labiatae family. The plant is native to North America, growing wild from Massachusetts and Vermont west to Wisconsin, and south to Florida and Arkansas.

Chemical components
The rhizome and roots of the *C. canadensis* contain saponins, tannins, mucilage, and resins.

Actions
The active chemical compounds of the plant show diuretic, astringent, and antifungal properties. The active ingredient responsible

for the diuretic action is not known. Tannins produce the character-istic astringent effect. In the treatment of burns, the proteins of ex-posed tissue are precipitated. An antiseptic, protective coat forms and allows for the regeneration of new tissue underneath (Tyler et al., 1988). Antifungal activity has been demonstrated in vitro using an alcoholic extract of the powdered roots.

Reported uses

Stoneroot is an herbal diuretic found in several OTC preparations claiming use for the treatment of menstrual distress, edema, and hypertension. The herb has also been reported as useful in the treat-ment of headaches and indigestion.

Its main use is claimed to be for the treatment of hemorrhoids, diarrhea, and varicose veins. These claims are made based on the herb's astringent properties. There appears to be no scientific evi-dence for any of these therapeutic claims.

Dosage

For diuretic action and in the treatment of stones in the bladder, 15 to 60 drops of the tincture P.O. t.i.d.

Adverse reactions

• Possible increased blood pressure (with chronic use)

Interactions

None reported; may potentially produce an additive effect with anti-hypertensives.

Contraindications and precautions

Contraindicated in pregnant or breast-feeding patients; effects are unknown. Use cautiously in patients with hypertension.

Special considerations

• Monitor liver function tests; prolonged use may lead to hepatotox-icity.
• Caution the patient to seek appropriate medical advice before self-medicating for high blood pressure or edema.

Points of interest

• An FDA advisory review panel on menstrual drug products found little scientific evidence to support the use of this herb.

Analysis

The major therapeutic claims for the use of stoneroot include its as-tringent and diuretic activities. However, none of the therapeutic claims have been substantiated in the scientific literature in either animal or human models and, thus, this herb cannot be recommended at this time.

References

Tyler, V.E., et al. *Pharmacognosy,* 9th ed. Philadelphia: Lea & Febiger, 1988.

SUNDEW

COMMON SUNDEW, DEW PLANT, RED ROT, ROUND-LEAVED SUNDEW, GREAT SUNDEW

Common trade names
None known.

Common forms
Available as a tincture and fluid or solid dried extract.

Source
Drosera rotundifolia is a carnivorous plant named for the sticky, dewlike substance produced on its leaves and used to trap insects. The entire flowering plant and leaves, excluding the roots, are the components most medicinally used.

Chemical components
The sundew plant, *D. rotundifolia,* contains droserone, flavonoids, tannins, glycosides, vitamin C, pigments, traces of essential oils, and organic acids. The exudate from the leaves contain proteolytic enzymes and plumbagin (Bienenfeld et al., 1966).

Actions
Although sundew is claimed to have expectorant, demulcent, and antispasmodic activities, there is no supporting evidence available. Some in vitro activity against *Staphylococcus* and *Pneumococcus* bacteria has been noted (Vinkenborg et al., 1969).

Reported uses
Traditionally, sundew has been used to treat pulmonary conditions such as bronchitis, whooping cough, asthmatic coughs, and pulmonary tuberculosis. It has also been used for the treatment of stomach ulcers. However, there are no human studies to support therapeutic use for any condition.

Dosage
The average daily dose is 3 g of herb.
Infusion: 1 cup of boiling water mixed with 1 teaspoon of dried

herb; let stand 15 minutes and take infusion P.O. t.i.d.
Tincture: 1 to 2 ml P.O. t.i.d.

Adverse reactions
• Urine discoloration (brownish orange; harmless)

Interactions
Disulfiram: disulfiram reaction may occur if herbal product contains alcohol. Don't use together.

Contraindications and precautions
Contraindicated in patients with tuberculosis or hypotension.

Special considerations
• Alert the patient and laboratory staff that the patient's urine may become discolored.
• Warn the patient taking disulfiram against use of the herbal product containing alcohol.
• Tell the patient with suspected tuberculosis to seek standard medical treatment. Persistent cough should be evaluated by the primary health care provider.

Analysis
There are insufficient data in humans to support any therapeutic use of sundew. Potential use in pulmonary conditions requires thorough clinical studies in humans.

References
Bienenfeld, W., et.al. "Flavonoids from *Drosera rotundifolia* L." *Arch Pharm Ber Dtsch Pharm Ges* 229:598-602, 1966.

Vinkenborg, J., et al. "The Presence of Hydroplumbagin Glucoside in *Drosera rotundifolia* L.," *Pharm Weekbl* 104:45-49, 1969.

SWEET CICELY
BRITISH MYRRH, (SWEET) CHERVIL, COW CHERVIL, ROMAN PLANT, SHEPHERD'S NEEDLE, SMOOTH CICELY, SWEET BRACKEN, SWEET FERN, SWEET HUMLOCK

Common trade names
None known.

Common forms
Available as an extract and ointment.

Source
The whole plant (roots, leaves, seeds) of the *Myrrhis odorata* is used for medicinal and culinary purposes.

Chemical components
None known.

Actions
Sweet cicely's main effect is to act as a GI stimulant. It is also claimed to have an antiseptic effect when used topically (Bunney, 1984).

Reported uses
Sweet cicely is claimed to be useful as a GI stimulant, antiflatulent, expectorant, and diuretic. The topical form is thought to be useful for treating small external bite wounds, and for treating ulcers and gout pain (Heinerman, 1996). There is a lack of scientifically based studies in the medical literature to support any of these claims. However, the plant is being studied in diabetes for use as an artificial sweetener in diabetic foods.

Dosage
No consensus exists.

Adverse reactions
None reported.

Interactions
Diuretics: possible increased effects of diuretic. Avoid concomitant use.

Contraindications and precautions
High doses of the herb are contraindicated in pregnant or breast-feeding patients. Use cautiously in patients with peptic ulcer disease or ulcerative colitis.

Special considerations
• Warn the patient receiving diuretics against use of this herb because of additive effects.

Points of interest
• The root from the *Ozmorrhiza longistylis,* also known as American sweet cicely, is claimed to have similar medicinal properties. The root of the plant is used to make a tea for the treatment of heartburn, acid indigestion, abdominal cramps, and flatulence, and for improving appetite.

Analysis

The entire sweet cicely plant is edible and considered safe for consumption. Thus, its use in medicine is likely harmless in moderate amounts. However, the medicinal claims have yet to be scientifically proven. To date, there are few data surrounding the use of this herb. Identification of any active ingredients, standardized formulations, and clinical trials are warranted to support current claims.

References

Bunney, S., ed. *The Illustrated Book of Herbs. Their Medicinal and Culinary Uses.* London: Octopus Books Ltd., 1984.

Heinerman, J. *Heinerman's Encyclopedia of Healing Herbs & Spices.* Englewood Cliffs, N.J.: Prentice Hall, 1996.

SWEET FLAG

BEE WORT, CALAMUS, RAT ROOT, SWEET MYRTLE, SWEET ROOT, SWEET SEDGE

Common trade names

Not commercially available.

Common forms

Available as dried powder, liquid extract, and tincture.

Source

The dried rhizome and roots of *Acorus calamus,* Araceae family, are used. Sweet flag is believed to have originated from India but now grows in most parts of the world, in wet soil or shallow water.

Chemical components

The active ingredients are the bicyclic sesquiterpines, alpha- and beta-asarone.

Actions

Asarone has been shown to be carcinogenic (Haseninejad and Caldwell, 1994). Sweet flag is claimed to have sedative (beta-asarone), anticholinergic, hypotensive, psychoactive (hallucinogenic), analgesic, stimulation (alpha-asarone), euphoric, and laxative activities. Asarone has some nematodocidal activity and anticoagulant effect in animals (Sugimoto et al., 1995); it is metabolically converted to TMA-2, a potent hallucinogen.

Reported uses

Native Americans of the Cree tribe chewed the root for its stimulant, euphoric, and hallucinogenic effects. They also used the drug as an analgesic and an antidiabetic agent. In Ayurvedic medicine, it is used mostly for digestive disorders. Current western herbalists recommend sweet flag as an antispasmodic for GI disturbances. Clinical human data supporting any claim in humans are lacking.

Dosage

Dried rhizome: 1 to 3 g P.O. t.i.d.
Liquid extract: 1 to 3 ml P.O. t.i.d.
Tincture: 2 to 4 ml P.O. t.i.d.

Adverse reactions

- Confusion
- Disorientation
- Hallucinations
- Mutagenic effects
- Nausea
- Vomiting

Interactions

Disulfiram: disulfiram reaction may occur if herbal product contains alcohol. Avoid use together.
Psychoactive, sedative, or stimulating agents: possible increased effects of these agents. Use cautiously.
Sedatives, other CNS depressants: antagonistic effects. Do not use together.

Contraindications and precautions

Contraindicated during pregnancy and in patients with psychiatric disorders. Use cautiously in patient at risk for hepatotoxicity.

Special considerations

- Monitor for adverse CNS reactions.
- Monitor for misuse or abuse of the herb.
- Advise the patient to avoid hazardous activities until the herb's CNS effects are known.
- Instruct the female patient to report planned or suspected pregnancy.
- Warn the patient taking disulfiram against use of an herbal product containing alcohol.

Points of interest

- Hepatocarcinogenicity associated with the asarones has been observed in animals (Hasheninejad and Caldwell, 1994).
- There are recent reports of sweet flag abuse by persons seeking the herb's psychoactive effects.
- The oil is used by the Cree for anointing in religious ceremonies.

Analysis

Sweet flag has been used for 2,000 years worldwide for several conditions and in religious ceremonies for its psychoactive properties. The United States, however, has banned its use as a food additive or supplement because of its mutagenic potential.

References

Hasheninejad, G., and Caldwell, J. "Genotoxicity of the Alkylbenzenes Alpha- and Beta-Asarone, Myristin and Elmicin as Determined by the UDS Assay in Cultured Rat Hepatocytes," *Food Chem Toxicol* 32:223-31, 1994.

Sugimoto, N., et al. "Mobility Inhibition and Nematocidal Activity of Asarone and Related Phenylpropanoids on Second-Stage Larvae of *Toxocara canis*," *Biol Pharm Bull* 18:605-09, 1995.

SWEET VIOLET

ENGLISH VIOLET, FLOR DE PROSEPINA, VIOLA, *VIOLA SUAVIS*, VIOLETA, *VIOLETA CHEIROSA*, *VIOLETA COMUN*

Common trade names

None known.

Common forms

Available as dried and fresh flowers and leaves.

Source

Active compounds have been derived from the roots, seeds, flowers, and leaves of *Viola odorata.*

Chemical components

Chemical compounds isolated from the seeds, roots, leaves, and flowers of *V. odorata* include saponin, myrosin, violamin, viola-quercetin, gaultherin, an emetine-like alkaloid (viola-emetin), 2-nitropropionic acid, and odoratine (alkaloid). Methylsalicyclic acid can be found after hydrolysis of gaultherin. Over 100 volatile oils have been isolated from the leaves.

Actions

Leaf extracts of *V. odorata* were found to be comparable with aspirin in reducing pyrexia in animals; a significant reduction in temperature was noted (Khattak et al., 1985).

Reported uses

V. odorata has been claimed to have several therapeutic uses. Decoctions and syrups made from the leaves and flowers have been used as a cough remedy and sedative, and applied topically as an anti-inflammatory agent. The dried root has been used for the treatment of constipation and as an emetic. Extracts of the leaves and flowers are also used in the manufacture of perfumes.

Dosage
No consensus exists. Various concentrations of extracts, decoctions, and powders have been used, making standardized dosage identification difficult.

Adverse reactions
• Possible cathartic effects

Interactions
Laxatives: additive effect. Monitor patient.

Contraindications and precautions
Contraindicated in pregnant or breast-feeding patients; effects are unknown.

Special considerations
• Explain that insufficient data exist for therapeutic use of this herb.

Points of interest
• *V. tricolor*, also known as the wild pansy, is a related species used for treating several skin conditions including eczema.

Analysis
There are few data about the pharmacologic or therapeutic effects of *V. odorata*. Studies in animals have shown that leaf extracts have antipyretic action comparable to aspirin. However, the therapeutic usefulness of *V. odorata* cannot currently be established.

References
Khattak, S.G., et al. "Antipyretic Studies on Some Indigenous Pakistani Medicinal Plants," *J Ethnopharmacol* 14:45-51, 1985.

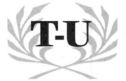

TANSY

BITTER BUTTONS, GOLDEN BUTTONS, YELLOW BUTTONS

Common trade names
Tansy Extract, Tansy Oil

Common forms
Available as an essential oil, fluid extract, and tea.

Source
Active components are derived from the dried leaves and flowering tops of *Tanacetum vulgare*, a member of the Compositae family. It should not be confused with other plants referred to as "tansy," including the tansy ragwort (*Senecio jacobaea*).

Chemical components
A range of tansy strains exist that yield extracts of varying chemical composition, which is determined more by the genetic makeup of the plant than environmental factors. Fresh tansy contains 0.12% to 0.18% volatile oil. Some strains yield an oil composed almost entirely of a toxic terpene, thujone, with several minor sesquiterpene and flavone components; others yield an oil that is nearly thujone-free. Besides thujone, these oils contain artemisia ketone, chysantheyl acetate, beta-caryophyllene, germacrene-D, borneol, camphor, isopinocamphone, isothujone, piperitone, gamma-terpinene, umbellulone, and other unidentified terpenes.

Actions
Tansy oil has shown in vitro activity against gram-positive bacteria, but not gram-negative bacteria. Toxic effects are likely attributable to thujone. The plants or extracts may cause contact dermatitis, possibly due to the sesquiterone lactones, arbusculin-A, or tanacetin components (Guin and Skidmore, 1987; Paulsen et al., 1993).

Reported uses
In ancient Greece, tansy was believed to impart immortality and was therefore used for embalming. It has been used as a stimulant, anthelmintic, menstrual stimulant, tonic, antispasmodic, and anti-inflammatory agent, and to treat bruises, swelling, fever, headaches,

sore throat, and diarrhea. The Micmac and Malecite Indians used tansy to prevent pregnancy (largely as an abortifacient) and as a diuretic (Chandler et al., 1982). Tansy leaves have been used to prepare a tea and as a food flavoring.

Dosage
No consensus exists. Because these plants vary considerably from one genetic "race" to another, it is not possible to predict the thujone content and the strength or toxicity of a given tansy preparation.

Adverse reactions
• Allergic rhinitis, sneezing
• Contact dermatitis
• Personality changes, renal damage (with chronic use)
⚠ Thujone, a relatively toxic compound, is likely responsible for the toxicity associated with tansy. As few as 10 drops of tansy oil has been reported to be fatal. Symptoms of tansy poisoning include rapid, weak pulse; seizures; severe gastritis; and violent muscle spasms.

Interactions
None reported.

Contraindications and precautions
Contraindicated in pregnant patients because of its potential abortifacient effects and in patients allergic to the herb or its components.

Special considerations
• Inform the patient wishing to use this herb that the chemical composition of the oil cannot be predicted unless specifically analyzed; thus, the safety profile is not known. Minute amounts of thujone have been fatal.
• Warn the patient about the risk of allergic dermatitis and rhinitis.
• Instruct the female patient to report planned or suspected pregnancy immediately.

Analysis
There are no clinical data to support use of this herb for any medical condition. The most frequent indication for tansy in folk medicine has been as an anthelmintic and insect repellent; however, safer and more effective products are available for these purposes. Because of the herb's unpredictable toxicity and allergenic properties, it cannot be recommended for use.

References

Chandler, R.F., et al. "Herbal Remedies of the Maritime Indians: Sterols and Triterpenes of *Tanacetum vulgare* L. (Tansy)," *Lipids* 17:102-106, 1982.

Guin, J.D., and Skidmore, G. "Compositae Dermatitis in Childhood," *Arch Dermatol* 123:500-02, 1987.

Paulsen, E., et al. "Compositae Dermatitis in a Danish Dermatology Department in One Year," *Contact Dermatitis* 29:6-10, 1993.

TEA TREE

AUSTRALIAN TEA TREE OIL, *MELALEUCA ALTERNIFOLIA*, MELALEUCA OIL, TEA TREE OIL

Common trade names
Jason Winter's Tea Tree Oil, Swanson Ultra Tea Tree Oil, Thursday Plantation Tea Tree Oil

Common forms
Available as creams, ointments, lotions, and soaps; also included in cosmetics, toiletries, and household products. Concentrations of melaleuca oil in these products range from less than 1% to 100%.

Source
Tea tree oil, or melaleuca oil, is an essential oil distilled from the leaves and branches of *Melaleuca alternifolia,* a member of the myrtle family (Myrtaceae) native to coastal areas of Australia.

Chemical components
The steam distillation of the leaves yields approximately 2% oil. The colorless to pale yellow oil is composed of terpene hydrocarbons (pinene, terpinene, cymene), cineol, and various minor sesquiterpenes and related alcohols. Composition of the extract, however, is varied; the oxygenated terpene, terpinen-4-ol, can constitute up to 60% of the total oil. Some oils contain high concentrations of 1,8-cineol, which is the main component of eucalyptus oil. Most commercially available tea tree oils contain little or no cineol. More than 100 different compounds (all plant terpenes) have been identified in melaleuca oil.

Actions
Terpinen-4-ol, a main component of tea tree oil, has significant antibacterial and antifungal activity in vitro; susceptible organisms include *Escherichia coli, Staphylococcus aureus, Proprionibacterium acnes, Pseudomonas aeruginosa, Streptococcus species,* and *Candida albicans.* Tea tree oil may also be effective against methicillin-resistant *S. aureus* (MRSA) carrier that has previously been treated with topical mupirocin (Carson et al., 1995).

In addition, there is some in vitro evidence that tea tree oil has antimicrobial activity against vancomycin-resistant enterococci (VRE) (Nelson, 1997). Development of microbial resistance to the oil has not been observed.

Reported uses
Tea tree oil has long been used primarily as a local antiseptic. Australian aborigines used it for burns, cuts, insect bites, and athlete's foot, among other disorders. Some studies indicate the oil is promising as a treatment for skin problems, including acne, eczema, lice infestation, furuncles, psoriasis, wound infections, vaginal candidiasis, chronic cystitis, and bacterial and fungal infections of the skin and oral mucosa (Nenoff et al., 1996). Melaleuca oil has also been compared with tolnaftate and clotrimazole solution for various skin conditions with some effect. It has also been studied against 5% benzoyl peroxide for the treatment of acne vulgaris (Bassett et al., 1990). More research is needed to prove its value in the treatment of skin infections, acne, and vaginal infections.

Dosage
Tea tree oil is applied locally in concentrations from 0.4% to 100%, depending on the type of product and nature and location of the skin disorder.

Adverse reactions
- CNS depression (ataxia, drowsiness)
- Dermatitis (in sensitive individuals)
- Diarrhea
- GI irritation
- Irritation of the oral and GI mucosa
- Vomiting

Interactions
None reported.

Contraindications and precautions
Use cautiously in patients with an allergy to any of the components of melaleuca oil, or in those prone to contact dermatitis. Avoid use in pregnant or breast-feeding patients; effects are unknown.

Special considerations
- Monitor for worsening of skin condition or infection.
- Advise the patient that melaleuca oil is ubiquitous in commercially available products, and concentration of the oil varies greatly.
- Because essential oils are more appealing to olfactory senses and exhibit more natural appeal than currently available topical drugs,

melaleuca may be preferred for antiseptic use. Encourage the patient to consider conventional therapy until substantial testing is done with the oil.

• Warn the patient that the oil should not be ingested, and should be kept out of the reach of small children. Even small amounts of oil taken internally may produce CNS depression. A 17-month-old child who ingested less than 10 ml of tea tree oil experienced ataxia and drowsiness, but recovered fully (Jacobs et al., 1994).

• Advise the female patient to avoid use of the herb during pregnancy or when breast-feeding.

Analysis

Interest in melaleuca oil has burgeoned with reports of favorable in vitro antimicrobial activity against MRSA and VRE, suggesting potential topical application. Although antimicrobial activity has been well documented, clinical trials and efficacy data are lacking for treatment of various skin disorders.

References

Bassett, I.B., et al. "A Comparative Study of Tea-Tree Oil Versus Benzoyl-peroxide in the Treatment of Acne," *Med J Aust* 153:455-58, 1990.

Carson, C.F., et al. "Susceptibility of Methicillin-Resistant *Staphylococcus aureus* to the Essential Oil of *Melaleuca alternifolia*," *J Antimicrob Chemother* 35:421-24,1995.

Jacobs, M.R., et al. "Melaleuca Oil Poisoning," *Clin Toxicol* 32:4:461-64, 1994.

Nelson, R.R.S. "In-Vitro Activities of Five Plant Essential Oils Against Methicillin-Resistant *Staphylcoccus aureus* and Vancomycin-Resistant *Enterococcus faecium*," *J Antimicrob Chemother* 40:305-06, 1997.

Nenoff, P., et al. "Antifungal Activity of the Essential Oil of *Melaleuca alternifolia* (Tea Tree Oil) Against Pathogenic Fungi In Vivo," *Skin Pharmacol* 9:388-94, 1996.

THUJA

EASTERN WHITE CEDAR, FALSE WHITE CEDAR, HACKMATACK, TREE-OF-LIFE, YELLOW CEDAR

Common trade names
None known.

Common forms
Available as liquid extract and tincture.

Source
Active components are obtained from the needles and young twigs of *Thuja occidentalis*, an evergreen conifer native to eastern North America. The tree belongs to the Cupressaceae family.

Chemical components
Thuja contains the volatile oil thujone, tannin, flavonoid glycoside, and a resin, thujin.

Actions
Thuja's actions appear related to its stimulating and blood-purifying volatile oil. Thuja has some mitogenic activity, inhibits HIV-1 antigens and HIV-1 specific reverse transcriptase, and is an inducer of a subset of T cells and various cytokinesin vitro (Offergeld et al., 1992). It has also been shown to be an immunostimulant in a rat liver model (Vomel, 1985). Thujone oil can cause seizures in animals (Elsasser-Beile et al., 1996).

Reported uses
Therapeutic claims for thuja include use as a diuretic, expectorant, astringent, and antiseptic. Although thuja has become popular as a cancer treatment, all the supporting data are from in vitro (Offergeld et al., 1992) or anecdotal case reports, and not from controlled human trials.

Dosage
Infusion: 1 teaspoon of dried herb in 1 cup boiling water, let stand 10 to 15 minutes and take P.O. t.i.d.
Tincture: 1 to 2 ml P.O. t.i.d.

Adverse reactions
• Asthma (Cartier et al., 1986)
• CNS stimulation
• Flatulence
• GI complaints
• Seizures
• Stomach irritation
• Uterine stimulation (may lead to spontaneous abortion)

Interactions
Anticonvulsants: lowered seizure threshold. Adjust anticonvulsant dosage as needed.
Caffeine, other stimulants: additive effect. Avoid concomitant use.

Contraindications and precautions
Contraindicated during pregnancy because of the risk of spontaneous abortion. Internal use is contraindicated in patients with seizure disorders. Use cautiously in patients with ulcers or gastritis because of its GI stimulating effects.

Special considerations

● Monitor for adverse reactions, such as excess stimulation.
● Warn the female patient to report planned or suspected pregnancy.
● Caution the patient against using this herb because little evidence regarding its medicinal use exists.

Analysis

Insufficient data exist in humans to support any medicinal use of thuja at this time. Further studies are needed to evaluate its effects in cancer and AIDS therapy. There are safer alternatives available for the traditional use of thuja as a diuretic and expectorant.

References

Cartier, A., et al. "Occupational Asthma Caused by Eastern White Cedar (*Thuja occidentalis*) with Demonstration that Plicatic Acid is Present in this Wood Dust and is the Causal Agent," *J Allergy Clin Immunol* 77: 639-45, 1986.

Elsasser-Beile, U., et al. "Cytokine Production in Leukocyte Cultures During Therapy with *Echinacea* Extract," *J Clin Lab Anal* 10: 441-45, 1996.

Offergeld, R., et al. "Mitogenic Activity of High Molecular Polysaccharide Fractions Isolated from the *Cuppressaceae Thuja occidentalis* L. Enhanced Cytokine-Production by Thyapolysaccharide, G-Fraction (TPSg)," *Leukemia* 6(Suppl 3):189S-91S, 1992.

Vomel, T. "Effect of a Plant Immunostimulant on Phagocytosis of Erythrocytes by the Reticulohistiocytary System of Isolated Perfused Rat Liver," *Arzneimittelforschung* 35:1437-39, 1985.

THYME

COMMON THYME, GARDEN THYME, RUBBED THYME, THYMI HERBA, TIMO

Common trade names
(Various manufacturers; available in combination)
Autussan "T," Olbas, Pertussin, Pertussin N

Common forms
Extract: 12% to 14%
Ointment: 1% to 2% thymol
Also available as an essential oil.

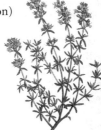

Source
Active components are derived from the dried leaves
and flowering tops of *Thymus vulgaris*, a member of the mint family (Labiatae); the plant is native to Spain and Italy and widely cultivated worldwide.

Chemical components

The composition of thyme essential or volatile oil is varied. Phenols, principally thymol, comprise 25% to 70% of the oils. Other components include carvacrol, camphene, sabinene, beta-pinene, 1,8-cineol, linalol, borneol, geraniol, geranyl acetate, sesquiterpine and alcohol.

Actions

Thyme extract contains thymol and other phenols, which have antiseptic, antitussive, and expectorant properties. Thymol acts as an expectorant by directly irritating gastric mucosa. It exerts antifungal action topically and systemically. It has been tested against actinomycosis in humans (Myers, 1937). However, its systemic action is greatly diminished in the presence of protein. Therefore, thymol is usually applied topically or taken orally. Thyme liquid extracts have shown spasmolytic action in animal models (van Den Broucke and Lemli, 1981).

Reported uses

Thyme products have been used most widely as food additives, flavoring agents, and condiments. Therapeutic claims include use as an antiflatulent, antifungal, anthelmintic, antitussive, antiseptic, antispasmotic, expectorant, diaphoretic, and digestive aid. It is commonly used as an antitussive in respiratory tract disorders. Its antiseptic properties are exploited in toothpastes, mouthwashes, and tooth fillings. Other anecdotal uses include treatment of dyspepsia, hysteria, dysmenorrhea, and headache.

Dosage

For itchy skin, 1% to 2% ointment applied topically as needed.
Cough syrup: 1 teaspoon P.O. every 2 hours as needed.
Essential oil: 5 to 10 drops in some water, P.O. b.i.d. or t.i.d.
Tea: 1.5 to 2 g dried herb P.O. t.i.d.

Adverse reactions

- Bradycardia
- Cheilitis, glossitis (with toothpaste)
- Dermatitis
- Diarrhea
- Dizziness
- Headache
- Muscle weakness
- Nausea
- Slow respirations
- Vomiting

⚠ Systemic allergic reactions have occurred when used as a flavoring agent. Symptoms include pruritus and swelling of the lips and tongue, dysphagia, dysphonia, progressive upper respiratory difficulty, edema, hypotension, nausea, and vomiting. Treatment involves epinephrine, corticosteroid, and antihistamine administration and fluid therapy (Benito et al., 1996).

Interactions
None reported.

Contraindications and precautions
Contraindicated in patients with a history of gastritis and intestinal disorders and in those with allergic sensitivity to various plants such as grass. Internal use is contraindicated in patients with enterocolitis or cardiac insufficiency and during pregnancy.

Special considerations
• Caution the patient with sensitive skin or known allergies to avoid this herb.
• Tell the patient that there are few clinical data to support thyme's use for any medical condition.

Analysis
Thyme preparations have been used for centuries to treat several disease states. In light of the limited availability of clinical studies that assess the safety and efficacy of thyme, these products cannot be recommended for therapeutic purposes. The use of thymol as an antiseptic may be useful in dental products, but well-designed studies are needed.

References
Benito, M., et al. "Labiatae Allergy: Systemic Reactions Due to Ingestion of Oregano and Thyme," *Ann Allergy Asthma Immunol* 76:416-18, 1996.
Myers, H.B. "Thymol Therapy in Actinomycosis," *JAMA* 108:1875, 1937.
van Den Broucke, C.O., and Lemli, J.A. "Pharmacological and Chemical Investigation of Thyme Liquid Extracts," *Planta Med* 41:129-35, 1981.

TONKA BEAN

CUMARU, TONKA SEED, TONQUIN BEAN, TORQUIN BEAN

Common trade names
Tonka Bean

Common forms
Tonka bean is difficult to obtain commercially; availability is rare.

Source
Active components are extracted from the fruits and seeds of *Dipteryx odorata*, a tree native to South America, specifically Brazil and Venezuela. The tonka bean tree belongs to the legume family (Leguminosae).

Chemical components
The primary chemical components of tonka bean are coumarin, dihydrocoumarin, and o-coumaric acid. Other components include melilotic acid, methyl melilotate, ethyl melilotate, 5-hydroxymethyl-furfural, fat, and starch.

Actions
Coumarin is metabolized within the body to 7-hydroxycoumarin, which then undergoes glucuronidation in the intestines and liver; this extensive first-pass metabolism results in a low absolute bio-availability of coumarin. Both coumarin and 7-hydroxycoumarin have inhibited growth of selected types of malignant human cell lines in vitro. The glucuronide metabolite of 7-hydroxycoumarin appears to be inactive (Marshall et al., 1994).

Reported uses
Tonka bean is claimed to relieve nausea and cramping; the fruit is also thought to act as an aphrodisiac. Coumarin has long been used as a flavoring agent in foods and a scent in pharmaceutical products. It has shown therapeutic benefit against lymphedema in recent clinical trials (Overik et al., 1995; Vettorello et al., 1996).

Dosage
Usual dose used is 60 mg P.O. coumarin daily. (Some studies have based doses on the coumarin content of the product.)

Adverse reactions
• Hepatotoxicity (possibly severe)

Interactions
Agents that cause hepatotoxicity: potential for additive toxicity. Avoid concomitant use.
Anticoagulants: may cause excessive bleeding. Avoid concomitant use.

Contraindications and precautions
Contraindicated in patients with any underlying hepatic dysfunction because of the potential for toxicity. Avoid use of the herb in pregnant or breast-feeding patients; effects are unknown.

Special considerations
• Monitor liver function tests.
• Advise the female patient to avoid use of the herb during pregnancy or when breast-feeding.
• Inform the patient that tonka bean is currently on the FDA's list of "unsafe" herbs.

Points of interest
• Do not confuse this herb with the synthetic anticoagulant, bis-hydroxycoumarin.

Analysis
Several tonka bean components, especially coumarin and 7-hydroxy-coumarin, show promise as future therapeutic agents. However, because efficacy and safety data are currently lacking, the herb cannot be recommended for any medicinal use

References
Marshall, M.E., et al. "Growth-Inhibitory Effects of Coumarin (1,2-Benzopyrone) and 7-Hydroxycoumarin on Human Malignant Cell Lines In Vitro," *J Cancer Res Clin Oncol* 120(Suppl):S3-S10, 1994.

Overvik, E., et al. "Activation and Effects of the Food-Derived Heterocyclic Amines in Extrahepatic Tissues," *Princess Takamatsu Symp* 23:123-33, 1995.

Vettorello, S., et al. "Contribution of a Combination of Alpha and Beta Benzpyrones, Flavonoids and Natural Terpenes in the Treatment of Lymphedema of the Lower Limbs at the 2d Stage of Surgical Classification," *Minerva Cardioangiol* 44:447-55, 1996.

TORMENTIL

BISCUITS, BLOODROOT, EARTHBANK, ENGLISH SARSAPARILLA, EWE DAISY, FIVE-FINGERS, FLESH AND BLOOD, SEPTFOIL, SEVEN LEAVES, SHEPHERD'S KNAPPERTY, SHEPHERD'S KNOT, THORMANTLE

Common trade names
None known.

Common forms
Available as rootstock, tincture, and powder.

Source
Active components are derived primarily from the rhizome and roots of *Potentilla tormentilla*, a perennial herb that belongs to the rose family (Rosaceae) and is native to Europe and Asia.

Chemical components

The rhizome contains mainly tannic acid, tormentol (a triterpine alcohol), a glycoside, tormentillin, starch, sugars, a bitter compound (chinovic acid), and essential oils (Stodola, 1984). Many other components have also been identified, such as adimericellagitannin, agrimoniin, gallic acid, ellagic acid, and catechol gallates.

Actions

Because it is rich in tannic acid, the herb is a strong astringent and also has some tonic properties. Tormentil has also been reported to have antiallergic, antiviral, and antihypertensive effects. In addition, it has demonstrated immunostimulant, antioxidant, and antielastase properties (Bos et al., 1996).

Reported uses

The astringent properties of *P. tormentilla* are reportedly useful topical agents as compresses or ointments for slow-healing wounds, rashes, grazes, burns, and sunburn. The tincture is claimed to be valuable as a gargle for throat and mouth inflammations (Grieve, 1997). Internal use of *P. tormentilla* has been touted as a treatment for diarrhea (Carr et al., 1987). Clinical trials are lacking for these indications and for its immunostimulant and antielastase properties.

Dosage

For diarrhea, mix 1 oz each of powdered tormentil, powdered galangal, and powdered marshmallow root with 240 grains powdered ginger and 1 pint of boiling water. Strain mixture, and take 5 to 10 ml (3 teaspoons) t.i.d. or q.i.d. Do not use for more than 3 to 4 days.

Gargle: boil 2 oz of bruised root in 50 oz water until reduced by one third. Strain cooled liquid and use as gargle.

Powder: ¼ to ½ teaspoon powder P.O. t.i.d.

Tea: 1 tablespoon rootstock in 1 cup of water, steep for 30 minutes, strain and drink during the day in "mouthful" doses.

Tincture: 20 to 30 drops P.O. b.i.d. or t.i.d.

Adverse reactions

• Acute ingestion of over 1 g tannins may cause nausea, vomiting, gastroenteritis, abdominal pain, constipation (with possible fecal impaction), and hepatic necrosis.

Interactions

Alkaloids, glycosides: precipitation and reduced absorption of drugs may occur. Avoid concomitant use internally.

Disulfiram: possible disulfiram reaction if tincture contains alcohol. Avoid concomitant use.

Contraindications and precautions

Avoid use of the herb in pregnant or breast-feeding patients; effects are unknown.

Special considerations

● Advise the female patient to avoid use of the herb during pregnancy or when breast-feeding.
● Warn the patient taking disulfiram not to use herbal product containing alcohol.

Points of interest

● In ancient Athens, Hippocrates used tormentil to treat malaria.
● The 17th-century British herbalist Nicholas Culpeper recommended packing tormentil root into a painful tooth. In the days before the discovery of dental plaque, the herb was used to dry up the "flux of humors" thought to cause toothaches (Carr et al., 1987).

Analysis

There are no clinical data to support taking this herb for any medical condition. Because little is known about its toxicologic properties, this herb is best avoided.

References

Bos, M.A., et al. "Procyanidins from Tormentil: Antioxidant Properties Towards Lipoeroxidation and Anti-Elastase Activity," *Biol Pharm Bull* 19:146-48, 1996.
Carr, A., et al. *Encyclopedia of Herbs.* Emmaus, Pa.: Rodale Press, 1987.
Grieve, M. *A Modern Herbal.* London: Tiger Books International, 1997.
Stodola, J. *The Illustrated Book of Herbs.* London: Octopus Books Ltd., 1984.

TRAGACANTH

ADRILEL, E413, GUM DRAGON, GOMA ALATIRA, GUM TRAGACANTH, HOG GUM, SHAGAL EL KETIRA, SYRIAN TRAGACANTH, TRAGACANTH TREE

Common trade names

None known; usually sold as tragacanth or gum tragacanth.

Common forms

Available as a gum, gel, viscous solution, and powder.

Source

Tragacanth is obtained by drying the gummy substance that exudes from the cut tap root and branches of *Astragalus gummifer* or other *Astragalus* species, low thorny shrubs belonging to the legume family (Leguminosae). The plants are native to the Middle East.

Chemical components

Tragacanth gum consists of two major fractions, tragacanthin and bassorin, with trace amounts of starch, a cellulose-like substance, amino acids, and amino acid derivatives. Tragacanthin is water-soluble and consists of an arabinogalactan and tragacanthic acid, whereas bassorin is a complex of methoxylated acids that swells to form a gel or viscous solution but is insoluble in water. Tragacanth may also contain some karaya, India gum, or acacia, other natural gums used for similar purposes.

Actions

When added to water, tragacanth swells to form a viscous jelly that is mixed with other ingredients to create the desired consistency in the final product. This action is likely attributable to the bassorin content; high-quality gums contain less tragacanthin. The herb also exerts a mild laxative effect (Iwu, 1993).

Tragacanth is an innocuous substance. Large doses (10 g) of tragacanth reduced intestinal transit time and increased fecal fat levels. However, plasma biochemistry, hematologic indices, urinalysis parameters, glucose tolerance, breath hydrogen, methane levels, and serum cholesterol, triglycerides, and phospholipids were not significantly changed. The quantity of tragacanth used in this study far exceeds the normal annual dietary intake (Eastwood et al., 1984). Other claims are that tragacanth stimulates phagocytosis, increases plasma cell counts of T lymphocytes, and acts against some experimental tumors (Iwu, 1993). Confirmatory data are lacking.

Tragacanth is not teratogenic, mutagenic, or allergenic. No adverse toxicologic effects have been observed in nonallergic persons (Eastwood et al., 1984).

Reported uses

FDA guidelines state that tragacanth may be used in concentrations of 0.2% to 1.3% to thicken, emulsify, stabilize, or flavor foods (Eastwood et al., 1984). The concentration in medicinal products ranges from 4.8% to 6% in oral liquids and 0.42 to 100 mg in tablets (Smolinske, 1992). Because of its action with water, tragacanth is used for preparing suspensions, emulsions, adhesives, and protective or lubricating barriers. It may be used in topical or oral products with glycerin to create suspensions or emulsions.

Tragacanth is more resistant to acid hydrolysis than other hydrocolloids, and is preferred in the preparation of acidic compounds. It has also been used as a binder and stabilizer in the preparation of cosmetics and hand lotions, to stiffen cloth, as a glue in bookbinding, and in the preparation of candy and other products (Smolinske, 1992).

The herb is also used in denture adhesives and toothpastes and as a bulk-forming laxative (Baker and Helling, 1986; Curry, 1986). In African folk medicine, tragacanth is used as a mild laxative; the leaves are used to prepare a first aid lotion (Iwu, 1993).

Dosage
FDA dietary guidelines allow concentrations of 0.2% and 1.3% as a thickener, stabilizer, and a flavoring agent in foods. Little consensus exists, although the usual recommended dose ranges from 0.42 to 100 mg tablets P.O. b.i.d. or t.i.d.

Adverse reactions
• Hypersensitivity reactions (abdominal pain, angioedema, arthralgia, asthma, dyspnea, fever, rash, pruritus, rhinitis, sneezing, urticaria) (Danoff et al., 1978; Smolinske, 1992)
• Allergic contact dermatitis (with topical jelly) (Smolinske, 1992)
⚠ The gum may contain microbial contaminants, such as coliform and salmonella bacteria (Farley and Lund, 1976).

Interactions
Fat, fat-soluble nutrients: may decrease absorption of these agents if taken in excess. Avoid excessive use.

Contraindications and precautions
Contraindicated in patients who have experienced hypersensitivity reactions when exposed to any of the natural gums used in food or pharmaceutical products. Avoid use of the herb in pregnant or breast-feeding patients; effects are unknown.

Special considerations
• Be aware that the gum may contain coliform bacteria. Monitor the patient closely for signs of infection.
• Monitor for hypersensitivity reactions.
• Advise the female patient to avoid use of the herb during pregnancy or when breast-feeding.

Points of interest
• The herb's use in foods, cosmetics, and pharmaceutical products has declined in favor of synthetic substances with similar physical properties.
• The FDA lists tragacanth as a generally safe food additive.
• Tragacanth gets its name from the Greek words *tragos* (goat) and *akantha* (horn), probably in reference to the curved or twisted appearance of the dried exudate.

Analysis

Because other natural and synthetic suspending and emulsifying agents are available, tragacanth is no longer widely used in U.S. pharmaceuticals, except in extemporaneous compounding and some commercial suspensions or tablets. The herb is regarded as safe for use in foods and other products, and there are no known reports of adverse effects in nonallergic individuals. Although it may be used as a mild bulk-forming laxative, safer and more effective products are readily available.

References

Baker, K.A., and Helling, D.K. "Oral Health Products," in *Handbook of Nonprescription Drugs*, 8th ed. Washington, D.C.: American Pharmaceutical Association, 1986.

Curry, C.E. "Laxative Products," in *Handbook of Nonprescription Drugs*, 8th ed. Washington, D.C.: American Pharmaceutical Association, 1986.

Danoff, D., et al. "Big Mac Attack," *N Engl J Med* 298:1095-96, 1978.

Eastwood, M.A., et al. "The Effects of Dietary Gum Tragacanth in Man," *Toxicol Lett* 21:73-81, 1984.

Farley, C.A., and Lund, W. "Suspending Agents for Extemporaneous Dispensing: Evaluation of Alternatives to Tragacanth," *Pharmaceutical J* 216:562-66, 1976.

Iwu, M.M. *Handbook of African Medicinal Plants*. Boca Raton, Fla.: CRC Press, 1993.

Smolinske, S.C. *Handbook of Food, Drug, and Cosmetic Excipients*. Boca Raton, Fla.: CRC Press, 1992.

TRUE UNICORN ROOT

AGUE GRASS, AGUE ROOT, ALOEROT, COLIC ROOT, CROW CORN, DEVIL'S-BIT, STAR GRASS, UNICORN ROOT, WHITETUBE STARGRASS

Common trade names
(Various manufacturers) Aletris-Heel, True Unicorn Root

Common forms
Available as a liquid and tea.

Source
Active components are derived from the rhizomes and roots of *Aletris farinosa,* a perennial herb of the lily family (Liliaceae) native to the eastern United States.

Chemical components
Unicorn root contains steroidal saponins—primarily diosgenin and gentrogenin—and alkaloids, essential oil, resin, and starch.

Actions
Diosgenin has been reported to have estrogen-like activity; hence, its use as a tonic. A famous patent medicine, "Lydia Pinkham's Vegetable Compound," (made of *A. farinosa*, pleurisy root [*Asclepias tuberosa*], other herbs, and alcohol) was said to be the cure for various gynecologic conditions. The alkaloids contribute to its CNS depressant effects (Lewis, 1977)

Reported uses
True unicorn root was popular with Native Americans. *A. farinosa* has been used to treat amenorrhea, dysmenorrhea, colic, diarrhea, flatulence, rheumatism, and snake bites. Other claims include its use as an antispasmodic, cathartic, diuretic, narcotic, and sedative, and to prevent habitual miscarriage (Duke, 1985; Horn, 1996).

Dosage
No consensus exists.

Adverse reactions
• GI disturbances (nausea, vomiting, diarrhea; with high doses)
• Stupor, balance disturbances (due to CNS depressant effects; in small doses)

Interactions
None reported; however, because of the herb's purported "narcotic effects," avoid use with CNS depressants or narcotics.

Contraindications and precautions
Avoid use in pregnant or breast-feeding patients; effects are unknown. Use cautiously in patients with GI disorders.

Special considerations
• Question the patient about need for herbal use.
• Warn the patient not to drive or perform activities that require alertness and coordination until CNS effects of the herb are known.
• Advise the female patient to avoid use of the herb during pregnancy or when breast-feeding.

Points of interest
• The true unicorn root should not be confused with false unicorn root (*Helonias luteum;* or *Chamaelirium luteum*). These herbs are different in chemical composition and claimed uses.

Analysis
True unicorn root has been used chiefly to treat gynecologic and GI conditions and rheumatism. Although little is known about the

chemical components, even small doses of the herb are associated with adverse effects. There are no clinical data to support use of this herb for any medical condition.

References

Duke, J.A., ed. *Handbook of Medicinal Herbs.* Boca Raton, Fla.: CRC Press, 1985.

Horn, V., and Weil, C., eds. *The Encyclopedia of Medicinal Plants.* New York: DK Publishing Inc., 1996.

Lewis, W.H. *Medical Botany: Plants Affecting Man's Health.* New York: John Wiley and Sons, 1977.

TURMERIC

CURCUMA, INDIAN SAFFRON, INDIAN VALERIAN, JIANG HUANG, RADIX, RED VALERIAN, TUMERIC

Common trade names
Turmeric Root

Common forms
Available as capsules, curry spices, dry rhizome, extract, oil, tincture, and turmeric spices.

Source
Active components are derived from the rhizome of *Curcuma longa,* a member of the ginger family (*Zingiberaceae*). Turmeric is grown and harvested commercially in many areas of India, China, Asia, Indonesia, and other tropical countries.

Chemical components
Turmeric contains an orange-yellow volatile oil, curcumin. Curcuminoid compounds include tumerone, atlantone, diaryl heptanoids, and zingiberone; these substances are considered the active component of the plant. Other compounds include sugars (glucose, fructose, arabinose), resins, proteins, vitamins, and minerals.

Actions
Turmeric compounds, especially curcumin, have been extensively studied. Curcumin appears to inhibit carcinogenesis at all steps of cancer formation; it promotes detoxification of carcinogens in vitro and in vivo (Stoner and Mukhtar, 1995). Antioxidant properties were noted in protein isolated from a liquid extract of turmeric (Selvam et al., 1995). Rats pretreated with curcumin had fewer and smaller tumors than controls when exposed to chemical carcinogens; this action was partially attributed to the antioxidant properties (Broadhurst, 1997; Hastak et al., 1997).

Curcumin shows promise in the treatment of cholelithiasis (Kiso et al., 1983). Intestinal cholesterol uptake was significantly reduced in rats given curcumin (Roa, 1970).

Curcumin is as effective as NSAIDs in the treatment of rheumatoid arthritis, osteoarthritis, and postoperative pain. It is thought to stimulate corticosteroid release, sensitize cortisol receptors, or increase the half life of cortisol through alteration of hepatic degradation processes (Broadhurst, 1997).

Turmeric extract inhibited gastric secretion and protected gastroduodenal mucosa against ulcer formation induced by stress, pyloric ligation, indomethacin, reserpine, and cysteamine in rats. However, in high doses it may be ulcerogenic (Rafatullah et al., 1990).

Curcumin has been used as an antiseptic and antiparasitic internally and externally; it has slowed the growth of most organisms associated with cholecystitis (Broadhurst, 1997). Curcumin has been found to interfere with the replication of viruses, including viral hepatitis and HIV. Curcumin has increased the CD4 count and inhibited the activity of enzymes that transport the virus into healthy cells (Broadhurst, 1997).

Reported uses

Turmeric has reportedly been used in cancer prevention and as a treatment adjunct. According to the American Institute for Cancer Research, curcumin prevents stomach, colon, oral, esophageal, breast, and skin cancers. It is also used in the treatment of inflammatory conditions (injuries, osteo- and rheumatoid arthritis), irritable bowel syndrome, atherosclerosis, liver disorders, cholelithiasis, GI diseases (ulcerations, gastritis, flatulence), and in infections caused by viruses, GI bacterial overgrowth, and parasitic infestation.

Traditional Chinese and Indian (Ayurvedic) philosophies of medicine involve the use of turmeric for flatulence, jaundice, menstrual problems, bloody urine, hemorrhage, toothache, bruises, chest pain, and colic. Poultices of turmeric have been used to relieve local pain and inflammation.

Dosage

The recommended dosage of curcumin is 400 to 600 mg P.O. t.i.d. For turmeric, an equivalent dosage of 8 to 60 g P.O. t.i.d. is necessary. Turmeric should be taken on an empty stomach.

Adverse reactions

- Allergic contact dermatitis
- Stomach ulcers (with high doses or prolonged use)

Interactions

Anticoagulants: possible additive effects on platelets. Avoid concomitant use.

Immunosuppressants: decreased effect. Use cautiously, if at all, in combination.

NSAIDs: may inhibit platelet function and increase the risk for bleeding. Avoid concomitant use.

Contraindications and precautions

Avoid use in pregnant or breast-feeding patients; effects are unknown. The American Herbal Products Association has classified turmeric as a menstrual stimulant; therefore, it may induce miscarriage. The herb is also contraindicated in patients with bleeding disorders and bile duct obstruction. Use cautiously in patients with a history of ulcers.

Special considerations

- Monitor bleeding studies if medicinal doses are being used.
- Tell the patient to report signs of unusual bruising or bleeding.
- Advise the female patient to avoid use of the herb during pregnancy or when breast-feeding.
- Warn the patient to keep turmeric preparations out of reach of children and pets.

Points of interest

- The antioxidant activity of curcumin is comparable with standard antioxidants, such as vitamins C and E, butylated hydroxyanisole, and butylated hydroxytoluene. Curcumin strongly inhibits the peroxidation of fats, thus helping to retard food spoilage. Because of its bright yellow color, curcumin is often added to butter, margarine, cheese, curry power, mustard, and other food products.

Analysis

Turmeric has shown potential as an anti-inflammatory agent because it appears to be as effective as NSAIDs and cortisol and has a lower incidence of the dangerous adverse effects associated with these agents. However, more clinical research is necessary to prove safety and efficacy in humans before turmeric can be recommended for any medical condition.

References

Broadhurst, L. "Curcumin, A Powerful Bioprotectant Spice, or…Curry Cures!" Botanical Medicine Conference. Philadelphia: May 15, 1997.

Hastak, K., et al. "Effect of Turmeric Oil and Turmeric Oleoresin on Cytogenic Damage in Patients Suffering from Oral Submucous Fibrosis," *Cancer Lett* 116:265-69, 1997.

Kiso, Y., et al. "Antihepatotoxic Principles of *Curcuma longa* Rhizome," *Planta Med* 49:185-87, 1983.

Rafatullah, S., et al. "Evaluation of Turmeric (*Curcuma longa*) for Gastric and Duodenal Antiulcer Activity in Rats," *J Ethnobotany* 29:25-34, 1990.

Roa, D.S. "Effect of Curcumin on Serum and Liver Cholesterol Levels in the Rat." *J Nutr* 100:1307-16, 1970.

Selvam, R., et al. "The Anti-oxidant Activity of Turmeric (*Curcuma longa*)," *J Ethnobotany* 47:59-67, 1995.

Stoner, G.D., and Mukhtar, H. "Polyphenols as Cancer Chemoprotective Agents," *J Cell Biochem* 22(Suppl):169-80, 1995.

VALERIAN

ALL HEAL, AMANTILLA, BALDRIANWURZEL, GREAT
WILD VALERIAN, HERBA BENEDICTA, KATZENWURZEL,
PHU GERMANICUM, PHU PARVUM, *PINNIS DENTATIS*,
SETEWALE CAPON'S TAIL, SETWELL, THERIACARIA,
VALERIANA, *Valeriana foliis pinnatis, Valeriana
radix*

Common trade names
Valerian Extract, Valerian Root,
Valerian Root Extract

Common forms
*Standardized capsules, tablets (0.8%
valerenic acid):* 250 mg, 400 mg, 450 mg, 493 mg, 530 mg, 550 mg
Standardized tinctures: 2% essential oil
Also available as tinctures and teas containing crude dried herb, and
in combination with other dietary supplements.

Source
Active components are derived from rhizomes and roots of *Valeriana officinalis,* a perennial herb native to Eurasia and naturalized
worldwide.

Chemical components
Valerian contains volatile oils, iridoid triesters known as valepotriates,
aliphatic acids, alkaloids, amino acids, aromatic acids, flavonoids, free
fatty acids, phenolic acids, sugars, and salts.

Actions
In vitro studies found that aqueous extracts of valerian inhibit the
uptake and stimulate the release of gamma-aminobutyric acid
(GABA), which may increase the extracellular concentration of
GABA in the synaptic cleft, thereby contributing to the herb's sedative effect. The increase in GABA release is independent of sodium-
potassium-ATPase activity. Most researchers attribute the sedative
effect more to the valepotriates and less to the sesquiterpene components of the volatile oils; others think it's due to the valepotriate
decomposition products (baldrinal and homobaldrinal). Because of

their epoxide structure, the valepotriates are cytotoxic in cell cultures. They are also highly unstable, decompose easily, and are not readily absorbed. Most preparations contain only small amounts.

The extract has weak anticonvulsant and antidepressant properties (Sakamoto et al., 1992). The herb also has antispasmodic effects on GI smooth muscle (Hazelhoff et al., 1982), produces coronary dilation, and has antiarrhythmic activity (Petkov, 1979).

Reported uses
Valerian is widely used in Europe, particularly in France and Germany, as a sedative and antispasmodic. The German Commission E recommends valerian for restlessness and nervous disturbances of sleep (Schulz et al., 1998). It is also used as a daytime sedative for restlessness and tension.

Dosage
The composition and purity of valerian preparations varies greatly.
For sleep disorders, 400 to 900 mg standardized valerian extract ½ to 1 hour before bedtime.
Tea: 2 to 3 g (1 teaspoon) of crude dried herb several times daily.
Tincture: 3 to 5 ml (½ to 1 teaspoon) several times daily.

Adverse reactions
With acute overdose or chronic use:
- Blurred vision
- Cardiac disturbance
- Excitability
- Headache
- Hypersensitivity reactions
- Insomnia
- Nausea

⚠ Risk of hepatotoxicity from combination products containing valerian (Shepard, 1993) and from overdosage averaging 2.5 g (Chan et al., 1995)

Interactions
Alcohol, CNS depressants: potential additive effects. Avoid concomitant use.
Disulfiram: disulfiram reaction if herbal product contains alcohol. Avoid concomitant use.

Contraindications and precautions
Contraindicated in patients with a history of allergy to valerian. Because of the risk of hepatotoxicity, avoid use in patients with hepatic impairment. Avoid use in pregnant or breast-feeding patients; effects are unknown.

Special considerations

- Monitor liver function tests periodically in patients with preexisting hepatic disease or with prolonged use.
- Inform the patient that many extract products contain 40% to 60% alcohol and may not be appropriate for all patients.
- Warn the patient taking disulfiram not to take an herbal form containing alcohol.
- Counsel the patient about the herb's sedative effects and to avoid hazardous activities until CNS effects of the herb are known.
- Advise the female patient to avoid use of the herb during pregnancy or when breast-feeding.
- Inform the patient that safety and efficacy data in children are lacking.

Analysis

Valerian appears to exert mild sedative-hypnotic effects; the extract improved the subjective-recalled quantity of sleep and decreased sleep latency without causing hangover effects. Most studies to date have been flawed methodologically: they were of short duration, used small sample sizes, and defined patient populations inadequately. Better planned and well-controlled studies are needed. A United States Pharmacopeia expert advisory panel has determined that there is insufficient evidence to support the use of valerian for treatment of insomnia.

References

Chan, T.Y.K., et al. "Poisoning Due To an Over-The-Counter Hypnotic, Sleep-Qik (Hyoscine, Cyprohepatadine, Valerian)," *Post Grad Med J* 71:227-28, 1995.

Hazelhoff, B., et al. "Antispasmodic Effects of *Valeriana* Compounds: An In-Vivo and In-Vitro Study on the Guinea Pig Ileum," *Arch Intern Pharmacodyn* 257:274-87, 1982.

Petkov, V. "Plants with Hypotensive Antiatheromatous and Coronarodilating Action," *Am J Chin Med* 7:197-236, 1979.

Sakamoto, T., et al. "Psychotropic Effects of Japanese Valerian Root Extract," *Chem Pharm Bull* 40:758-61, 1992.

Schulz, V., et al. *Rational Phytotherapy: A Physicians' Guide to Herbal Medicine,* 3rd ed. New York: Springer Publishing Co., 1998.

Shepard, C. "Sleep Disorders. Liver Damage Warning with Insomnia Remedy," *BMJ* 306:1472, 1993.

VERVAIN

AMERICAN VERVAIN, BLUE VERVAIN, ENCHANTER'S HERB, EUROPEAN VERVAIN, HERBA VENERIS, HERBE SACRÉE, HERB OF THE GRACE, HOLY HERB, PIGEON GRASS, PURVAIN, SIMPLER'S JOY, WILD HYSSOP

Common trade names
Blue Vervain

Common forms
Capsules: 360 mg

Source
Active components are obtained from the leaves and flowering heads of European vervain, *Verbena officinalis,* a member of the vervain or verbena family (Verbenaceae). Originally native to the Mediterranean, the herb is now cultivated widely throughout Europe, Asia, and North America. A related species, the American vervain, *V. hastata,* is native to the central and eastern United States and is also used medicinally.

Chemical components
Vervain contains tannin, flavonoids (mainly luteolin 7-diglucuronide), glycosides (verbenalin, hastatoside, verbenin), and volatile oils (geraniol, limonene, verbenone). The leaves contain adenosine and beta-carotene. The roots and stems contain stachyose.

Actions
In large doses, the glycoside verbenin has been thought to stimulate milk excretion in low doses and inhibit sympathetic nerve endings on the heart, blood vessel, intestine, and salivary glands. Two studies failed to show antidiarrheal, antithyrotropic, or antigonadotropic activity (Almeida et al., 1995; Auf'Mkolk et al., 1984).

Reported uses
Traditionally, vervain has been claimed to be useful in rheumatism, ocular disease, fever, anemia, bronchitis, kidney stones, tumors, colds, cramps, dysuria, eczema, edema, hemorrhoids, insomnia, malaria, neuralgia, pertussis, pleurisy, tympany, ulcers, and uterine disorders. It has also been used as an analgesic, anthelmintic, antispasmodic, aphrodisiac, astringent, diaphoretic, diuretic, emetic, and expectorant. However, clinical data are lacking. One study of vervain for use against kidney stones concluded that more effective pharmacologic therapies are available (Grases et al., 1994).

Dosage

As a purgative and for bowel pain, a decoction of 2 oz to 1 quart P.O. daily has been used (Almeida et al., 1995).
As a sedative, 360 mg (1 capsule) P.O. at bedtime.

Adverse reactions

• Contact dermatitis
• CNS paralysis followed by stupor and clonic and tetanic seizures (with large doses)

Interactions

Anticoagulants: possible enhanced effect. Avoid concomitant use.

Contraindications and precautions

Use cautiously in patients with multiple allergies or those with asthma or other respiratory disorders. Also use with caution in patients with a history of seizure disorders. In large doses, vervain is capable of inducing seizures.

Special considerations

• Explain that vervain may exacerbate seizure activity if taken in excessive amounts by patients with seizure disorders.
• Advise the patient that there are no clinical data to support use of this herb for any medical condition.
• Tell the patient receiving anticoagulants that even though vervain has been known in folk medicine to slow blood coagulation, it should still be used with caution until more data are available.

Points of interest

⚠ The FDA has classified vervain as an herb of undefined safety.

Analysis

Although vervain has had many traditional uses, there are few, if any, clinical data to support its use for any medical condition. Therefore, it cannot be recommended for use.

References

Almeida, C.E., et al. "Analysis of Antidiarrheic Effects of Plants Used in Popular Medicine," *Revista De Saude Publica* 29:428-33, 1995.

Auf'Mkolk, M., et al. "Inhibition by Certain Plant Extracts of the Binding and Adenylate Cyclase Stimulatory Effect of Bovine Thyrotropin in Human Thyroid Membranes," *Endocrinology* 115:527-34, 1984.

Grases, F., et al. "Urolithiasis and Phytotherapy," *Int Urol Nephrol* 26:507-11, 1994.

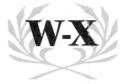

WAHOO

ARROWWOOD, BITTER ASH, BLEEDING HEART, BURNING-BUSH, BURSTING HEART, FISH-WOOD, INDIAN ARROWWOOD, PEGWOOD, PRICKWOOD, SKEWERWOOD, SPINDLETREE, STRAWBERRY BUSH, STRAWBERRY TREE

Common trade names
(Available in combination) GB Tablets, Indigestion Mixture, Jecopeptol, Ludoxin, Stago, Stomachiagil

Common forms
Available as tablets, extracts, tinctures, dried powders, syrups, and teas.

Source
Active components are obtained from the dried bark of the root, and sometimes the stem, of *Euonymus atropupureus,* a shrub or tree native to the central eastern United States and Canada.

Chemical components
Wahoo bark and extracts contain euonymol, euonysterol, atropurol, atropurpurin, asparagine, homoeuonysterol, phytosterol, galactitol, triacetin, citrullol, dulcitol, and various tartaric acids.

Actions
The herb is said to promote biliary function and intestinal secretions by acting as a direct bile stimulant. It also acts as a mild laxative and also increases capillary circulation (Grieve, 1997). Other *Euonymus* species appear to have attracted more attention from investigators than wahoo. The bark of *E. sieboldianus* yields euonymoside, a cytotoxic cardenolide glycoside that may prove to be active against human lung and ovary carcinomas (Baek et al., 1994).

Reported uses
Wahoo is claimed to be useful as a diuretic, emetic, expectorant, cathartic, menstrual stimulant, tonic, liver stimulant, antipyretic, and digestive aid. An oil or powder form of wahoo has been used to kill head lice.

Dosage
Dried root: 1 oz added to 1 pint water, simmered slowly; 1 cup taken b.i.d. or t.i.d.
Euonymin extract: 1 to 4 grains.

Adverse reactions
• Chills
• Diarrhea
• Seizures
• Syncope
• Vomiting
• Weakness

Interactions
None reported.

Contraindications and precautions
Avoid use in pregnant or breast-feeding patients; effects are unknown.

Special considerations
• Advise the patient that there are no clinical data to support use of this herb for any medical condition.
• Discourage the patient from consuming wahoo because of its potential toxicity.
• Advise the female patient to avoid use of the herb during pregnancy or when breast-feeding.

Analysis
This herb has been used to treat several conditions. Because clinical data are lacking and the ingestion of large quantities of wahoo may be hazardous, this herb cannot be recommended for any indication.

References
Baek, N.I., et al. "Euonymoside: A New Cytotoxic Cardenolide Glycoside from the Bark of *Euonymus sieboldianus,*" *Planta Med* 60:26-29, 1994.
Grieve, M. *A Modern Herbal.* London: Tiger Books International, 1997.

WATERCRESS
GARDEN CRESS, SCURVY GRASS, WASSERKRESSE

Common trade names
None known.

Common forms

Available as whole plant, tea, and juice from the leaves.

Source

All plant parts of *Nasturtium officinale* are used for medicinal purposes. The plant is a low-growing aquatic belonging to the mustard family (Cruciferae or Brassicaceae) and native to Europe. It is naturalized in the United States and should not be confused with the garden nasturtium or Indian cress (*Tropaeolum majus*), a popular annual flower that belongs to a different plant family.

Chemical components

Watercress contains gluconasturtiin, the glucosinolate precursor of phenethyl isothiocyanate, benzyl glucosinolate, benzyl isothiocyanate (BITC), vitamins A and C, iron, phosphates, and oils.

Actions

The body converts gluconasturtiin to phenethyl isothiocyanate (PEITC). PEITC is also released when the fresh plant is chewed. The N-acetylcysteine metabolite of PEITC is detectable in human urine (Chung et al., 1992, 1997). PEITC and synthetic isothiocyanates acted as inhibitors of the tobacco-specific carcinogen nitrosamine 4-(methylnitrosamino)-1-(3-pyridyl)-1-butanone (NNK) in animal models. PEITC is thought to inhibit the metabolic activation NNK and inhibit lung tumorigenesis (Hecht et al., 1995). In animals, BITC has demonstrated some ability to inhibit lung tumor formation induced by NNK. However, doses of 200 mg/kg in rats did not reduce tumor mass and caused toxic effects. (Pintao et al., 1995).

Reported uses

The plant is a popular salad green. It has been used as an anti-inflammatory and antimicrobial, and the juice of the leaves has been used to treat acne, eczema, rashes, and topical infections.

Dosage

A dose of 2 oz fluid extract (juice) P.O. t.i.d. was used in a human clinical study (Hecht et al., 1995).

Adverse reactions

None reported in humans.

Interactions

Acetaminophen: watercress plants may inhibit the oxidative metabolism of acetaminophen (Chen et al., 1996). Avoid concomitant use.

Contraindications and precautions
Avoid use in pregnant or breast-feeding patients; effects are not clearly documented in humans.

Special considerations
• Several reports of fascioliasis of the liver (parasitic fluke infection) have been reported after ingesting wild watercress (Rivera et al., 1984).
• Advise the female patient to avoid use of the herb during pregnancy or when breast-feeding.
• Instruct the patient to carefully wash the fresh herb before use if collecting from the wild, to reduce the risk of ingesting water-borne parasites or pathogens.
• Inform the patient using other medications to use watercress cautiously because drug interactions with watercress are largely unknown.
• Tell the patient that more safety and efficacy data for watercress are needed.

Points of interest
• Because it contains vitamin C, watercress was once used to prevent scurvy. The use of watercress in salads has been popular for centuries.

Analysis
Although recent research has shown watercress compounds to be promising anticancer agents, further research is needed. The role of PEITC as a protective agent in human cancers remains to be established. Watercress has no apparent activity against currently existing tumors. The fact that very few reports of toxicity exist despite the consumption of watercress over a long period of time indicates that this herb is safe. Recommendations for consumption await additional safety research.

References
Chen, L., et al. "Decrease of Plasma and Urinary Oxidative Metabolites of Acetaminophen after Consumption of Watercress by Human Volunteers," *Clin Pharmacol Ther* 60:651-60, 1996.

Chung, F.L., et al. "Quantification of Human Uptake of the Anticarcinogen Phenethyl Isothiocyanate after a Watercress Meal," *Cancer Epidemiol Biomarkers Prev* 1:383-88, 1992.

Chung, F.L., et al. "Chemopreventative Potential of Thiol Conjugates of Isothiocyanates for Lung Cancer and a Urinary Biomarker of Dietary Isothiocyanates," *J Cell Biochem Suppl* 27:76-85, 1997.

Hecht, S.S., et al. "Effects of Watercress Consumption on Metabolism of a Tobacco-Specific Lung Carcinogen in Smokers," *Cancer Epidemiol Biomarkers Prev* 4:877-84, 1995.

Pintao, A.M., et al. "In Vitro and In Vivo Antitumor Activity of Benzyl Isothiocyanate: A Natural Product from *Tropaeolum majus*," *Planta Med* 61:233-36, 1995.

Rivera, J.V., et al. "Radionuclide Imaging of the Liver in Human Fascioliasis," *Clin Nucl Med* 9:450-53, 1984.

WILD CHERRY

BLACK CHOKE, CHOKECHERRY, RUM CHERRY

Common trade names
Wild Cherry Bark, Wild Cherry Bark Compound

Common forms
Available as liquid extract (1 oz, 2 oz) and as teas.

Source
Active components are derived from the dried bark of *Prunus virginiana or P. serotina,* which are found in the woods and fields throughout the northern United States. The fruit is edible, but the seeds should be discarded.

Chemical components
The bark, seeds, and leaves of wild cherry trees contain amygdalin, a cyanogenic glycoside. Beta-glucosidase, present in the human gastrointestinal tract, converts amygdalin to hydrogen cyanide (HCN). Wild cherry also contains emulsin, b-methylaesculetin, phytosterol, L-mandelic acid, oleic acid, p-coumaric acid, trimethyl gallic acid, ipuranol, dextrose, sugar, tannin, starch, and calcium oxalate (Ellenhorn, 1997).

Actions
Wild cherry has been touted to possess astringent, sedative, analgesic, and antitussive properties.

Reported uses
Wild cherry has been used to treat coughs and colds, respiratory problems, diarrhea, and certain cancers.

Dosage
Liquid extract: 1 to 2 g in 1 cup of boiling water P.O. t.i.d.

Adverse reactions
The following reactions are the result of cyanide poisoning:
• Headache
• Muscle weakness
• Nausea

- Respiratory failure
- Spasms, tremors
- Stomach ulcers
- Vomiting

⚠ Stupor, coma, and death

⚠ Because all plant parts contain HCN, wild cherry is considered to be toxic. Death has occurred in children who ate seeds, drank tea made from the plant, or chewed on the leaves. Ingestion of the leaves by livestock has also resulted in death. There is more HCN in wilted than dried leaves. Symptoms of HCN poisoning include difficulty breathing, paralysis of the voice, twitching, spasms, stupor, and coma leading to death. In mild cases, symptoms include nausea, vomiting, headache, muscle weakness, and irregular heartbeat (Ellenhorn, 1997).

Interactions
None reported.

Contraindications and precautions
Contraindicated in pregnant or breast-feeding patients because of the presence of cyanogenic glycosides and its possible teratogenic effect.

Special considerations
- Explain that consumption of wild cherry extracts can be dangerous and may cause death from cyanide poisoning.
- Keep wild cherry plant parts out of reach of children.
- Tell the patient that there are insufficient data to support any therapeutic use of the extracts.

Points of interest
- Congenital malformations due to cyanogenic glycosides in a related species, black cherry (*P. serotina*) have been reported in animals (Selby et al., 1971).
- The lethal adult dose of HCN is 50 mg. Lethal doses for cyanogenic plants cannot be predicted because of variations in content, extraction methods, and metabolism (Ellenhorn, 1997).
- Application of some chemical herbicides have been shown to reduce the amount of hydrocyanic acid content in wild cherry (Williams and James, 1983).

Analysis
Although the herb has been used for various conditions, wild cherry bark, seeds, and leaves are potentially toxic. There are insufficient clinical data to substantiate use of wild cherry extracts for any medical condition.

References

Ellenhorn, M.J., ed. *Ellenhorn's Medical Toxicology: Diagnosis and Treatment of Human Poisoning.* Baltimore: Williams & Wilkins, 1997.

Selby, L.A., et al. "Outbreak of Swine Malformations Associated with the Wild Black Cherry, *Prunus serotina*," *Arch Environ Health* 22:496-501, 1971.

Williams, M.C., and James, L.F. "Effects of Herbicides on the Concentration of Poisonous Compounds in Plants: A Review," *Am J Vet Res* 44:2420-22, 1983.

WILD GINGER

Canada snakeroot, colic root, false coltsfoot, Indian ginger, Vermont snakeroot

Common trade names
None known.

Common forms
Available as the whole root.

Source
Active components are derived from the dried rhizome and roots of *Asarum canadense,* a low-growing perennial herb native to the northern and central United States and southern Canada.

Chemical components
Wild ginger contains 2.5% volatile oil, which contains terpenoids such as methyl eugenol, borneol, linalool, geraniol, and pinene. Other compounds include a pungent resin, starch, gum, a fragrant principle called asarol, and traces of a fixed oil.

Actions
Volatile oil components linalool, geraniol, and eugenol have demonstrated antibacterial and antifungal activity (Pattnaik et al., 1997). Geraniol inhibited pancreatic tumor growth in animals receiving this agent as part of their diet (Burke et al., 1997).

Reported uses
Wild ginger reportedly has been used as an aromatic stimulant, antiflatulent, and a tonic, and for treating angina and arrhythmias. Methyl eugenol is a rapid-acting anodyne used in dentistry.

Dosage
No consensus exists.

Adverse reactions
- Cheilitis and stomatitis; burning sensation
- Contact dermatitis

Interactions
Conflicting reports exist on the effects of certain terpenoids (citral, linool) on hepatic metabolism. Some reports indicate that they may induce the hepatic oxidative pathway (Roffey et al., 1990). Effects on specific isoenzymes and on particular medications are unknown, but these terpenoids could potentially lower levels of other hepatically eliminated medications.

Contraindications and precautions
Avoid use in pregnant or breast-feeding patients; effects are unknown. Use with caution, if at all, in patients with a history of allergic contact dermatitis, especially to any of the volatile oils or terpenoid compounds.

Special considerations
• Inform the patient that there are no clinical data to support use of this herb for any medical condition.
• Advise the female patient to avoid use of the herb during pregnancy or when breast-feeding.
• Instruct the patient with a history of allergic contact dermatitis to avoid use of wild ginger.

Analysis
Preliminary data appear to warrant further study of components of wild ginger as antimicrobial and potential anticancer agents. Insufficient evidence exists to support any therapeutic application at this time.

References
Burke, Y.D., et al. "Inhibition of Pancreatic Cancer Growth by the Dietary Isoprenoids Farnesol and Geraniol," *Lipids* 32:151-56, 1997.
Pattnaik, S., et al. "Antibacterial and Antifungal Activity of Aromatic Constituents of Essential Oils," *Microbios* 89:39-46, 1997.
Roffey, S.J., et al. "Hepatic Peroxisomal and Microsomal Enzyme Induction by Citral and Linalool in Rats," *Food Chem Toxicol* 28:403-08, 1990.

WILD INDIGO
FALSE INDIGO, HORSE FLY WEED, INDIGO WEED, *PODALYRIA TINCTORIA*, RATTLEBUSH, RATTLESNAKE WEED, *SOPHORA*, YELLOW INDIGO

Common trade names
Wild Indigo

Common forms
Available as a tincture.

Source
Active components are derived from the leaves and dried roots of *Baptisia tinctoria,* a perennial herb belonging to the legume family (Leguminosae) and native to central and eastern United States and Canada.

Chemical components
Wild indigo contains glycoproteins containing arabinose, arabino-galactans, and alkaloids (baptitoxine, baptisine, baptisin, and quino-lizindine). The root of the plant contains gum, albumen, starch, a yellowish resin, and a crystalline substance.

Actions
Wild indigo is claimed to act as an antiseptic, emetic, and astringent. Immunomodulating properties are attributed to the plant's arabino-galactan components and other glycoproteins (Beuscher et al., 1989; Beuscher and Kopanski, 1985; Egert and Beuscher, 1992). When used in combination with other plant extracts, a stronger phagocytic stimulant activity than Echinacea extract alone was noted in mice (Wagner and Jurcic, 1991).

Reported uses
This herb has been claimed to be useful as an antimicrobial and laxative. Evidence surrounding therapeutic effects is sparse and poorly documented.

Dosage
Tincture: 10 to 20 drops P.O. t.i.d.

Adverse reactions
• Although there are no reports of toxic ingestion in humans, the alkaloids have toxic potential.
• Vomiting (with high doses)

Interactions
None reported.

Contraindications and precautions
Contraindicated in patients with allergies to this or related plant species. Avoid use in pregnant or breast-feeding patients; effects are unknown.

Special considerations
• Explain that there is little information about the herb's therapeutic benefit or risk.

- Advise the female patient to avoid use of the herb during pregnancy or when breast-feeding.
- Inform the patient with allergies to wild indigo or related plant species not to use this herb.

Analysis
Despite the folkloric use of wild indigo as an antiseptic, safety and efficacy data in humans are lacking. Immunomodulating properties of wild indigo are based on in vitro experiments, but appear promising and warrant additional investigation.

References
Beuscher, N., and Kopanski, L. "Stimulation of Immunity by the Contents of *Baptisia tinctoria*," *Planta Med* Oct(5):381-84, 1985.

Beuscher, N., et al. "Immunologically Active Glycoproteins of *Baptisia tinctoria*," *Planta Med* 55:358-63, 1989.

Egert, D., and Beuscher, N. "Studies on Antigen Specificity of Immunoreactive Arabinogalactan Proteins Extracted from *Baptisia tinctoria* and *Echinacea purpurea*," *Planta Med* 58:163-65, 1992.

Wagner, H., and Jurcic, K. "Immunologic Studies of Plant Combination Preparations. In-Vitro And In-Vivo Studies on the Stimulation of Phagocytosis," *Arzneimittelforschung* 41:1072-76, 1991.

WILD LETTUCE

BITTER LETTUCE, GERMAN LACTUCARIUM, LETTUCE OPIUM

Common trade names
Lactucarium, Lettuce Hash, Lettucine, Lopium

Common forms
Available as dried juice (sap) from stems, dried leaves, lettuce leaf cigarettes, and tincture.

Source
The dried leaves of *Lactuca virosa* are rolled (with tobacco or other additives) into a cigarette and smoked. The stem juice may be taken directly from the plant for various purposes. The plant should not be confused with the garden lettuce, *L. sativa.*

Chemical components
The plant contains flavonoids (apigenin, luteolin), terpenoids (lactucin, lactupicrin, germanicol), lactucone (lactucerin), coumarins (aesculin, cichoriin), various acids (citric, malic, cichoric, and oxalic), mannitol, proteins, resins, and carbohydrates. The milky white latex sap contains lactucin and lactucopicrin. The leaves contain

polycyclic aromatic hydrocarbons and two isoenzymes of carbonate dehydratase (Wickstrom et al., 1986).

Actions
Lactucin and lactucopicrin are claimed to produce CNS depression and sedative effects. A study in rabbits concluded that wild lettuce has no hypoglycemic activity (Roman-Ramos et al., 1995). Another study showed that the latex of *L. sativa* had mild antifungal activity against *Candida albicans* (Giordani et al., 1991).

Reported uses
Smoking lettuce leaf cigarettes has been used to produce a euphoric effect (Huang et al., 1982). The sap of the plant has been used to induce sleep and treat coughs.

Dosage
Dried leaves (tea): 0.5 to 3 g t.i.d.
Lactucarium (dried latex extract): 0.3 to 1 g t.i.d.
Liquid extract (1:1 in 25% alcohol): 0.5 to 30 ml t.i.d.
Tincture: 2 to 4 ml t.i.d.

Adverse reactions
• Contact dermatitis (Krook, 1977)
⚠ Smoking large quantities of wild lettuce may be potentially toxic. Overdoses may be characterized by stupor, shallow breathing, and coma; death may occur (Huang et al., 1982).

Interactions
None reported.

Contraindications and precautions
Avoid use in pregnant or breast-feeding patients; effects are unknown. The herb is also contraindicated in patients allergic to any member of the lettuce family.

Special considerations
• Inform the patient that there are no clinical data to support use of this herb for any medical condition.
• Advise the female patient to avoid use of the herb during pregnancy or when breast-feeding.
• Warn the patient about the risk of hallucinogenic effects from smoking wild lettuce leaves.

Points of interest
• Ancient Egyptians used wild lettuce for its supposed ability to induce sleep.

- During the 1970s, wild lettuce was smoked in the United States as an "alternative hallucinogen."
- Although some sources state that trace amounts of morphine exist in some *Lactuca* species, there is not enough to exert any clinical pharmacological effect (Huang et al., 1982).

Analysis

Claims of hallucinogenic effects from smoking wild lettuce leaves are unsubstantiated. Because little is known about potential toxicity from the use of this herb, the use of wild lettuce is not recommended.

References

Giordani, R., et al. "Glycosidic Activities of *Candida albicans* After Action of Vegetable Latex Saps (Natural Antifungals) and Isoconazole (Synthetic Antifungal)," *Mycoses* 34:67-73, 1991.

Huang, Z.J., et al. "Studies on Herbal Remedies I: Analysis of Herbal Smoking Preparations Alleged To Contain Lettuce (*Lactuca sativa* L.) and Other Natural Products," *J Pharm Sci* 71:270-71, 1982.

Krook, G. "Occupational Dermatitis from *Lactuca sativa* (Lettuce) and *Cichorium* (Endive): Simultaneous Occurrence of Immediate and Delayed Allergy as a Cause of Contact Dermatitis," *Contact Dermatitis* 3:27-36, 1977.

Roman-Ramos, R., et al. "Anti-hyperglycemic Effect of Some Edible Plants," *J Ethnopharmacol* 48:25-32, 1995.

Wickstrom, K., et al. "Polycyclic Aromatic Compounds (PAC) in Leaf Lettuce," *Z Lebensum Unters Forsch* 183:182-85, 1986.

WILD YAM

COLIC ROOT, MEXICAN WILD YAM, RHEUMATISM ROOT

Common trade names

None known.

Common forms

Available as a liquid extract, tincture, topical oil, tea, powder, DHEA powder for extemporaneous compounding in 25-mg and 50-mg capsules, and chewing gum containing 25 mg DHEA.

Source

Wild yam, *Dioscorea villosa* L., belongs to the family Dioscoreaceae and grows wild in the damp woodlands of North America and Central America. It is a deciduous perennial vine that often climbs to 20 feet and is characterized by heart-shaped leaves and tiny green flowers.

Chemical components

Wild yam contains steroidal saponins, diosgenin, dioscenin, DHEA, phytosterols (beta-sitosterol), alkaloids, and tannins.

Actions

This herb was historically the sole source of the raw materials for manufacturing contraceptive hormones, cortisone, and anabolic hormones. Wild yam contains large amounts of dioscin, which has anti-inflammatory activity.

DHEA, a constituent of wild yam, is a steroid hormone produced in the adrenal gland in humans; it is the most abundant adrenocorticoid hormone in the body. DHEA is believed to be useful in several conditions, including AIDS, Alzheimer's disease, CV disease, cancer, hypercholesterolemia, multiple sclerosis, obesity, psychological disorders, and systemic lupus erythematosus.

Some studies suggest that very low DHEA levels in the body may contribute to the development of an AIDS-defining condition or opportunistic infection. Recently, a noncontrolled study found that patients with AIDS taking DHEA had reductions in viral load (Salvato et al., 1996). Open, uncontrolled studies of patients with multiple sclerosis showed DHEA had a beneficial effect on subjective feelings of strength, stamina, and well-being but did not improve disability.

In a double-blind study, patients with systemic lupus erythematosus given DHEA for 3 months showed marked improvement compared with placebo (Morales et al., 1994). Wild yam has not been proven to promote anabolic effects in humans.

Reported uses

Wild yam is claimed to be useful in the treatment of adrenal exhaustion, inflammatory rheumatism, rheumatoid arthritis, dysentary, diverticulosis, stomach and muscle cramps, spasmodic asthma, intermittent claudication, menopausal symptoms, pain in the womb and ovaries, gall or biliary stones, and as an antispasmodic or diaphoretic.

Dosage

Average dose is 2 to 4 g or fluid equivalent P.O. t.i.d.

As a food supplement, DHEA dosage should not exceed 50 mg daily; medical approval is required for higher doses. DHEA doses over 25 mg daily should be avoided in women because of reports of irreversible voice changes and hirsutism.

Liquid extract: 2 to 4 ml in water P.O. t.i.d., or 5 to 30 drops P.O. t.i.d.

Tincture (1:5 in 45% alcohol): 2 to 10 ml in water P.O. t.i.d.

Oil: external use only.

Tea: ¼ teaspoon to 1 cup boiling water, steep 15 minutes; ¼ to 1 cup P.O. t.i.d.
Powder: 0.5 to 2 g P.O. t.i.d.

Adverse reactions
- Acne
- Hair loss
- Headache
- Hirsutism
- Menstrual irregularities
- Oily skin
- Potential for stimulating growth of prostate cancer

Interactions
None reported.

Contraindications and precautions
Avoid use in pregnant patients because of the possibility of fetal masculinization. Use cautiously in patients with hepatic disease because of liver damage with high doses in animal models.

Also avoid use of the herb in patients with a family history of hormone-induced malignancies, including breast, ovarian, uterine, and prostate cancer.

Special considerations
- Advise the patient to acquire DHEA, or any other natural product, from reliable sources to ensure quality, purity, and strength.
- Advise the patient about the different formulations of DHEA and their potential adverse effects.
- Tell the female patient to avoid use of wild yam during pregnancy.
- Inform the female patient that irreversible voice changes and hirsutism may occur if more than 25 mg of DHEA is taken daily.

Analysis
DHEA in wild yam is touted to be useful for several conditions. Data are lacking about the proper dose and long term effects of this agent. There are no studies to date that provide convincing evidence that DHEA has any appreciable benefit on any disease state.

References
Morales, A.J., et al. "Effects of Replacement Dose Dihydroepiandrosterone in Men and Women of Advancing Age," *J Clin Endocrinol Metab* 78:1360-67, 1994.

Salvato, P., et al. Viral load response to augmentation of natural dihydroepiandrosterone (DHEA). XI International Conference on AIDS, 1996.

WILLOW
BLACK WILLOW, WHITE WILLOW

Common trade names
(Various manufacturers; available in combination) Aller g Formula 25, White Willow Bark, Willowprin

Common forms
Capsules: 379 mg, 400 mg
Liquid extract: 1 oz

Source
Active components are derived from the bark of various willows such as the white willow (*Salix alba)* and black willow *(S. nigra).* White willow is native to Europe and naturalized in the United States, whereas black willow is native to North America.

Chemical components
Willow bark contains phenolic glycosides (salicin, salicortin, salireposide, and picein), esters of salicylic acid and salicyl alcohol, tannins, catechins, and flavonoids. Concentrations of the salicylate-like agent, salicin, ranges from 0.5% to 10% in the bark, depending on the species.

Actions
The salicylate-like compounds exert anti-inflammatory, analgesic, antipyretic, and uricosuric effects. Tannins exert astringent effects. Flowers of a Russian species (*S. daphnoïdes)* have yielded thromboplastin-like agents that trigger procoagulant effects in animals.

Reported uses
In ancient Egypt, extracts of willow bark were commonly used to treat inflammatory conditions. Willow is claimed to be an effective analgesic and antipyretic, and is thought to be useful in the treatment of rheumatism, other systemic inflammatory diseases, and influenza.

Dosage
Average daily dose of salicin is 60 to 120 mg P.O.
Dried bark: 1 to 3 g as a decoction (cold tea), P.O. t.i.d.
Liquid extract (1:1 in 25% alcohol): 1 to 3 ml P.O. t.i.d.

Adverse reactions
• Asthma exacerbations, allergic rhinitis from aerosolized willow pollen
• Contact dermatitis, local irritation

- GI bleeding
- Hepatic dysfunction
- Increased bleeding time
- Renal damage
- Salicylate toxicity (nausea, vomiting, dizziness, tinnitus, CNS confusion, lethargy, metabolic acidosis, diarrhea)

⚠ Anaphylaxis

Interactions

Anticoagulants: may enhance the risk of bleeding. Avoid concomitant use.

Antihypertensives: may reduce effectiveness. Avoid concomitant use.

Diuretics: enhanced risk for salicylate toxicity; may reduce effectiveness. Avoid concomitant use.

NSAIDs: may increase the risk of stomach ulceration and bleeding. Avoid concomitant use.

Contraindications and precautions

Contraindicated in patients with salicylate hypersensitivity. Avoid use in pregnant or breast-feeding patients; effects are unknown.

Use cautiously in patients with asthma, allergic rhinitis, or prior history of plant allergy, and in those prone to systemic thromboembolism, such as those with prior venous thromboembolic disease or thromboembolic stroke, previous MI, poor ejection fraction, or atrial fibrillation. Also use cautiously in patients with renal insufficiency, prior history of GI bleeding, peptic ulcers, and in patients with bleeding tendencies.

Special considerations

- Counsel the patient with history of allergy or asthma to avoid use of willow products.
- Advise the patient taking anticoagulants to avoid use of willow due to risk of increased bleeding.
- Inform the patient that insufficient evidence exists to confirm a therapeutic application for willow. Commercial products containing salicylic acid are readily available. Tell the patient to use standardized products.

Points of interest

- Autopsy reports of the great composer, Ludwig von Beethoven, suggest a probable link between his chronic use of powdered willow bark and the development of renal papillary necrosis (Schwarz, 1993).
- In a Norwegian study, cadmium was found to accumulate in some bird species who fed on willow seeds and insects (Hogstad, 1996).

Analysis

Willow has a long history as an analgesic and anti-inflammatory agent. However, there are few, if any, clinical data to support use of this herb for any medical condition. Because salicylate-like compounds occur in widely varying strengths in the plant, only standardized salicylate products are recommended.

References

Hogstad, O. "Accumulation of Cadmium, Copper, and Zinc in the Liver of Some Passerine Species Wintering in Central Norway," *Sci Total Environ* 183:187-94, 1996.

Schwarz, A. "Beethoven's Renal Disease Based on His Autopsy: A Case of Papillary Necrosis," *Am J Kidney Dis* 21:643-52, 1993.

WINTERGREEN

BOXBERRY, CANADA TEA, CHECKERBERRY, DEERBERRY, GAULTHERIA OIL, MOUNTAIN TEA, OIL OF WINTERGREEN, PARTRIDGEBERRY, TEABERRY

Common trade names

Koong Yick Hung Fa Oil (KYHFO); Wintergreen Altoids; Wintergreen Sucrets

Common forms

Available as teas, lotions, liniments, ointments, lozenges, creams, and oil.

Source

The active component is obtained from the leaves and bark of *Gaultheria procumbens*, a low-growing herb belonging to Ericaceae family and native to parts of Canada and the eastern United States.

Chemical components

Wintergreen contains less than 1% of wintergreen oil. This oil is approximately 98% methyl salicylate. No drug product should contain more than 5% methyl salicylate. Other compounds include gaultherin and carbohydrates (D-glucose, D-xylose).

Actions

Methyl salicylate produces counterirritant and skin reddening effects. Analgesia may result from the masking of pain due to counterirritation or the analgesic properties of the salicylate itself. Antiflatulent effects occur when taken internally.

Reported uses

Wintergreen has been used to treat inflamed and swollen muscles, ligaments, and joints. It is also claimed to provide relief for neurologic pain from sciatica and trigeminal neuralgia.

Dosage

Apply 10% to 30% wintergreen oil or methyl salicylate product to the skin, not to exceed t.i.d. or q.i.d.

Adverse reactions

● GI irritation, vomiting, lethargy, hyperpnea (with oral use)
⚠ Methyl salicylate is highly soluble in lipids, and may cause salicylate poisoning from overgenerous topical application. Heat and physical activity increase its absorption through the skin. Symptoms of salicylate poisoning include acid-base disturbances, endocrine abnormalities, fluid and electrolyte disturbances, bleeding, pulmonary edema, rhabdomyolysis, hepatitis, coagulopathy, tinnitus, nausea, vomiting, and CNS toxicity. Death may occur (Chan, 1996).

Interactions

Anticoagulants: combined use with the topical wintergreen oil may result in increased INR with subsequent bleeding (Chow et al., 1989; Yip et al., 1990).

Contraindications and precautions

Contraindicated for internal use in patients with gastroesophageal reflux disease. Avoid use in pregnant or breast-feeding patients; effects are unknown. Use cautiously in patients receiving anticoagulants.

Special considerations

● Tell the patient who is sensitive to aspirin to avoid wintergreen.
● Advise the patient receiving oral anticoagulants to reduce use of wintergreen.
● Remind the patient not to use topical wintergreen agents with heating devices or warmed towels, to avoid skin irritation.
● Advise the patient to avoid using the oil topically after strenuous exercise or in hot humid weather to avoid toxic effects.
● Keep wintergreen (methyl salicylate) products out of the reach of children. (See *Wintergreen toxicity.*)
● Advise the female patient to avoid use during pregnancy or when breast-feeding.

RESEARCH FINDINGS
Wintergreen toxicity

Because products containing wintergreen oil have a tantalizing, candylike aroma, small children are at risk for ingesting potentially lethal quantities. The aroma, together with unprotected packaging and lack of knowledge about its potential hazards, makes wintergreen dangerous. As little as 4 ml has caused extreme illness and death.

In one report, a 21-month-old infant ingested wintergreen oil, which was labeled as a flavoring or candy. Although only one swallow was witnessed by the child's parents, the salicylate concentration was 81 mg/dl 6 hours after ingestion. The infant experienced repeated vomiting, lethargy, and hyperpnea. Emergency treatment consisted of I.V. bicarbonate and fluids and supportive care; the recovery was uneventful (Howrie and Moriarty, 1985).

This toxic hazard can be minimized by restricting bottle size and methyl salicylate concentration; mandating FDA regulation of labeling with clear, concise descriptions of ingredients and adverse effects; and providing warnings about the risks if the herb is misused. In addition, the use of child-resistant containers should be used for all liquid products containing more than 5% wintergreen by weight.

Points of interest
- Oil from sweet birch (*Betula lenta*) is also rich in methyl salicylate.
- An old folk remedy for children who developed "bad chests" during the winter months involved their wearing a paper "jacket" made from a large brown paper bag, with holes cut in it for the head and arms, and coated with camphor and wintergreen oil (Watson, 1992).
- Commercial products containing methyl salicylate generally use the synthetic compound.

Analysis
There are no efficacy data for wintergreen in any medicinal capacity, so its use cannot be recommended. Wintergreen oil should not be taken internally.

References
Chan, T.Y. "Potential Dangers from Topical Preparations Containing Methyl Salicylate," *Hum Exp Toxicol* 15:747-50, 1996.
Chow, W.H., et al. "Potentiation of Warfarin Anticoagulation by Topical Methyl Salicylate Ointment," *J Soc Med* 82:501-02, 1989.
Howrie, D.L., and Moriarty, R. "Candy Flavoring as a Source of Salicylate Poisoning," *Pediatrics* 75:869-71, 1985.

Watson, R. "Senna-Pod and Wintergreen," *Nursing Times* 88:64, 1992.

Yip, A.S.B., et al. "Adverse Effects of Topical Methyl Salicylate Ointment on Warfarin Anticoagulation: An Unrecognized Potential," *Postgrad Med J* 66:367-69, 1990.

WITCH HAZEL

HAMAMELIS, SNAPPING HAZEL, SPOTTED ALDER, TOBACCO WOOD, WINTERBLOOM

Common trade names
Witch Doctor, Witch Hazel Cream, Witch Hazel Liquid, Witch Hazel Pads, Witch Stik

Common forms
Available as liquid extract, witch hazel water (milder form of extract), cream, and medicated pads.

Source
The active components are derived from the leaves and bark of *Hamamelis virginiana,* a shrub native to America. Witch hazel is prepared by distilling twigs of the plant and adding alcohol to the distillate. Commercial sources originate from the Blue Ridge Mountain region (Virginia), North Carolina, and Tennessee. Witch hazel water distillate is prepared from wintergreen twigs and contains 13% to 15% alcohol in water with a trace of volatile oil.

Chemical components
Witch hazel contains tannins, flavonoids (kaempferol, quercetin and others), traces of volatile oil (eugenol, safrole, sesquiterpenes), a bitter principle, calcium oxalate, fixed oil, resin, wax, saponins, and gallic acid.

Actions
Witch hazel is reported to exert astringent, antihemorrhagic, and anti-inflammatory effects. Some studies have shown that witch hazel distillate reduces swelling and inflammation of skin after exposure to ultraviolet B radiation (Hughes-Formella et al., 1998; Masaki et al., 1995); however, another study failed to show this effect (Duwieija et al., 1994). Other components from witch hazel bark have demonstrated antimutagenic properties (Dauer et al., 1998).

Reported uses
Witch hazel has long been used to relieve anal or vaginal itching and irritation, hemorrhoids, and postepisiotomy or hemorrhoidectomy discomfort. It is also claimed to be useful for treating varicose veins,

bruises, and local swelling. Witch hazel has been used as a gargle to decrease inflammation of mucous membranes of the mouth, gums, and throat.

Dosage
Dried leaves: 2 g as a tea t.i.d. as a gargle.
Liquid extract (1:1 in 45% alcohol): 2 to 4 ml t.i.d.
Witch hazel water: apply topically t.i.d. or q.i.d.

Adverse reactions
• Carcinogenic (controversial; related to safrole component [Dauer et al., 1998])
• Contact dermatitis
• Hepatotoxicity (tannin component)
• Nausea, vomiting, constipation (over 1,000 mg)

Interactions
None reported.

Contraindications and precautions
Avoid use of the herb in pregnant or breast-feeding women; effects are unknown.

Special considerations
• Warn the patient not to consume witch hazel internally.
• Advise the patient to consult a primary health care provider if condition does not improve or worsens after a few days of topical use of witch hazel.
• Warn the patient to keep witch hazel out of the reach of children.

Analysis
Witch hazel products are known to be effective astringents and possess hemostatic effects. Although they are apparently safe for external use, witch hazel products are not for internal use.

References
Dauer, A., et al. "Proanthocyanidins from the Bark of *Hamamelis virginiana* Exhibit Antimutagenic Properties Against Nitroaromatic Compounds," *Planta Med* 64:324-27, 1998.

Duwieja, M., et al. "Anti-inflammatory Activity of *Polygonum bistorta, Guaiacum officinale* and *Hamamelis virginiana* in Rats," *J Pharm Pharmacol* 46:286-90, 1994.

Hughes-Formella, B.J., et al. "Anti-inflammatory Effects of Hamamelis Lotion in a UV-B Erythema Test," *Dermatology* 196 316-22, 1998.

Masaki, H., et al. "Protective Activity of Hamamelitannin on Cell Damage of Murine Skin Fibroblasts Induced By UVB Irradiation," *J Dermatol Sci* 10:25-34, 1995.

WORMWOOD

ABSINTHE, ABSINTHIUM

Common trade names
None known.

Common forms
Available as an essential oil.

Source
Active components of wormwood are extracted
from the leaves and flowering tops of *Artemisia
absinthium,* a shrubby perennial herb native to Europe,
northern Africa and western Asia.

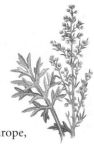

Chemical components
Extracts of *A. absinthium* contain the glucosides absinthin and
anabsinthin, lactones (including santonin), and other compounds.
The plant contains a sweet-smelling volatile oil consisting of terpenes, primarily thujone, with smaller amounts of phellandrene,
pinene, and azulene.

Actions
Santonin has shown anti-inflammatory, antipyretic, and analgesic
activity in mice (al-Harbi et al., 1994). Thujone exerts narcotic-like
analgesic effects (Rice and Wilson, 1976); it is believed to be responsible for causing the symptoms associated with absinthism. This
syndrome is marked by digestive disorders, sleeplessness, trembling,
paresthesia, loss of intellect, hallucinations, psychosis, seizures,
paralysis, and possible brain damage.

Crude extracts of *A. absinthium* have also demonstrated preventative and curative effects on acetaminophen hepatotoxicity in mice
(Gilani and Janbaz, 1995).

Reported uses
Common therapeutic claims for wormwood include use as a sedative, antipyretic, and anthelmintic. Lay publications promote wormwood as an insect repellent. These sources encourage the planting of
wormwood hedges or use of powders and infusions around gardens
and other areas where insects may be a problem (Sherif et al., 1987).

Dosage
No consensus exists.

FOLKLORE
Wormwood and van Gogh

Wormwood extract was the main ingredient in absinthe, a toxic emerald green liqueur that was popular until its ban in the early 20th century. Vincent van Gogh was believed to be addicted to absinthe and craved other substances containing terpenes such as paints. It is now believed that the predominance of yellow in his paintings and the hallucinations he experienced were related to his consumption of absinthe and other thujone-related compounds (Arnold and Loftus, 1991; Bonkovsky et al., 1992).

Adverse reactions
• Allergic reactions (with topical use in sensitized persons)
• Anion gap acidosis, rhabdomyolysis, and subsequent renal failure (Weisbord et al., 1997)
• Porphyria (Bonkovsky et al., 1992)
• Seizures
• Xanthopsia (Arnold and Loftus, 1991)
⚠ Absinthism may result from chronic intake of wormwood compounds. (See *Wormwood and van Gogh.*)

Interactions
None reported.

Contraindications and precautions
Avoid use in pregnant or breast-feeding patients; effects are unknown. Internal and long-term use is contraindicated.

Special considerations
• Monitor the patient who uses wormwood for symptoms of absinthism.
• Explain that wormwood should not be taken internally.

Points of interest
• Wormwood, derived from *A. absinthium*, should not be confused with other substances termed "wormwood." Sweet wormwood or Chinese wormwood, derived from *A. annua*, has been used in China for almost 2,000 years for fever, and the active component, artemisinin, recently has received much attention as an antimalarial (van Geldre et al., 1997).
• A thujone-free extract of wormwood is used as a flavoring agent for alcoholic beverages such as vermouth.

Analysis

Wormwood shows some promise as an anti-inflammatory, antipyretic, anthelmintic, and hepatoprotective agent; however, more animal and human clinical data are needed. Because wormwood extract has been associated with potentially serious CNS toxicity, the herb cannot be recommended for internal use at this time.

References

al-Harbi, M.M., et al. "Studies on the Antiinflammatory, Antipyretic and Analgesic Activities of Santonin," *Jpn J Pharmacol* 64:135-39, 1994.

Arnold, W.N., and Loftus, L.S. "Xanthopsia and van Gogh's Yellow Palette," *Eye* 5:503-10, 1991.

Bonkovsky, H.L., et al. "Porphyrogenic Properties of the Terpenes Camphor, Pinene, and Thujone (with a Note on Historic Implications for Absinthe and the Illness of Vincent van Gogh)," *Biochem Pharmacol* 43:2359-68, 1992.

Gilani, A.H., and Janbaz, K.H. "Preventative and Curative Effects of *Artemisia absinthium* on Acetaminophen and CCl4-Induced Hepatotoxicity," *Gen Pharmacol* 26:309-15, 1995.

Rice, K.C., and Wilson, R.S. "(-)-3-Isothujone, a Small Nonnitrogenous Molecule with Antinociceptive Activity in Mice," *J Med Chem* 19:1054-57, 1976.

Sherif, A., et al. "Drugs, Insecticides and Other Agents from *Artemisia*," *Med Hypotheses* 23:187-93, 1987.

van Geldre, E., et al. "State of the Art Production of the Antimalarial Compound Artemisinin in Plants," *Plant Mol Biol* 33:199-209, 1997.

Weisbord, S.D., et al. "Poison on Line: Acute Renal Failure Caused by Oil of Wormwood Purchased Through the Internet," *N Engl J Med* 337:825-27, 1997.

WOUNDWORT

HEDGE WOUNDWORT, MARSH WOUNDWORT

Common trade names

None known.

Common forms

Available as tea, ointment, and tincture.

Source

Active components are derived from the leaves and stems of *Stachys palustris* and *S. sylvatica*, members of the mint family (Labiatae).

Chemical components

Woundwort contains various flavonoids and iridoids.

Actions

Mechanisms of action are not well described for this herb. Investigations have focused on other species of *Stachys*. *S. sieboldii* may contain a promising agent (acteoside) for the prevention of glomer-ulonephritis (Hayashi et al., 1996).

Reported uses
Both varieties of woundwort have been used to stop bleeding and promote healing of wounds. It has also been used as an astringent and antiseptic. Internally, woundwort is claimed to be useful as an antispasmodic, to ease cramps and joint pain, and to treat vertigo, diarrhea, and dysentery.

Dosage
For stomach cramps or diarrhea, 1 to 2 ml of tincture P.O. t.i.d.
Tea: steep 1 teaspoon dried herb in 1 cup boiling water for 10 to 15 minutes; drink tea t.i.d.
Poultice: apply bruised leaves to wound.
Ointment: incorporate dried leaves into an ointment base, and apply topically.

Adverse reactions
None reported.

Interactions
None reported.

Contraindications and precautions
Avoid use in pregnant or breast-feeding patients; effects are un-known.

Special considerations
• Advise the patient that there are no clinical data to support taking this herb for any medical condition.
• Advise the female patient to avoid use of woundwort during preg-nancy or when breast-feeding.

Analysis
Although woundwort has traditionally been used to promote wound healing and has been taken internally for other complaints, there is no scientific evidence to support these uses. This herb cannot be rec-ommended for use until safety and efficacy data become available.

References
Hayashi, K., et al. "Acteoside, a Component of *Stachys sieboldii* MIQ, May Be a Promising Antinephritic Agent (3): Effect of Acteoside on Expression of Intercellular Adhesion Molecule-1 in Experimental Nephritic Glomeruli in Rats and Cultured Endothelial Cells," *Jpn J Pharmacol* 70:157-68, 1996.

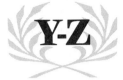

Y-Z

YARROW

ACHILLEA MILLEFOLIUM, BLOODWORT, GORDALDO, MILFOIL, NOSEBLEED, OLD MAN'S PEPPER, SANGUINARY, SOLDIER'S WOUNDWORT, STANCHGRASS, THOUSAND-LEAF

Common trade names
Diacure, Lasadoron, Rheumatic Pain Remedy, Yarrow Flowers

Common forms
Capsules: 320 mg, 340 mg
Liquid extract: 1 oz, 2 oz
Also available as a tincture and powder.

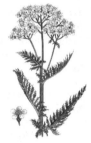

Source
The drug is extracted from the dried leaves and flowering tops of *Achillea millefolium*, a plant native to Europe and Asia and naturalized in North America. The plant is a member of the daisy family (Compositae).

Chemical components
Yarrow contains tannins, amino acids, fatty acids, sesquiterpene lactones, and peroxides.

Actions
Yarrow is claimed to have antispasmodic and anti-inflammatory actions. It is also believed to have vasodilatory, diaphoretic, astringent, and GI stimulatory effects. Some sesquiterpenoid compounds isolated from the herb have been reported to display activity against mouse P-388 leukemia cells in vivo (Tozyo et al., 1994).

Reported uses
Yarrow has been used as an emergency styptic applied externally to heal skin wounds and as an external wash for eczema. Taken internally, the herb is thought to reduce phlegm and other symptoms associated with respiratory infections; it has also been used in disorders of the digestive, urinary, and female reproductive systems.

Dosage

Dried herb: 2 to 4 g as a tea P.O. t.i.d.
Liquid extract (1:1 in 25% alcohol): 2 to 4 ml P.O. t.i.d.
Tincture (1:5 in 45% alcohol): 2 to 4 ml P.O. t.i.d.

Adverse reactions

• Allergic contact dermatitis in up to 50% of patients (Hausen et al., 1991; Rucker et al., 1991)
• Photosensitivity (conflicting reports)
• Uterine stimulant (with increased doses)

Interactions

Anticoagulants: may increase anticoagulant effect. Use together cautiously.
Antihypertensives: may enhance hypotensive effect. Monitor patient.
CNS depressants: may enhance sedative effect. Use together cautiously.
Disulfiram: possible disulfiram reaction if the herbal product contains alcohol. Avoid concomitant use.

Contraindications and precautions

Contraindicated in patients with a history of allergy to yarrow or other members of the Compositae family. Avoid use in pregnant or breast-feeding patients; effects are unknown.

Special considerations

• Monitor for adverse CNS effects.
• Monitor blood pressure of patients also taking antihypertensive agents.
• Warn the patient taking disulfiram to avoid use of an herbal product containing alcohol.
• Advise the female patient to avoid use of the herb during pregnancy or when breast-feeding.
• Advise the patient to avoid hazardous activities until effects on CNS are known.
• Warn the patient with known skin allergies to avoid handling the plant.
• Warn the patient to discontinue the drug if rash, bleeding, or any unusual signs or symptoms occur.

Points of interest

• Yarrow obtained its scientific name, *Achillea*, from the warrior Achilles of Homeric legend. At the battle of Troy, a Greek god appeared and showed Achilles how to stop bleeding by applying yarrow leaves.

Analysis

Although yarrow has many folk uses, there are no clinical studies for any disease state in humans. Therefore, it should be used cautiously in view of its apparent tendency to cause contact dermatitis.

References

Hausen, B.M., et al. "Alpha-Peroxyachifolid and Other New Sensitizing Sesquiterpene Lactones from Yarrow (*Achillea millefolium* L., Compositae)," *Contact Dermatitis* 24:274-80, 1991.

Rucker, G., et al. "Peroxides As Plant Constituents. 8. Guaianolide-Peroxides from Yarrow, *Achillea millefolium* L., a Soluble Component Causing Yarrow Dermatitis." *Arch Pharm* 324:979-81, 1991.

Tozyo, T., et al. "Novel Antitumor Sesquiterpenoids in *Achillea millefolium*," *Chem Pharm Bull (Tokyo)* 42:1096-1100, 1994.

YERBA MATÉ

ARMINO, BARTHOLOMEW'S TEA, BOCA JUNIORS, CAMPECHE, EL AGRICULTOR, ELACY, FLOR DE LIS, GAUCHO, JAGUAR, JESUIT'S TEA, LA HOJA, LA MULATA, LA TRANQUERA, LONJAZO, MADRUGADA, MATÉ, MATÉ BULK LOOSE TEA, NOBLEZA GAUCHA, ORO VERDE, PARAGUAY TEA, PAYADITO, ROSAMONTE, SAFIRA, UNION, YERBA-DE-MATÉ, YI-YI, ZERBONI

Common trade names

None known.

Common forms

Available as leaves, tea, and liquid extract

Source

Yerba maté is a drink made from the dried leaves of *Ilex paraguariensis* of the holly family (Aquifoliaceae), an evergreen tree native to Paraguay, Argentina, and Brazil.

Chemical components

The leaves of yerba maté contain tannin, methylxanthines (including caffeine, theobromine, and theophylline), resin, and crude fiber. Other compounds include the antitumor compound ursolic acid, sterols (related to cholesterol and ergosterol), fats, carotene, vitamins A and B, riboflavin, ascorbic acid, and nicotinic acid. Pyrrolizidine alkaloids have also been detected (McGee et al., 1976).

Actions

The pharmacological properties of caffeine, theophylline, and theobromine have been evaluated in humans and are well documented.

Unlike caffeine and theophylline, theobromine has no stimulant effects on the CNS. Theobromine also has a weaker diuretic effect and is a less powerful stimulant of smooth muscle than theophylline. Large doses of theobromine may result in nausea and vomiting.

Reported uses

Aside from its popularity as a tea drink in South America, many therapeutic claims have been made for yerba maté; these include use as a diuretic, antirheumatic, analgesic, antidepressant, cathartic, and CNS stimulant. It has been promoted for the management of diabetes, as well as heart, nerve, and stomach disorders. In Germany, yerba maté is used for the management of physical and mental fatigue because of its purported analeptic properties. In China, yerba maté is reportedly given parenterally for its hypotensive effect and is also used as an appetite suppressant.

Dosage

Fluid extract (1:1 in 25% alcohol): 2 to 4 ml P.O. t.i.d.
Tea: 2 to 4 g dried leaf P.O. t.i.d.

Adverse reactions

- Flushing
- Hepatotoxicity
- Irritability
- Muscle twitching
- Nausea
- Nervousness
- Palpitations
- Vomiting
- Withdrawal headache

⚠ Prolonged consumption of yerba maté has been linked to increased cancer risk. (See *Yerba maté drinking and increased cancer risk,* page 684.)

Interactions

Benzodiazepines, other CNS depressants: may counteract effects of these drugs. Avoid concomitant use.
Caffeine, other CNS stimulants including smoking: additive effects. Monitor patient.
Disulfiram: possible disulfiram reaction if herbal product contains alcohol. Avoid concomitant use.
Diuretics: may have an additive effect. Do not use together.
Hepatic microsomal enzyme inhibitors (cimetidine, ciprofloxacin, verapamil): may decrease clearance of yerba maté methylxanthines and cause toxicity. Use together cautiously.

RESEARCH FINDINGS
Yerba maté drinking and increased cancer risk

Consumption of large quantities of yerba maté has been associated with increased risk of esophageal and bladder cancers. A recent case-control study showed an association between yerba maté drinking and mouth, laryngeal, and pharyngeal cancers.

The unadjusted relative risk for all upper digestive tract cancers was 2.1. After controlling for tobacco smoking, alcohol use, and coffee or tea drinking, the relative risk was 1.6. Most of the excess risk for yerba maté drinkers was for oral and pharyngeal cancers (Pintos et al., 1994).

In another case-control study, yerba maté was linked to increased risk of bladder cancer. After adjustment for age, social class, and tobacco smoking, a sevenfold increase in risk of bladder cancer was seen among the heavy tea drinkers (De Stefani et al., 1991).

Contraindications and precautions

Contraindicated in patients with hypertension and anxiety. Avoid use in pregnant or breast-feeding patients; effects are unknown. The herb is also contraindicated in children, who may be especially susceptible to the toxic effects of yerba maté.

Special considerations

• Explain that heavy consumption of yerba maté may increase the risk of liver disease, upper digestive tract cancers, and bladder cancer.
• Monitor liver function tests, and observe for signs and symptoms of methylxanthine toxicity.
• Warn the patient taking disulfiram to avoid use of an herbal form that contains alcohol.
• Advise the patient to avoid caffeine and other CNS stimulants while using this herb.
• Counsel the patient to report any unusual signs or symptoms.

Points of interest

• Yerba maté is a popular beverage, much like coffee or tea, in parts of South America (primarily Brazil, Paraguay, and Argentina).
• Yerba maté was originally served in a small gourd (maté) and sipped through a filter straw to prevent ingestion of plant material. Burnt sugar, lemon juice, or milk are sometimes added to the drink.

Analysis

Yerba maté is a popular beverage, but little evidence exists to support its medicinal uses. Risks appear to outweigh any potential benefits. The herb contains methylxanthines and potentially hepatotoxic compounds that could have detrimental effects in patients with chronic medical conditions. Chronic consumption of yerba maté has been linked to increased risk of certain cancers.

References

De Stefani, E., et al. "Black Tobacco, Maté, and Bladder Cancer. A Case-Control Study from Uruguay," *Cancer* 67:536-40, 1991.

McGee, I., et al. "A Case of Veno-Occlusive Disease of the Liver in Britain Associated With Herbal Tea Consumption," *J Clin Pathol* 29:788-94, 1976.

Pintos, J., et al. "Maté, Coffee, and Tea Consumption and Risk of Cancers of the Upper Aerodigestive Tract in Southern Brazil," *Epidemiology* 5:583-90, 1994.

YERBA SANTA

BEAR'S WEED, CONSUMPTIVE'S WEED, GUM PLANT, HOLY WEED, MOUNTAIN BALM, TARWEED

Common trade names
Respirtone

Common forms
Available as a liquid extract (1 oz), liniment, powder, syrup, and tea.

Source
Active components are derived from the leaves and roots of *Eriodictyon californicum,* an evergreen shrub belonging to the waterleaf family (Hydrophyllaceae) and native to the mountains of California and northern Mexico.

Chemical components
The plant contains various acids (cerotinic, formic, and butyric); a resin consisting of pentacontane, xanthoeriodictyol, priodonal, and chrysoeriodictyol; a phenol; eriodictyonone; tannins; and a volatile oil; sugar; fixed oil; and gum.

Actions
Physiologic mechanisms of action are poorly described. It is reported that yerba santa exerts an expectorant effect. Two flavonoids recently isolated from the plant, cirsimaritin and chrysoeriol, show some promise as anticancer agents (Liu et al., 1992).

Reported uses

Native Americans used yerba santa externally for bruises and inflammation, and they smoked or chewed the leaves for asthma. The herb has also been used to treat tuberculosis, the common cold, rheumatic pain, bronchial conditions, and hay fever.

Dosage

A tea is made from the leaves for coughs, colds, asthma, and tuberculosis. Powdered leaves are used as a stimulating expectorant. A liniment formulation of the leaves is applied topically to reduce fever. Fresh leaves are applied as poultices for bruises, and younger leaves are applied to relieve rheumatism.

Adverse reactions

None reported.

Interactions

None reported.

Contraindications and precautions

Avoid use in pregnant or breast-feeding patients; effects are unknown.

Special considerations

● Advise the patient not to chew yerba santa leaves because they leave a gummy residue on the teeth.
● Inform the patient that there are no clinical data to support use of this herb for any medical condition.
● Advise the patient not to depend on this herb alone to treat such conditions as asthma or tuberculosis.

Points of interest

● Yerba santa is available in several OTC herbal preparations and as a pharmaceutical flavoring to mask the flavor of bitter drugs. The fluid extract is also used in foods and beverages.

Analysis

Information regarding the safety and efficacy of this agent is scant. No clinical trials or published case reports are available for evaluation. As a result, its use cannot be recommended.

References

Liu, Y.L., et al. "Isolation of Potential Cancer Chemopreventative Agents from *Eriodictyon californicum*," *J Natl Prod* 55:357-63, 1992.

YEW

AMERICAN YEW, CALIFORNIA YEW, CHINWOOD, GLOBE-
BERRY, GROUND HEMLOCK, OREGON YEW, WESTERN
YEW

Common trade names
Yew Tea

Common forms
Available as an extract (concentrated tincture), salve, and capsules
(with olives)

Source
Active components are derived from the bough tips and bark of the
Pacific or Western Yew (*Taxus brevifolia*), native to the northwestern
United States and British Columbia.

Chemical components
Several alkaloids are found in yew plants. The most notable include
taxine (a mixture of alkaloids), taxol (or paclitaxel, a diterpenoid
taxane), taxicatin, milossine, and ephedrine. Other compounds include lignans, tannins, and resin.

Actions
Paclitaxel inhibits cell division by interfering with microtubule formation. Microtubules are necessary for proper division of cellular
genetic information (O'Leary et al., 1998).

Reported uses
Herbal extracts of yew were used by Native Americans for rheumatism, fever, and arthritis. The plant's toxicity is well recognized; all
parts of the plant are poisonous except the succulent red outer cov-
ering of the seeds (Howard and DeWolf, 1974).

Paclitaxel is FDA labeled for metastatic ovarian cancer after failure of first-line chemotherapy. Numerous studies have documented
its effectiveness in metastatic ovarian and breast cancer (O'Leary et
al., 1998).

Paclitaxel has been identified in lesser quantities in other yew
species such as the American yew and *T. cuspidata*, the Japanese yew.
The English yew contains a similar compound called docetaxel, also
known as taxotere.

Dosage
Consumption of this herb can be highly hazardous. Use only under
the supervision of a qualified health care professional.

Tincture: 10 to 60 drops P.O. b.i.d. to q.i.d.
Tea: 1 cup P.O. daily.
Salve: apply as needed.

Adverse reactions

The following have been reported with paclitaxel; some or all may also appear with ingestion of large amounts of yew products.

- Alopecia
- Anemia
- Arthralgias
- Arrhythmias
- Elevated lipids
- Elevated liver function tests
- Hypersensitivity reactions, rash
- Hypotension
- Leukopenia
- Myalgias
- Nausea
- Neutropenia
- Peripheral neuropathy
- Thrombocytopenia
- Vomiting

Interactions

Chemotherapeutic agents: may potentiate myelosuppressive effects. Do not use together unless the benefits outweigh possible harmful effects.
Ketoconazole: inhibits paclitaxel metabolism. Avoid concomitant use.

Contraindications and precautions

Avoid use in pregnant or breast-feeding patients; effects are unknown.

Special considerations

- Monitor liver function tests.
- Although paclitaxel (and its derivative, docetaxel) are highly effective anticancer drugs, consumption of yew products (as entire plant or whole plant extracts) has not been studied for the treatment of cancer. These agents are also toxic. Thus, patients with cancer should avoid using nonpharmaceutical yew products for treatment.
- Be aware that some patients have attempted to abuse yew plants to intentionally harm themselves (Stebbing et al., 1995).

Points of interest

- Paclitaxel was formerly referred to as taxol. Subsequently, Bristol-Myers Squibb named their brand of paclitaxel Taxol, after approval by the FDA for chemotherapy-refractive metastatic ovarian cancer.

• Other chemical components of yew species are being studied for their chemotherapeutic potential (Huxtable 1995; O'Leary et al., 1998; von Hoff, 1997).

Analysis
There are no clinical data to support taking this herb (as derived from raw plant parts) for any medical condition. However, paclitaxel and other components of yew are effective chemotherapeutic agents that can be used only under medical supervision.

References
Howard, R.A., and DeWolf, G. "Poisonous Plants," *Arnoldia* 34:41-96, 1974.

Huxtable, R.J. "Regional Sources of Natural Products: *Taxomyces andreanae*," *Proc West Pharmacol Soc* 38:1-4, 1995.

O'Leary, J., et al. "Taxanes in Adjuvant and Neoadjuvant Therapies for Breast Cancer," *Oncology* 12:23-27, 1998.

Stebbing, J., et al. "Deliberate Self-Harm Using Yew Leaves (*Taxus baccata*)," *Br J Clin Pract* 49:101, 1995.

von Hoff, D.D. "The Taxoids: Same Roots, Different Drugs," *Semin Oncol* 24:S13:3-10; 1997.

YOHIMBE

APHRODIEN, *CORYNANTHE YOHIMBE*, CORYNINE, *PAUSINYSTALIA YOHIMBE*, QUEBRACHINE, YOHIMBEHE, YOHIMBENE, YOHIMBIME, YOHIMBINE

Common trade names
(Also available in combination) Aphrodyne, Dayto Himbin, Potensan, Vikonon Combination, Yobinol, Yocon, Yohimbine HCl, Yohimex

Common forms
Tablets: 3 mg, 5.4 mg

Source
Active components are derived from the bark of *Pausinystalia yohimbe,* a West African tree native to Congo, Cameroon, and Gabon. The main agent, yohimbine, is also found in the roots of *Rauwolfia serpentina.*

Chemical components
Yohimbe bark contains a mixture of approximately 6% alkaloids, of which yohimbine hydrochloride is most important. Chemically, yohimbine possesses some structural similarity to reserpine and lysergic acid.

Actions

The alkaloid yohimbine is relatively selective for alpha$_2$-adrenoceptors. In high concentrations, yohimbine may also interact with alpha$_1$-adrenoceptors, serotonin, and dopamine receptors. Yohimbine is also an MAO inhibitor that acts centrally and peripherally. CNS effects include excitation, irritability, tremor, elevated blood pressure, and increased heart rate. It also produces antidiuresis due to the release of antidiuretic hormone in the CNS. Peripherally, yohimbine affects autonomic nervous system activity by reducing adrenergic activity and increasing cholinergic activity.

Reported uses

Yohimbe has long been used in Africa as an aphrodisiac; it has also been used as an hallucinogenic agent (Siegel, 1976). Yohimbine has been used for orthostatic hypotension and clonidine overdose (Roberge et al., 1996). However, yohimbe has been most heavily studied for possible use in treating vasculogenic male impotence. The mechanism of action is believed to be improved cavernous arterial blood flow and corporeal smooth muscle relaxation. Clinical trials have produced contradictory results.

One study demonstrated a positive benefit from yohimbine in male patients, some of whom were diabetic (Morales et al., 1982). Two other studies found no improvement. No significant benefit was found when yohimbine was compared with placebo in patients with organic erectile dysfunction (Teloken et al., 1998). A randomized crossover study of patients treated with yohimbine and isoxsuprine in combination, and pentoxifylline alone, found neither regimen effective against mixed vasculogenic erectile dysfunction (Knoll et al., 1996).

Dosage

For male impotence, 5.4 mg P.O. t.i.d. based on clinical studies. If adverse effects occur, reduce to 2.7 mg P.O. t.i.d. and gradually increase to 5.4 mg. Dosage of 20 to 30 mg daily may cause increased heart rate and blood pressure. However, one trial used a single daily dose of 100 mg.

For orthostatic hypotension, 12.5 mg P.O. daily; however more research is needed on the use and dosage of yohimbe for orthostatic hypotension (Roberge et al., 1996).

Adverse reactions

- Acute renal failure
- Anorexia
- Anxiety
- Diarrhea
- Dizziness

- Dysuria, genital pain
- Headache
- Hypertension
- Irritability
- Nausea
- Nervousness
- Skin flushing
- Tachycardia
- Tremor

⚠️Manic reactions occurred when an average daily dose of 12.5 mg yohimbe was given to psychiatric patients experiencing orthostatic hypotension from psychotropic drugs (Price et al., 1984).

Interactions

OTC stimulants (caffeine, phenylephedrine, phenylpropanolamine): causes additive effects. Decrease dose or avoid concomitant use.
Selective serotonin reuptake inhibitors, venlafaxine: increased stimulation. Do not use together.
Tricyclic antidepressants: increased concentration. Lower dose of these agents with concomitant use.
Tyramine-containing foods (cheese, wine, liver): may cause high blood pressure. Avoid concomitant use.

Contraindications and precautions

Contraindicated in patients with psychiatric disorders, renal or hepatic disease, hypersensitivity to yohimbe, or a history of gastric or duodenal ulcer. Also contraindicated in children and in pregnant or breast-feeding patients. Use cautiously in patients with hypertension.

Special considerations

- Know that yohimbe is usually not used by women.
- Monitor for adverse CNS and cardiac effects.
- Explain that the effects of long-term use of yohimbe for over 10 weeks is not known.
- Tell the patient to avoid caffeine.

Points of interest

- The herb has no FDA-sanctioned use in humans.
- Yohimbe has been on the USDA unsafe herb list since March 1977.

Analysis

Yohimbe has been used primarily as an aphrodisiac and for the treatment of male erectile impotence. However, clinical trials have produced contradictory results. The most convincing data suggest a role in male organic impotence associated with diabetes. To date, no studies have compared yohimbe with other currently available treatments for male impotence. Until further studies define the precise role of yohimbe in this disorder, the drug cannot be recommended.

References

Knoll, L.D., et al. "A Randomized Crossover Study using Yohimbine and Isoxsuprine versus Pentoxifylline in the Management of Vasculogenic Impotence," *J Urol* 155:144-46, 1996.

Morales, A., et al. "Nonhormonal Pharmacological Treatment of Organic Impotence," *J Urol* 128:45-47, 1982.

Price, H.L., et al. "Three Cases of Mania Symptoms Following Yohimbine Administration," *Am J Psychiatry* 141:1267-68, 1984.

Roberge, R.J., et al. "Yohimbine as an Antidote for Clonidine Overdose," *Am J Emerg Med* 14:7:678-80, 1996.

Siegel, R.K. "Herbal Intoxication: Psychoactive Effects from Herbal Cigarettes, Tea, and Capsules," *JAMA* 236:473-76, 1976.

Teloken, C., et al. "Therapeutic Effects of High Dose Yohimbine Hydrochloride on Organic Erectile Dysfunction," *J Urol* 159:124, 1998.

Additional references

Bisset, N.G., ed. *Herbal Drugs and Phytopharmaceuticals.* Boca Raton, Fla.: CRC Press, 1994.

Blumenthal, M., ed. *The Complete German Commission E Monographs: Therapeutic Guide to Herbal Medicines.* Austin, Tex.: American Botanical Council, 1998.

Brinker, F. *Herb Contraindications and Drug Interactions.* Sandy, Oreg: Eclectic Institute Inc., 1997.

Brinker, F. *The Toxicology of Botanical Medicines,* rev. 2nd ed. Sandy, Oreg.: Eclectic Medicinal Publications, 1996.

British Herbal Pharmacopoeia, Consolidated ed. London: British Herbal Medicine Association, 1983.

Budavari, S. *The Merck Index: An Encyclopedia of Chemicals, Drugs, and Biologicals.* 12th ed. Whitehouse Station, N.J.: Merck & Co., 1996.

Chevallier, A. *The Encyclopedia of Medicinal Plants.* New York: DK Pub., 1996.

Claus, E.P. *Pharmacognosy,* 4th ed. Philadelphia: Lea & Febiger, 1961.

Covington, T.R., ed. *Handbook of Nonprescription Drugs,* 11th ed. Washington, D.C.: American Society of Hospital Pharmacists, 1993.

Crellin, J.K., and Philpott, J. *Herbal Medicine Past and Present. A Reference Guide to Medicinal Plants,* Vol. 2. Durham, N.C.: Duke University Press, 1990.

der Marderosian, A.H., and Liberti, L.E. *Natural Product Medicine: A Scientific Guide to Foods, Drugs, Cosmetics.* Philadelphia: G.F. Stickley Co.,1988.

Dobelis, I.N., ed. *Magic and Medicine of Plants.* Pleasantville, N.Y.: Reader's Digest Association, Inc., 1986.

Duke, J.A. *The Green Pharmacy.* Emmaus, Pa.: Rodale Press, 1997.

Evans, W.C. *Trease and Evan's Pharmacognosy,* 13th ed. New York: Bailliere Tindall, 1989.

Gennaro, A.R., ed. *Remington's Pharmaceutical Sciences,* 17th ed. Easton, Pa.: Mack Publishing Company, 1985.

Goodman, L.S., et al. *Goodman and Gilman's: The Pharmacological Basis of Therapeutics,* 7th ed. New York: Macmillan Publishing Company, 1985.

Graf, A.B. *Hortica: A Color Cyclopedia of Garden Flora.* East Rutherford, N.J.: Roehrs Company, 1992.

Graf, A.B. *Tropica: A Color Cyclopedia of Exotic Plants and Trees,* 4th ed. East Rutherford, N.J.: Roehrs Company, 1992.

Haddad, L.M., and Winchester, J.F. *Clinical Management of Poisoning and Drug Overdose,* 2nd ed. Philadelphia: W.B. Saunders Co., 1990.

Hoffman, D. *The Complete Illustrated Holistic Herbal*. Rockport, Md.: Element Books Inc., 1996.

Kowalchik, C., and Hylton, W.H., eds. *Rodale's Illustrated Encyclopedia of Herbs.* Emmaus, Pa.: Rodale Press Inc., 1987.

Lacy, C., et al: *Drug Information Handbook,* 4th ed. Cleveland: Lexi-Comp, Inc., 1996.

Lampe, K.E., and McCann, M.A. *AMA Handbook of Poisonous and Injurious Plants.* Chicago: American Medical Association, 1985.

Leung, A.Y., and Foster, S. *Encyclopedia of Common Natural Ingredients Used in Food, Drugs and Cosmetics.* New York: John Wiley and Sons, Inc., 1980.

McEvoy, G.K., ed. *American Hospital Formulary Service Drug Information.* Bethesda, Md.: American Society of Health-System Pharmacists, 1998.

McGuffin, M., et al. *The American Herbal Products Association's Botanical Safety Handbook.* Boca Raton, Fla.: CRC Press, 1997.

Millspaugh, C.F. *American Medicinal Plants.* New York: Dover Publications, Inc., 1974. Reprint of 1892 edition.

Newall, C.A., et al. *Herbal Medicines. A Guide for Health-Care Professionals.* London: The Pharmaceutical Press, 1996.

Ody, P. *The Complete Medicinal Herbal.* New York: Dorling-Kindersley, 1993.

Olin, B.R., ed. *The Lawrence Review of Natural Products.* St. Louis: Facts and Comparisons, 1991.

Osol, A., et al.: *The United States Dispensatory,* 27th ed. Philadelphia: Lippincott-Raven Pubs., 1973.

Reynolds, J., et al., eds. *Martindale—The Extra Pharmacopoeia,* 31st ed. London: The Royal Pharmaceutical Society, 1996.

Rumack, B.H., et al., eds. *POISINDEX System.* Englewood, Colorado: MICROMEDEX, Inc., 1998.

Trease, G.E., and Evans, W.C.: *Pharmacognosy.* London: Bailliere Tindall, 1972.

Tyler, V. E. *The Honest Herbal. A Sensible Guide to the Use of Herbs and Related Remedies.* Binghamton, N. Y.: Pharmaceutical Product Press, 1993.

Tyler, V.E., et al. *Pharmacognosy,* 9th ed. Philadelphia: Lea & Febiger, 1988.

United States Pharmacopeia-23: National Formulary-18: Rockville, Md.: United States Pharmacopeial Convention Inc., 1995.

Weiss, R.F. *Herbal Medicine.* Beaconsfield, England: Beaconsfield Publishers Ltd., 1988.

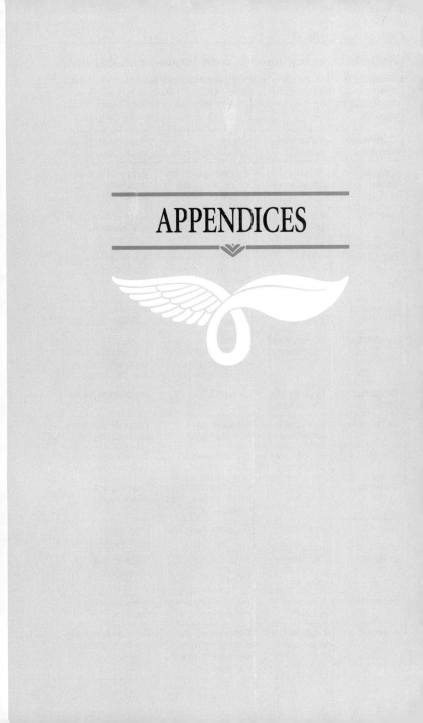

APPENDICES

Selected herbal agents with limited clinical data

Scientific and clinical data for some herbal agents are severely limited even though the agents are currently in use. This chart lists some of these agents and their uses as they have been described in anecdotal reports.

Common name	Botanical name	Other pseudonyms	Reported uses
balm of gilead	*Populus gileadensis*	Fir balsam, fir pine, silver pine, silver fir, balsam Canada	Antipyretic, anti-rheumatic, anal-gesic
balmony	*Chelone glabra*	Chelone, snake-head, turtle-bloom	Used in hepatobil-iary disease
bittersweet nightshade	*Solanum dul-camara*	European bitter-sweet, felonwood, felonwort, scarlet berry, violet bloom, woody nightshade	Pain, gout, fever, rheumatism, asth-ma, whooping cough, skin dis-eases
burr marigold	*Bidens tripartita*	Water agrimony	Astringent, dia-phoretic, diuretic
calabar bean	*Physostigma venenosum*	Chop nut, esere nut, faba calabari-ca, ordeal bean, Physostigma	Used in Alzheim-er's disease, anti-cholinergic rever-sal, glaucoma
California poppy	*Eschscholzia californica*	None	Sedative/hypnotic
camphor tree	*Cinnamomum camphora*	Laurel camphor, kamphor balm	Used for damaged or abraded skin
chervil	*Anthriscus cerefolium*	Garden chervil, salad chervil	Diuretic, expecto-rant, hypotensive
cleavers	*Galium aparine*	Bedstraw, catch-weed, goose grass, clives	Diuretic, anti-inflammatory
corn silk	*Zea mays*	Stigmata maydis	Hypoglycemic, diuretic, antilithic
costmary	*Chrysanthe-mum balsa-mita*	Bible leaf	Spice in foods or beverages
cramp bark	*Viburnum opulus*	Snowball tree, high cranberry	Antispasmodic, sedative
cudweed	*Gnaphalium uliginosum*	Cottonweed, life everlasting, march everlasting, marsh cudweed	Astringent, antisep-tic, decongestant

Selected herbal agents with limited clinical data

(continued)

Common name	Botanical name	Other pseudonyms	Reported uses
fringe tree	*Chionanthus virginicus*	Poison ash, snow-drop tree, snow-flower, graybeard, white fringe	Bile stimulant
gravel root	*Eupatorium purpureum*	Trumpet-weed, Joe-pye weed	Antilithic, anti-rheumatic
grindelia	*Grindelia camporum; Grindelia spp.*	Hardy grindelia, gum plant, rosin weed	Smooth muscle relaxant
guaiacum	*Guaiacum officinale*	Lignum vitae, guaiac	Anti-inflammatory, diuretic
hydrangea	*Hydrangea arborescens*	Seven barks, mountain hydrangea	Antilithic, tonic, duiretic, antiprosta-tic
Jamaica quassia	*Pacrasma excelsa*	Quassia wood, bit-ter wood	Gastric stimulant, amebicidal
kousso	*Hagenia abyssinica*	Kousso tree	Cathartic, anthelmintic
lemon balm	*Melissa offici-nalis*	Balm, melissa, sweet balm, balm-mint	Antithyroid, antiviral
lemon verbena	*Aloysia triphylla*	Louisa	Antispasmodic, sedative
lime blossom	*Tilia vulgaris*	Linden	Antispasmodic, diaphoretic, diuretic
lungwort moss	*Lobaria pul-monaria*	Oak lungs, lung moss	Expectorant, demulcent
mouse ear	*Pilosella offic-inarum, Hieracium pilosella*	Felon herb, hawk-weed, pilosella, mouse-ear hawk-weed	Antispasmodic, expectorant
pellitory of the wall	*Parietaria dif-fusa*	Lichwort	Diuretic, antilithic
pennywort	*Umbilicus rupestris*	Navelwort	Used for earache
pilewort	*Ranunculus ficaria*	Ficaria, lesser celandine	Astringent, demul-cent

(continued)

Selected herbal agents with limited clinical data

(continued)

Common name	Botanical name	Other pseudonyms	Reported uses
pleurisy root	*Asclepias tuberosa*	Butterfly weed, tuber root	Diuretic, expectorant
queen's delight	*Stillingia sylvatica*	Queen's root, silverleaf, yawroot	Expectorant, astringent, cathartic
sage, wood	*Teucrium scorodonia*	Large-leaved germander, hind heal, garlic sage	Antibacterial, antiflatulent, antirheumatic
salad burnet	*Sanguisorba officinalis*	Lesser burnet, burnet saxifrage, pimpinella sanguisorba	Treatment of excessive bleeding (menstrual, uterine, or wound), fever, or burns; antiseptic; antimicrobial
savory	*Satureja hortensis*	Summer savory	Spasmolytic, antibacterial, antidiuretic, antiflatulent
Scotch pine	*Pinus sylvestris*	Scot's pine, scotch fir	Antiseptic, antimicrobial
silverweed	*Potentilla anserina*	Argentine, crampweed, goosewort, moon grass, wild tansy	Anti-inflammatory, diuretic
smooth strophanthus	*Strophanthus gratus*	Ouabain	Cardiac stimulant
sweet woodruff	*Galium odoratum, Asperula odorata*	Waldmeister, master of the wood	Anti-inflammatory
tarragon	*Artemisia dracunculus*	Dragon's mugwort, French tarragon	Antibacterial, diuretic, hypnotic
Virginia snakeroot	*Aristolochia serpentaria*	Birthwort, pelican flower, sangrel, snakeweed	Stimulant, digestive, diaphoretic

Herbal agents listed as unsafe by the FDA

The FDA categorizes herbal agents according to their relative safety. This list outlines the common and botanical names of herbal agents listed by the FDA as unsafe.

Common name	Botanical name
American mistletoe	Phoradendron flavescens
arnica	Arnica montana
bittersweet nightshade*	Solanum dulcamara
bloodroot	Sanguinaria canadensis
broom	Cytisus scoparius
deadly nightshade*	Atropa belladonna
Dutch tonka bean*	Dipteryx odorata
English tonka bean*	Dipteryx oppositifolia
European mistletoe	Viscum album
heliotrope*	Heliotropium europaeum
horse chestnut	Aesculus hippocastanum
jimsonweed	Datura stramonium
lily of the valley	Convallaria majalis
lobelia	Lobelia inflata
Madagascar periwinkle*	Catharanthus roseus
mandrake*	Mandragora officinarum
mayapple	Podophyllum peltatum
morning glory*	Ipomoea purpurea
periwinkle*	Vinca rosea
snakeroot	Eupatorium spp.
spindle tree*	Euonymus europaeus
St. John's wort	Hypericum perforatum
sweet flag	Acorus calamus
true jalap*	Exagonium purga
wahoo	Euonymus atropurpureus
wormwood	Artemisia absinthium
yohimbe	Corynanthe yohimbe, Pausinystalia yohimbe

* Not specifically discussed in earlier chapters.

Potentially unsafe plants

Numerous plants have been identified as being potentially harmful. This chart lists the common and botanical names of unsafe plants and the more serious adverse reactions that can occur from their use.

Common name	Botanical name	Serious adverse reactions
American mistletoe	Phoradendron flavescens	Hypertension, hypertensive crisis
American yew	Taxus canadensis	Cytotoxicity
arnica	Arnica montana	Violent gastroenteritis, nervous disorder, muscle weakness, collapse
autumn crocus	Colchicum autumnale	GI toxicity, vomiting, neurologic toxicity, renal failure
belladonna	Atropa beladonna	Anticholinergic toxicity
betel palm	Areca catechu	Teratogenesis
bird's foot trefoil	Lotus corniculatus	Cyanide poisoning: seizures, paralysis, coma, death
bittersweet nightshade	Solanum dulcamara	Cardiac toxicity
black nightshade	Solanum americanum	Cardiac toxicity
black locust	Robina pseudo acacia	Bradycardia, nausea, vomiting, dizziness
bloodroot	Sanquinaria canadensis	Destruction of tissue on application
blue flag	Iris versicolor	Severe nausea, vomiting, diarrhea
broom	Cytisus scoparius	GI toxicity or dehydration
calabar bean	Physostigma venenosum	Cholinergic toxicity
castor oil plant	Ricinus communis	GI toxicity or dehydration
chaparral	Larrea trindentata	Fulminant hepatic failure
comfrey	Symphytum officinale	Hepatotoxicity
cotton	Gossypium hirsutum	Hypokalemia, male sterility, heart failure at high doses
daffodil	Narcissus pseudonarcissus	CNS depression, carcinogenicity, coma, death

Potentially unsafe plants *(continued)*

Common name	Botanical name	Serious adverse reactions
ergot	*Claviceps purpurea*	Hallucinations, hypertension, tissue ischemia, acute infection of the skin involving lymphatic vessels
foxglove	*Digitalis purpurea*	Bradycardia, heart block, arrhythmias
germander	*Teucrium scorodonia*	Hepatotoxicity
goldenseal	*Hydrastis candensis*	Hyperreflexia, hypertension, seizures, respiratory failure
heliotrope	*Heliotropium europaeum*	Hepatotoxicity
hedge mustard	*Sisymbrium officinale*	Cardiac toxicity, heart failure
hemp dogbane	*Apocynum cannabinum*	Cardiac stimulant, arrhythmias
henbane	*Hyoscyamus niger*	Anticholinergic toxicity
horse chestnut	*Aesculus hippocastanum*	Bleeding
Indian pink	*Spigelia marilandica*	Death (from overdose)
Indian tobacco	*Lobelia inflata*	Paralysis, hypothermia, cardiovascular collapse, coma, death
jalap root	*Exagonium purga*	Dramatic purgative cathartic
jimsonweed	*Daturia stramonium*	Anticholinergic toxicity, hallucinations
life root	*Senecio longilobus*	Hepatic failure from hepatic venoocclusive disease
lily of the valley	*Convallaria majalis*	Cardiac toxicity
marsh marigold	*Caltha palustris*	Inflammation of mucosal tissues and bronchospasm
mayapple	*Podophyllum peltatum*	Severe GI irritation
monkshood, wolfsbane	*Aconitum spp.*	Cardiotoxicity, neurotoxicity, hypotension, arrhythmias

(continued)

Potentially unsafe plants *(continued)*

Common name	Botanical name	Serious adverse reactions
moonseed	*Menispermum canadense*	Tachycardia, severe vomiting or diarrhea
morning glory	*Ipomoea purpurea*	Potential for hallucinations, psychosis
periwinkle	*Vinca major, V. minor*	Cytotoxicity, renal failure, hepatic failure, neurologic damage
poison hemlock	*Conicum maculatum*	Birth defects
queen's delight	*Stillingia sylvatica*	GI toxicity, mutagenesis
strychnine tree	*Strychnos nux-vomica*	CNS stimulation leading to seizures and cardiac arrest
wallflower	*Cheiranthus cheiri*	Cardiac toxicity, heart failure, bradycardia
wild cherry	*Prunus virginiana*	Dyspnea, vertigo, seizures
wild licorice	*Glycyrrhiza lepidota*	Hypotension, hypernatremia, hypertension, muscle weakness
wintercress	*Barbarea vulgaris*	Renal damage
wormseed	*Chenopodium ambrosioides*	Seizures, paralysis
wormwood	*Artemisia absinthium*	Rhabdomyolysis, renal failure, seizures, mental deterioration, optic neuritis
yellow jessamine	*Gelsemium sempervirens*	Paralysis, death

Herbal agents to avoid during pregnancy

Certain herbal agents pose risk to pregnant women. This chart lists common and botanical names of proven or suspected uterine stimulants and teratogens.

Common name	Botanical name
aloe	*Aloe vera*
arnica	*Arnica montana*
barberry, common	*Berberis vulgaris*
betel palm	*Areca catechu*
borage	*Borago officinalis*
bloodroot	*Sanguinaria canadensis*
burdock	*Arctium lappa*
butterbur	*Petasites hybridus*
catnip	*Nepeta cataria*
celandine	*Chelidonium majus*
celery	*Apium graveolens*
chamomile	*Chamaemelum nobile*
chaparral	*Larrea tridentata*
chicory	*Chicorium intybus*
coltsfoot	*Tussilago farfara*
comfrey	*Symphytum officinale*
damiana	*Turnera diffusa var aphrodisiaca*
devil's claw	*Harpagophytum procumbens*
fenugreek	*Trigonella foenum-graecum*
feverfew	*Chrysanthemum* or *Tanacetum parthenium*
garlic	*Allium sativum*
ginger	*Zingiber officinale*
goldenseal	*Hydrastis canadensis*
gotu kola	*Centella asiatica, Hydrocotyle asiatica*
hawthorn	*Crataegus monogyma, C. oxyacantha, C. laevigata*
hops	*Humulus lupulus*

(continued)

Herbal agents to avoid during pregnancy *(continued)*

Common name	Botanical name
horehound, black and white	*Marrubium vulgare, Ballota nigra*
hyssop	*Hyssopus officinalis*
jaborandi tree	*Pilocarpus jaborandi*
Jamaican dogwood	*Piscidia piscipula*
juniper	*Juniperus communis*
licorice	*Glycyrrhiza glabra*
madder	*Rubia tinctorium*
male fern	*Dryopteris filix-mas*
mayapple	*Podophyllum peltatum,* other *Podophyllum spp.*
meadowsweet	*Filipendula ulmaria*
milk thistle	*Silybum marianum*
mistletoe	*Viscum alba, Phoradendron serotinum*
motherwort	*Leonurus cardiaca*
mugwort	*Artemisia vulgaris*
mustard	*Brassica nigra*
myrrh	*Commiphora molmol,* other *Commiphora spp.*
nettle	*Urtica dioica*
nutmeg	*Myristica fragrans*
papaya	*Carica papaya*
parsley	*Petroselinum crispum,* other *Petroselinium spp.*
passion flower	*Passiflora incarnata,* other *Passiflora spp.*
peach	*Prunus persica*
pennyroyal	*Hedeoma pulegioides, Mentha pulegium* (mint)
plantains	*Plantago major, P. lanceolata, P. media, P. psyllium*
pokeweed	*Phytolacca americana*
poplars	*Populus spp.*

Herbal agents to avoid during pregnancy *(continued)*

Common name	Botanical name
prickly ash	*Zanthoxylum americanum*
Queen Anne's lace	*Daucus carota*
ragwort	*Packera aurea, Senecio aureus*
raspberry	*Rubus idaeus*
rauwolfia	*Rauvolfia serpentina*
red clover	*Trifolium pratense*
rue	*Ruta graveolens*
saffron	*Crocus sativus*
sage	*Salvia officinalis*
St. John's wort	*Hypericum perforatum*
sassafras	*Sassafras albidum*
senega	*Polygala senega*
senna	*Cassia senna, C. acutifolia*
shepherd's purse	*Capsella bursa-pastoris*
skullcap	*Scutellaria laterifolia*
skunk cabbage	*Symplocarpus foetidus*
squill	*Urginea maritima*
tansy	*Tanacetum vulgare*
turmeric	*Curcuma longa*
vervain	*Verbena officinalis*
watercress	*Tropaeolum majus*
wild cherry	*Prunus virginiana, P. serotina*
wild ginger	*Asarum canadense*
willow	*Salix nigra, other Salix spp.*
wormwood	*Artemisia absinthum*
yarrow	*Achillea millefolium*

Potential drug–herbal agent interactions

Herbal agents can interact with other drugs, increasing or decreasing their effects or causing toxic reactions related to the drugs. This chart lists known interactions between selected herbs and commonly used drugs or drug classes.

	ACE inhibitors	acetaminophen	alpha blockers	anticholinergics	anticoagulants	antidepressants	antihypertensives	beta blockers	caffeine	carbamazepine	CNS depressants	
aloe												
angelica					I							
arnica							D					
basil												
bee pollen												
betony							I					
black cohosh							I					
black haw					I							
blue cohosh							D					
bogbean					I							
broom						I		I				
buchu					I							
bugleweed												
butcher's broom			D									
cacao tree												
capsicum							D					
cat's-claw					I		I					
celandine												
chamomile					I							
charcoal												
chondroitin					I							
cowslip												
creatine										D		
cucumber												

I = increased effects   D = decreased effects   T = toxicity

	CNS stimulants	corticosteroids	digoxin	diuretics	doxorubicin	hypoglycemics	iron	lithium	MAO inhibitors	nicotine	oral contraceptives	sedatives	sulfonamides	theophylline	thyroid hormones
			I												
						I									
						D									
										I					
															D
									T						
									T						
									T						
						I							D		
														D	
				I								I			
				I											

(continued)

Potential drug–herbal agent interactions *(continued)*

	ACE inhibitors	acetaminophen	alpha blockers	anticholinergics	anticoagulants	antidepressants	antihypertensives	beta blockers	caffeine	carbamazepine	CNS depressants
dandelion							I				
deadly nightshade				I							
dong quai					I						
fenugreek					I						
fumitory							I	I			
galanthamine											
garlic					I						
ginger					I						
ginkgo					I						
ginseng											
goldenseal							I				
gotu kola											
green tea											
guarana											
hops											I
horse chestnut					I						
horsetail											
Irish moss					I		I				
jaborandi tree				D							
Jamaican dogwood											I
jimsonweed				I							
kava											I
kelp					I		I				
khella					I		I				
lavender											I
licorice											

I = increased effects   D = decreased effects   T = toxicity

	CNS stimulants	corticosteroids	digoxin	diuretics	doxorubicin	hypoglycemics	iron	lithium	MAO inhibitors	nicotine	oral contraceptives	sedatives	sulfonamldes	theophylline	thyroid hormones
				I		I									
						I									
			I												
									T						
						I			T						
			I												
						D									
					I										
														I	
	I			I											
			I												

(continued)

Potential drug–herbal agent interactions *(continued)*

	ACE inhibitors	acetaminophen	alpha blockers	anticholinergics	anticoagulants	antidepressants	antihypertensives	beta blockers	caffeine	carbamazepine	CNS depressants	
lily of the valley												
lungwort					I							
marshmallow												
melatonin												
mistletoe											I	
myrrh												
myrtle												
night-blooming cereus												
opium											I	
oregano												
pau d'arco					I							
pill-bearing spurge	I			D								
plantain										D		
poplar					I							
prickly ash					I							
Queen Anne's lace							I			I		
red clover					I							
sage												
Siberian ginseng												
St. John's wort												
tonka bean					I							
valerian											I	
watercress		I										
wintergreen					I							
yarrow					I		I					
yohimbe						I						

I = increased effects   D = decreased effects T = toxicity

	CNS stimulants	corticosteroids	digoxin	diuretics	doxorubicin	hypoglycemics	iron	lithium	MAO inhibitors	nicotine	oral contraceptives	sedatives	sulfonamides	theophylline	thyroid hormones
			I												
						I									
												I			
						I									
						I									
			I												
							D								
								D							
			I												
											I				
						I									
			I												
								T	T						
												I			

Therapeutic monitoring guidelines

As with traditional medicines, many herbal agents require close monitoring to detect adverse reactions. This chart lists tests that should be monitored for selected herbal agents.

	Complete blood count	Liver function tests	Renal function/ electrolytes	Coagulation studies	Blood glucose
aloe			x		
angelica				x	
basil					x
bayberry		x			
bearberry			x		
bee pollen					x
betony		x			
bistort		x			
black haw				x	
blackroot		x			
blue cohosh					x
boneset		x			
borage		x			
buchu		x			
cascara			x		
castor bean			x		
cat's-claw				x	
chaparral		x			
chondroitin	x			x	
condurango		x			
cowslip		x			
cucumber			x		
dandelion					x
dock, yellow			x		
dong quai				x	
fenugreek				x	x

Therapeutic monitoring guidelines *(continued)*

	Complete blood count	Liver function tests	Renal function/ electrolytes	Coagulation studies	Blood glucose
garlic	x				
ginger				x	
gingko				x	
ginseng					x
gotu kola					x
horse chestnut				x	
jaborandi tree		x			
kava	x				
kelp				x	
kelpware			x	x	x
khella		x			
lovage			x		
lungwort				x	
marshmallow					x
mayapple	x	x	x		
myrrh					x
myrtle					x
pau d'arco				x	
pennyroyal oil		x	x		
pomegranate		x			
poplar		x		x	
ragwort		x			
red clover				x	
rhatany		x			
royal jelly					x
sage					x
sarsaparilla			x		
shark cartilage		x			

(continued)

Therapeutic monitoring guidelines *(continued)*

	Complete blood count	Liver function tests	Renal function/ electrolytes	Coagulation studies	Blood glucose
skullcap		x			
soapwort		x	x		
sorrel		x	x		
squaw vine		x			
tonka bean		x		x	
turmeric				x	
valerian		x			
willow		x	x	x	
wintergreen				x	
wormwood			x		

Study data on herbal agents by disorder

Many studies conducted on herbal agents involve in vitro or animal studies but not necessarily clinical trials in humans. This chart lists, by disorder, commonly used herbal agents and the types of studies that have been performed to date.

Disorder	Herbal agent	In vitro studies	Animal studies	Human studies
Allergic rhinitis	nettle			x
Anxiety	kava			x
	pill-bearing spurge		x	
Arrhythmia	angelica		x	
	broom	x	x	
Arthritis	angelica	x		
	avens	x		
	bogbean	x		
	borage		x	x
	capsicum	x		x
	centaury	x		
	chondroitin			x
	cloves	x		
	evening primrose oil			x
	ginger		x	x
	glucosamine	x	x	x
	goldenrod		x	
	jambul		x	
	Juniperus communis	x		
	marigold	x		
	mullein	x		
	myrrh	x		
	nutmeg		x	
	papaya			x
	pill-bearing spurge		x	
	plantain		x	

(continued)

Study data on herbal agents by disorder *(continued)*

Disorder	Herbal agent	In vitro studies	Animal studies	Human studies
Arthritis *(continued)*	rose hips	x		
	sarsaparilla		x	
	skullcap	x		
	turmeric	x		x
Asthma	pill-bearing spurge		x	
Benign prostatic hypertrophy	nettle		x	x
	pumpkin			x
	saw palmetto			x
Cancer	angelica	x		
	burdock	x	x	
	caraway		x	
	celandine			x
	chaparral	x		
	condurango		x	
	evening primrose oil	x		
	garlic		x	
	goldenrod	x		
	green tea	x	x	x
	Iceland moss	x	x	
	kelp		x	
	lavender		x	x
	mayapple			x
	melatonin			x
	mistletoe	x	x	x
	mullein	x		
	pau d'arco	x		
	red clover	x		
	rose hips	x		
	rosemary	x		

Study data on herbal agents by disorder *(continued)*

Disorder	Herbal agent	In vitro studies	Animal studies	Human studies
Cancer*(continued)*	self-heal	x		
	shark cartilage			x
	skullcap		x	x
	soapwort	x		
	turmeric		x	
	watercress		x	x
Constipation	caraway			x
	cascara sagrada			x
	castor bean			x
	senna			x
Dementia	chaparral		x	
	galanthamine			x
	ginkgo			x
Dental diseases	bloodroot	x		x
	gum arabic			x
Depression	DHEA			x
	St. John's wort			x
Diabetes	basil			x
	burdock		x	
	dandelion		x	
	fenugreek	x	x	
	ginseng			x
	Juniperus communis	x	x	
	myrrh	x		
Diarrhea	barberry			x
	evening primrose oil			x
Dyspepsia	caraway			x
Eczema	evening primrose oil			x
Edema	tonka bean			x

(continued)

Study data on herbal agents by disorder *(continued)*

Disorder	Herbal agent	In vitro studies	Animal studies	Human studies
Glaucoma	jaborandi tree		x	x
Graves' disease	bugleweed	x		
Headache	feverfew	x		x
Heart failure	coenzyme Q-10			x
Hemostasis	Chinese rhubarb			x
HIV, AIDS	cat's-claw	x		
	chaparral	x		
	daffodil	x		
	Iceland moss	x		
	marigold	x		
	schisandra	x		
	self-heal	x		
	skullcap	x		
	spirulina	x		
	thuja	x		
Hyperlipidemia	fenugreek		x	x
	flax			x
	garlic		x	x
	royal jelly		x	
	safflower			x
	saffron		x	
	turmeric		x	
Impotence	yohimbe			x
Infection	chaparral	x		
	cloves	x		
	cranberry	x	x	x
	echinacea	x		x

Study data on herbal agents by disorder *(continued)*

Disorder	Herbal agent	In vitro studies	Animal studies	Human studies
Infection *(continued)*	Juniperus communis	x		
	marjoram	x		
	oregano	x		
	pill-bearing spurge	x		
	pomegranate	x		
	sage	x		
	squalamine	x		
	tea tree	x		
	turmeric	x		
Insomnia	chamomile			x
	melatonin			x
	valerian			x
Liver disorders	dandelion		x	x
	evening primrose oil	x		
	milk thistle			x
	Queen Anne's lace		x	
	schisandra		x	
	turmeric	x	x	
Menopause	black cohosh		x	x
Nausea and vomiting	ginger			x
Parasite infection	male fern			x
	pumpkin		x	
Peptic ulcer disease	butterbur	x	x	
	ginger	x	x	
	Iceland moss	x		
	licorice			x
	nutmeg		x	

(continued)

Study data on herbal agents by disorder *(continued)*

Disorder	Herbal agent	In vitro studies	Animal studies	Human studies
Peripheral arterial insufficiency	butcher's broom		x	x
	ginkgo			x
	gotu kola			x
	grapeseed			x
	horse chestnut			x
Poor exercise performance	creatine			x
Premenstrual syndrome	evening primrose oil			x
Psoriasis	sarsaparilla			x
Renal disease	Chinese rhubarb		x	x
Thrombosis	angelica	x	x	
	guarana	x		
	kelpware	x		
Warts	mayapple			x
Wounds	aloe	x	x	x
	comfrey		x	
	echinacea	x		x
	gotu kola			x
	marigold		x	

Herbal agents resource list

Health care professionals wishing to obtain more information on herbal
agents or the status of complementary and alternative medicine in general can consult the following list of related resources. Keep in mind that
specific Internet addresses sometimes change without notice. The sites
listed here are home pages for their respective organizations.

●

American Botanical Council
PO Box 201660
Austin, TX 78720-1660
Tel: (512) 331-8868
Fax: (512) 331-1924
www.herbs.org

●

American Foundation of Traditional Chinese Medicine
505 Beech Street
San Francisco, CA 94133
Tel: (415) 776-0502
Fax: (415) 776-9053

●

APRALERT
College of Pharmacy
The University of Illinois at Chicago
Contact: Mary Lou Quinn
Tel: (312) 996-2246
Fax: (312) 996-7107
www.pmmp.uic.edu

●

The Australasian College of Herbal Studies
USA Office
PO Box 57
530 First Street
Lake Oswego, OR 97034
Tel: (503) 635-6652 or (800) 48-STUDY
FAX: (503) 636-0706
www.achs@herbed.com

Herbal agents resource list *(continued)*

Botanical Society of America
Office of Publications
1735 Neil Avenue
Columbus, OH 43210-1293
Tel: (614) 292-3519

Centers for Disease Control and Prevention
Public Health Service
US Department of Health and Human Services
1600 Clifton Road NE
Atlanta, GA 30333
Tel: (404) 639-3311
www.cdc.gov

Lloyd Library
917 Plum Street
Cincinnati, OH 45202
Tel: (513) 721-3707
www.libraries.uc.edu/lloyd

Office of Dietary Supplements
National Institutes of Health
Building 31, Room 1B25
31 Center Drive, MSC 2086
Bethesda, MD 20892-2086
Tel: (301) 435-2920
www.odp.od.nih.gov

Office of Alternative Medicine
OAM Clearinghouse
PO Box 8218
Silver Spring, MD 20907-8218
Tel: (888) 644-6226
Fax: (301) 495-4957
www.altmed.od.nih.gov

●
US Food and Drug Administration
Public Health Service
Department of Health and Human Services
5600 Fishers Lane
Rockville, MD 20857
www.fda.gov

●
US National Library of Medicine
National Institutes of Health
8600 Rockville Pike
Bethesda, MD 20894
Tel: (888) 346-3656
www.nlm.nih.gov

Herbal agent information sheet

Patient _____ **Date** _____

Health care provider _____ **Phone** _____

Dear Patient,

When taking a herbal agent keep in mind the following general tips.

• Be sure to tell your health care provider about _all_ the medicines you take, including herbal agents and vitamins.

• Make sure your primary health care provider is aware of your medical history, including allergies.

• Women of childbearing age should consider using appropriate contraception because little is known about the effects of herbal agents on a fetus.

• Purchase your herbal agent from reputable sources such as a pharmacy.

• Read labels carefully when purchasing herbal products. Check that the term "standardized" is on the label. Standardized means that the dose of medicine in each tablet or capsule in that package is the same. Also check that the label states specific percentages, amounts, and strengths of active ingredients.

• When taking herbal agents, follow the prescription exactly. Taking too much of an herbal agent or taking it inappropriately may not only diminish its effectiveness but also increase the risk of dangerous side effects.

• Never ignore symptoms you may be experiencing.

• Never use herbal agents to delay seeking more appropriate therapy.

• Be aware that herbal agents are not necessarily a substitute for traditional, proven medical therapy.

• Contact your primary health care provider if you experience side effects of this herbal agent or if you have other health concerns that would normally require medical attention.

Professional's Handbook of Complementary & Alternative Medicines
© Springhouse Corporation, 1999.

• Call your primary health care provider if you experience abdominal cramping; abnormal bleeding or bruising; changes in heart rate or rhythm; changes in vision; dizziness or fainting; hair loss; hallucinations, inability to concentrate or other mental changes; hives, itching, rash, or other allergic symptoms; loss of appetite; or dramatic weight loss.

• Never allow other people to take your medicine. Store these herbal agents out of the reach of children and pets.

• If you have questions about the herbal agent you're taking, seek advice from a qualified health care provider. If your primary health care provider isn't knowledgeable about herbal medicines, ask for a referral to someone experienced in using these agents.

About this herbal agent

This agent is called _____

You are taking this agent to _____

The dosage you should take is _____

Special instructions for how to take or store this agent include _____

_____

Side effects of this agent include _____

_____

_____

Other instructions _____

_____

_____

_____

_____

INDEX

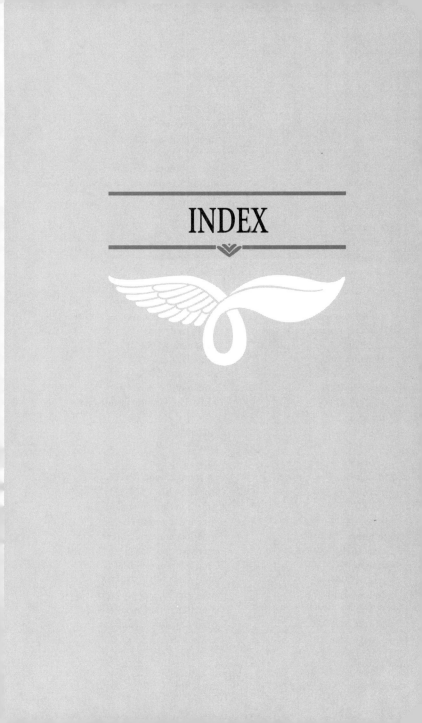

Index

t refers to a table

t refers to a table

B

t refers to a table

C

D

t refers to a table

E

F

fairy cup, 199-201
fairywand, 247-248
false cinnamon, 170-172
false coltsfoot, 661-662
false hellebore, 326-329
false indigo, 662-664
false saffron, 561-562
false unicorn root, 247-248
false valerian, 538-539
false white cedar, 633-635
farasyon maiy, 108-110
farfara, 186-188
featherfew, 253-256
featherfoil, 253-256
febrifuge plant, 253-256
Federal Food, Drug, and Cosmetic
        Act, 5, 6
felon herb, 132-133, 441-443
felonwort, 144-147
feltwort, 272-274
fenchel, 248-250
fenchelholz, 576-578
fennel, 248-250
fenouil, 248-250
fenouille, 248-250
fenugreek, 250-253
feverfew, 253-256
    and migraine prophylaxis, 255
fevertree, 243-244
feverwort, 96-98
field balm, 138-141
fieldhove, 186-188
field lady's mantle, 487-488

field mallow, 412-413
field pansy, 478-479
field poppy, 547-548
figwort, 256-258
filfil, 500-503
Filipendula, 423-426
filius ante patrem, 186-188
finocchio, 248-250
first-aid plant, 25-29
fishfuddle, 358-360
fish poison tree, 358-360
fish-wood, 655-656
five-fingers, 282-286, 639-641
flag lily, 88-90
flanders poppy, 547-548
flannel-leaf, 443-445
Flatulence
    allspice for, 24
    caraway for, 128
    juniper for, 368
flax, 258-261
    uses of, 261
flaxseed, 258-261
fleaseed, 512-514
flesh and blood, 639-641
fleur de coucou, 211-213
fleur-de-lis, 88-90
fleur d'ulmaire, 423-426
fleurs de mauve, 412-413
flor de lis, 682-685
flor de prosepina, 627-628
Florence fennel, 248-250
flores ulmariae, 423-426
flower-de-luce, 88-90
foalswort, 186-188
Food and Drug Administration, 5-6

t refers to a table

t refers to a table

J

M

N

Z

Notes

Notes

Notes